W9-CHP-801

Transplantation Immunology

METHODS IN MOLECULAR BIOLOGY™

John M. Walker, SERIES EDITOR

352. Protein Engineering Protocols, edited by *Kristian Müller and Katja Arndt, 2006*

351. *C. elegans:* *Methods and Applications,* edited by *Kevin Strange, 2006*

350. Protein Folding Protocols, edited by *Yawen Bai and Ruth Nussinov 2006*

349. YAC Protocols, *Second Edition,* edited by *Alasdair MacKenzie, 2006*

348. Nuclear Transfer Protocols: *Cell Reprogramming and Transgenesis,* edited by *Paul J. Verma and Alan Trounson, 2006*

347. Glycobiology Protocols, edited by *Inka Brockhausen-Schutzbach, 2006*

346. *Dictyostelium discoideum* Protocols, edited by *Ludwig Eichinger and Francisco Rivero-Crespo, 2006*

345. Diagnostic Bacteriology Protocols, *Second Edition,* edited by *Louise O'Connor, 2006*

344. Agrobacterium Protocols, Second Edition: *Volume 2,* edited by *Kan Wang, 2006*

343. Agrobacterium Protocols, Second Edition: *Volume 1,* edited by *Kan Wang, 2006*

342. MicroRNA Protocols, edited by *Shao-Yao Ying, 2006*

341. Cell–Cell Interactions: *Methods and Protocols,* edited by *Sean P. Colgan, 2006*

340. Protein Design: *Methods and Applications,* edited by *Raphael Guerois and Manuela López de la Paz, 2006*

339. Microchip Capillary Electrophoresis: *Methods and Protocols,* edited by *Charles Henry, 2006*

338. Gene Mapping, Discovery, and Expression: *Methods and Protocols,* edited by *M. Bina, 2006*

337. Ion Channels: *Methods and Protocols,* edited by *J. D. Stockand and Mark S. Shapiro, 2006*

336. Clinical Applications of PCR: *Second Edition,* edited by *Y. M. Dennis Lo, Rossa W. K. Chiu, and K. C. Allen Chan, 2006*

335. Fluorescent Energy Transfer Nucleic Acid Probes: *Designs and Protocols,* edited by *Vladimir V. Didenko, 2006*

334. PRINS and *In Situ* PCR Protocols: *Second Edition,* edited by *Franck Pellestor, 2006*

333. Transplantation Immunology: *Methods and Protocols,* edited by *Philip Hornick and Marlene Rose, 2006*

332. Transmembrane Signaling Protocols: *Second Edition,* edited by *Hydar ali and Haribabu Bodduluri, 2006*

331. Human Embryonic Stem Cell Protocols, edited by *Kursad Turksen, 2006*

330. Embryonic Stem Cell Protocols, Second Edition, *Vol. II: Differentiation Models,* edited by *Kursad Turksen, 2006*

329.Embryonic Stem Cell Protocols, Second Edition, *Vol. I:* *Isolation and Characterization,* edited by *Kursad Turksen, 2006*

328. New and Emerging Proteomic Techniques, edited by *Dobrin Nedelkov and Randall W. Nelson, 2006*

327. Epidermal Growth Factor: *Methods and Protocols,* edited by *Tarun B. Patel and Paul J. Bertics, 2006*

326. *In Situ* Hybridization Protocols, *ThirdEdition,* edited by *Ian A. Darby and Tim D. Hewitson, 2006*

325. Nuclear Reprogramming: *Methods and Protocols,* edited by *Steve Pells, 2006*

324. Hormone Assays in Biological Fluids, edited by *Michael J. Wheeler and J. S. Morley Hutchinson, 2006*

323. Arabidopsis Protocols, *Second Edition,* edited by *Julio Salinas and Jose J. Sanchez-Serrano, 2006*

322. *Xenopus* Protocols: *Cell Biology and Signal Transduction,* edited by *X. Johné Liu, 2006*

321. Microfluidic Techniques: *Reviews and Protocols,* edited by *Shelley D. Minteer, 2006*

320. Cytochrome P450 Protocols, *Second Edition,* edited by *Ian R. Phillips and Elizabeth A. Shephard, 2006*

319. Cell Imaging Techniques, *Methods and Protocols,* edited by *Douglas J. Taatjes and Brooke T. Mossman, 2006*

318. Plant Cell Culture Protocols, *Second Edition,* edited by *Victor M. Loyola-Vargas and Felipe Vázquez-Flota, 2005*

317. Differential Display Methods and Protocols, *Second Edition,* edited by *Peng Liang, Jonathan Meade, and Arthur B. Pardee, 2005*

316. Bioinformatics and Drug Discovery, edited by *Richard S. Larson, 2005*

315. Mast Cells: *Methods and Protocols,* edited by *Guha Krishnaswamy and David S. Chi, 2005*

314. DNA Repair Protocols: *Mammalian Systems, Second Edition,* edited by *Daryl S. Henderson, 2005*

313. Yeast Protocols: *Second Edition,* edited by *Wei Xiao, 2005*

312. Calcium Signaling Protocols: *Second Edition,* edited by *David G. Lambert, 2005*

311. Pharmacogenomics: *Methods and Protocols,* edited by *Federico Innocenti, 2005*

310. Chemical Genomics: *Reviews and Protocols,* edited by *Edward D. Zanders, 2005*

309. RNA Silencing: *Methods and Protocols,* edited by *Gordon Carmichael, 2005*

308. Therapeutic Proteins: *Methods and Protocols,* edited by *C. Mark Smales and David C. James, 2005*

307. Phosphodiesterase Methods and Protocols, edited by *Claire Lugnier, 2005*

306. Receptor Binding Techniques: *Second Edition,* edited by *Anthony P. Davenport, 2005*

305. Protein–Ligand Interactions: *Methods and Applications,* edited by *G. Ulrich Nienhaus, 2005*

304. Human Retrovirus Protocols: *Virology and Molecular Biology,* edited by *Tuofu Zhu, 2005*

303. NanoBiotechnology Protocols, edited by *Sandra J. Rosenthal and David W. Wright, 2005*

METHODS IN MOLECULAR BIOLOGY™

Transplantation Immunology

Methods and Protocols

Edited by

Philip Hornick

National Heart and Lung Institute, London, UK

Marlene Rose

National Heart and Lung Institute, Harefield, UK

HUMANA PRESS TOTOWA, NEW JERSEY

999 Riverview Drive, Suite 208
Totowa, New Jersey 07512

www.humanapress.com

This publication is printed on acid-free paper. ∞
ANSI Z39.48-1984 (American Standards Institute)

Permanence of Paper for Printed Library Materials.
Cover illustration: From Fig. 3, Chapter 17, "Experimental Models of Graft Arteriosclerosis," by Bezhad Soleimani and Victor C. Shi.

Production Editor: Robin B. Weisberg

Cover design by Patricia F. Cleary

For additional copies, pricing for bulk purchases, and/or information about other Humana titles, contact Humana at the above address or at any of the following numbers: Tel.: 973-256-1699; Fax: 973-256-8341; E-mail: orders@humanapr.com; or visit our Website: www.humanapress.com

Printed in the United States of America. 10 9 8 7 6 5 4 3 2 1

eISBN: 1-59745-049-9

ISSN: 1064-3745

Library of Congress Cataloging-in-Publication Data

Transplantation immunology : methods and protocols / edited by Philip Hornick, Marlene Rose.
p. ; cm. -- (Methods in molecular biology, ISSN 1064-3745 ; v. 333)
Includes bibliographical references and index.
ISBN 1-58829-544-3 (alk. paper)
1. Transplantation immunology. I. Hornick, Philip. II. Rose, Marlene L. III. Series: Methods in molecular biology (Clifton, N.J.) ; v. 333.
[DNLM: 1. Graft Rejection--diagnosis. 2. Graft Rejection--immunology. 3. Laboratory Techniques and Procedures. 4. Organ Transplantation --adverse effects. 5. Transplantation, Homologous--immunology.
W1 ME9616J v.333 2006 / WO 680 T7725 2006]
QR188.8T732 2006
617.9'5--dc22

2005028830

Preface

Our understanding of the immunological mechanisms of rejection has greatly improved over the past 10 years. Much of this is the result of technical innovations in the laboratory, resulting in more detailed analysis of experimental graft rejection and better ways of detecting and monitoring the patients' immune response to the allografted organ. *Transplantation Immunology: Methods and Protocols* focuses, in the main, on practical methods of detecting the immune response to the allografted organ. The first six chapters are, however, more theoretical. They provide an update on current practices of renal, liver, islet, and lung transplantation, and pathways of antigen presentation and chronic rejection. A possible novel therapy of transplant rejection involves the overexpression of molecules of interest in donor or recipient tissues, the issues of the best vectors, whether viral or nonviral is reviewed in Chapters 8 and 9. Methods of HLA typing and methods of detecting HLA antibodies have considerably changed in recent years and current methods are described in two chapters. More specialized methods, generally confined to research labs at present, such as proteomics, laser dissection microscopy, and real-time polymerase chain reaction, are described. Whereas monitoring the antibody response to transplantation has been performed by many laboratories in the past, monitoring the T-cell response is still laborious and hence the province of very specialized laboratories. The traditional method, quantitative limiting dilution analysis, is described and compared with new techniques. The area of tolerance induction and reprogramming of the immune system is covered in Chapter 11, and current practices of organ preservation and immunosuppressive drugs (Chapters 15 and 16) are also included. Finally, chronic rejection has been difficult to mimic in experimental models, all models are limited, and this subject is updated in the final chapter.

Transplantation Immunology: Methods and Protocols is intended for clinicians and scientists interested in the practice of solid organ transplantation. The chapters all give broad overviews and as such will be suitable for relative newcomers to the field. For those already familiar or expert in certain laboratory methods, we hope they find the chapters about the newer techniques of interest and value.

Philip Hornick
Marlene Rose

Contents

Contributors

PAUL J. R. BARTON • *National Heart and Lung Institute, Imperial College London, Heart Science Centre, Harefield Hospital, Harefield, Middlesex, England*

J. ANDREW BRADLEY • *Department of Surgery, University of Cambridge, Cambridge, Cambridgeshire, England*

CHRISTOPHER J. CALLAGHAN • *Wellcome Trust Research Training Fellow, University Department of Surgery, Addenbrooke's Hospital, Cambridge, England*

LOUISE COLLINS • *Clinical Sciences, GKT School of Medicine, Kings College; The Rayne Institute, London, England*

AYESHA DE SOUZA • *Transplant Immunology, National Heart and Lung Institute, Imperial College London; Heart Science Centre, Harefield Hospital, Harefield, Middlesex, England*

LEANNE E. FELKIN • *National Heart and Lung Institute, Imperial College London, Heart Science Centre, Harefield Hospital, Harefield, Middlesex, England*

PETER J. FRIEND • *Nuffield Department of Surgery, John Radcliffe Hospital, Oxfordshire, Oxford, England*

LING GAO • *Transplant Programme, Victor Chang Cardiac Research Institute, Sydney, Australia*

ALLAN R. GLANVILLE • *Department of Thoracic Medicine, St. Vincent's Hospital, Darlinghurst, New South Wales, Australia*

LUIS GRACA • *Therapeutic Immunology Group, Sir William Dunn School of Pathology, Oxfordshire, Oxford, England*

MARIA P. HERNANDEZ-FUENTES • *Immunoregulation Laboratory, Department of Nephrology and Transplantation, School of Medicine, Kings College London, University of London, London, England*

MARK HICKS • *Heart and Lung Transplant Unit and Department of Clinical Pharmacology, St. Vincent's Hospital, Sydney and Department of Physiology and Pharmacology, University of New South Wales, Australia*

ALFRED HING • *Transplant Programme, Victor Chang Cardiac Research Institute, Sydney, Australia*

PHILIP HORNICK • *Cardiothoracic Surgery, National Heart and Lung Institute, Imperial College Hammersmith Campus, London, England*

PETER MARK ANTHONY HOPKINS • *Queensland Heart-Lung Transplant Unit, The Prince Charles Hospital, Chermside, Brisbane, Queensland, Australia*

CHARLES J. IMBER • *Queen Elizabeth Liver Unit, Queen Elizabeth Hospital, Birmingham, England*

JONATHAN R. T. LAKEY • *Department of Surgery, Faculty of Medicine and Dentistry, University of Alberta, Edmonton, Alberta, Canada*

CHARLOTTE LAWSON • *Veterinary Basic Sciences, The Royal Veterinary College, London, England*

PETER S. MACDONALD • *Heart and Lung Transplant Unit, St. Vincent's Hospital, Sydney and Transplant Programme, Victor Chang Cardiac Research Institute, Sydney, Australia*

EMMA MCGREGOR • *Department of Vascular Surgery, Imperial College School of Medicine, Charing Cross Hospital, London, England*

MOHAMMADREZA MIRBOLOOKI • *Department of Surgery, Faculty of Medicine and Dentistry, University of Alberta, Edmonton, Alberta, Canada*

KAY POULTON • *Transplantation Laboratory, Central Manchester and Manchester, Children's University Hospitals NHS Trust, Manchester Royal Infirmary, Manchester, England*

MARLENE ROSE • *Heart Science Centre, National Heart and Lung Institute, Imperial College, Harefield Hospital, Harefield, England*

JONATHON RYAN • *Heart and Lung Transplant Unit, St. Vincent's Hospital, Sydney, Australia*

ALAN SALAMA • *Renal Section, Division of Medicine, Hammersmith Hospital, Imperial College London, London, England*

A. M. JAMES SHAPIRO • *Department of Surgery, Faculty of Medicine and Dentistry, University of Alberta, Edmonton, Alberta, Canada*

STEPHEN SHELDON • *Transplantation Laboratory, Central Manchester and Manchester, Children's University Hospitals NHS Trust, Manchester Royal Infirmary, Oxford Road, Manchester, England*

VICTOR C. SHI • *Transplantational Research, Novartis Pharmaceutical Corp., Summit, NJ*

JOHN D. SMITH • *Tissue Typing Laboratory, Royal Brompton and Harefield NHS Trust, Harefield Hospital, Harefield, Middlesex, England*

BEZHAD SOLEIMANI • *Cardiothoracic Surgery, National Heart and Lung Institute, London, England*

ANNE B. TAEGTMEYER • *National Heart and Lung Institute, Imperial College London, Heart Science Centre, Harefield Hospital, Harefield, Middlesex, England*

HERMAN WALDMANN • *Therapeutic Immunology Group, Sir William Dunn School of Pathology, Oxfordshire, Oxford, England*

1

Current Status of Renal Transplantation

Christopher J. Callaghan and J. Andrew Bradley

Summary

Renal transplantation is the best treatment for most patients with end-stage renal failure. It markedly improves quality of life and in some cases increases life expectancy. Advances in immunosuppression and other areas of practice have led to an incremental improvement in outcome; 1- and 5-yr graft survival after cadaveric renal transplantation is now around 90 and 70%, respectively. This success has led to increased demand for transplantation that cannot be met by cadaveric heart-beating donors, numbers of which have remained relatively static. Increasing use is now being made of kidneys from so-called "marginal" or "extended criteria" cadaveric donors and from non-heart-beating donors. More reliance is also being placed on living kidney donation, which accounts for around 25% of kidney transplants in the United Kingdom and 50% of transplants in the United States. Much effort in renal transplantation is now being directed toward improving long-term outcomes. This chapter provides an overview of these and other issues in renal transplantation, focusing on some of the topics of current interest.

Key Words: Renal transplantation; immunosuppression; organ donation; long-term outcomes.

1. Introduction

The first kidney transplant that was successful in the long term was performed in Boston in 1954 between genetically identical twins. The immunological barrier between genetically unrelated individuals was then overcome in the 1960s, when azathioprine and steroids were used with moderate success. Cyclosporine was introduced in the late 1970s and heralded the modern era of kidney transplantation *(1)*. Renal transplantation is now the optimal therapy for the majority of patients with end-stage renal disease (ESRD). Not only does renal transplantation provide a better quality of life than either peritoneal dialysis or hemodialysis *(2,3)* but there is increasing evidence that it offers a survival advantage

From: *Methods in Molecular Biology, vol. 333: Transplantation Immunology: Methods and Protocols*
Edited by: P. Hornick and M. Rose © Humana Press Inc., Totowa, NJ

Table 1
Underlying Renal Disease in UK Adult Kidney-Only Transplants, 2003–2004

Not reported[a]	37.3%
Polycystic kidneys, adult type	10.4%
Pyelonephritis/interstitial nephritis	8.4%
Glomerulonephritis	7.7%
Diabetes mellitus (types 1 and 2)	6.7%
IgA nephropathy	6.6%
Renovascular disease	5.7%
Other diseases	17.2%

[a]A high proportion of this group is made up of patients with end-stage renal disease of unknown cause.

Personal communication, UK Transplant, July 2004.

IgA, immunoglobulin A.

over dialysis *(4)*. Transplantation is also the most cost-effective treatment for ESRD *(5,6)*.

This chapter aims to provide a brief overview of renal transplantation, with emphasis on issues of current interest. For a more complete account of the field, the reader is directed to one of the comprehensive textbooks available *(7)*.

1.1. Current UK Activity and Results

The majority of patients with ESRD should be considered for renal transplantation. The most common underlying diagnoses in adults undergoing renal transplantation are glomerulonephritis, diabetes, pyelonephritis, renovascular disease, and polycystic kidney disease (**Table 1**).* Contraindications to renal transplantation are listed in **Table 2**. The success of renal transplantation is reflected in the ever-growing numbers of patients waiting for a transplant. In March 2003, 6447 people were on the active waiting list for a renal transplant in the United Kingdom (**Fig. 1**), with a median waiting time for adults of approx 500 d. Although 1667 kidney transplants were performed in 2002, an increase of 5% from the previous year, the disparity between demand and supply continues to grow (**Fig. 1**).

The total number of renal transplants performed annually in the United Kingdom has remained relatively static since the mid-1990s, despite recent improvements in the number of living donor kidneys used. This is owing to reductions

* Statistics prepared by UK Transplant from the National Transplant Database maintained on the behalf of transplant services in the United Kingdom and Republic of Ireland. UK Transplant statistics can be found at http://www.uktransplant.org.uk/ukt/statistics/statistics.jsp.

Table 2
Contraindications to Renal Transplantation

Predicated patient survival <5 yr
Malignancy
Severe refractory disease elsewhere
AIDS
Predicted graft loss >50% at 1 yr
Patients unable to comply with immunosuppressive medication
History of noncompliance
Poorly controlled psychosis or regular use of class A drugs
Immunosuppression predicted to cause life-threatening complications

AIDS, acquired immunodeficiency syndrome.

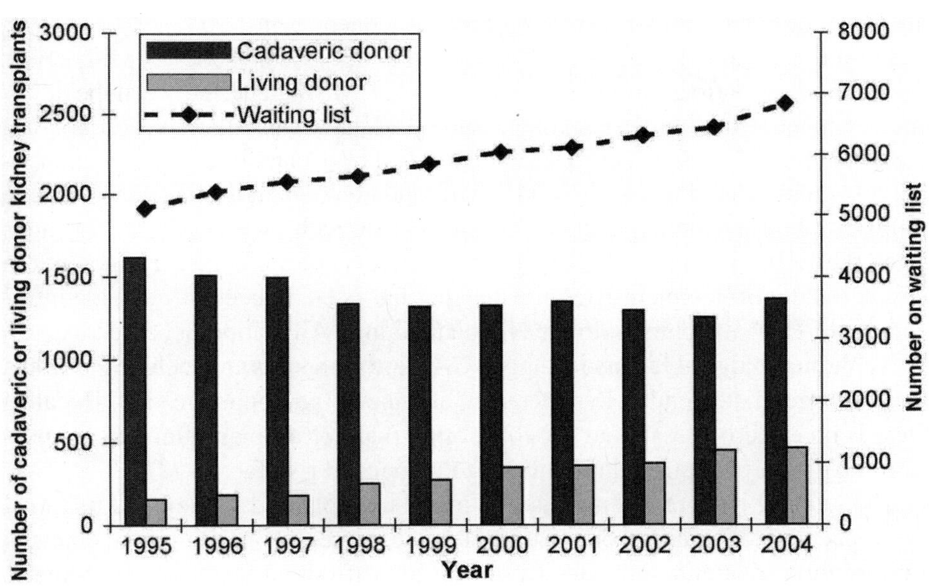

Fig. 1. Kidney-only transplants and active transplant list at year end in the United Kingdom, 1995–2004. (Courtesy of UK Transplant.)

in road traffic accidents and cerebrovascular accidents, the two leading causes of death of cadaveric heart-beating donors (Renal Transplant Audit 1990–1998, UK Transplant, Bristol).

Kidney transplant survival is improving year after year *(8)*, as a result of refinements in immunosuppression, postoperative management, and laboratory support services. Ninety percent of cadaveric grafts survive to 1 yr, with 5- and 10-yr allograft survival rates of approx 70% and 50%, respectively.

1.2. Determinants of Long-Term Outcome

Improvements in long-term graft survival are mainly a result of better outcomes in the first year posttransplantation *(8,9)*. It is disappointing to note that the rate of graft loss after 1 yr has remained relatively unchanged since the 1980s, at 3–5% per year. Long-term graft loss is primarily the result of chronic allograft nephropathy (CAN) (40%) or death with a functioning graft (40%). Recurrence of the initial renal disease in the renal transplant is also an important cause of graft failure (10% of late graft loss). CAN is characterized histologically by intimal hyperplasia in small- and medium-sized arteries, interstitial fibrosis, glomerulosclerosis, and tubular atrophy. Both immunological (chronic rejection) and nonimmunological factors contribute to the development of CAN *(10)*. The clinical manifestations of CAN are a progressive decline in renal function with proteinuria and hypertension. The precise mechanisms are poorly understood, but a number of risk factors have been identified.

Immunological risk factors for CAN include previous episodes of acute rejection *(8)* and suboptimal immunosuppression *(11)*. Mismatches between the donor and recipient at the human leukocyte antigen (HLA)-DR, HLA-A, and HLA-B loci also reduce long-term graft survival in renal transplantation *(12)*. Mismatching is expressed as a mismatch (MM) grade, and the MM grade may vary between 0-0-0 (full house match) and 2-2-2 (complete mismatch), with each integer signifying the HLA-A, -B, and -DR locus, respectively. In the United Kingdom, the number of donor–recipient HLA mismatches has been reduced through the introduction of HLA matching into the National Kidney Allocation Scheme.

Nonimmunological factors leading to CAN are numerous and include increased recipient age, male gender, hypertension, and increased donor age *(12)*. Because there is no effective treatment for CAN other than retransplantation, it is important to try wherever possible to minimize associated risk factors *(11)*.

The rates of recurrent renal disease in the transplanted kidney and its clinical impact vary depending on the underlying disease *(13)*. Histological changes suggestive of diabetic nephropathy can be identified in most grafts in diabetic recipients, but clinically overt diabetic nephropathy is uncommon. In contrast, up to 50% of patients with focal segmental glomerulosclerosis experience disease recurrence, and there is a 50% chance of graft loss within 2 yr.

Death with a functioning graft is most commonly the result of cardiovascular disease (CVD) in the recipient *(14)*. This is discussed in more detail later.

2. Recipient Evaluation

Evaluation of a prospective recipient for renal transplantation should be performed as soon as it becomes apparent that therapy for ESRD will be required. Early transplantation is desirable in patients with ESRD, and there is evidence that pre-emptive transplantation (i.e., transplantation in the months preceding the need for dialysis) is associated with a particularly good outcome ***(15)***. Patients with ESRD secondary to diabetic nephropathy may, if sufficiently fit, be suitable candidates for simultaneous pancreas and kidney transplantation ***(16)***.

With improvements in anesthetic, surgical, and HLA typing techniques, renal transplantation can now be offered to groups of patients previously considered to be at an unacceptably high risk. This includes older patients, those with significant comorbidities such as diabetes mellitus or ischemic heart disease, and highly sensitized patients requiring retransplantation. Advanced age alone is not a contraindication to receiving a renal transplant because improvements in graft survival now mean that survival benefits outweigh potential risks to elderly patients ***(17,18)***. In practice, however, transplantation is rarely considered in those over 75 yr of age.

Evaluation of renal transplant candidates should be undertaken to determine that the risks of surgery and immunosuppression are acceptable to both the patient and the transplant team. Clinical assessment should focus on assessing general fitness (especially of the cardiovascular and respiratory systems), excluding concurrent malignancy and infection, and identifying any psychosocial issues that may interfere with compliance with immunosuppressive therapy ***(19)***. Screening for CVD is a vital component of the assessment process because of its high prevalence in patients with ESRD (*see* **Subheading 9.**). Patients with diabetes and older patients require particularly rigorous screening for cardiovascular pathology.

3. Expansion of the Donor Pool

The majority of donor kidneys in the United Kingdom come from cadaveric heart-beating (brain-stem-dead) donors declared dead using well-recognized criteria ***(20,21)***. The steady decrease in the number of these donors has led to the need to improve organ utilization and to investigate other potential sources of donor kidneys such as marginal donors, non-heart-beating donors (NHBDs), and living donors.

3.1. Marginal Donors

The lengthening waiting list for renal transplantation has led to a relaxation in the selection criteria for kidney donors and the use of kidneys from so-called marginal donors. There is no widely accepted definition of what constitutes a marginal kidney, but examples include donors at the extremes of age, those with longstanding hypertension or diabetes, or donors where there is an increased risk of disease transmission. As might be expected, the results of transplantation with marginal kidneys are inferior to those with standard kidneys ***(22)***.

Transplanting both kidneys from a very marginal donor into one recipient is a potential option and may result in better renal function in the recipient. Dual kidney transplants from marginal donors has been reported to give similar results to single kidney transplants from nonmarginal donors *(23)*, and dual transplantation does not appear to increase the rate of surgical complications *(24)*. This procedure is rarely undertaken in the United Kingdom, with only one dual transplant performed in 2002–2003.

Objective methods of assessing donor kidney quality are necessary to enable rational decision making about organ usage, but none are in widespread use. Scoring systems using donor variables such as age, history of hypertension, renal function, kidney biopsy findings, cause of death, and HLA mismatch may provide a quantitative approach to identifying marginal kidneys *(25,26)*. Until scoring systems become widespread, careful consideration is required as to how best to allocate these organs from marginal donors. It is also important that potential recipients offered kidneys from marginal donors receive careful counseling to enable informed consent to be given *(27)*.

3.2. Living Donors

The outcome of kidney transplantation from living donors has been shown to be superior to that of kidney transplantation from cadaveric donors *(8)*. Although they are usually poor matches for HLA, grafts from living unrelated donors have 3-yr survival rates equivalent to those from living related organs *(28)*. Concerns surrounding living donor transplantation center on the potential risks to the donor and on the possibility of coercion, which may be difficult to detect.

The peri-operative mortality rate for live donor nephrectomy is in the region of 0.03% *(29)*, and the peri-operative major complication rate is approx 2%. There is no long-term increase in mortality after kidney donation, but donors may develop asymptomatic proteinuria and hypertension more often than the general population *(30)*. In addition to a rigorous health screen, potential donors must be carefully questioned by the transplant team about their motives for donation and all attempts must be made to ensure that coercion does not occur.

Medical evaluation of the prospective donor is extensive and can be divided into different phases *(31)*. ABO blood grouping and cross-match testing are performed first to establish that living donor transplantation is feasible. This is followed by a complete medical assessment, including assessment of renal function, and radiological definition of the renal vascular anatomy. If both kidneys have single renal arteries, the left kidney is usually selected for donation because the longer left renal vein makes the recipient operation marginally technically easier.

Removal of the donor's kidney has traditionally been performed through a 15- to 20-cm-long flank incision (open-donor nephrectomy). Postoperative wound pain, which may be chronic in around 5% of donors, and poor cosmesis are potential problems with this approach. Advances in surgical techniques and fiber-optic technology have enabled the introduction of laparoscopic (keyhole) live donor nephrectomy (LLDN) *(32)* in an attempt to reduce postoperative morbidity. Instrument access to the kidney is gained through four abdominal ports requiring 1- to 2-cm incisions each, and the donor kidney is then removed after mobilization through a 6-cm abdominal incision.

Although no large randomized controlled trials have been performed, long-term graft function after LLDN is similar to that after open nephrectomy. Some studies have suggested that early graft function may be marginally delayed after LLDN *(33,34)*. The laparoscopic approach requires a longer operative time *(35)*, although this disadvantage is counterbalanced by improved cosmesis, shorter postoperative stay, reduced analgesic requirement, and earlier return to work *(36)*. Morbidity is similar for the two approaches, although LLDN may leave the donor at long-term risk of small bowel obstruction from adhesions. Some centers offering LLDN have observed increases in donation rates *(37)*, although it difficult to know whether LLDN *per se* is responsible for this.

Although the number of living donor transplants in the United Kingdom is increasing (**Fig. 1**), it makes up only 21% of total kidney transplant activity (UKT 2003 data). This compares poorly with North America, Scandinavia, and Australia, all of which have higher rates of living donation. United Network for Organ Sharing data for 2001 showed, for the first time, that the number of living-donor kidney transplants in the United States exceeded the number of cadaveric transplants undertaken. There is, therefore, considerable scope for further increasing the living kidney donor rate in the United Kingdom.

3.3. Non-Heart-Beating Donors

NHBDs are donors from whom organs are retrieved following declaration of death by conventional means, that is, irreversible cessation of circulatory and respiratory function. NHBDs were the main source of organs before the widespread acceptance of brainstem death criteria in the late 1970s but then declined markedly owing to less favorable results. In recent years, the use of NHBDs has increased in many centers in an attempt to offset the severe shortage of kidneys from cadaveric heart-beating donors.

NHBDs can be separated into categories on the basis of their mode of death *(38)* (**Table 3**). Uncontrolled NHB donations (categories 1 and 2) occur in emergency settings, and because the process of seeking consent from relatives is often protracted, warm ischemic times must be minimized by inserting a double-balloon triple-lumen catheter via the femoral artery, allowing selective perfusion of the renal arteries with cooled organ-preservation solution *(39)*. Controlled NHB donations (categories 3 and 4) are derived from critically ill patients who have died in an intensive care setting. This allows time for con-

Table 3
Maastricht Categories of Non-Heart-Beating Donors

Maastricht category	Description	Location
1	Dead on arrival	Outside hospital, emergency room
2	Unsuccessful resuscitation	Emergency room, intensive care, general ward
3	Treatment withdrawn, awaiting cardiac arrest	Intensive care
4	Cardiac arrest while brainstem dead	Intensive care

From **ref.** ***38***.

sent to donation to be taken from relatives. Once medical intervention has been withdrawn and death has been declared by the medical staff, the transplant team waits a further 5–10 min before starting the organ-retrieval operation.

The insertion of medical devices into uncontrolled NHBDs before consent has been obtained from the relatives raises ethical and legal questions ***(40)***. In the United Kingdom, the acceptance of this technique in potential uncontrolled donors has been achieved by discussions with the local ethics committee and by requesting the coroner's permission before inserting a double-balloon triple-lumen catheter ***(41)***.

The principal concern relating to renal transplants from NHBDs is the higher rates of delayed graft function (DGF) and primary nonfunction (PNF) when compared to kidneys from cadaveric heart-beating donors ***(42,43)***. Careful donor selection may minimize PNF ***(44,45)***, and despite a higher incidence of DGF than after transplantation with kidneys from cadaveric heart-beating donors, the long-term survival of heart-beating and NHBD kidneys is very similar ***(43–45)***. Other trials report similar PNF rates between the two groups. Although DGF after transplantation of kidneys from cadaveric heart-beating donors may be associated with reduced long-term graft survival ***(46)***, the long-term graft survival of NHBD grafts appears comparable to cadaveric heart-beating grafts.

There are significant logistical difficulties in instituting a NHBD program. Referrals of potential uncontrolled donors call for enthusiasm and dedication from accident and emergency department staff and a rapid response from the transplant team. Controlled NHBDs often require the surgical team and operating room nursing staff to wait for prolonged periods for the patient to develop asystole once ventilation has been discontinued.

Although the use of kidneys from NHBDs is increasing, the number performed in the United Kingdom remains relatively small. Only 103 transplants from NHBDs were performed in 2002–2003 (6% of the total kidney transplants undertaken). This low level of utilization reflects the medical, ethical, legal, and logistical hurdles that need to be overcome before the concept of NHB donation is widely accepted. NHBDs have the potential to make a major contribution to the organ donor pool. A 40% increase in the overall supply of cadaveric kidneys has been reported from a Dutch center using NHBD kidneys ***(47)***; if maintained, this would substantially reduce the renal transplant waiting list ***(42)***.

3.4. ABO-Incompatible Renal Transplants

Traditionally, ABO blood group compatibility is considered an essential prerequisite for successful kidney transplantation. ABO-incompatible kidney transplants are likely to be rapidly destroyed by hyperacute rejection owing to anti-A and/or anti-B antibodies binding to A and/or B antigens on the graft endothelium, activating the complement cascade and inducing platelet aggregation and intravascular thrombosis ***(48,49)***.

Graft loss is not inevitable, however, and in 1981 Slapak and colleagues observed that plasmapheresis overcame rapid rejection in an accidental ABO-incompatible renal transplant that resulted from a blood typing error ***(50)***. There has recently been increased interest in the use of ABO-incompatible living donor kidney transplants, particularly in countries where, because cadaveric donation is rare for cultural reasons, there is no alternative donor source. Japanese surgeons have reported that selected subgroups of patients can achieve acceptable outcomes following transplantation of ABO-incompatible kidneys if pretransplant anti-ABO antibody reduction is combined with splenectomy and/or postoperative anticoagulation and high-dose immunosuppression.

Pretransplant anti-A/anti-B immunoglobulin (Ig)G and IgM antibody titers are reduced by either plasma exchange or immunoabsorption, with subsequent replacement with type AB plasma. Splenectomy is performed in an attempt to reduce the recipient's ability to produce anti-A/anti-B antibodies once the ABO-incompatible living donor kidney transplant has been performed ***(51)***. Anticoagulation with platelet aggregation inhibitors is used to prevent the initiation of intra-renal disseminated intravascular coagulation due to humoral rejection. The need for time-consuming preoperative treatment means that this approach is readily applicable only to recipients of living donor and not cadaveric donor organs.

From 1989 to 1998, a total of 312 ABO-incompatible living kidney transplants were performed in Japan ***(52)***, approx 10% of all living donor grafts. The procedure has shown the most promise for recipients younger than 15 yr, with progressively less favorable results in older age groups. The largest study of pediatric recipients of ABO-incompatible living kidney transplants reported actuarial 1- and 5-yr graft survival rates of 87% and 85%, respectively, with 100% patient survival ***(53)***. There are no significant differences in graft survival between A- and B-incompatible transplants ***(52)***.

Blood group A can be subdivided into A_1 and A_2 types on the basis of the degree of expression of the A epitope by tissues. Type A_1 is strongly expressed, and A_2 is only weakly expressed. In Europeans, A_1 is the dominant A blood group and makes up approx 80% of the total type A population ***(54)***. In contrast to A_1-incompatible kidney transplantation, A_2-incompatible transplants do not require pretransplant antibody removal if recipients with low anti-A serum titers are selected. This means that A_2-incompatible cadaveric renal transplants can potentially be undertaken. One single-center series of A_2-incompatible cadaveric kidney transplants reported an actuarial 2-yr graft survival of 94% for those patients with a low pretransplant anti-A IgG titer ***(55)***. These results have been difficult to replicate ***(56)***, and therefore this approach remains confined to a small number of units.

At present, a number of factors prevent A_1BO-incompatible living kidney transplants from achieving widespread acceptance in the Western transplantation community. These include the relative availability of ABO-compatible cadaveric and living grafts, the complex and expensive pretransplant plasmapheresis required, and the inferior early graft survival rates when compared to ABO-compatible kidney transplants. An alternative approach to dealing with ABO-incompatible living donors and recipients is to undertake paired donation. This involves an exchange agreement between two donor–recipient pairs such that kidneys from two living donors who are both ABO incompatible with their intended recipients are donated to the reciprocal ABO-compatible recipients. This has been practiced successfully in South Korea for many years and is also undertaken in a small number of American centers. Under current UK legislation, paired donation is illegal ***(57)***, but there is hope that new legislation might enable this approach to be used for ABO-incompatible living donor kidney transplantation.

4. Recipient Operative Technique

Operative techniques for renal transplantation have remained relatively constant for the last 40 yr (**Fig. 2**). The donor kidney is placed extraperitoneally in either iliac fossa. The renal vein is anastomosed to the external iliac vein, and the donor renal artery is anastomosed to either the external or internal iliac artery. Once the venous and arterial anastomoses have been completed, the vascular clamps are removed to allow perfusion of the graft, and the ureter–bladder anastomosis is then performed. Insertion of a double-J ureteric stent has been shown to reduce urological complications, particularly urine leaks ***(58)***.

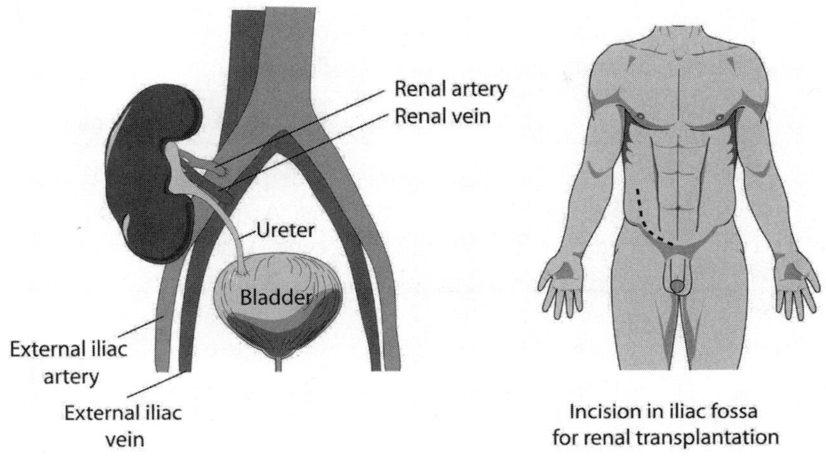

Fig. 2. Schematic view of right iliac fossa renal transplant. Anastomosis of renal vessels to external iliac vessels.

5. Current Immunosuppressive Strategies

The commonly used oral immunosuppressive agents are of broadly three classes: calcineurin inhibitors (cyclosporine, tacrolimus), antiproliferative agents (azathioprine, mycophenolate mofetil), and steroids (prednisolone). Combined use of a single agent from each class is known as triple therapy, the standard regime of immunosuppression in early to midterm posttransplantation. This provides broad immunosuppression based on the differing mechanisms of action of each class. Additional immunosuppression at the time of renal transplantation (induction therapy) is common practice because the risk of acute rejection highest in first 6 mo. Induction therapy usually consists of antibody prophylaxis with either daclizumab (Zenapax®, Roche) or basiliximab (Simulect®, Novartis) (*see* below).

Cyclosporine (CyA, Sandimmun®, Novartis) was introduced in the late 1970s by Sir Roy Calne in Cambridge and resulted in a marked improvement in graft-survival rates ***(59)***. CyA combined with azathioprine (AZA) and prednisolone became the standard immunosuppressive regime during the 1980s. The mid-1990s saw the introduction of a CyA microemulsion formulation (Neoral®, Novartis), resulting in better absorption and more consistent dosing ***(60)***. Other new drugs to emerge at this time were tacrolimus (Prograf®, Fujisawa) and mycophenolate mofetil (MMF, CellCept®, Roche). Substitution of tacrolimus for CyA in the triple therapy protocol led to a significant reduction in acute rejection ***(61)***, as did MMF when compared to azathioprine in CyA-based triple therapy ***(62)***.

Table 4
Adverse Cardiovascular Risk Profiles of Common Immunosuppressant Medications

Medication	Diabetes	Hypertension	Hyperlipidemia
Corticosteroids	+++	++	+++
Cyclosporine	++	++	++
Tacrolimus	+++	++	+
Sirolimus	–	–	+++

Within each of the three main classes of immunosuppressive drugs, the side-effect profiles are similar. The calcineurin inhibitors, although chemically unrelated, are associated with hypertension, hyperlipidemia, and the development of diabetes to varying degrees (**Table 4**). Of most concern are the nephrotoxic effects of calcineurin inhibitors, which can cause permanent renal damage and contribute to CAN. The antiproliferative agents lead to dose-related nonspecific bone marrow suppression, and MMF causes gastrointestinal disturbances. The debilitating side effects of steroids are well known and include osteoporosis, cataracts, hypertension, adrenal suppression, skin atrophy, neuropsychiatric changes, and peptic ulceration. Also, the continued use of steroids may be associated with poorer long-term graft outcome ***(12)***. Posttransplant immunosuppressive protocols have been developed that are entirely steroid-free ***(63)***, but in most centers steroids are given at the time of transplantation and then slowly tapered to the minimal required dose. In some patients steroids can be stopped completely, but unfortunately steroid withdrawal can initiate an episode of acute rejection, especially in black recipients ***(64)***.

A new class of immunosuppressants, the mammalian target of rapamycin (mTOR) inhibitors, was launched in the late 1990s. The first member of the mTOR inhibitor class to enter clinical practice was rapamycin (sirolimus, Rapamune®, Wyeth). The main side effects of sirolimus are hyperlipidemia and myelosuppression. An advantage of the mTOR inhibitors is their lack of nephrotoxicity. Cyclosporine withdrawal from a sirolimus–CyA–steroid regimen has been shown to lead to improved graft function and reduction in hypertension ***(65)***. There is hope that the calcineurin-sparing effects of sirolimus may lead to decreased rates of CAN in the long-term. At present the optimal role of sirolimus in renal transplantation is unknown and the long-term results of trials are awaited ***(66)***.

As acute rejection rates have dropped and the number of clinically effective immunosuppressant agents has increased, the clinical focus has moved towards optimizing long-term outcomes and tailoring immunosuppressive regimes to the needs of the individual patient. Tacrolimus should be avoided in patients with diabetes, and sirolimus should be used with caution in patients with preexisting CVD. Steroid use should be minimized for both groups. Patients who are at particularly high risk of an acute rejection episode may benefit from more potent immunosuppression.

6. Acute Rejection Monitoring and Management

Acute rejection occurs in approx 30% of renal transplant recipients within the first 6 mo postoperatively, depending on the immunosuppressive regime and the immunological risk profile of the patient. In the majority of cases, acute rejection is reversible and results in early graft loss in less than 10% of rejection episodes. Acute rejection may, however, be an important predictor of chronic rejection ***(67)*** and therefore of long-term function and graft survival ***(8)***. Acute vascular rejection and rejection episodes that are severe, recurrent, or of late onset are associated with an increased risk of chronic rejection ***(67)***. The prevention, early diagnosis, and effective management of acute rejection are therefore vital.

Acute rejection is recognized clinically by a rapid deterioration in graft function (i.e., increased creatinine) after exclusion of alternative diagnoses such as dehydration, urinary tract infection, calcineurin-inhibitor toxicity, or inflow/outflow obstruction. Percutaneous ultrasound-guided biopsy is often valuable and can be performed under local anesthetic with a major complication rate of 0.5% ***(68)***. Histological analysis enables the diagnosis, classification, and scoring of acute rejection according to the Banff criteria ***(69,70)***.

Recognition that the prevention of clinical acute rejection may result in improved long-term graft outcomes has led to an interest in detecting subclinical rejection with serial biopsies (protocol biopsies). Subclinical rejection is defined as the presence of histological changes meeting the criteria for acute rejection in patients with stable graft function ***(71)***. The incidence of subclinical rejection in the first 3 mo posttransplant varies from 5 to 50% ***(71)***. In one small study its presence was shown to be associated with increased rates of CAN at 2 yr ***(72)***, and treatment with methylprednisolone correlated with improved 2-yr graft outcomes ***(73)***. In an era of increasing graft survival and decreasing acute rejection rates, subjecting patients to protocol biopsies and the potential morbidity of high-dose steroids may be inappropriate given that the natural history of subclinical rejection is not known with certainty ***(74)***. A prospective randomized trial with long-term follow-up is needed to resolve this issue.

Noninvasive methods to detect imminent acute rejection are also being developed. Techniques include measurement of perforin and granzyme B gene expression in peripheral blood ***(75,76)***, and measurement of soluble C4d and adhesion molecules in the urine by enzyme-linked immunosorbent assay *(77)*. Noninvasive tests for CAN are also being investigated *(78,79)*, but none have undergone large-scale trials or entered routine clinical use.

6.1. Management of Acute Rejection

First-line treatment of acute rejection is with high-dose intravenous steroid (e.g., methylprednisolone 0.5–1 g daily for 3 d). In up to 50% of cases, acute rejection is steroid resistant and treatment with polyclonal antithymocyte globulin (ATG) is required *(80)*. This is given under close supervision as a result of the risk of pulmonary edema from cytokine release syndrome. Anti-CD3 monoclonal antibody (muromonab-CD3, Orthoclone OKT®3, Ortho Biotech) has also been used with similar efficacy and side effects *(81)*. Early reports have suggested that high-dose pooled human immunoglobulin may be superior because of its relatively benign side-effect profile *(82)*.

As already noted, both daclizumab and basiliximab, monoclonal antibodies directed against the interlukin-2 receptor α chain (CD25), reduce the incidence of acute rejection by approx 30% when given prophylactically around the time of transplantation *(83,84)*. These agents, which are widely used, appear to be free from significant side effects, and their ability to reduce acute rejection makes them cost-effective *(85)*.

6.2. C4d Staining and Antibody-Mediated Rejection

Since the mid-1990s, it has become increasingly apparent that antibody may mediate allograft rejection in settings other than hyperacute rejection. This has occurred through the recognition that C4d deposition in graft peritubular capillaries is a reliable marker of antibody-mediated acute rejection *(86)*. C4d is a stable inactive degradation product of complement factor C4, formed when the classical complement cascade is activated by the binding of antidonor antibodies to the endothelium of the allograft.

Capillary C4d staining has been found in 30% of biopsies performed for renal graft deterioration *(87)* and has been found to be 95% sensitive and specific for the presence of antidonor antibodies *(88)*. The definitive diagnosis of acute antibody-mediated rejection requires morphological evidence of acute tissue injury with immunopathological evidence for antibody action (C4d staining or immunoglobulin and complement in arterial fibrinoid necrosis) and serological evidence of antidonor antibodies *(69)*.

C4d staining may also occur in CAN, mildly altered graft function, or with normal histology. In these settings, the clinical significance of C4d staining remains unclear. However, when features of acute cellular or humoral rejection are present, C4d staining appears to be a marker of severity *(89)*. Therefore, anti-B-cell therapy (antithymocyte globulin, intravenous immunoglobulin, mycophenolate mofetil) or removal of antibody (plasmapheresis, immunoabsorption) should be considered ***(90)***.

7. Management of the Sensitized Patient

Exposure to foreign HLA leads to immunological sensitization and the generation of lymphocyte cytotoxic or binding antibodies in the recipient's serum. Sensitization to alloantigens may result from previous failed grafts, pregnancies, and blood transfusions. Preexisting antibodies against a donor's HLA may cause hyperacute rejection and immediate graft loss; to avoid this problem, a crossmatch test, in which serum of the prospective recipient is tested against donor lymphocytes plus complement, is routinely performed before making the final decision to carry out transplantation. In general, a positive T-cell cross-match test (donor cell lysis) is a contraindication to renal transplantation.

Sensitization is reported as the panel-reactive antibody (PRA). This is the percentage of panel cells, selected to include common HLA antigens, which are lysed by the patient's serum. Highly sensitized patients are arbitrarily defined as those with a PRA of 85% or greater. Such patients are more likely to have a positive lymphocyte cross-match test and will thus wait longer for a transplant if this is not taken into account in allocation systems. This will tend to disadvantage young patients requiring multiple transplants. Management of the sensitized patient involves techniques to reduce PRA as well as organ allocation schemes to prevent excessively long waiting times. Strategies to reduce the incidence of sensitization by minimizing exposure to alloantigens in the transplant population are also important. The UK kidney allocation scheme avoids, wherever possible, poorly HLA-matched kidney transplants, especially in younger recipients.

The introduction of recombinant human erythropoietin has revolutionized the treatment of the anemia of chronic renal failure by reducing the need for blood transfusion. This has also reduced sensitization ***(91)***. Despite the introduction of leucocyte-depleted blood products in the United Kingdom in 1999 to minimize the risk of variant Creutzfeldt-Jakob disease (vCJD) transmission, studies elsewhere have not demonstrated the expected reduction in allosensitization ***(92)***.

Organ-allocation schemes play the major role in managing highly sensitized patients. Under the UK National Kidney Allocation Scheme, highly sensitized patients are given priority over patients with PRAs of less than 85% such that blood-group-compatible kidneys are allocated to 0-0-0 mismatched highly sensitized patients. Eurotransplant has similar programs and has demonstrated reduced waiting time to transplantation for highly sensitized patients ***(93)***. The recent publication of HLAMatchmaker, an algorithm that determines

HLA compatibility at the level of amino acid triplets in antibody-accessible regions of HLA molecules, may also be valuable in identifying more HLA-matched donors for this group of patients ***(94)***.

Clinical strategies to decrease PRAs, and thus increase the chances of a negative crossmatch, include administration of intravenous gammaglobulin ***(95)***, induction immunosuppression with antithymocyte globulin ***(96)***, plasma exchange/immunoabsorption ***(97)***, or a combination of the above ***(98)***.

8. BK-Virus-Associated Nephropathy

Renal transplant recipients are, like all transplant recipients, at increased risk of infection, particularly viral infections such as cytomegalovirus infection ***(99)***. A review of infectious complications after renal transplantation is beyond the scope of this chapter. However, since it was first reported in 1995, BK-virus-associated nephropathy (BKVN) has emerged as an important cause of renal allograft loss and is therefore highlighted here.

BK virus (also known as polyomavirus hominis 1) is an unenveloped double-stranded DNA virus that infects 75% of the general population. Primary infection occurs in childhood, resulting in a vague flu-like illness. The route of transmission is unclear. BK virus then persists in the urinary tract, from where it may undergo asymptomatic reactivation in immunocompetent individuals. In the immunocompromised the disease is more virulent, especially in kidney transplant patients ***(100)***.

In renal transplant recipients, BK viral disease has a wide variety of manifestations, including ureteric stenosis, transient graft dysfunction, or irreversible allograft failure secondary to BKVN. BKVN is defined as deterioration of graft function associated with histologically apparent BK virus allograft infection ***(101)***. It occurs in approx 8% of renal transplant patients ***(102)***, and the incidence appears to be rising. This may be the result of the use of more potent immunosuppressants, increased awareness, and better diagnostic tools.

Definitive diagnosis of BKVN requires allograft biopsy ***(103)***. BKVN is seen as intranuclear inclusion bodies in tubular epithelial cells with enlarged nuclei. Ongoing viral replication leads to an accompanying inflammatory response with fibrosis and eventually atrophic tubules. Infected cells shed into the urine are known as decoy cells. Quantitative polymerase chain reaction (PCR) of BKV DNA in serum is the most commonly used noninvasive test, with sensitivity and specificity of 100% and 88%, respectively ***(102)***.

In the absence of rejection, which is often coexistent, management consists of immunosuppressant reduction. If rejection is present, management is difficult—a two-step protocol of antirejection treatment followed by lowered immunosuppression has been advocated ***(100)***. Antiviral treatment with cidofivir may be of use, but it is potentially nephrotoxic and has not yet been evaluated in randomized trials. Much remains to be learned about the natural history, diagnosis, and optimum treatment of this disease.

9. Cardiovascular Disease in the Renal Transplant Patient

As short-term success rates in kidney transplantation improve, clinical attention is focusing increasingly on maximizing long-term survival. Death with a functioning graft causes 40% of late graft losses, with CVD accounting for approximately half of all deaths after renal transplantation ***(14)***. CVD includes ischemic heart disease, peripheral vascular disease, cerebrovascular disease, and cardiac failure. A recipient aged 25–34 yr has a 10 times higher relative risk of dying of CVD than an age- and gender-matched control ***(104)***. Overall, kidney recipients have a prevalence of CVD five times that of the general population ***(105)***. Prevention and management of CVD and its risk factors is therefore a high priority.

Studies on the general population such as the Framingham Heart Study have identified risk factors for the development of CVD and ischemic heart disease in particular. Modifiable risk factors include hypertension, hypercholesterolemia, obesity, sedentary lifestyle, smoking, and diabetes; age, gender, ethnic group, and family history of CVD are unmodifiable risk factors. Although these traditional risk factors also apply to renal transplantation patients, they tend to underestimate the prevalence of CVD ***(106)***. Proteinuria, chronic immunosuppression, infections, and hyperhomocysteinemia may help to explain the higher than predicted CVD burden of the transplant population (**Fig. 3**).

CVD is often already present prior to transplantation. ESRD and hemodialysis are associated with hypertension, fluid overload, anemia, and the metabolic effects of chronic uremia on the cardiovascular system ***(107)***. In addition, diabetes or renovascular disease may be the underlying cause of ESRD, placing the patient in a very high-risk group. All patients referred for consideration of renal transplantation should therefore undergo screening and management for both CVD risk factors and overt CVD ***(19)***. Smoking cessation advice and support is especially important, as is encouragement to exercise regularly.

Once transplantation has occurred, screening should continue in the outpatient clinic because calcineurin inhibitors (tacrolimus, cyclosporine) and corticosteroids are associated with the development of hypertension, diabetes, and hyperlipidemia to differing degrees. Hypertension should be treated initially with general measures such as weight reduction, salt restriction, and exercise. However, antihypertensive drugs are often necessary. In patients with uncontrollable hypertension, renal artery stenosis should be excluded. Hyperlipidemia is commonly treated with diet control and HMG-CoA reductase inhibitors (statins). In addition, statins may have a role in the primary prevention of CVD ***(108)*** as well as a potential immunosuppressant action ***(109,110)***.

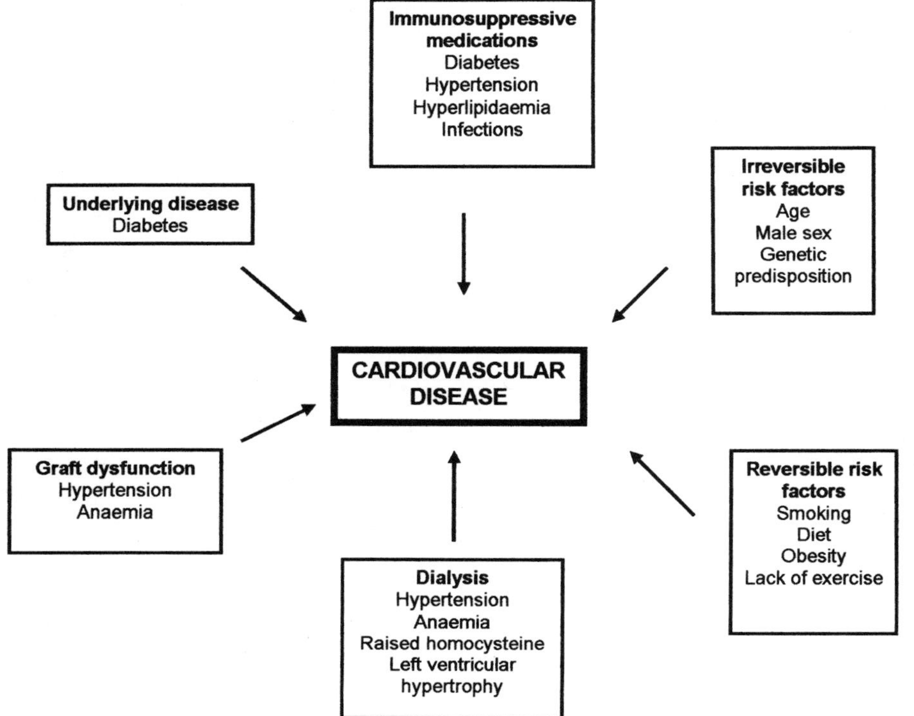

Fig. 3. Cardiovascular disease risk factors in renal transplant recipients.

In practice, the majority of renal transplant recipients receive statins and antiplatelet agents such as aspirin in an attempt to reduce cardiovascular morbidity and mortality. Postttransplant diabetes mellitus (PTDM) has an incidence of 4–18% ***(111)***, and fasting blood glucose tests should be undertaken every 3 mo ***(112)***. Initial treatment is with dietary modification, although oral hypoglycemics or even insulin may be necessary. Preexisting diabetes requires intensive monitoring and blood glucose control. Control of hypertension, hyperlipidemia, and PTDM may also require modifications to the patient's immunosuppressive regime.

Other risk factors may also play a part in the development of CVD in the renal transplant recipient. Elevated plasma homocysteine has been identified as an independent factor for CVD in the renal transplant population ***(113)***, but as yet there is no evidence that reduction of homocysteine levels reduces the incidence of CVDs. Routine homocysteine measurement and the use of folate supplements are therefore currently not recommended ***(114)***. Systemic inflammation or low-grade infection may also play a role in the development of CVD because C-reactive protein, a marker of inflammation, is associated with an increased risk of ischemic heart disease in renal transplant recipients ***(115)***. Proteinuria has been shown to be an independent risk factor for both cardiovascular and noncardiovascular death ***(116)***. Treatment with an angiotensin-converting enzyme inhibitor, even in normotensive patients, should be considered ***(117)***.

10. Conclusion

As with other types of organ transplantation, the major problem facing the field of renal transplantation is a shortage of organs due to declining rates of cadaveric heart-beating donors. Although the use of alternative sources of organs such as living donors and NHBDs is rising, at present this increase is only sufficient to keep the overall number of transplants performed static. Techniques to enable ABO-incompatible renal transplantation are expected to widen access to living donor kidneys, a high-quality source of grafts. With advances in immunosuppression and increasing long-term graft survival, the clinical focus is shifting to improving the quality of life of renal transplant recipients by minimizing immunosuppression-related side effects and preventing cardiovascular diseases. Despite this progress, CAN remains a significant problem. Further work on the prevention and early detection of CAN is essential if the significant gains in long-term renal graft survival seen over the last 20 yr are to continue.

References

1. Bradley, J. A. and Hamilton, D. N. H. (2001) Organ transplantation: an historical perspective, in *Transplantation Surgery* (Hakim, N. S. and Danovitch, G. M, eds.), Springer, London, p. 1.
2. Evans, R. W., Manninen, D. L., Garrison, L. P., Jr., et al. (1985) The quality of life of patients with end-stage renal disease. *N. Engl. J. Med.* **312**, 553–559.
3. Valderrabano, F., Jofre, R., and Lopez-Gomez, J. M. (2001) Quality of life in end-stage renal disease patients. *Am. J. Kidney Dis.* **38**, 443–464.
4. Wolfe, R. A., Ashby, V. B., Milford, E. L., et al. (1999) Comparison of mortality in all patients on dialysis, patients on dialysis awaiting transplantation, and recipients of a first cadaveric transplant. *N. Engl. J. Med.* **341**, 1725–1730.
5. Eggers, P. (1992) Comparison of treatment costs between dialysis and transplantation. *Semin. Nephrol.* **12**, 284–289.
6. Croxson, B. E. and Ashton, T. (1990) A cost effectiveness analysis of the treatment of end stage renal failure. *NZ Med. J.* **103**, 171–174.
7. Morris, P. J. (2001) *Kidney Transplantation. Principles and Practice,* W.B. Saunders, Philadelphia.
8. Hariharan, S., Johnson, C. P., Bresnahan, B. A., Taranto, S. E., McIntosh, M. J., and Stablein, D. (2000) Improved graft survival after renal transplantation in the United States, 1988 to 1996. *N. Engl. J. Med.* **342**, 605–612.

9. Hariharan, S., McBride, M. A., Cherikh, W. S., Tolleris, C. B., Bresnahan, B. A., and Johnson, C. P. (2002) Post-transplant renal function in the first year predicts long-term kidney transplant survival. *Kidney Int.* **62**, 311–318.
10. Pascual, M., Theruvath, T., Kawai, T., Tolkoff-Rubin, N., and Cosimi, A. B. (2002) Strategies to improve long-term outcomes after renal transplantation. *N. Engl. J. Med.* **346**, 580–590.
11. Monaco, A. P., Burke, J. F. Jr., Ferguson, R. M., et al. (1999) Current thinking on chronic renal allograft rejection: issues, concerns, and recommendations from a 1997 roundtable discussion. *Am. J. Kidney Dis.* **33**, 150–160.
12. Opelz, G. (2000) Factors influencing long-term graft loss. The Collaborative Transplant Study. *Transplant. Proc.* **32**, 647–649.
13. Denton, M. D. and Singh, A. K. (2000) Recurrent and de novo glomerulonephritis in the renal allograft. *Semin. Nephrol.* **20**, 164–175.
14. Briggs, J. D. (2001) Causes of death after renal transplantation. *Nephrol. Dial. Transplant.* **16**, 1545–1549.
15. Papalois, V. E., Moss, A., Gillingham, K. J., Sutherland, D. E., Matas, A. J., and Humar, A. (2000) Pre-emptive transplants for patients with renal failure: an argument against waiting until dialysis. *Transplantation* **70**, 625–631.
16. White, S. A., Nicholson, M. L., and London, N. J. (1999) Vascularized pancreas allotransplantation—clinical indications and outcome. *Diabet. Med.* **16**, 533–534.
17. Roodnat, J. I., Zietse, R., Mulder, P. G., Rischen-Vos, J., van Gelder, T., Ijzermans, J. N., and Weimar, W. (1999) The vanishing importance of age in renal transplantation. *Transplantation* **67**, 576–580.
18. Schaubel, D., Desmeules, M., Mao, Y., Jeffery, J., and Fenton, S. (1995) Survival experience among elderly end-stage renal disease patients. A controlled comparison of transplantation and dialysis. *Transplantation* **60**, 1389–1394.
19. Kasiske, B. L., Cangro, C. B. , Hariharan, S., et al.; American Society of Transplantation (2002) The evaluation of renal transplantation candidates: clinical practice guidelines. *Am. J. Transplant.* **1 (Suppl. 2)**, 3–95.
20. (1995) Criteria for the diagnosis of brain stem death. Review by a working group convened by the Royal College of Physicians and endorsed by the Conference of Medical Royal Colleges and their Faculties in the United Kingdom. *J. R. Coll. Physicians Lond.* **29**,381–382.
21. Wijdicks, E. F. (2001) The diagnosis of brain death. *N. Engl. J. Med.* **344**, 1215–1221.
22. Ojo, A. O., Hanson, J.A., Meier-Kriesche, H., et al. (2001) Survival in recipients of marginal cadaveric donor kidneys compared with other recipients and wait-listed transplant candidates. *J. Am. Soc. Nephrol.* **12**, 589–597.
23. Jerius, J. T., Taylor, R. J., Murillo, D., and Leone, J. P. (2000) Double renal transplants from marginal donors: 2-year results. *J. Urol.* **163**, 423–425.
24. Remuzzi, G., Grinyo, J., Ruggenenti, P., et al. (1999) Early experience with dual kidney transplantation in adults using expanded donor criteria. Double Kidney Transplant Group (DKG). *J. Am. Soc. Nephrol.* **10**, 2591–2598.

25. Nyberg, S. L., Matas, A. J., Kremers, W. K., et al. (2003) Improved scoring system to assess adult donors for cadaver renal transplantation. *Am. J. Transplant.* **3**, 715–721.
26. Perico, N., Ruggenenti, P., Scalamogna, M., Locatelli, G., and Remuzzi, G. (2002) One or two marginal organs for kidney transplantation? *Transplant. Proc.* **34**, 3091–3096.
27. Persson, M. O., Persson, N. H., Kallen, R., Ekberg, H., and Hermeren, G. (2002) Kidneys from marginal donors: views of patients on informed consent. *Nephrol. Dial. Transplant.* **17**, 1497–1502.
28. Terasaki, P. I., Cecka, J. M., Gjertson, D W., and Takemoto, S. (1995) High survival rates of kidney transplants from spousal and living unrelated donors. *N. Engl. J. Med.* **333**, 333–336.
29. Najarian, J. S., Chavers, B. M., McHugh, L. E., and Matas, A. J. (1992) 20 years or more of follow-up of living kidney donors. *Lancet* **340**, 807–810.
30. Kasiske, B. L., Ma, J. Z., Louis, T. A., and Swan, S. K. (1995) Long-term effects of reduced renal mass in humans. *Kidney Int.* **48**, 814–819.
31. (2000). *UK Guidelines for Living Donor Kidney Transplantation,* British Transplantation Society, London, p. 1.
32. Ratner, L. E., Ciseck, L. J., Moore, R. G., Cigarroa, F. G., Kaufman, H. S., and Kavoussi, L. R. (1995) Laparoscopic live donor nephrectomy. *Transplantation* **60**,1047–1049.
33. Waller, J. R., Hiley, A. L., Mullin, E. J., Veitch, P S., and Nicholson, M. L. (2002) Living kidney donation: a comparison of laparoscopic and conventional open operations. *Postgrad. Med. J.* **78**, 153–157.
34. Ratner, L. E., Montgomery, R A., and Kavoussi, L. R. (1999) Laparoscopic live donor nephrectomy: the four year Johns Hopkins University experience. *Nephrol. Dial. Transplant.* **14**, 2090–2093.
35. Velidedeoglu, E., Williams, N., Brayman, K. L., et al. (2002) Comparison of open, laparoscopic, and hand-assisted approaches to live-donor nephrectomy. *Transplantation* **74**, 169–172.
36. Lind, M. Y., Ijzermans, J. N., and Bonjer, H. J. (2002) Open vs. laparoscopic donor nephrectomy in renal transplantation. *BJU Int.* **89**,162–168.
37. Kuo, P. C. and Johnson, L. B. (2000) Laparoscopic donor nephrectomy increases the supply of living donor kidneys: a center-specific microeconomic analysis. *Transplantation* **69**, 2211–2213.
38. Kootstra, G. (1995) Statement on non-heart-beating donor programs. *Transplant Proc.* **27**, 2965–2965.
39. Garcia-Rinaldi, R., Lefrak, E. A., Defore, W. W., et al. (1975) In situ preservation of cadaver kidneys for transplantation: laboratory observations and clinical application. *Ann. Surg.* **182**, 576–584.
40. Bos, M. A. (1995) Legal issues concerning the use of non-heart-beating donors. *Transplant. Proc.* **27**, 2929–2931.
41. Dunlop, P., Varty, K., Veitch, P. S., Nicholson, M. L., and Bell, P. R. (1995) Non-heart-beating donors: the Leicester experience. *Transplant. Proc.* **27,** 2940–2941.

42. Cho, Y. W., Terasaki, P. I., Cecka, J. M., and Gjertson, D. W. (1998) Transplantation of kidneys from donors whose hearts have stopped beating. *N. Engl. J. Med.* **338**, 221–225.
43. Nicholson, M. L., Metcalfe, M. S., White, S. A., et al. (2000) A comparison of the results of renal transplantation from non-heart-beating, conventional cadaveric, and living donors. *Kidney Int.* **58**, 2585–2591.
44. Weber, M., Dindo, D., Demartines, N., Ambuhl, P. M., and Clavien, P. A. (2002) Kidney transplantation from donors without a heartbeat. *N. Engl. J. Med.* **347**, 248–255.
45. Metcalfe, M. S., Butterworth, P. C., White, S. A., et al. (2001) A case-control comparison of the results of renal transplantation from heart-beating and non-heart-beating donors. *Transplantation* **71**,1556–1559.
46. Pirsch, J. D., Ploeg, R. J., Gange, S., et al. (1996) Determinants of graft survival after renal transplantation. *Transplantation* **61**, 1581–1586.
47. Kootstra, G. (1997) The asystolic, or non-heartbeating, donor. *Transplantation* **63**, 917–921.
48. Hume, D. M., Merrill, J. P., Miller, B. F., and Thorn, G. W. (1955) Experiences with renal homotransplantation in the human: report of nine cases. *J. Clin. Invest.* **34**, 327–382.
49. Starzl, T. E., Marchioro, T. L., Holmes, J. H., et al. (1964) Renal homografts in patients with major donor-recipient blood group incompatibilities. *Surgery* **55**,195–200.
50. Slapak, M., Naik, R. B., and Lee, H. A. (1981) Renal transplant in a patient with major donor-recipient blood group incompatibility: reversal of acute rejection by the use of modified plasmapheresis. *Transplantation* **31**, 4–7.
51. Alexandre, G. P. J., Squifflet, J. P., Bruyere, M. D., et al. (1985) Splenectomy as a prerequisite for successful human ABO-incompatible renal transplantation. *Transplant. Proc.* **17**, 138–143.
52. Takahashi, K. (2001) *ABO-Incompatible Kidney Transplantation*, Elsevier, Amsterdam.
53. Shishido, S., Asanuma, H., Tajima, E., et al. (2001) ABO-incompatible living-donor kidney transplantation in children. *Transplantation* **72**, 1037–1042.
54. Daniels, G. (1995) *Human Blood Groups*, Blackwell Science, Oxford.
55. Nelson, P. W., Landreneau, M. D., Luger, A. M., et al. (1998) Ten-year experience in transplantation of A2 kidneys into B and O recipients. *Transplantation* **65**, 256–260.
56. Schnuelle, P. and van der Woude, F. J. (1998) Should A2 kidneys be transplanted into B or O recipients? *Lancet* **351**, 1675–1676.
57. Sells, R. A. (1997) Paired-kidney-exchange programs. *N. Engl. J. Med.* **337**, 1392–1393.
58. Pleass, H. C., Clark, K. R., Rigg, K. M., et al. (1995) Urologic complications after renal transplantation: a prospective randomized trial comparing different techniques of ureteric anastomosis and the use of prophylactic ureteric stents. *Transplant Proc.* **27**, 1091–1092.

59. Calne, R. Y. (1987) Cyclosporin in cadaveric renal transplantation: 5-year follow-up of a multicentre trial. *Lancet.* **2**, 506–507.
60. Curtis, J. J., Barbeito, R., Pirsch, J., Lewis, R. M., Van Buren, D. H., and Choudhury, S. (1999) Differences in bioavailability between oral cyclosporine formulations in maintenance renal transplant patients. *Am. J. Kidney Dis.* **34**, 869–874.
61. Knoll, G. A. and Bell, R. C. (1999) Tacrolimus versus cyclosporin for immunosuppression in renal transplantation: meta-analysis of randomised trials. *BMJ* **318**, 1104–1107.
62. Halloran, P., Mathew, T., Tomlanovich, S., Groth, C., Hooftman, L., and Barker, C. (1997) Mycophenolate mofetil in renal allograft recipients: a pooled efficacy analysis of three randomized, double-blind, clinical studies in prevention of rejection. The International Mycophenolate Mofetil Renal Transplant Study Groups. *Transplantation* **63**, 39–47.
63. Birkeland, S. A. (2001) Steroid-free immunosuppression in renal transplantation: a long-term follow-up of 100 consecutive patients. *Transplantation* **71**, 1089–1090.
64. Ahsan, N., Hricik, D., Matas, A., et al. (1999) Prednisone withdrawal in kidney transplant recipients on cyclosporine and mycophenolate mofetil—a prospective randomized study. Steroid Withdrawal Study Group. *Transplantation* **68**, 1865–1874.
65. Oberbauer, R., Kreis, H., Johnson, R. W., et al.; Rapamune Maintenance Regimen Study Group. (2003) Long-term improvement in renal function with sirolimus after early cyclosporine withdrawal in renal transplant recipients: 2-year results of the Rapamune Maintenance Regimen Study. *Transplantation* **76**, 364–370.
66. Watson, C. J. (2001) Sirolimus (rapamycin) in clinical transplantation. *Transplant. Rev.* **15**, 165–168.
67. Humar, A., Kerr, S., Gillingham, K. J., and Matas, A. J. (1999) Features of acute rejection that increase risk for chronic rejection. *Transplantation* **68**, 1200–1203.
68. Furness, P. N., Philpott, C. M., Chorbadjian, M. T., et al. (2003) Protocol biopsy of the stable renal transplant: a multicenter study of methods and complication rates. *Transplantation* **76**, 969–973.
69. Racusen, L. C., Colvin, R. B., Solez, K., et al. (2003) Antibody-mediated rejection criteria—an addition to the Banff 97 classification of renal allograft rejection. *Am. J. Transplant.* **3**, 708–714.
70. Racusen, L. C., Solez, K., Colvin, R. B., et al. (1999) The Banff 97 working classification of renal allograft pathology. *Kidney Int.* **55**, 713–723.
71. Roberts, I. S., Reddy, S., Russell, C., et al. (2004) Subclinical rejection and borderline changes in early protocol biopsy specimens after renal transplantation. *Transplantation* **77**, 1194–1198.
72. Legendre, C., Thervet, E., Skhiri, H., et al. (1998) Histologic features of chronic allograft nephropathy revealed by protocol biopsies in kidney transplant recipients. *Transplantation* **65**, 1506–1509.
73. Rush, D., Nickerson, P., Gough, J., et al. (1998) Beneficial effects of treatment of early subclinical rejection: a randomized study. *J. Am. Soc. Nephrol.* **9**, 2129–2134.

74. Matas, A. J., Gillingham, K. J., Payne, W. D., and Najarian, J. S. (1994) The impact of an acute rejection episode on long-term renal allograft survival (t1/2). *Transplantation* **57**, 857–859.
75. Simon, T., Opelz, G., Wiesel, M., Ott, R. C., and Susal, C. (2003) Serial peripheral blood perforin and granzyme B gene expression measurements for prediction of acute rejection in kidney graft recipients. *Am. J. Transplant.* **3**, 1121–1127.
76. Vasconcellos, L. M., Schachter, A. D., Zheng, X. X., et al. (1998) Cytotoxic lymphocyte gene expression in peripheral blood leukocytes correlates with rejecting renal allografts. *Transplantation* **66**, 562–566.
77. Lederer, S. R., Friedrich, N., Regenbogen, C., Getto, R., Toepfer, M., and Sitter, T. (2003) Non-invasive monitoring of renal transplant recipients: urinary excretion of soluble adhesion molecules and of the complement-split product C4d. *Nephron Clin. Pract.* **94**, 19–26.
78. Magee, C. C., Denton, M. D., Womer, K. L., Khoury, S. J., and Sayegh, M. H. (2004) Assessment by flow cytometry of intracellular cytokine production in the peripheral blood cells of renal transplant recipients. *Clin. Transplant.* **18**, 395–401.
79. Hricik, D. E., Rodriguez, V., Riley, J., et al. (2003) Enzyme linked immunosorbent spot (ELISPOT) assay for interferon-gamma independently predicts renal function in kidney transplant recipients. *Am. J. Transplant.* **3**, 878–884.
80. Gaber, A. O., First, M. R., Tesi, R. J., et al. (1998) Results of the double-blind, randomized, multicenter, phase III clinical trial of thymoglobulin versus Atgam in the treatment of acute graft rejection episodes after renal transplantation. *Transplantation* **66**, 29–37.
81. Midtvedt, K., Fauchald, P., Lien, B., et al. (2003) Individualized T cell monitored administration of ATG versus OKT3 in steroid-resistant kidney graft rejection. *Clin. Transplant.* **17**, 69–74.
82. Casadei, D. H., del C Rial, M., Opelz, G., et al. (2001) A randomized and prospective study comparing treatment with high-dose intravenous immunoglobulin with monoclonal antibodies for rescue of kidney grafts with steroid-resistant rejection. *Transplantation* **71**, 53–58.
83. Vincenti, F., Kirkman, R., Light, S., et al. (1998) Interleukin-2-receptor blockade with daclizumab to prevent acute rejection in renal transplantation. Daclizumab Triple Therapy Study Group. *N. Engl. J. Med.* **338**,161–165.
84. Nashan, B., Moore, R., Amlot, P., Schmidt, A. G., Abeywickrama, K., and Soulillou, J. P. (1997) Randomised trial of basiliximab versus placebo for control of acute cellular rejection in renal allograft recipients. CHIB 201 International Study Group. *Lancet* **350**, 1193–1198.
85. Chilcott, J. B., Holmes, M. W., Walters, S., Akehurst, R. L., and Nashan, B. (2002) The economics of basiliximab (Simulect) in preventing acute rejection in renal transplantation. *Transplant. Int.* **15**, 486–493.
86. Lederer, S. R., Kluth-Pepper, B., Schneeberger, H., Albert, E., Land, W., and Feucht, H. E. (2001) Impact of humoral alloreactivity early after transplantation on the long-term survival of renal allografts. *Kidney Int.* **59**, 334–341.

87. Nickeleit, V., Zeiler, M., Gudat, F., Thiel, G., and Mihatsch, M. J. (2002) Detection of the complement degradation product C4d in renal allografts: diagnostic and therapeutic implications. *J. Am. Soc. Nephrol.* **13**, 242–251.
88. Mauiyyedi, S., Crespo, M., Collins, A. B., et al. (2002) Acute humoral rejection in kidney transplantation: II. Morphology, immunopathology, and pathologic classification. *J. Am. Soc. Nephrol.* **13**, 779–787.
89. Nickeleit, V. and Mihatsch, M. J. (2003) Kidney transplants, antibodies and rejection: is C4d a magic marker? *Nephrol. Dial. Transplant.* **18**, 2232–2239.
90. Shah, A., Nadasdy, T., Arend, L., et al. (2004) Treatment of C4d-positive acute humoral rejection with plasmapheresis and rabbit polyclonal antithymocyte globulin. *Transplantation* **77**, 1399–1405.
91. Vella, J. P., O'Neill, D., Atkins, N., Donohoe, J. F., and Walshe, J. J. (1998) Sensitization to human leukocyte antigen before and after the introduction of erythropoietin. *Nephrol. Dial. Transplant.* **13**, 2027–2032.
92. Karpinski, M., Pochinco, D., Dembinski, I., Laidlaw, W., Zacharias, J., and Nickerson, P. (2004) Leukocyte reduction of red blood cell transfusions does not decrease allosensitization rates in potential kidney transplant candidates. *J. Am. Soc. Nephrol.* **15**, 818–824.
93. Doxiadis, I. I., De Meester, J., Smits, J. M., et al. (1998) The impact of special programs for kidney transplantation of highly sensitized patients in Eurotransplant. *Clin. Transplant.* 115–120.
94. Duquesnoy, R. J., Howe, J., and Takemoto, S. (2003) HLAmatchmaker: a molecularly based algorithm for histocompatibility determination. IV. An alternative strategy to increase the number of compatible donors for highly sensitized patients. *Transplantation* **75**, 889–897.
95. Jordan, S. C., Vo, A., Bunnapradist, S., et al. (2003) Intravenous immune globulin treatment inhibits crossmatch positivity and allows for successful transplantation of incompatible organs in living-donor and cadaver recipients. *Transplantation* **76**, 631–636.
96. Thibaudin, D., Alamartine, E., de Filippis, J. P., Diab, N., Laurent, B., and Berthoux, F. (1998) Advantage of antithymocyte globulin induction in sensitized kidney recipients: a randomized prospective study comparing induction with and without antithymocyte globulin. *Nephrol. Dial. Transplant.* **13**, 711–715.
97. Higgins, R. M., Bevan, D. J., Carey, B. S., et al. (1996) Prevention of hyperacute rejection by removal of antibodies to HLA immediately before renal transplantation. *Lancet* **348**, 1208–1211.
98. Montgomery, R. A., Zachary, A. A., Racusen, L. C., et al. (2000) Plasmapheresis and intravenous immune globulin provides effective rescue therapy for refractory humoral rejection and allows kidneys to be successfully transplanted into crossmatch-positive recipients. *Transplantation* **70**, 887–895.
99. Brennan, D. C. (2001) Cytomegalovirus in renal transplantation. *J. Am. Soc. Nephrol.* **12**, 848–855.
100. Hirsch, H. H., and Steiger, J. (2003) Polyomavirus BK. *Lancet Infect. Dis.* **3**, 611–623.

101. Kazory, A., and Ducloux, D. (2003). Renal transplantation and polyomavirus infection: recent clinical facts and controversies. *Transplant. Infect. Dis.* **5**, 65–71.
102. Hirsch, H. H., Knowles, W., Dickenmann, M.,et al. (2002) Prospective study of polyomavirus type BK replication and nephropathy in renal-transplant recipients. *N. Engl. J. Med.* **347**, 488–496.
103. Lin, P. L., Vats, A. N., and Green, M. (2001) BK virus infection in renal transplant recipients. *Pediatr. Transplant.* **5**, 398–405.
104. Foley, R. N., Parfrey, P. .S, and Sarnak, M. J. (1998) Clinical epidemiology of cardiovascular disease in chronic renal disease. *Am. J. Kidney Dis.* **32(5 Suppl. 3)**, S112–S119.
105. Raine, A. E., Margreiter, R., Brunner, F. P., et al. (1992) Report on management of renal failure in Europe, 22, 1991. *Nephrol. Dial. Transplant.* **7(Suppl. 2)**, 7–35.
106. Kasiske, B. L., Chakkera, H. A., and Roel, J. (2000) Explained and unexplained ischemic heart disease risk after renal transplantation. *J. Am. Soc. Nephrol.* **11**, 1735–1743.
107. Foley, R. N. (2003) Clinical epidemiology of cardiac disease in dialysis patients: left ventricular hypertrophy, ischemic heart disease, and cardiac failure. *Semin. Dial.* **16**, 111–117.
108. Holdaas, H., Fellstrom, B., Jardine, A. G., et al.; Assessment of LEscol in Renal Transplantation (ALERT) Study Investigators (2003) Effect of fluvastatin on cardiac outcomes in renal transplant recipients: a multicentre, randomised, placebo-controlled trial. *Lancet* **361**, 2024–2031.
109. Kwak, B., Mulhaupt, F., Myit, S., and Mach, F. (2000) Statins as a newly recognized type of immunomodulator. *Nat. Med.* **6**, 1399–1402.
110. Holdaas, H. and Jardine, A. (2003) Acute renal allograft rejections, a role for statins? *Minerva Urol. Nefrol.* **55**, 111–119.
111. Kasiske, B. L., Vazquez, M. A., Harmon, W. E., et al. (2000) Recommendations for the outpatient surveillance of renal transplant recipients. American Society of Transplantation. *J. Am. Soc. Nephrol.* **11 (Suppl. 15)**, S1–86.
112. EBPG Expert Group on Renal Transplantation (2002) European best practice guidelines for renal transplantation. Section IV: long-term management of the transplant recipient. IV.5.4. Cardiovascular risks. Post-transplant diabetes mellitus. *Nephrol. Dial. Transplant.* **17 (Suppl. 4)**, 28.
113. Ducloux, D., Motte, G., Challier, B., Gibey, R., and Chalopin, J. M. (2000) Serum total homocysteine and cardiovascular disease occurrence in chronic, stable renal transplant recipients: a prospective study. *J. Am. Soc. Nephrol.* **11**,134–137.
114. EBPG Expert Group on Renal Transplantation (2002). European best practice guidelines for renal transplantation. Section IV: Long-term management of the transplant recipient. IV.5.5. Cardiovascular risks. Hyperhomocysteinaemia. *Nephrol. Dial. Transplant.* **17 (Suppl. 4)**, 28.
115. Ducloux, D., Kazory, A., and Chalopin, J. M. (2004) Predicting coronary heart disease in renal transplant recipients: a prospective study. *Kidney Int.* **66**, 441–447.

116. Roodnat, J. I., Mulder, P. G., Rischen-Vos, J., van Riemsdijk, I. C., van Gelder, T., Zietse, R., IJzermans, J. N., and Weimar, W. (2001) Proteinuria after renal transplantation affects not only graft survival but also patient survival. *Transplantation* **72**, 438–444.
117. Bostom, A. D., Brown, R. S. Jr., Chavers, B. M., et al. (2002) Prevention of post-transplant cardiovascular disease—report and recommendations of an ad hoc group. *Am. J. Transplant.* **2**, 491–500.

2

Current Status of Liver Transplantation

Peter J. Friend and Charles J. Imber

Summary

Liver transplantation has become the treatment of choice for a wide range of end-stage liver disease. As outcomes have improved, so the demand for this therapy has increasingly exceeded the availability of donor organs. Access to liver transplantation is controlled such that donor organs are generally allocated to the patients who are likely to benefit most, although if all patients who might benefit were placed on the waiting list, the donor shortage would be greatly increased.

Recurrence of the original liver disease is emerging as an important issue. Fewer patients are transplanted for liver tumors, as earlier results showed a very high rate of recurrence. In recent years there has been a change in the underlying conditions of patients on the waiting list, and a preponderance of patients now present with hepatitis C and alcoholic cirrhosis.

Increasingly, transplant units are looking to sources of donor organs that would previously have been deemed unsuitable—such marginal donors include non-heart-beating donors (NHBDs). Results from controlled NHBDs—those cases in which cardiac arrest is predicted—suggest that this is a good source of viable organs.

Splitting a donor liver to provide two grafts has successful enabled the transplantation of a child and an adult from one organ. The transplantation of two adults from a single organ remains a greater challenge.

Transplantation from living donors has been practiced increasingly over the last decade, although anxieties have been expressed over donor safety. In many countries this now represents a significant contribution to overall liver transplant activity.

Key Words: Liver; transplantation; donor; allocation; indications.

1. Historical Perspective

The first human liver transplant was performed on March 1, 1963, at the University of Colorado on a 3-yr-old boy suffering with biliary atresia *(1)*. He died before the operation was completed; it was not until 1967 that the first

From: *Methods in Molecular Biology, vol. 333: Transplantation Immunology: Methods and Protocols*
Edited by: P. Hornick and M. Rose © Humana Press Inc., Totowa, NJ

meaningful survival was reported *(2)*. Between 1967 and 1980, 170 liver transplants were performed at the University of Colorado, and between 1968 and 1983, 138 transplants took place in Cambridge, England *(2)*, with 1-yr survival rates of approx 30%. With the emergence of cyclosporine, pioneered by Borel and Calne, as well as gradual refinements of various technical aspects, particularly bile duct reconstruction and coagulation support, outcome figures improved.

In 1983, a National Institutes of Health (NIH) Consensus Conference concluded that liver transplantation was now a therapeutic option for patients with end-stage liver disease, rather than an experimental procedure *(3)*. This led to a rapid expansion of the number of patients referred for liver transplantation worldwide. Five years after the NIH conference, 616 patients awaited liver transplants in the United States. Ten years later, this number had increased to 12,056.

Since the early 1980s, there have been significant advances in all aspects of liver transplantation, including recipient selection, donor management, operative technique, immunosuppression, and postoperative management of liver recipients. These changes, which have marked the evolution from an experimental technique to established and routine therapy, have resulted in enormous improvements in outcome. The overall 1-yr survival for adults and pediatric orthotopic liver transplants is now expected to be in excess of 85%, with 5- and 10-yr survival in excess of 70 and 60%, respectively *(4–7)*. Partly as a consequence of this improved outcome, the selection criteria have broadened, leading to changes in the demographics of the patient population.

2. Current Indications for Liver Transplantation

The goal of liver transplantation is not only to prolong life, but also to improve the quality of life. The selection of patients to achieve these goals and the ideal time at which to intervene during the course of chronic liver disease remain among the greatest challenges for the transplant team. The current indications for liver transplantation can be categorized as follows: advanced chronic liver disease, fulminant hepatic failure, inherited metabolic liver disease, and liver tumors.

Controversy exists over transplantation for alcoholic liver disease, hepatitis B, hepatitis C, and hepatic malignancy because of the risk of recurrent disease and consequent reduced long-term survival. There has been much ethical debate in relation to the use of a scarce resource in both patients with self-inflicted diseases and conditions with a high probability of recurrence. Neuberger and colleagues clearly demonstrated the difficulties faced in attempting to allocate such a scarce resource *(8)*. This study showed that the priorities of the public differed from those of the medical profession. The former placed greater emphasis on factors such as age of recipient, whereas doctors felt that outcome and value to society were a greater priority. Patients who displayed traits consistent with antisocial behavior (e.g., alcoholism) were given a low level of importance by all. In general, the indications for liver transplantation can be defined as either an intolerable quality of life (because of the liver disease) or an anticipated length of life of less than 1 yr because of liver failure.

3. Organ-Allocation Policies

Various schemes have evolved to allocate organs with some reference to urgency. In the United States, the Model for End-Stage Liver Disease (MELD) score, based on serum creatinine, bilirubin, and international normalized ratio (INR), was developed initially during a retrospective study at the Mayo Clinic of patients undergoing transhepatic portosystemic shunts (TIPS). It was subsequently validated as a determinant of short-term prognosis in patients with chronic liver disease ***(9)*** and utilized as a disease severity index. In February 2002, the MELD score was implemented by the United Network for Organ Sharing (UNOS) as a criterion for organ allocation to adult patients with chronic liver disease followed the ruling of the Department of Health that allocation be conducted according to medical urgency. Priority is still given to status 1 patients (fulminant hepatic failure or early graft failure following transplantation requiring emergency re-transplantation); these remain a local and regional priority. After these patients, livers are offered to patients based upon their probability of candidate death derived from MELD scores. With a MELD score of 6 or less, the time on the waiting list is also used as a prioritization factor ***(10)***. Early reports indicate that this allocation system based on medical severity may reduce the number of deaths on the waiting list ***(11)***.

In the United Kingdom, four fundamental concepts underpin the allocation policy, as agreed at the Edinburgh colloquium in 1996 ***(12)***. First, guidelines need to be drawn up and agreed on by all those involved. Second, the main criteria for selection must be based on quality of life and anticipated life expectancy. Third, patients selected for transplantation should have a more than a 50% probability of being alive 5 yr after the transplant. Finally, livers are allocated to give the maximum outcome (in preference to every potential recipient having equal share of the donor pool by right). Thus, it is generally agreed that organ allocation should be based on utilitarian rather than deontological principles.

In UK practice, certain patients (those with either fulminant liver failure or primary nonfunction of a transplant—the equivalent of UNOS status 1) have national priority (these patients are deemed "super-urgent"). Thereafter, livers are offered first to the retrieving unit and then, if there is no suitable recipient locally, around the rest of the country on a continually rolling priority based on the balance of net export at each individual center. Thus, livers are allocated to the most urgent patients on an individual basis (i.e., *ad hominem*), but otherwise all livers are allocated to the transplant unit (rather than to the individual patient). At a local level, individual patient prioritization is usually established at a multidisciplinary meeting. These difficult decisions are based on the principles outlined above, with general co-morbidity of the recipient, length of time on the waiting list, as well as disease progression all taken into account. If a patient's condition deteriorates while on the list, it may be necessary to consider removing him or her from the active waiting list. Effective communication not only between members of the medical team but also with the patient and his or her family is clearly essential at every level of the process.

In addition to blood group matching and, to some extent, size matching, the selection of the recipient for a particular donor organ may also be affected by the quality of the liver on offer. In the interests of obtaining the maximum benefit for the maximum number of patients, there is a strong argument to utilize organs from the better donors in the sicker recipients—the patients who are least able to tolerate a poorly functioning transplant in the immediate postoperative period. Healthier recipients are more able to cope with the period of poor initial graft function that can be associated with the use of a marginal liver (*see* below). This is now a generally accepted principle in the interests of obtaining the maximum benefit from the limited donor supply, but one that clearly poses ethical issues on occasions.

4. Hepatitis C/HIV Infection

There has been a clear shift in indications for transplantation in the last 15 yr, with a continued increase in non-cholestatic liver diseases predominantly made up of hepatitis C and alcoholic liver disease. In the United States, the proportion of recipients with hepatitis C virus (HCV) infection increased from 12 to 37% between 1990 and 2000, with a similar increase in the number and proportion of liver transplant candidates registered with hepatitis C on the waiting list ***(13)***. According to the UNOS, in 2001 there were 9783 patients with hepatitis C awaiting a cadaveric liver transplant. Combined infection with hepatitis B or C and HIV (contracted together through either sexual or intravenous routes) has led to a cohort of such patients with chronic liver failure being considered for transplantation. Reservations have been voiced because of the potential for reemergence of hepatitis in CD4-deficient recipients, as well as the use of a scarce resource in an individual with a preexisting life-limiting disease. However, with continual improvements in anti-retroviral medication in HIV (the use of protease inhibitors in combination with non-nucleoside reverse-transcriptase inhibitors), there is now a greatly improved life expectancy with this condition. This allows many patients coinfected with HIV and hepatitis B/C to be considered for liver transplantation with reasonable prospects for survival.

A recent report on HCV-infected liver transplant recipients estimated the risk of developing recurrent cirrhosis to be as high as 44% at 5 yr posttransplant ***(14)***. Berenguer et al. reported data from the UNOS registry demonstrating that 5-yr graft survival in recipients transplanted for hepatitis C was 56.8%, the worst of all indications with the exception of malignancy ***(14)***. Antiviral agents (interferon, including pegylated interferons, ribavarin, or combinations) have a low rate of success because of poor patient tolerance, side effects, or a limited and/or transient response.

In contrast, significant progress has been achieved in the outcome of hepatitis B virus (HBV)-infected liver recipients with the use of current HBV antiviral agents. Han and colleagues reported negative hepatitis B surface antigen serology in 98.3% of patients after transplantation using intramuscular anti-hepatitis B immunoglobulin and lamivudine ***(15)***.

5. Tumors

Another major demographic shift is the reduction in the proportion of patients transplanted for primary liver cancer. This diagnosis is clearly associated with poor outcome because of recurrent disease. In the European Liver Transplant Registry (ELTR) data, the 1-, 5-, and 9-yr patient survivals for patients with cirrhosis (79, 69, and 62%) are significantly better than for patients treated for primary liver cancer (67, 40, and 26%). With improvements in imaging technology, as well as the adoption of defined selection policies, the proportion of livers being transplanted for cancer is falling.

6. Retransplantation

In recent years there has been a significant decrease in the number of retransplants performed. This reflects improvements in every step of the transplant process, including choice of donors, preservation fluids, surgical techniques, and, perhaps most important, postoperative recipient management and immunosuppressive protocols. This issue was addressed by Clemente et al. ***(16)*** in a large retrospective analysis covering more than a decade. They demonstrated a shift in the major cause of retransplantation from chronic rejection to primary graft failure, with 5-yr actuarial survival rates dependent on the cause of graft failure (45.5% for chronic rejection and 19.4% for primary failure) ***(16)***. Graft loss caused by rejection is now uncommon after liver trans-plantation. The incidence of chronic rejection in 1048 liver recipients followed for a mean period of more than 6 yr was only 3% ***(17)***. In a randomized trial comparing cyclosporine with tacrolimus after liver transplantation (the Tacrolimus vs Microemulsified Ciclosporin [TMC] study), the incidence of chronic rejection was only 0.3% in the tacrolimus group ***(18)***. Another study concluded that chronic rejection does not occur in the pediatric liver recipient population as long as baseline immunosuppression with tacrolimus is maintained *(19)*.

7. Immunosuppression

The mainstay of post-liver-transplant immunosuppression is triple therapy with a calcineurin inhibitor (usually tacrolimus), together with an anti-proliferative agent (mycophenolate or azathioprine) and a corticosteroid (prednisolone). Increasingly, clinicians are tailoring the immunosuppressive regimen to the individual recipient. For example, faster withdrawal of corticosteroids has been shown to be efficacious in recipients transplanted for hepatitis B, where the drug is known to increase viral replication *(20)*. In contrast, prolonged low-dose steroid use in autoimmune hepatitis has been shown to reduce disease recurrence in the graft *(21)*.

Particularly since publication of the TMC study in October 2002, the large majority of liver units have preferentially used tacrolimus over cyclosporine as a first-line calcineurin inhibitor *(18)*. This randomized prospective multicenter study of 606 patients demonstrated a significantly better graft and patient survival at 1 yr in patients on tacrolimus. The combined primary endpoint of death, retransplantation, or treatment failure (owing to rejection) was reached in 21% patients on the tacrolimus arm and 32% in the cyclosporine arm of the trial—a significant difference.

Tolerance remains the goal of the transplant physician. There is evidence that some patients are able to have immunosuppression withdrawn and yet maintain adequate graft function. Starzl's group in Pittsburgh have proposed that dissemination of donor leukocytes (including pluripotent stem cells) occurs from allografts inducing donor/recipient nonreactivity. A series of 95 recipients was reported in which weaning from immunosuppression was attempted *(22)*. These patients were all more than 5 yr from transplant and had stable graft function. At the time of the report, 20% were drug free up to 4.5 yr later, and 39% remained in the weaning process. Twenty-six percent of patients required reinstitution of their immunosuppression for biopsy-proven or presumed acute rejection. Chronic rejection was not seen. This group has also described specific genetic polymorphisms of tumor necrosis factor (TNF)-α and interleukin (IL)-10 in children that have been successfully weaned from immunosuppression after liver transplantation *(23)*.

Other tolerance-induction strategies have been attempted in animals, including total body irradiation, costimulation blockade, development of chimerism, and lymphocyte depletion using a variety of monoclonal and polyclonal antibodies. Buhler and colleagues recently published a case report of combined human leukocyte antigen (HLA)-matched donor bone marrow and renal allotransplantation. This is the first example of an intentional and clinically applicable approach to inducing renal allograft tolerance achieving potent and sustained antitumor effects in patients with multiple myeloma ***(24)***.

8. Donors

The biggest obstacle to the continued expansion of liver transplantation is the increasing gap between waiting lists and organ availability. If localized primary liver tumors, alcoholic liver disease, and allograft failure are accepted as indications, the demand for liver transplants has been calculated to be 25 per million population ***(25)***. Using current donor criteria, no more than 80% of all donor livers can be used ***(25)***; thus, depending on donor incidence, between 30 and 80% of the patient demand can be met. In 2001, 1978 potential liver recipients died on the waiting list in the United States without receiving a graft (UNOS database).

On first consideration, the prospects for the future are not encouraging. Donor numbers have decreased because of a progressive (and welcome) fall in the two leading causes of brain death in the United Kingdom: head injury from road traffic accidents and intracranial hemorrhage ***(26)***. Between 1989 and 1992, the annual number of donors in the United Kingdom resulting from road traffic accidents fell from 279 to 194, a decrease of 30%. The situation is further complicated by changes in neurosurgical practice. Improvements in imaging and shortage of intensive care beds have resulted in a more restrictive policy in the transfer of patients to regional neurosurgical units: patients with a very poor prognosis can now be identified at an early stage. For this reason many patients who would previously have been assessed in a neurosurgical intensive care unit are no longer identified as potential donors ***(27)***.

A number of strategies are evolving to address the current situation. These include the use of organs from marginal donors (those outside the criteria previously used in respect to age, co-morbid condition, and cardiovascular stability), organs from NHBDs, the more extensive use of liver splitting (to obtain two transplants from one donor liver), and the transplantation of organs from living donors. Each of these potential solutions raises specific clinical and ethical issues.

9. Marginal Donors

What constitutes a "marginal donor" remains controversial, and different transplant units have developed their own arbitrary policies to determine whether a liver is used or discarded based on broadly accepted guidelines. A selection of 10 major studies in the last decade on this subject includes no less than 32 separate parameters in the various definitions. These include preexisting liver damage (steatosis, obesity, alcohol, deranged liver function tests), adverse lifestyle (drug abuse, homosexual practice), age, hemodynamic instability (hypotension, inotrope use, cardiac arrest, NHBDs), risks of sepsis and malignancy, and others (length of stay on intensive therapy unit [ITU], malnutrition, hypernatremia).

Widening the acceptance criteria in an effort to expand the donor pool has become a necessity. The use of livers from marginal donors has been shown in several studies to lead to an increased risk of primary graft dysfunction *(28–31)*. This term encompasses both catastrophic primary nonfunction, resulting in death or retransplantation in the first week, or impaired primary function manifest as a coagulation disturbance and increased transaminase levels and resulting in prolonged ITU stay and increased requirement for renal support (and greatly increased cost).

Both primary nonfunction and impaired primary function represent the clinical manifestations of cumulative injury derived from the period of brain death within the donor, subsequent warm/cold ischemia during preservation, and reperfusion at the time of transplantation.

A recent study from Birmingham suggested that the two most important independent donor variables that correlate with graft dysfunction are macrosteatosis (>30% on histopathological analysis) and donor age *(32)*. In the study the outcome with such marginal organs could be dramatically improved if cold ischemia time was restricted to no more than 12 h. Strasberg et al. reaffirmed this association by describing cold preservation time, steatosis, and donor age as the only three parameters with a proven relationship to early graft outcome, the others having an uncertain relationship that required further evaluation *(33)*.

10. Reduced-Size Liver Transplantation

Size reduction of an adult liver was implemented initially to overcome the need for size-matched grafts in pediatric recipients. The technique was introduced clinically in 1981, and the first successful transplant of part of a liver was reported by Bismuth and Houssin, who transplanted the left lobe from an adult to a child in 1984 *(34)*. Further experience at several centers suggested that the use of the left lateral segment (segments II and III) taken from an adult donor would provide an ideal-sized graft for a small child and that the results were comparable to whole size-matched grafts *(35)*. An additional refinement, reported from both Europe and Australia, was the retention of the recipient vena cava, to which the venous outflow (the left hepatic vein) of the graft was anastomosed *(36,37)*. This allowed even larger donor-to-recipient size mismatches as well as retaining a right hemi-liver with intact vena cava. This enabled the concept of liver splitting and, subsequently, living donation.

10.1. Liver Reduction

Liver reduction involves transplantation of part of the liver, the remaining liver being discarded. It is a solution to size discrepancy, but does not affect the overall availability of donor organs. Liver transplantation from reduced livers (as opposed to split livers) is now usually restricted to left liver grafts (segments I–IV), usually including the donor cava, and left lateral segmental grafts (segments II–III), excluding the vena cava. Generally, if a right lobe graft would fit, then the entire liver would be suitable. The technique has been developed further by the transplantation of a single hepatic segment—either segment II or segment III ***(38)***.

Patient and graft survival is equivalent to, and in some circumstances better than, survival after full-size grafting ***(39)***. Rates of arterial thrombosis are lower when a pediatric recipient receives a reduced adult graft rather than a cadaveric whole pediatric graft, presumably because of the larger caliber of the donor vessel ***(40)***. Conversely, the presence of a cut surface increases the rate of bleeding and bile leaks in the reduced grafts. The development of liver reduction has made possible a reduction in pretransplant deaths in small children from 25% in 1989 to less than 10% today ***(41)***. This technique also led directly to the surgical techniques necessary for liver splitting and living donor transplants.

11. Split Liver Transplantation

Split liver transplantation, first reported by Pichlmayr et al. in 1988 ***(42)***, has the advantage of providing not only organs suitable for small children, but also additional transplants suitable for small adults. Usually, the adult would receive the right-liver graft including segment IV with the inferior vena cava attached and a child the left lateral segment. Segment I (the caudate lobe) is either preserved or discarded, depending on local preference.

Transplants have also been performed of two adult recipients using a single split liver. In these cases, segment IV is retained with the left lobe. The main technical challenge is to provide an adequate mass of liver tissue to both recipients: the left lobe (typically 40% of the liver mass) is sufficient only for a recipient of small body mass. Postoperative liver function can be predicted based on the transplanted liver mass as a proportion of the weight of the recipient. A proportion of 1% (transplantation of a 700-g liver lobe into a 70-kg patient) is considered a safe limit.

Although usually performed as an ex vivo procedure (the operation is performed on the explanted, cooled liver), the splitting procedure can also be performed *in situ* during the donor-procurement procedure. This has the advantages of less preservation injury (shorter cold ischemia time) and improved hemostasis of the cut surface ***(25)***. Ex vivo splitting is also associated with a higher rate of biliary complications (22% vs 27%) compared with whole-organ (4%) or *in situ* split grafts (0% vs 3%) ***(43)***. However, the logistics are complex because of the considerably prolonged donor operation and the necessity of a very experienced retrieval team. It places enormous additional strain on the already stretched resources of liver-retrieval teams, other transplant teams, and donor hospitals. The *ex situ* technique is therefore generally employed, with the procedure performed once the liver has been returned to the transplanting center.

The early experience of liver splitting involved application of the new procedure in high-risk patients, often as a desperate measure; this was reflected in a high morbidity rate ***(44)***. Between January 1987 and June 1999 a total of 1036 split grafts (mostly *ex situ*) was transplanted in 898 patients. In adults, the 1-yr patient and graft survival rates were 68 and 60%, respectively. In children (<15 yr), the corresponding figures were 75 and 59%. Survival rates were significantly better in centers that had performed more than 40 split transplants, suggesting a significant learning curve (European Liver Transplant Registry. Custodian: R Adam, Villejuif, France).

12. Living-Related Transplantation (LRT)

One of the most challenging and controversial developments devised as a means of reducing waiting list deaths is the use of partial liver grafts from living donors. The first clinical success was reported in 1989 ***(45)***, and since that time the technique has been adopted in many centers with great success. Initially, the major proponents were the Japanese liver units where legal and cultural issues render cadaveric donation rare.

The use of living donors has enormous potential advantages in terms of organ quality (absence of the adverse effects of brain death, short cold ischemia time), which reduce the risk of early dysfunction. Also, it enables the transplant to be carried out as a planned procedure at a time optimal to the patient and suitable for the donor and the transplant team. However, although increasingly widely performed not only in Japan, but also in North America and Europe, living donor liver transplantation has yet to make a major impact in the United Kingdom. This reflects unresolved anxieties about donor safety as well as the basic ethical dilemma of putting a healthy individual's life at risk. Living donation must meet three major ethical requirements if it is to succeed: (1) a convincing need for the technique, (2) acceptable risk and benefit to the participants, and (3) a satisfactory process for ensuring adequate informed consent and protection of the donor. It is yet to be seen whether this technique will become widely practiced in Britain.

13. NHBDs

The use of organs from NHBDs is increasingly seen as an important solution to the discrepancy between the supply and demand for donor livers. This is accentuated by the changes in neurosurgical practice (described above) whereby patients with catastrophic cerebral injury are identified at an early stage and allowed to die following withdrawal of medical support. These patients, therefore, are usually not diagnosed as brain dead, and death occurs and is defined by cardiac arrest. Because cardiac arrest in these donors is predicted, it is possible to prepare the transplant team and to await the moment of death. Such donors are, therefore, termed "controlled" NHBDs. Other situations are unpredictable (e.g., the cardiac arrest that occurs outside the hospital or in the emergency department), usually preceded by an unsuccessful attempt at cardiac resuscitation. The logistics of organ retrieval in such cases are more complex. These organ donors are termed "uncontrolled" NHBDs.

Many ethical issues are involved in retrieval of organs from NHBDs. The points of potential conflict of interest (between care of the donor and recipient) include intervention prior to declaration of death and the duration of mandatory no-touch period after cardiac arrest before organ retrieval. The clinical and moral requirements governing NHBD cadaveric organ-procurement policy can be summarized as follows: (1) organs can only be taken from donors who are dead; (2) the care of the living must never be compromised in favor of potential recipients; and (3) informed consent must be obtained prior to retrieval.

In HBDs death is defined by neurological criteria, whereas in NHBDs death is declared only after cardiac arrest. Thus, a fundamental difference between HBDs and NHBDs is that, until the moment after cardiac arrest, the NHBD is alive. The rationale for the mandatory "hands-off period" is to delay any intervention until such time as any central neurological activity, present before cardiac arrest, will have ceased beyond doubt.

The time between cardiac arrest and the start of the organ-retrieval process varies in different institutions: intervals ranging from no waiting to 10 min have been reported. The first international workshop in Maastricht, Netherlands, held in 1995 recommended that a 10-min period after cardiopulmonary arrest be allowed before intervention by the transplant team. However, there is evidence that the 10-min no-intervention period contributes to an increased incidence of primary nonfunction and delayed graft function.

Clinical experience with NHBD liver transplantation is limited ***(46–48)***. Under controlled circumstances, with shorter warm ischemia times, the results are acceptable ***(49)***. In an uncontrolled setting, when cardiac arrest occurs outside the operating room, results have been poor with a high rate of primary nonfunction ***(47)***. Otero and colleagues reported a primary nonfunction rate of 20% in 20 grafts from Maastricht category 2 (uncontrolled) NHBDs ***(50)***; the corresponding primary nonfunction rate in 40 HBDs was 2%. Most of the successful cases reported from this group utilized continuous in vivo perfusion with cardiopulmonary bypass or chest compressions with oxygenation. It is likely that this provides some recovery of cellular energy stores prior to cold storage.

14. Auxiliary Liver Transplantation

There are two situations in which it is logical to transplant a donor liver but to preserve part of the patient's own liver: transplantation for fulminant liver failure and transplantation for metabolic liver disease.

In many patients with fulminant liver failure, regeneration of hepatocytes leads to recovery and avoids the need for transplantation—the operation is indicated in those patients who are unlikely to survive long enough for adequate regeneration to occur. The objective in auxiliary liver transplantation is to transplant enough healthy functioning liver tissue to bridge the patient over the period of acute liver failure while allowing the native liver time to recover.

In patients with certain metabolic disorders, liver transplantation has been recommended in order to provide one liver-specific enzyme—the function of the liver is otherwise normal. It may be possible to provide adequate levels of enzyme function by transplanting part of a donor liver *(34)*. Examples of such metabolic defects include Crigler–Najjar syndrome type I *(51)*, ornithine transcarbamylase deficiency *(52)*, and propionic acidemia *(53)*.

The advantages of auxiliary transplantation in these circumstances are clear—the patient is largely spared the risks normally associated with graft failure due to rejection and other causes. Importantly, in the case of fulminant liver failure, if the native liver recovers, immunosuppression can be gradually withdrawn, sparing the patients all the long-term morbidity of immunosuppression, including infection, malignancy, and nephropathy.

Currently most groups performing auxiliary partial orthotopic liver transplants (APOLTs) use right, left, or left lateral splits/reduced grafts. Technical problems include compression of major venous vessels into and out of the graft, inadequate portal flow into the donor graft and subsequent thrombosis, inadequate graft size, and toxic liver syndrome in patients with acute failure. These problems have largely been overcome, and satisfactory results have been reported *(54)*; auxiliary transplantation is being considered by a number of centers as a potential adjunct to orthotopic transplant *(55)*. Experience with immunossuppression withdrawal is limited; however, the collected European experience found that 65% of patients surviving more than 1 yr with a successful auxiliary liver transplant were free of immunossuppression *(54)*. In this series the overall 1-yr patient survival rate of 62% in auxiliary liver transplantation was similar to that for orthotopic liver transplantation (61%).

15. Xenotransplantation

The use of animals, particularly pigs, as an organ source presents a very attractive alternative to human organs. Pigs can be bred and raised under very clean and controlled conditions. The anatomy and physiology is similar to human counterparts, and the waiting list could be cleared with huge expansion of the potential donor pool. Before this can become a clinical reality, however, problems relating to immunological, microbiological, and physiological barriers need to be overcome.

In 1992 and 1993, two orthotopic xenotransplantations were performed, placing baboon livers into patients with liver failure secondary to hepatitis B infection. These patients survived 70 and 26 d ***(56)***. The livers worked, but not normally, with levels of proteins including albumin remaining in the normal range for baboons and not humans.

No long-term pig-to-primate liver transplants have been performed, although porcine livers transgenic for human complement regulatory proteins have functioned successfully in the short term. Patients with acute liver failure have been supported for a few hours to days with extracorporeal liver perfusion (ECLP) while a human donor liver is sought ***(57)***. These procedures have indicated the pig liver to be functional in the short term, with improvements in clinical status and reduction of blood ammonia and lactic acid levels. Whether genetic engineering would be able to "humanize" a pig liver adequately remains to be seen. The major porcine complement factors are only 70% homologous with human factors, and pig and human albumin 65% homologous, discrepancies that may be exaggerated in cascade or regulatory systems.

Pigs and humans represent discordant species, and xenografts from one to the other would be expected to undergo hyperacute rejection because of the presence of preformed antibodies to the α-gal epitope on vascular endothelium leading to activation of the classical complement pathway. Transgenic techniques have been developed to prevent the hyperacute response. These include the production of pigs transgenic for a human complement regulatory proteins—the introduction of a single human complement regulator gene has been shown to abolish the immediate, complement-mediated hyperacute xenograft rejection. However, induced antibodies and subsequent cellular mechanisms are not controlled by this means ***(58)***.

Having controlled the immediate effect of complement activation caused by preformed antibodies, a xenograft is at risk of damage from induced antibodies (delayed xenograft rejection). This has proved difficult to control using conventional immunosuppressive drugs. McGregor and colleagues recently reported that by combining the use of organs that express human decay accelerating factor (hDAF) with the administration of a soluble Gal glyco-conjugate and other immunosuppressive agents, the survival of pig hearts in baboons is extended to a median of 76 d ***(59)***. The recent generation of pigs that do not express the main target antigen ***(60)*** (α1,3-galactosyltransferase gene–knockout pigs [GT-KO]) might prevent the antibody response.

Safety issues include concern about transmission of exogenous viral infections, such as cytomegalovirus, from donor pig to recipient. Early weaning and subsequent isolation can lead to an absence of virus in these piglets. The presence of endogenous retroviruses in all pig cells has also led to concern. Oldmixon et al. showed that certain pigs lack the capacity to transmit porcine endogenous retrovirus to human cells in vitro ***(61)***.

However, even if the safety and immunological barriers to porcine xenotransplantation were overcome, there are real doubts as to the potential value of liver xenotransplantation. Although probably useful in the short-term treatment of liver failure (as a liver-assist device), it is widely agreed that there would be large-scale incompatibilities involving many enzyme systems within the pig liver and proteins synthesized by the liver. It is unlikely, therefore, that the pig liver will prove to be a good substitute for the human liver in clinical transplantation, at least without major genetic engineering.

16. The Future

The practice of liver transplantation has become a victim of its own success, with an inexorable rise in patients waiting for surgery and a donor pool that remains static. The future must involve improved utilization of potential organ donors—current initiatives within the British transplant community are addressing this. Optimization of donors including improvements in nutrition as well as possible techniques for ameliorating reperfusion injury are being investigated, as are improvements in preservation techniques and viability assessment (including normothermic extracorporeal perfusion). Living donor transplantation remains a controversial technique, but one that could go a long way to redressing the shortage of donors. Improvements in immunosuppression have had a major effect on the survival of liver-transplant patients, a trend that is likely to continue. A clinically applicable means of achieving immunological tolerance would radically reduce the short- and long-term risks of liver transplantation. Although clearly desirable, this would have the effect of expanding still further the population of patients for whom transplantation is the preferred treatment.

References

1. Starzl, T. M., Marchioro, T. L., and Von Kaulia, K. N. (1963) Homotransplantation of the liver in humans. *Surg. Gynecol. Obstet.* **117**, 659–676.
2. Starzl, T. E., Iwatsuki, S., Van Thiel, D. H., et al. (1982) Evolution of liver transplantation. *Hepatology* **2**, 614–636.
3. (1984). National Institute's of Health Consensus Development Conference Statement: Liver Transplantation. *Hepatolog*; **4**, 107S–110S.
4. Jain, A., Reyes, J., Kashyap, R., et al. (2000) Long-term survival after liver transplantation in 4,000 consecutive patients at a single center. *Ann. Surg.* **232**, 490–500.
5. Gordon, R. D., Fung, J., Tzakis, A. G., et al. (1991) Liver transplantation at the University of Pittsburgh, 1984 to 1990. *Clin. Transplant.* 105–117.

6. Abbasoglu, O., Levy, M. F., Brkic, B. B., et al. (1997) Ten years of liver transplantation: an evolving understanding of late graft loss. *Transplantation* **64**, 1801–1807.
7. Asfar, S., Metrakos, P., Fryer, J., et al. (1996). An analysis of late deaths after liver transplantation. *Transplantation* **61**, 1377–1381.
8. Neuberger, J., Adams, D., Macmaster, P., Maidment, A., and Speed, M. (1998) Assessing priorities for allocation of donor liver grafts: survey of public and clinicians. *BMJ* **317**,172–175.
9. Kamath, P. S., Wiesner, R. H., Malinchoc, M., et al. (2001) A model to predict survival in patients with end stage liver disease. *Hepatology* **33**, 464–470.
10. UNOS. Policy 3.6.: Allocation of livers. Available at: http://www.org/organDatasource/OrganSpecificPolicies.asp?display=Liver., Accessed August 13, 2003.
11. Freeman, R. B., Rohrer, R. J., Katz, E., et al. (2001) Preliminary results of a liver allocation plan using a continuous medical severity score that de-emphasizes waiting time. *Liver Transplant.* **7**, 173–178.
12. Select Committee of Experts on the Organisational Aspects of Cooperation in Organ Transplantation. Meeting the organ shortage: current status and strategies for improvement of cadaveric organ donation. Madrid: ONT, 1996.
13. Kim, W. R. (2002) The burden of hepatitis C in the United States. *Hepatology* **36**, S30–S34.
14. Berenguer, M.., Prieto, M., Rayon, J. M., et al. (2000) Natural history of clinically compensated HCV-related graft cirrhosis following liver transplantation. *Hepatology* **32**, 852–858.
15. Han, S. H., Martin, P., Edelstein, M., et al. (2003) Conversion from intravenous to intramuscular hepatitis B immune globulin in combination with lamivudine is safe and cost-effective in patients receiving long term prophylaxis to prevent hepatitis B recurrence after liver transplantation. *Liver Transplant.* **9**, 182–187.
16. Clemente, G., Duran, F., Loinaz, C., et al. (1999) Late orthotopic liver retransplant indications and survival. Liver Transplant Spanish Group. *Transplant Proc.* **31**, 511–514.
17. Jain, A., Demetris, A. J., Kashyap, R,. et al. (2001) Does tacrolimus offer virtual freedom from chronic rejection after primary liver transplantation? Risk and prognosic factors in 1048 liver transplants with a mean follow-up of 6 years. *Liver Transplant.* **7**, 623–630.
18. O'Grady, J.G., Burroughs, A., Hardy, P., Elbourne, D., Troesdale, A., and the UK and Republic of Ireland Liver Transplant Study Group (2002) Tacrolimus versus microemulsified ciclosporine in liver transplantation: the TMC randomised controlled trial. *Lancet* **360**, 1119–1125.
19. Jain, A., Mazariegos, G., Polzharna, R., et al. (2003) The absence of chronic rejection in paediatric primary liver transplant patients who are maintained on tacrolimus based immunosuppression: a long-term analysis. *Transplantation* **75**, 1020–1025.
20. Yokosuka, O. (2000) Role of steroid priming in the treatment of chronic hepatitis. *Br. J. Gastroenterol. Hepatol.* (**Suppl.**), E41–45.

21. Heffron, T.G., Smallwood, G.A., Oakley, B., et al. (2002) Autoimmune hepatitis following liver transplantation: relationship to recurrent disease and steroid weaning. *Transplant. Proc.* **34**, 3311–3312.
22. Mazariegos, G., Reyes, J., Marino, I.R., et al. (1997) Weaning of immunosuppression in liver transplant recipients. *Transplantation* **63**, 243–249.
23. Mazariegos, G. V., Reyes, J., Webber, S. A., et al. (2002) Cytokine gene polymorphisms in children successfully withdrawn from immunosuppression after liver transplantation. *Transplantation* **73**, 1432–1435.
24. Buhler, L. H., Spitzer, T. R., Sykes, M., et al. (2002) Induction of kidney allograft tolerance after transient lymphohematopoietic chimerism in patients with multiple myeloma and end-stage renal disease. *Transplantation* **74**, 1405–1409.
25. Busuttil, R. W. and Goss, J. A. (1999) Split liver transplantation. *Ann. Surg.* **229**, 313–321.
26. New, W., Solomon, M., Dingwall, R., and McHale, J. (1994) A question of give and take: improving the supply of donor organs for transplantation. Research report, Kings Fund Institute, **18**.
27. Briggs, J. D., Crombie, A., Fabre, J., Major, E., Thorogood, J., and Veitch, P. S. (1997) Organ donation in the UK: a survey by a British Transplantation Society working party. *Nephrol. Dial. Transplant.* **12**, 2251–2257.
28. Ploeg, R. J., D'Alessandro, A. M., Knechtle, S. J., et al. (1993) Risk factors for primary dysfunction after liver transplantation—a multivariate analysis. *Transplantation* **55**, 807–813.
29. Makowka, L., Gordon, R. D., Todo, S., et al. (1987) Analysis of donor criteria for the prediction of outcome in clinical liver transplantation. *Transplant. Proc.* **19**, 2378–2382.
30. Rull, R., Vidal, O., Momblan, D., et al. (2003) Evaluation of potential liver donors: Limits imposed by donor variables in liver transplantation. *Liver Transplant.* **9**, 389–393.
31. Salizzoni, M., Franchello, A., Zamboni, F., et al. (2003) Marginal grafts: finding the correct treatment for fatty livers. *Transplant. Int.* **16**, 486–493. Epub 2003 Mar 28.
32. Tekin, K., Imber, C. J., Atli, M., et al. (2004) A simple scoring system to evaluate the effects of cold ischaemia on marginal donors. *Transplantation* **77**, 411–416.
33. Strasberg, M., Howard, T. K., Molmenti, E. P., and Hertl, M. (1994) Selecting the donor liver: risk factors for poor function after orthotopic liver transplantation [see comments]. *Hepatology* **20**, 829–838.
34. Bismuth, H. and Houssin, D. (1984) Reduced size orthotopic liver graft in hepatic transplantation in children. *Surgery* **95**, 367–370.
35. Broelsch, C. E., Emond, J. C., andThistlewaite, J. R. (1988) Liver transplantation including the concept of reduced size liver transplants in children. *Ann. Surg.* **208**, 410–420.
36. Ringe, B., Pichlmayr, R., andBurdelski, M. (1988) A new technique of hepatic vein reconstruction in partial liver transplantation. *Transplant. Int.* **1**, 3035.

37. Strong, R., Ong, T. H., Pillayb, P., Wall, D., Balderson, G., and Lynch, S. (1988) A new method of segmental orthotopic liver transplantation in children. *Surgery* **104**, 104–107.
38. de Santibanes, E., McCormack, L., and Mattera, J. (2000) Partial left lateral segment transplant from a living donor. *Liver Transplant.* **6**, 108–112.
39. Badger, I. L., Czerniak, A., and Beath, S. (1992) Hepatic transplantation in children using reduced size grafts. *Br. J. Surg.* **79**, 47–49.
40. Houssin, D., Soubrane, O., Boillot, O., et al. (1992) Orthotopic liver transplantation with a reduced-size graft: an ideal compromise in paediatrics? *Surgery* **111**, 532–542.
41. Malatack, J. J., Schaid, D. J., Urbach, A. H., et al. (1987) Choosing a paediatric recipient for orthotopic liver transplantation. *J. Pediatr. Surg.* **111**, 479–489.
42. Pichlmayr, R., Ringe, B., Gubernatis, G., and Hauss, J. (1988) Transplantation of a donor liver to two recipients (splitting transplantation)—a new method in the further development of segmental liver transplantation. *Langenbecks Arch. Chir.* **373**, 127–130.
43. Rogiers, X., Malago, M., Gawad, K., et al. (1996) In situ splitting of cadaveric livers. The ultimate expanion of a limited donor pool. *Ann. Surg.* **224**, 331–339.
44. Bismuth, H, Morino, M, Castaing, D, et al. (1989) Emergency orthotopic liver transplantation in two patients using one donor liver. *Br. J. Surg.* **76**, 722–724.
45. Strong, R. W., Lych, S. V., Hin Ong, T. H., Matsunami, H., and Koido, Y. (1990) Successful liver transplantation from a living donor to her son. *N. Engl. J. Med.*. **322**, 1505–1507.
46. Gomez, M., Garcia-Buitron, J. M., Fernandez-Garcia, A, et al. (1997) Liver transplantation with organs from non-heart-beating donors. *Transplant. Proc.* **29**, 3478–3479.
47. Casavilla, A., Ramirez, C., Shapiro, R., et al (1995) Experience with liver and kidney allografts from non-heart-beating donors. *Transplantation* **59**, 197–203.
48. D'Alessandro, A. M., Hoffmann, R. M., Knechtle, S. J., et al. (1995) Successful extrarenal transplantation from non-heart-beating donors. *Transplantation* **59**, 977–982.
49. Reich, D. J., Munoz, S. J., Rothstein, K. D., et al. (2000) Controlled non-heart-beating donor liver transplantation: a successful single centre experience, with topic update. *Transplantation* **70**, 1159–1166.
50. Otero, A., Gomez-Gutierrez, M., Suarez, F., et al. (2003) Liver transplantation from Maastricht category 2 non-heart-beating donors. *Transplantation* **76**, 1068–1073.
51. Rela, M., Muiesan, P., Vilca-Melendez, H., et al. (1999) Auxiliary partial orthotopic liver transplantation for Crigler-Najjar syndrome type I. *Ann. Surg.* **229**, 565–569.
52. Uemoto, S., Yabe, S., Inomata, Y., et al. (1997) Coexistenct of a graft with the preserved native liver in auxiliary partial orthotopic liver transplantation from a living donor for ornithine transcarbamylase deficiency. *Transplantation* **63**, 1026–1028.

53. Saudubray, J. M., Touati, G., Delonlay, P., et al. (1999) Liver transplantation in propionic acidaemia. *Eur J Pediatr.* **158**, S65–S69.
54. van Hoek, B., de Boer, J., Boudjema, K., Williams, R., Corsmit, O., et al (1999) Auxiliary versus orthotopic liver transplantation for acute liver failure. *J. Hepatol.* **30**, 699–705.
55. Langnas, A. N., Fox, I. J., Heffron, T. G., et al. (1995) University of Nabraska Medical Centre Liver Transplant Program. *Clin. Transplant.* 177–185.
56. Starzl, T. E., Fung, J. J., Tzakis, A. G., et al. (1993) Baboon-to-human liver transplantation. *Lancet* **341**, 65–71.
57. Makowka, L., Cramer, D. V., Hoffman, A., et al. (1995) The use of a pig liver xenograft for temporary support of a patient with fulminant hepatic failure. *Transplantation* **59**, 1654–1659.
58. Waterworth, P. D., Cozzi, E., and Tolan, M. J. (1997) Pig-to-primate cardiac xenotransplantation and cyclophosphamide therapy. *Transplant. Proc.* **29**, 899–900.
59. McGregor, C. G., Teotia, S. S., and Schirmer, J. M. (2003) Advances in preclinical cardiac xenotransplantation [abstr 47]. *J. Heart Lung Transplant.* **22**, S89–S89.
60. Phelps, C. J., Koike, C., Vaught, T. D., et al. (2003) Production of alpha-1,3 galactosyltransferase-deficient pigs. *Science.* **299**, 411–414.
61. Oldmixon, B., Wood, J. C., Ericsson, T. A., et al. (2002) Porcine endogenous retrovirus transmission characteristics of an inbred herd of miniature swine. *J. Virol.* **76**, 3045–3048.

3

Current Status of Clinical Islet Cell Transplantation

Jonathan R. T. Lakey, Mohammadreza Mirbolooki, and A. M. James Shapiro

Summary

Clinical outcomes of pancreas transplantation were superior to that of islet transplantation until the introduction of the Edmonton protocol. Significant advances in islet isolation and purification technology, novel immunosuppression and tolerance strategies, and effective antiviral prophylaxis have renewed interest in clinical islet transplantation for the treatment of diabetes mellitus. The introduction of a steroid-free antirejection protocol and islets prepared from two donors led to high rates of insulin independence. The Edmonton protocol has been successfully replicated by other centers in an international multicenter trial. A number of key refinements in pancreas transportation, islet preparation, and newer immunological conditioning and induction therapies have led to continued advancement through extensive collaboration between key centers. This chapter provides an overview of the history of islet transplantation followed by a discussion of the state of the art of clinical islet transplantation. The challenges facing the clinician–scientist in the 21st century are also presented in this review.

Key Words: Type 1 diabetes; transplantation; islet cell; islet isolation; Edmonton protocol.

1. Introduction

Diabetes mellitus (DM) is a clinical syndrome of abnormal carbohydrate, lipid, and protein metabolism characterized by hyperglycemia and glucosuria owing to the inadequate secretion and/or utilization of insulin. Insulin-dependent diabetes mellitus (IDDM) is an autoimmune disease caused by the progressive destruction of the insulin-secreting β-cells in the islets of Langerhans *(1)*. The loss of more than 90% of the β-cell mass, triggered by unknown environmental factors and mediated by cytotoxic T cells, condemns genetically susceptible individuals to a lifelong dependence on insulin therapy *(2,3)*.

From: *Methods in Molecular Biology, vol. 333: Transplantation Immunology: Methods and Protocols*
Edited by: P. Hornick and M. Rose © Humana Press Inc., Totowa, NJ

There are an estimated 177 million diabetics worldwide. Of the 8 million patients in North America, 1 million have type 1 diabetes and 7 million have type 2 diabetes; and another 8 million are believed to be undiagnosed. About 30,000 new type 1 cases are diagnosed each year in North America, and the incidence is rising annually ***(4)***. According to the Diabetic Resources Network, there are an estimated 1.5 million diabetics in Canada, and this number is expected to double by 2010. It is the leading cause of death by disease and the number one cause of adult blindness ***(5)***. Diabetes is responsible for 25% of cardiac surgeries, 40% of end-stage renal disease (ESRD), and approx 50% of nontraumatic amputations. The economic costs and its burden on Canadian society are staggering, consuming in excess of 10% of health care expenditures, or about $9 billion in 2000 ***(6)***.

1.1 Diabetes and the Quest for a Cure

The Diabetes Control and Complications Trial (DCCT) of 1993 and its follow-up report in 1997 established that aggressive control of blood glucose lowered (but did not correct) glycated hemoglobin (HbA_{1C}) values and significantly delayed the progression of chronic diabetic complications ***(7,8)***. The United Kingdom Prospective Diabetes Study Group (UKPDS) of type 2 diabetics with microvasculature disease reported similar findings ***(9)***. These studies confirmed unequivocally that tight control of blood glucose is essential if the microvascular complications are to be prevented.

Intensive therapy is based on frequent self-monitoring of capillary blood glucose (four or more times each day) using skin puncture sampling and analysis with a portable glucose meter ***(10)***. Insulin can be self-administered by multiple injections (three or more times a day) or by pump therapy ***(11,12)***. The penalty for this optimal metabolic control is an alarming threefold increase in severe hypoglycemia. Even with aggressive medical management, exogenous (subcutaneous) insulin therapy will never recreate the real-time variation of blood glucose. The effects of chronic hyperglycemia and peripheral hyperinsulinemia are believed to accelerate diabetic microangiopathy ***(13,14)***. These observations have prompted researchers to explore alternative methods to restore physiological blood glucose regulation.

β-Cell replacement is the only treatment that reestablishes and maintains long-term glucose homeostasis with near-perfect feedback controls ***(15)***. Pancreas transplantation is the standard therapy for insulin-dependent diabetics with established or imminent ESRD ***(16)***. Pancreas transplantation is also an option for patients who (1) require urgent third-party intervention for frequent, acute, and severe metabolic complications (hypoglycemia, hyperglycemia, ketoacidosis), (2) have incapacitating clinical and emotional problems with exogenous insulin therapy, or (3) exhibit frequent acute complications despite strict compliance with optimal medical management. Normalization of blood glucose can reverse diabetic nephropathy ***(17)*** and stabilize or improve neuropathy ***(18)*** and cardiovascular status, but not advanced retinopathy ***(19)***. Clinical outcomes have improved dramatically since the first cadaveric pancreas–kidney transplant in 1966 by Kelly and Lillehei at the University of Minnesota ***(20)***. The procedure is technically demanding and continues to have significant peri-operative mortality and morbidity despite refined surgical techniques, effective immunosuppression modalities, antiviral prophylaxis, and posttransplant monitoring ***(21,22)***. Although graft rejection rates are low, the risks associated with pancreas transplantation have generally limited its use to co-transplantation with other organs. The current 1-yr graft and patient survival rates are 80–90% and as high as 95%, respectively ***(23)***. In contrast, islet transplantation with its reduced antigen load, technical simplicity, and low morbidity has the potential to prevent chronic complications and improve quality of life. From a research perspective, islet transplantation is the ideal model for testing novel immunosuppression and tolerance, and cytoprotection protocols. It has several advantages over other experimental models because (1) unlike failed heart, lung, and liver transplants, which require life-saving emergency retransplantation, a diabetic would resume insulin therapy if the islet graft fails, (2) retransplantation is associated with low morbidity, (3) allogeneic and autoimmune barriers must be neutralized, and (4) islets can be cryopreserved or manipulated in vitro to reduce immunogenicity or to induce cellular expansion.

The potential of pancreas transplantation for the treatment of diabetes began in 1889 when Minkowski and von Mering unexpectantly discovered that removal of the canine pancreas resulted in hyperglycemia and glucosuria, followed by ketoacidosis and death ***(24)***. The first clinical attempt to transplant the pancreas was performed 5 yr later by Williams, who implanted fragments of freshly slaughtered sheep's pancreas in the subcutaneous tissues of a 13-yr-old boy dying of diabetic ketoacidosis ***(25)***. Although there was temporary improvement in glucosuria before his death 3 d later, it was inevitable that the xenograft would fail without the benefit of immunosuppression. Pioneering experiments by Minkowski, Ssobolew, Barron, and others quickly gave rise to the realization that the exocrine pancreas was not necessary to treat diabetes ***(26)***. In 1902, Ssobolew proposed transplanting only the endocrine tissue, but he had no practical means to separate the islets from the acinar tissue. Consequently, this approach would lie in a near-dormant state for more than 60 yr ***(27,28)***.

The discovery of insulin by Banting and Best in 1922 transformed diabetes from an inevitably fatal disease following the onset of ketoacidosis to that of a chronic incurable illness with debilitating comorbidities and premature death ***(29,30)***. Clinicians were eager to declare that insulin therapy would cure diabetes, a fact that was not overlooked by Banting, who concluded his 1923 Nobel laureate lecture with: "Insulin is not a cure but is a treatment; it enables the diabetic to burn sufficient carbohydrates, so that proteins and fats may be added to the diet in sufficient quantities to provide energy for the economic burdens of life" ***(31)***. Meanwhile, surgeons continued to refine pancreas and vascular surgery techniques that would eventually set the stage for future breakthroughs in organ transplantation and transplantation immunology. However, it was obvious by the 1930s that exogenous insulin therapy did not prevent the progression of the clinical syndromes now known as the complications of diabetes. It was not until the late 1940s that the scope and severity of the disease was really known. The consequences of 15–20 yr of persistent hyperglycemia resulted in renal failure, blindness, heart disease, neuropathy, and atherosclerosis ***(32)***. The clinical introduction of glucocorticoids and azathioprine (and later cyclosporine) coupled with the success of kidney transplantation in the early 1960s provided the impetus to once again explore the possibility of pancreas transplantation as a treatment for insulin-dependent diabetes ***(33)***. Canine and clinical studies of vascularized pancreas transplantation in the late 1960s and early 1970s were disastrous. While organ procurement and preservation were major obstacles, peritonitis, graft rejection, and septicemia secondary to the breakdown of the duodenal anastomosis in the presence of high-dose corticosteroids were largely responsible for a mortality rate in excess of 60% and a dismal 1-yr graft-survival rate of 3% ***(20)***. Because some of these problems resulted from contaminated exocrine tissue in the graft, efforts were undertaken to determine the feasibility and efficacy of grafting only the insulin-producing tissue.

1.2. The Evolution of Clinical Islet Transplantation

Prior to the late 1960s, the harvesting of islets for morphological and physiological studies required the meticulous microdissection of rodent pancreata ***(27)***. Lacy and Kostianovsky extensively refined Moskalewski's technique of dispersing minced rodent pancreatic tissue into fragments from which large numbers of islets could then be separated ***(34,35)***. Briefly, the pancreas was distended with a balanced salt solution via the pancreatic duct, which was then chopped into small fragments and mechanically agitated with bacterial collagenase enzyme. In 1970, Younoszai et al. demonstrated some amelioration of glucosuria and glycemia in diabetic rats by intraperitoneal implantation of allografted islets ***(28)***. The first reports of successful islet transplantation in rats with chemically induced diabetes were published in 1972 by Ballinger and Lacy and others. Kemp et al. demonstrated that the liver was the most effective environment for islet implantation in rodents ***(36)***. The islets undergo a process of angiogenesis and neovascularization to form a rich nutritional blood supply and a core-to-mantle microvascular network that optimizes intercellular β-to-α/δ signaling for precise insulin and glucagon secretion. Transportal embolization is the method of choice in clinical islet transplantation, although there is some debate as to whether the liver is the best site ***(37)***. In 1977, Najarian et al. at the University of Minnesota performed the first successful clinical islet allotransplant under protective cover with azathioprine and corticosteroids ***(38)***. One year later Largiader et al. reported the first C-peptide-negative diabetic to achieve insulin independence at 1 yr after simultaneous kidney transplant and intrasplenic infusion of nonpurified pancreatic tissue from a single donor ***(39)***. Researchers prematurely predicted that islet transplantation would cure diabetes and that vascularized pancreas transplantation would only be a footnote in the history books. However, the extrapolation of rodent islet transplant technology into the clinical arena proved to be very problematic. This was due in part to the inability to prepare an adequate islet implant mass from the more fibrous human pancreas. Little attention was given to the composition, purity, and viability of the pancreatic digest or the consequences of transplanting such tissue into human subjects ***(40)***. Most attempts were disappointing and very often catastrophic, with hepatic infarction, portal vein thrombosis, disseminated intravascular coagulation, and splenic infarction accounting for much of the morbidity and mortality ***(21)***. These events and ineffective immunosuppression would critically hinder the development of clinical islet transplantation for the next 20 yr ***(41)***. Methods would eventually be developed that enabled the isolation of islets from dogs, pigs, primates, and humans ***(42,43)***. Indeed, the present-day concept of clinical islet transplantation is based on techniques developed in large animal models ***(41)***.

There were sporadic reports in the 1990s of insulin independence following islet allotransplantation for extended periods ***(44–48)***. In 1992, Pyzdrowski at the University of Minnesota reported a series of five patients (ages 12–37 yr) who became insulin independent after intrahepatic islet autotransplantation following total or near-total pancreatectomy (>99%) for severe chronic pancreatitis ***(49)***. Other autotransplant studies demonstrated that a critical mass of 300,000 islets could reestablish and maintain insulin independence beyond 2 yr ***(50,51)***. These were the first studies to prove that islet autotransplantation was feasible and safe. More than 240 autotransplants have been performed worldwide in the last 15 yr ***(52)***. Most recipients had undergone total or near-total pancreatectomy for intractable pain and/or failure to thrive secondary to chronic pancreatitis. Oberholzer et al. recently reported long-term insulin independence in two patients who underwent islet autotransplantation following distal pancreatectomy for insulinomata well localized to the surgical neck of the pancreas, with no signs of recurrence at 3 and 6 yr posttransplant, respectively ***(53)***. To date, the longest period of insulin independence following autotransplantation is more than 13 yr ***(54)***.

Of the 237 well-documented allotransplants recorded in the Islet Transplant Registry (ITR) database in Giessen, Germany, from January 1, 1990 to December 31, 2000, less than 12% of recipients were insulin-free at 1 yr posttransplant. Graft survival, defined as basal C-peptide less than 0.5 ng/mL, was 41% ***(48,52)***. The majority were islet–kidney transplants. Tolerance was induced with either antilymphocyte globulin (ALG) or antithymocyte globulin (ATG). Cyclosporine, azathioprine, and glucocorticoids were used for maintenance immunosuppression. Although these disappointing results were in sharp contrast to those of clinical autotransplantation, there were two notable exceptions. In 1990, Tzakis et al. at the University of Pittsburgh reported a small series of nondiabetics who had undergone islet and co-transplantation of a liver, kidney, and bowel following multivisceral resection for primary or secondary hepato-biliary malignancies ***(44)***. Two years later, Ricordi et al. reported a follow-up series of 22 cluster organ–islet allotransplants ***(45)***. Most grafts were from a single pancreas of a multi-visceral donor and were implanted in the liver via the portal vein following reperfusion. More than 50% of recipients were able to remain insulin-free (the longest >5 yr) before succumbing to recurrent metastatic disease. These studies provided a unique opportunity to study islet allografts in the absence of autoimmune reactivity. Other factors believed to contribute to the success of these multivisceral organ–islet transplants were as follows: (1) the use of partially purified preparations allowed a greater number of islets to be implanted ***(55)***; (2) the patients who were able to achieve insulin independence had a larger implant mass relative to their body weight ***(48)***; (3) tacrolimus monotherapy in the absence of corticosteroids provided effective immunosuppression ***(56)***; (4) experimental studies have shown that liver transplantation improves immunological tolerance to other organs from the same donor when simultaneously transplanted ***(57)***; and (5) cachectic individuals are known to be very sensitive to insulin ***(58)***.

1.3. Early Clinical Trials: Prelude to the Edmonton Protocol

In 1989, the first two of seven patients in an early cohort received approx 260,000 islets isolated from two cadaveric donor pancreata. A kidney from the first donor was also implanted ***(59)***. Intravenous insulin was administered for 10–14 d with intensive blood glucose monitoring to maintain normoglycemia and preserve β-cell function. Immunosuppressive therapy included Minnesota antilymphoblast globulin (MALG), corticosteroids, azathioprine, and cyclosporine. Posttransplant C-peptide production gradually declined over 1–3 mo. Graft failure coincided with cytomegalovirus (CMV) infection, with neither patient achieving insulin independence. Subsequently, four patients were transplanted with fresh allografts supplemented with cryopreserved islets to create a total islet mass of more than 10,000 IE/kg (islet equivalent [IE]: standardized to the volume of an islet 150 μm in diameter per kilogram body weight of the recipient) ***(60)***. One patient remained insulin-free for more than 2 yr ***(48)***. The seventh patient underwent a simultaneous liver and islet transplant. Embolization of partially purified pancreatic tissue into the liver via the portal vein resulted in complete portal vein thrombosis and required emergency retransplantation ***(55,56)***. All patients eventually required insulin therapy. Two allografts remained C-peptide positive, the longest for more than 9 yr. Researchers from Pittsburgh, St. Louis, Milan, and Miami also reported some early success with islet allotransplants, but technical problems, particularly with the collagenase, would temporarily dampen enthusiasm for developing islet transplantation ***(47,61,62)***.

These data demonstrated that most patients were unable to achieve or maintain insulin independence because (1) the islet implant mass was subtherapeutic ***(63)***, (2) a high proportion of the islets failed to engraft ***(64)***, (3) the islets were damaged in the liver (the site of implantation) by direct, local toxic effects of the immunosuppressants ***(65)***, and (4) ineffective immunosuppression failed to prevent acute or chronic rejection or the recurrence of autoimmune diabetes ***(66)***. The high metabolic demand of preexisting insulin resistance in patients with incipient renal failure also placed undue stress on the islets ***(67,68)***. Implanted islets were also lost owing to functional exhaustion ***(69)***. Four criteria have been identified with insulin independence: (1) the critical islet implant mass was 6000 IE/kg or more; (2) the critical cold ischemia (preservation) time (CIT) was less than 8 h; (3) polyclonal antibodies such as ALG or ATG were very effective in depleting cytotoxic T cells; and (4) the liver was the favored implantation site ***(70–72)***.

By the late 1990s, controlled pancreas distension with low-endotoxin Liberaseô (Roche, Indianapolis, IN), automated tissue dissociation, and purification on continuous Ficoll gradients made it possible to manufacture high-yield islet preparations suitable for experimental and clinical transplantation ***(73,74)*** (**Fig. 1**). The Giessen protocol employed endotoxin-free reagents during processing and intravenous insulin, parenteral hyperalimentation, and antioxidant therapy (nicotinamide, pentoxifylline, vitamin D) to improve islet engraftment and overcome early graft rejection ***(75,76)***. Insulin independence was achieved in about 25% of patients with ATG induction and maintenance immunosuppression with methylprednisolone, azathioprine, and cyclosporine. Maffi et al. of Milan reported that mycophenolate mofetil (MMF), vitamin D, cyclosporine, steroids, and metformin enhanced islet allograft survival from 33% to more than 50% ***(77)***.

Using a similar strategy that emphasized strict quality-control criteria and aggressive peri-transplant management, Oberholzer et al. reported improved islet allograft function in 13 patients with IDDM followed over a period of 3 mo to 5 yr under cover of basiliximab (a chimeric anti-interleukin ([IL]-2 receptor-α monoclonal antibody [anti-IL-2R-α MAb]), steroids, cyclosporine, and MMF ***(46)***. Based on these data, the Swiss-French (GRAGIL) consortium, using a cen-

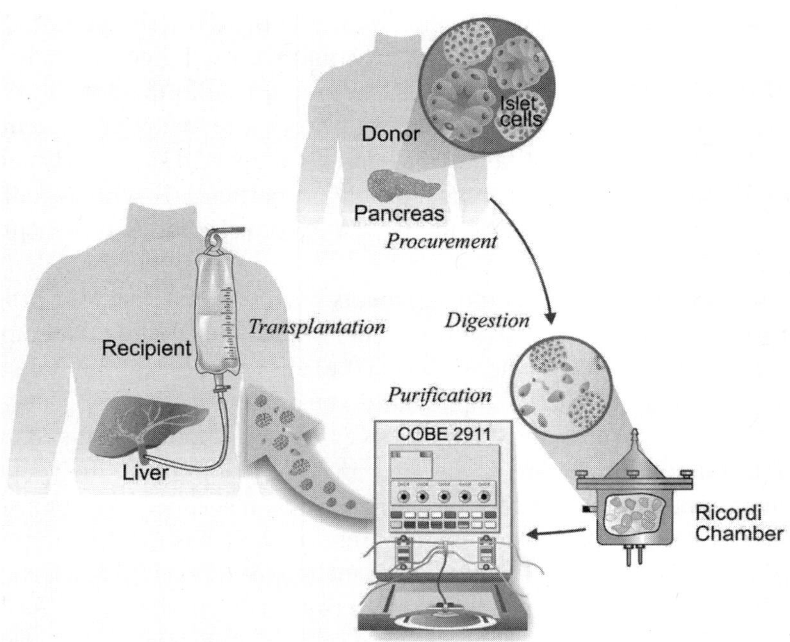

Fig. 1. Schematic view of clinical islet cell transplantation.

tral processing facility and refined peri-transplant management protocols, reported a 1-yr allograft survival rate of 50%. Two of five patients with single-donor allografts achieved insulin independence after 6–8 mo. Interestingly, both recipients received islets shipped from another center *(78)*. Three individuals eventually resumed insulin therapy but remained C-peptide positive. There were no episodes of primary graft failure (PGF). The remaining five allografts eventually lost all function.

1.4. Development of Steroid-Free Immunosuppression

The resurgence of autoimmune activity is an ominous sign indicative of impending graft failure. The importance of an effective immunosuppressive regimen is well demonstrated by the fact that autoimmune recurrence following identical twin-to-twin segmental pancreas transplantation can be prevented *(79)*. The limited success of early clinical islet transplants revealed that conventional immunosuppressants were relatively ineffective in preventing allograft rejection when compared to their effect on vascularized pancreas grafts. Most if not all agents were associated with impaired β-cell function, reduced graft revascularization, or serious long-term side effects such as nephrotoxicity and malignancy *(80)*. Cyclosporine and glucocorticoids exert their diabetogenic synergism through reduced insulin secretion, increased peripheral insulin resistance, and direct toxicity to the fl cell *(81)*. Azathioprine, a purine analog originally developed as an anticancer agent, revolutionized renal transplantation in the early 1960s. It inhibits T-cell proliferation by blocking DNA and RNA synthesis. Leukopenia is the most common side effect. Azathioprine toxicity is dose dependent and often reversible. Azathioprine monotherapy does not appear to adversely affect β-cell function or insulin sensitivity. MMF provides more specific potent immunosuppression by inhibiting the *de novo* synthesis of guanosine nucleotides in T and B cells. Unlike azathioprine, MMF is not teratogenic *(82)*. MMF also potentiates the antiviral effects of ganciclovir and inhibits the upregulation of adhesion molecules on the surface of cytotoxic T cells. Overimmunosuppression can result in life-threatening opportunistic infections and malignancy, particularly lymphoma *(83,84)*. Polyclonal antibodies such as ATG and ALG are very effective in high-immunological-risk patients *(85)*.

The introduction of sirolimus was a major key to the development of steroid-free immunosuppression *(23,86)*. Unlike other immunosuppressants, sirolimus interrupts cell-cycle kinetics late in the G_1 phase, prior to entry into the S phase. The specific inhibition of the lymphocyte response (growth factor mediated) to mitogenic stimuli leaves other proliferative pathways unaffected. Thus, sirolimus blocks T- and B-cell recruitment, activation, and clonal expansion by inhibiting IL-2 and other cytokine production. Its low diabetogenic potential, minimal nephrotoxicity, and synergism with tacrolimus and other calcineurin inhibitors has been responsible for very low rejection rates in clinical liver, kidney, and pancreas transplantation *(87)*. Sirolimus-based protocols have demonstrated prolonged islet graft survival and improved function through enhanced insulin half-life and increased insulin sensitivity *(88)*. Tacrolimus is a more potent calcineurin inhibitor, and, like cyclosporine, its inhibitory effects on insulin secretion are dose-dependent *(89)*. Low-dose tacrolimus combined with sirolimus and corticosteroids have resulted in unprecedented low rejection rates in liver, kidney, and pancreas transplantation *(90)*. Daclizumab (Zenapax®, Roche Pharmaceuticals) is a recombinant MAb engineered to specifically target the α-chain of the IL-2 IL-2R-α, which is expressed only by activated lymphocytes. It provides potent immunosuppression by inhibiting both T- and B-cell proliferation and inhibiting interferon-γ secretion *(91,92)*. It has been very effective in renal transplants. Its safety profile is unmatched by any other immunosuppressive agent currently in use. Thus, triple therapy with tacrolimus, sirolimus, and daclizumab prevents activation of the immune cascade at several sites by inhibiting (1) T-cell activation, (2) IL-2 and other pro-inflammatory cytokine production, and (3) IL-2α receptor ligand engagement and T-cell proliferation and clonal expansion *(93)*. This steroid-free strategy is particularly advantagous in the setting of a marginal islet engraftment mass in that it reduces β-cell toxicity substantially.

Table 1
Effect of Islet Cell Transplantation

	Islet transplant recipients	Type 1diabetic subjects	Nondiabetic control subjects
n	7	7	7
Sex (M/F)	6/1	4/3	3/4
BMI (kg/m²)	23.0 ± 1.2	24.3 ± 1.4	24/2 ± 0.8
Age (yr)	43 ± 3	39 ± 3	37 ± 5
Duration of daibetes (yr)	27 ± 6	26 ± 3	—
Total islets transplanted per patient	840,155 ± 52,943	—	—
HbA_{1c} (%)	5.8 ± 0.1	9.7 ± 0.6	5.4 ± 0.1

2. The Edmonton Protocol

In 2000, we reported that seven consecutive nonuremic patients with type 1 DM transplanted with an average of approx 800,000 islets were insulin independent beyond 1 yr ***(94)***. The Edmonton protocol, a glucocorticoid-free immunosuppression regimen combined with an optimal islet engraftment mass, was a dramatic departure from previous attempts. The protocol addressed specific barriers to insulin independence identified by Hering and Ricordi. Autoimmune recurrence and allograft rejection were counteracted with the novel cocktail of daclizumab, sirolimus, and low-dose tacrolimus. This landmark study confirmed for the first time in the history of clinical islet transplantation that long-term islet function and excellent blood glucose control could be achieved with results similar to that of vascularized pancreas transplantation ***(66)***. Expeditious graft processing followed by immediate transplantation, the limitation of prolonged cold ischemia, the avoidance of culture and cryopreservation, and the elimination of exposure to xenoproteins, such as fetal calf serum (FCS), further optimized the recovery of functionally viable islets. Subsequent follow-up of the original cohort confirmed that long-term insulin independence was possible and that the therapy was safe and well tolerated ***(95–97)*** **(Table 1)**.

2.1. Patient Selection and Preoperative Evaluation

The benefits of insulin-free status must be carefully weighed against the potential risks of long-term immunosuppression on an individual basis. Most early islet transplants were combined with a kidney transplant in patients with end-stage diabetic nephropathy ***(52)***. These individuals often have significant peripheral insulin resistance, which can be very slow to reverse after successful transplantation ***(67,98)***. This problem and the concomitant nephrotoxicity of the calcineurin inhibitors can be easily overcome by transplanting only C-peptide-negative diabetics who have adequate renal reserve (creatinine clearance >80 mL/min/1.73 m² or microproteinuria <300 mg/24 h) ***(99)***.

We select adults (18–65 yr) with type 1 DM for more than 5 yr who are at greatest risk and exhibit one or more of the following: (1) at least two episodes of severe hypoglycemia with reduced awareness during the preceding 12 mo, (2) marked glycemic lability ("brittle diabetes") characterized by erratic blood glucose levels that interfere with daily activities and/or requiring third-party intervention on two or more occasions during the previous 12 mo ***(100)***, and (3) the presence of early but progressive secondary diabetic complications that fail to stabilize with intensive insulin therapy ***(7,8)***. Diabetics with severe coronary artery disease are excluded. Patients with unstable retinopathy should not be transplanted because sudden changes in blood glucose can precipitate retinal hemorrhage ***(101)***. Diabetics with a recent or active history of substance abuse (including smoking), daily insulin requirements of more than 0.7 IU/kg, body weight greater than 90 kg, BMI higher than 28 kg/m^2, active infection (including hepatitis B and C, AIDS, and tuberculosis), or a history of malignancy (except basal cell carcinoma or squamous cell carcinoma) are not eligible. A positive pregnancy test, intention of future pregnancy, or failure to practice effective contraception also preclude enrollment. Only 10% of the more than 1500 Canadians with DM we have evaluated are suitable candidates for islet-alone transplantation.

A thorough and independent review of potential candidates was performed by two diabetologists and a multidisicplinary transplant team. Upon enrollment, each patient gave written informed consent and underwent the following baseline tests: a complete blood count (CBC), liver function tests (LFTs), electrolytes, calcium, magnesium, thyroid function, lipid panel, renal function tests (RFTs), and coagulation profile. Patients with labile diabetes or recurrent hypoglycemia secondary to adrenal insufficiency and celiac disease were excluded. Prostate-specific antigen (PSA) levels were determined in men older than 40 yr. Women older than 40 yr underwent mammograms. Eye assessment, chest X-ray, dental assessment, abdominal ultrasound, and an electrocardiogram (and other cardiac tests, if warranted) were also performed. All patients were screened for CMV, HIV, hepatitis, Epstein-Barr nuclear antigen (EBNA), varicella-zoster, syphilis, tuberculosis, and toxoplasmosis. Lymphocytotoxic antibody screens were performed. Blood glucose and C-peptide levels before and after 90 min of ingesting a standard mixed meal were recorded. Serum was analyzed for anti-insulin antibodies and islet autoantibodies.

2.2. Pancreas Procurement

We process organs that the Human Organ Procurement Exchange (HOPE) program does not allocate for pancreas transplantation. In 2000, Health Canada reported that only 65 organs from 473 donors were used for vascularized pancreas transplantation ***(102)***. Two-thirds of the pancreata were never recovered from suitable donors, and a significant number arrived at the isolation laboratory with CITs exceeding 8 h. Donor pancreata were selected according to factors known to have a positive influence on islet yield and subsequent insulin independence: age over 20 yr, high BMI, blood glucose greater than 10 mMol/L, and no history of prolonged cardiac arrest or severe hypotension requiring inotropic support. Mean donor age was 44 ± 11 yr. Islet injury from excessive cold storage (mean CIT 7.5 ± 4 h) was minimized whenever possible by employing chartered jet transport.

The pancreas is a difficult organ to procure for transplantation ***(103)***. Surgical expertise, procurement technique, and minimal warm ischemia time (WIT) of less than 20 min have a major impact on the recovery of functionally viable islets and posttransplant clinical outcomes ***(104)***. Most reports describe methods for the combined removal of the pancreas and liver ***(105)***. Until recently, the harvesting of the pancreas specifically for islet transplantation had not been addressed ***(106,107)***. The whole pancreas or a segmental graft can either be resected *en bloc* with the liver as part of the multiorgan retrieval process or removed while the liver is perfused with University of Wisconsin (Viaspan or Belzer UW; Barr Laboratories, Inc. Pomona, NY) solution ***(107)***. The following surgical principles are of paramount importance: (1) atraumatic handling of the pancreas (a damaged pancreatic capsule leads to enzyme leakage, loss of ductal integrity and, ultimately, poor islet yields) ***(108)***, (2) rapid *in situ* cooling to minimize WIT and stabilize endogenous enzyme activity ***(107)***, and (3) immediate processing to minimize cold ischemic injury. We have demonstrated that rapid mobilization of the spleen to the midline after cross-clamping the aorta and embedding the entire pancreas in iced saline-slush led to a doubling of islet yield and a significant improvement in islet viability ***(106,107)***. Ideally, the pancreas should be removed *en bloc* with the spleen and a stapled cuff of proximal and distal duodenum.

2.3. Islet Preparation

The islets were prepared using controlled pancreas perfusion with Liberase HIô, automated tissue dissociation in a modified Ricordi chamber, and osmotic stabilization with chilled UW solution for 30 min prior to purification on continuous Ficoll gradients using a refrigerated COBE 2991 cell apheresis system (COBE BCT, Inc. Lakewood, CO) ***(71)***. More recently, the islets were cultured in modified insulin-transferrin-selenium (ITS) medium containing hydroxyethyl piperazine ethane sulfonate (HEPES) buffer and nicotinamide for 48 h ***(97,109)***. Insulin independence is rarely achieved with less than 9000 IE/kg (about 640,000 islets) ***(52)***. The mean cumulative islet mass transplanted at our institution is currently 13,000 IE/kg. Although we usually do not use preparations with less than 250,000 IE, the smallest islet mass that has secured insulin independence in our series is 230,000 IE. Islets were prepared from two (and sometimes three or four) sequential donors in the majority of cases. The mean time between the first and second implants was 70 d. Each preparation was matched to the recipient's blood type and cross-matched for lymphocytoxic antibodies but not HLA phenotypes. Samples of the final preparation were submitted for signal transduction and activation of transcription (STAT) Gram stain and aerobic, anaerobic, fungal, and *Mycoplasma* culture. Islet viability was determined by the membrane dye exclusion technique. Islet function was assessed using static incubation in low- and high-glucose media. The endocrine composition of the grafts was determined by immunohistochemistry ***(110)***.

2.4. Islet-Alone Transplantation

Preoperatively, blood glucose was maintained between 6 and 10 mMol/L using a 10% dextrose infusion supplemented with potassium chloride and insulin ***(7,8)***. The islets were transplanted in the liver by percutaneous transhepatic intraportal embolization using the modified Seldinger technique ***(111)***. Performed under local anesthesia with conscious sedation, the procedure was usually completed within 15 –30 min. A portal venogram was used to visualize the intraparenchymal venous architecture and to confirm the position of the needle and catheter tip within the main vein. Some centers prefer direct visualization of the portal (or mesenteric) vein to minimize the risk of hemorrhage and portal vein thrombosis. This can be safely accomplished by either mini-laparotomy or hand-assisted laparoscopic surgery in conjunction with therapeutic heparinization. These methods may be more suitable for centers with little or no experience in islet transplantation. The transjugular route offers an alternate means of avoiding multiple punctures. However, serious complications such as biliary rupture, capsular puncture, and extrahepatic portal vein puncture have been reported ***(112)***. The majority of patients (>90%) were safely discharged within 12–24 h.

2.5. Pretransplant Conditioning and Posttransplant Therapy

Posttransplant blood glucose was maintained between 4 and 10 mMol/L. Blood glucose is often normal for the first 16–24 h, after which time it is usually necessary to resume insulin therapy (Lispro preprandial and neutral Protamine Hagedora at bedtime), albeit at much lower doses. Daily insulin requirements were about one-half that of pretransplant ***(7,8)***. Daclizumab (1 mg/kg) was given intravenously at the time of transplant and repeated at 2-wk intervals for a total of five doses ***(91,92,113)***. This method allows time for a supplemental transplant procedure. The induction course was repeated if another transplant was required beyond 10 wk. Sirolimus was given orally as a loading dose of 0.2 mg/kg orally immediately pretransplant. The maintenance dose (initially 0.1 mg/kg/d) was adjusted to 24-h target serum trough levels of 12–15 ng/mL (as determined by high-performance liquid chromatography) for 3 mo and were then reduced to 7–10 μg/L thereafter ***(87,114)***. To minimize the risk of drug-induced islet injury, low-dose tacrolimus (at one-quarter to one-half the standard dose for other organ transplants) was administered beginning on d 10 at 2 mg orally twice daily and adjusted to target 12-h serum trough levels of 3–6 μg/L ***(87,115)***. All patients received ganciclovir (1 g orally three times a day) for 3 mo for CMV and posttransplant lymphoproliferative disorder (PLPD) prophylaxis ***(84,116)***, preemptive oral trimethoprimsulfamethoxazole if the white blood cell (WBC) count was less than 2.5×10^9/L (target range 5–10 $\times 10^9$/L), and pentamidine (300 mg/mo) for prevention of *Pneumocystis carinii* pneumonia (PCP) ***(84)***.

Campath-1H, a humanized MAb (Millennium Pharmaceuticals, Cambridge, MA) directed against the surface antigen CD52 expressed by lymphocytes and monocytes, has been proven to be highly effective in the treatment of many hematological malignancies and autoimmune diseases ***(117)***. To date, there have been no reports of increased risk of malignancy, posttransplant lymphoma, or life-threatening infections among the more than 200 kidney transplant recipients worldwide ***(118,119)***. Despite its excellent safety profile and its ability to induce profound lymphocyte depletion, the use of campath-1H and sirolimus without calcineurin inhibitor therapy has raised some concern. Kirk et al. treated seven living-related kidney transplant recipients with only campath-1H ***(110,118)***. In the absence of maintenance immunosuppression, acute rejection was evidenced by an increase in the number of circulating monocytes, an atypical monocytic infiltrate in the graft, and augmented tumor necrosis factor (TNF)-α expression. Low-dose sirolimus reversed graft rejection and provided excellent renal function in all cases. After careful consideration, it was felt that the risk of endothelium-directed monocyte-mediated rejection would be much less likely in the islet setting. Although most donor-derived endothelial cells are removed during the purification process, we felt it prudent to add a micro-dose of tacrolimus. Micro-dosing without drug-level monitoring (0.5 mg orally once every other day or about 10% of the low dose currently used in Edmonton protocol) was delayed until d 7 posttransplant to minimize toxicity to the freshly transplanted islets. Unlike previous trials, which relied on extensive preconditioning with corticosteroids, only campath-1H (20 mg iv) was given on d 2 and 1. Complement-mediated cytokine "storm," a toxic condition characterized by low-grade fever, mild hypertension, nausea, vomiting, and urticaria, was avoided by predosing campath-1H on d 2 with a single dose (10 mg/kg iv) of anti-TNF-α (infliximab [Remicade]).

Abdominal ultrasound with Doppler interrogation of the portal vein was conducted within 24 h of transplantation. Postoperative hemorrhage was detected in 9 of 98 procedures by the presence of free fluid and/or a drop in hemoglobin. Five patients required transfusion for non-life-threatening hemorrhage, while

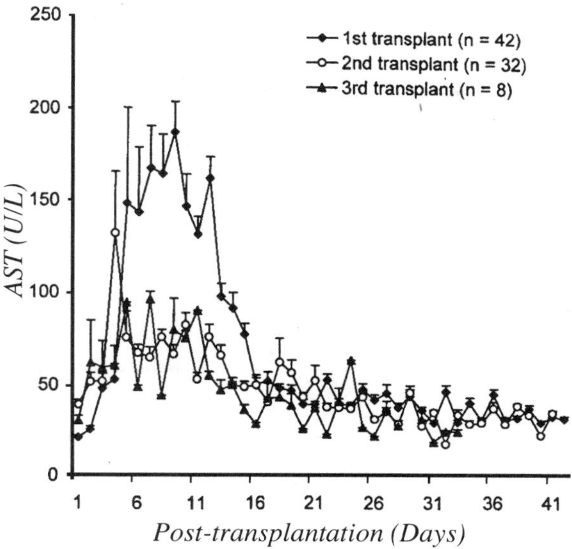

Fig. 2. Peak aspartate aminotransferase (AST) after sequential islet transplantation.

another experienced a rise in portal pressure following infusion of the final (less pure) layer of islets. The patient was anticoagulated and transfused and underwent successful decompression of a subcapsular hematoma and partial hepatectomy because of an expanding intrahepatic hematoma. These risks are potentially avoidable, particularly if the procedure is performed under ultrasound, computed tomography (CT), or fluoroscopic guidance, and the catheter tract is plugged with Gelfoam (Pharmacia and Upjohn, Mississauga, ON) after islet infusion. Hemostatic gelatin-sponge embolization was abandoned early in the study when a customized stiffened 4-Fr micropuncture catheter became available (Cook Canada Inc., Stouffville, ON). The percutaneous transhepatic intraportal approach has a proven safety record and remains our method of choice. We are currently evaluating the efficacy of catheter tract ablation with laser photocoagulation and mini-laparotomy in conjunction with full-dose heparinization and preemptive anti-inflammatory treatment with anti-TNF-α (infliximab) ***(120)***.

Postoperative liver enzyme levels were elevated in about 50% of procedures. This phenomenon is self-limiting and resolves within 3 wk posttransplant. Although the exact cause is unknown, islet embolization most likely induces hepatic injury by obstructing peripheral portal inflow. Liver transaminase levels were lower following subsequent transplants, suggesting that immunosuppression may have a protective effect ***(121)***. The difference in the median peak aspartate aminotransferase (AST) after sequential islet transplantation was not statistically significant **(Fig. 2)**. Even though portal venous pressures returned

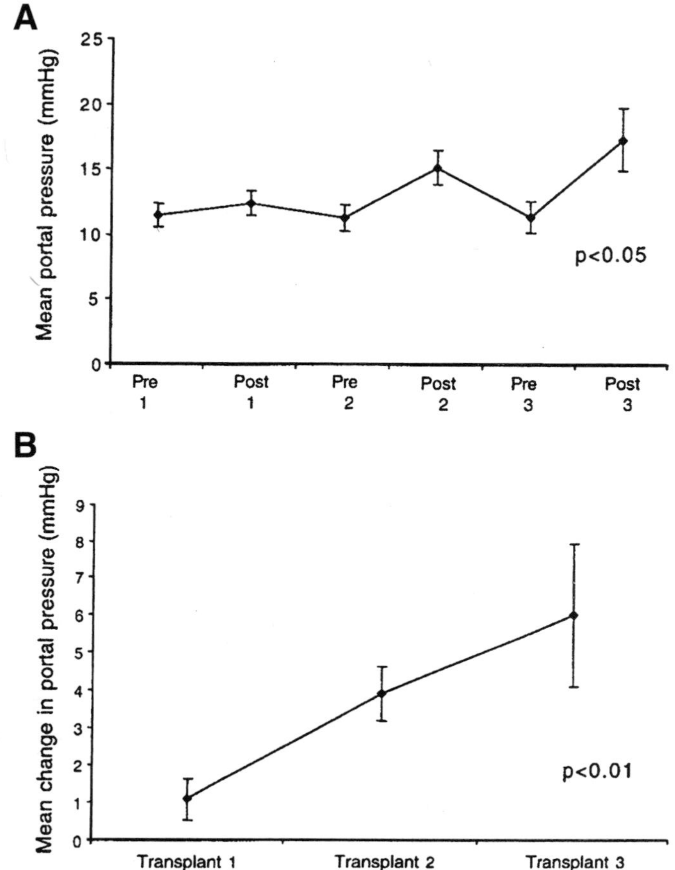

Fig. 3. **(A)** Mean portal pressures measured during first, second, and third islet infusions. **(B)** The mean acute change in portal pressure increases as patients receive more than one islet transplant.

to baseline between procedures, the incremental rise in peak postinfusion portal pressure with successive transplants suggests that the elasticity of the portal system is limited **(Fig. 3)**. It is unknown at this time whether these acute changes will have any long-term significance; however, multiple (two to four) sequential islet transplants can be performed safely if only highly purified islets are implanted and portal venous pressure is carefully monitored ***(122)***. The risk of portal vein thrombosis can be minimized even further by using a closed-bag gravity infusion system, graded low-dose intraportal heparinization (35 U/kg body weight if the packed cell volume [PCV] is <5 mL or 70 U/kg if >5 mL), and smaller infusion volumes (<10 mL and preferably <5 mL) ***(123)***.

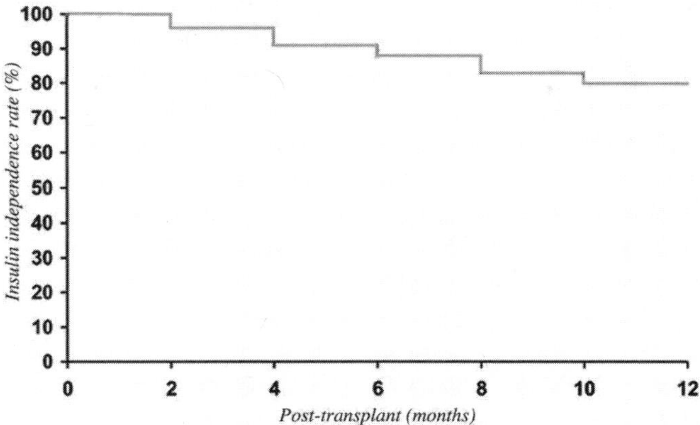

Fig. 4. Kaplan–Meier survival curves showing a mean 82% insulin independence in 118 cosecutive islet-alone transplantations.

2.6. Clinical Outcomes

Our latest series includes data from 48 consecutive C-peptide-negative patients and 98 percutaneous transhepatic procedures and is the largest single-center series worldwide ***(97)***. All patients had chronic complications including metabolic lability (86%), microalbuminuria (64%), retinopathy (50%), neuropathy (29%), and vasculopathy (7%). As of January 2003, 34 patients have received completed transplants (mean cumulative islet mass 369,940 ± 130,000 IE), whereas another 14 await a second transplant. Gender was well matched (21 males, 27 females). The mean recipient age was 42 ± 9 yr. Mean duration of type 1 diabetes was 25 ± 11 yr. Mean pretransplant recipient weight was 70 ± 9 kg. Daily mean pretransplant insulin requirement was 0.6 ± 0.2 IU/kg. The transplant is considered to be a success if there is restoration of sustained euglycemia either without any exogenous insulin or with reduced insulin requirement. Independence from insulin injections is defined by (1) fasting glucose levels of more than 7.8 *mM*l/L more than three times a week (using the morning fasting glucose level) and (2) 2-h postprandial glucose values (using any postmeal glucose) of more than 10 *mM*/L more than four times a week. The transplant is also considered to be a success even if an intercurrent illness or other event (such as high tacrolimus levels) requires insulin for more than 14 d, provided medical assessment after the event demonstrates insulin independence and adequate glucose control.

Islets were transplanted under either the original or modified Edmonton protocol incorporating infliximab and/or campath-1H. Using Kaplan–Meyer survival analysis, the rate of insulin independence at 1-yr post-transplant is 82%. **(Fig. 4)** This compares favorably with previous reports by our group ***(94–96)***.

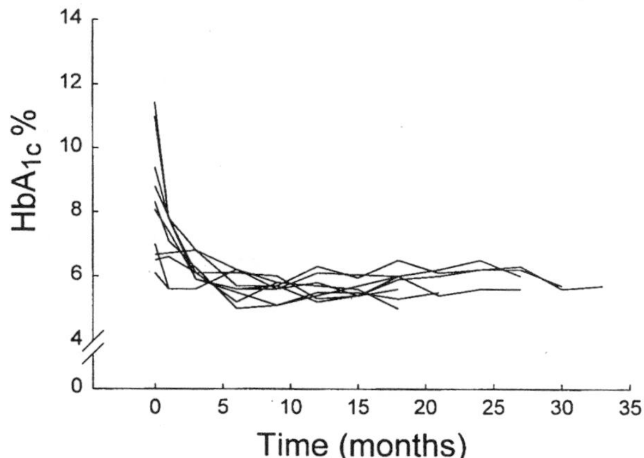

Fig. 5. HbA1c at 3-mo intervals after islet transplantation in subjects who remained insulin independent.

The majority of grafts remain functional beyond 3 yr. Micro anti-insulin antibody (MIAA) concentrations generally returned to normal after the discontinuation of insulin therapy ***(124)***. It is interesting to note, however, that even with effective immunosuppression, the presence of autoimmune reactivity in some autoantibody-negative recipients with vascularized pancreas allografts suggests that an increase in autoantibodies (glutamic acid decarboxylase [GAD] and ICA 512 [islet cell antibodies]) and not their presence pretransplant may be a better predictor of pancreas and islet graft failure ***(125)***. In our latest series, prophylactic immunosuppression failed to prevent autoimmune recurrence in two cases (at 8.5 and 9 mo, respectively). Both individuals had GAD levels in excess of 30 times the upper limit of normal. We intend to retransplant these patients using protocols that specifically inhibit the autoimmune pathway ***(126)***. Tacrolimus toxicity and islet "burnout" (complete loss of insulin reserve) resulted in PGF in two patients at 9.5 and 11 mo, respectively. Most patients have excellent glycemic control and exhibit normal or improved HbA_{1C} values. Mean HbA_{1C} values fell significantly from 8.0% pretransplant to 6.0% posttransplant **(Fig. 5)**. Graft survival (as defined by detectable C-peptide >0.5 ng/mL) is 88% over 3 yr, confirming that islet allografts can retain long-term function. C-peptide secretion (fasting 2.3 ng/mL vs stimulated 5.8 ng/mL) remained stable over 3 yr. Mean body weight was reduced by 6%.

The treatment has been generally safe and well tolerated. To date there have been no deaths, life-threatening infections, malignancies (including posttransplant lymphoproliferative disorder [PTLD]), CMV infections, or CMV seroconversions despite the use of multiple donor/recipient mismatches, presumably because the infected lymphocytes are removed during the purification process. Two patients developed potentially fatal neutropenia (<5 × 10^3/L), requiring hospitalization and temporary granulocyte-colony stimulating factor (G-CSF) therapy ***(127)***. Most patients developed painful superficial mouth ulcers, but these resolved when the target sirolimus level was lowered and the liquid form was changed to a capsule formulation. About 60% of patients developed sirolimus-related dyslipidemia and required statin therapy ***(128)***. About 50% of recipients required either starting or increasing antihypertensive therapy following transplantation. Intestinal upset was an inconvenience in about 50% of cases but gradually settled down over time. One patient with preexisting coronary artery disease required an angioplasty. (Cardiac disease amenable to medical or surgical intervention should be corrected before transplant.) Three patients who achieved insulin independence required photocoagulation therapy for retinal hemorrhages. This emphasizes the importance of stable retinopathy pre-transplant. Retinopathy has stabilized in all patients. Other minor complaints included headache, diarrhea, and tremor.

All patients remain unsensitized except for one recipient, who had detectable donor-specific panel reactive antibodies (PRA) after 2 yr following the complete withdrawal of all immunosuppressants. This is an important factor to consider for patients who may eventually require a kidney, liver, or heart transplant.

Campath-1H was well tolerated, and profound lymphocyte depletion was maintained for more than 230 d (absolute lymphocyte count [ALC]: 11%; CD3 marker: 5–10%). Infliximab therapy lowered serum TNF-α levels, lowered peak liver enzyme rise, and improved islet engraftment significantly when compared to untreated controls.

Three patients were successfully converted from tacrolimus and sirolimus to tacrolimus and MMF. One patient had severe diltiazem-induced ileal ulceration posttransplant, whereas another developed intractable gastroparesis. Both patients remain insulin-free, and despite high tacrolimus levels (10 ng/mL), one patient continues to have normal glucose tolerance, confirming our previous findings that in the absence of corticosteroids, high-dose tacrolimus therapy outside the engraftment window is safe and effective ***(115)***. Renal function remains unchanged in all but two cases, even after conversion from tacrolimus and sirolimus to MMF and sirolimus. Both patients require small amounts of insulin, despite relatively high C-peptide levels (which are likely the result of inadequate renal clearance). This observation suggests that sirolimus interferes with islet neovascularization early in the engraftment phase ***(129)***. MMF and sirolimus may therefore not provide adequate protection against autoimmune recurrence and allograft rejection during the conversion phase. A third patient was converted to MMF and sirolimus because of tacrolimus-induced diarrhea and headache.

All patients enjoy a marked improvement in overall quality of life. The elimination of glycemic lability and the life-threatening consequences of unrecognized hypoglycemia have been the most obvious benefits ***(94–97,130)***. Despite prolonged insulin independence and near-normal glycemic control, islet transplantation does not restore hypoglycemic counterregulation or symptom recognition in recipients with longstanding diabetes and loss of hypoglycemic awareness ***(131)***. While robust glucagon response to arginine stimulation confirms the presence of functioning β-cells, the absence of glucagon and epinephrine response to a stepwise hypoglycemic clamp suggests that islets implanted in the liver do not function in a physiological manner. This abnormal metabolic sensing and signaling may be due to the influence of an unidentified soluble factor in the liver or an acquired defect following transplantation such as the loss of β-cells during processing. Because the liver is the site of endogenous glucose production, higher intrahepatic glucose levels could potentially prevent transplanted islets from sensing peripheral hypoglycemia, thus impairing glucagon secretion ***(132)***. However, this explanation is not satisfactory, as intrahepatic islets are implanted on the portal venous side, which has a slightly lower ambient glucose level as a result of the mixture of portal vein and hepatic artery blood ***(133,134)***. The absence of the recovery of epinephrine response to glucose and symptom recognition may reflect posttransplant subclinical hypoglycemia or the incomplete renervation of the islets in the presence of an underlying chronic autonomic neuropathy ***(133)***. Tacrolimus, like cyclosporine, has been shown to have a direct negative effect on β-cell function, but its effect on α-cell function is unclear ***(87)***. Although sirolimus has little diabetogenic potential, its effect on α-cell function is also unknown ***(139)***. The correction of hypoglycemic awareness, even in patients with partial grafts, appears to have little or no impact on clinical outcomes. However, the failure to restore counterregulatory responsiveness has the potential to jeopardize susceptible recipients to recurrent episodes of hypoglycemia, especially in individuals who may require temporary insulin therapy for an intercurrent illness. Long-term prospective studies are therefore needed to determine the significance of this defect and whether it regresses over time.

Metabolic tests have confirmed that graft function remains relatively stable over time, but mean insulin reserve is only about 20% of normal. Unfortunately, the onset of hyperglycemia often heralds the irreversible destruction of more than 90% of the β-cell mass. Glucose tolerance is markedly impaired in most patients. To date, only one patient has normal glucose tolerance ***(95–97)***. There is no simple test to detect islet graft rejection, unlike the situation in patients with kidney grafts, where a progressive rise in serum creatinine is indicative of organ dysfunction and impending graft failure. The acute insulin response to arginine correlated better with transplanted islet mass than acute insulin response to glucose (AIR_g) and area under the curve for insulin (AUC_i). The AIR_g and AUC_i were more closely related to glycemic control. The AUC_i directly posttransplant was lower in those individuals who eventually became C-peptide deficient. Therefore, a reduction in AIR_g as well as proinsulin levels and split-proinsulin levels over time may be an early indicator of graft dysfunction ***(136,137)***. Preliminary findings in our series suggest that both total intact and split-proinsulin levels and total intact and total split- proinsulin–to–insulin ratios are significantly lower in transplanted patients. Low proinsulin levels may reflect a suboptimal β-cell mass. Low proinsulin-to-insulin ratios strongly suggest that intrahepatic islets release insulin into the systemic circulation via the hepatic vein rather than into the portal venous system. It is unknown at this time whether impaired glucose tolerance with insulin independence and a normal HbA_{1C} will be adequate protection against secondary complications of diabetes. Thus, the long-term outcome of islet transplantation remains under proactive review.

2.7. International Multicenter Trial of the Edmonton Protocol

The Immune Tolerance Network (ITN) is a collaborative international agency dedicated to developing clinical tolerance therapies for a wide range of immune-related conditions, including transplantation and autoimmune diseases ***(138)***. The ITN, with generous financial support from the Juvenile Diabetes Research Foundation (JDRF) and the National Institutes of Health (NIH), is committed to implementing (1) novel short-term immunotherapeutic strategies that involve gradual weaning and complete withdrawal of all immunosuppressants by 1 yr and (2) tolerance protocols incorporating hemopoietic chimerism with an emphasis on T-cell depletion and irradiation-free regimens.

The Edmonton protocol and its minor variants have been successfully replicated in more than 25 centers worldwide, with cumulative data from more than 300 patients. Encouraging findings from the ongoing (3-yr) ITN international multicenter trial include the following:

1. Insulin independence has been achieved in 75% of single-donor islet transplants using a protocol of perfluorochemical-based (two-layer) preservation, short-term culture, and preemptive co-stimulatory signal blockade ***(139,140)***.
2. Islets cultured for 24–48 h in antioxidant-enriched Miami medium improves the quality of islet preparations and facilitates the shipment of islets between centers ***(141)***.
3. Perfluorochemical (PFC)-based preservation optimizes islet recovery and post-transplant graft function without inducing oxidative stress ***(142–147)***.
4. Rescue gradients improve the recovery of trapped islets lost during purification (C. Ricordi, personal communication).
5. Insulin independence has been achieved with islet grafts derived from NHBDs ***(148)***.

6. Sirolimus-based therapy can induce insulin independence following sequential kidney–islet transplants ***(149)***.
7. Anti-inflammatory and calcineurin-inhibitor-free strategies with profound T-cell depletion have been shown to improve islet engraftment ***(97,150)***.

3. In Search of the Elusive Islet

The Collaborative Islet Transplant Registry (CITR), funded by the NIH and administered by the EMMES Corporation of Rockville, Maryland, is collecting comprehensive data from centers in the United States and Canada and will share this information with the ITR ***(151)***.

3.1. Technical Challenges in Clinical Islet Transplantation

Many technical and ethical challenges must be addressed if clinical islet transplantation is to move forward ***(152)***. Cooperation between organ transplant centers, the procurement team, and the isolation laboratory is crucial if all available cadaveric pancreata are to be referred appropriately and expeditiously. Islet yields remain quite variable (typically 25–75% of the potential islet mass). Clinical results vary considerably across centers despite comprehensive efforts to standardize isolation/purification procedures and establish strict quality control criteria in accordance with World Health Organization (WHO) Good Manufacturing Practice (GMP) guidelines ***(153)***. The production of high-quality islets is expensive, labor-intensive, and time-consuming. Because the process has a steep learning curve and has yet to be standardized, the technology would be best served by establishing centralized processing facilities and regional networks dedicated to recruiting potential recipients and procuring and transplanting organs ***(78)***.

Efforts to manufacture high-yield preparations suitable for clinical transplantation have been challenging. Numerous methods have been attempted, including continuous or discontinuous density (isopygnic) gradients, magnetic microspheres coated with islet or cytotoxic antiacinar MAbs, photothermolysis of exocrine tissue by antibody-mediated radiosensitization, exploitation of the osmotic permeability differential between the exocrine and endocrine tissues, fluorescence-activating cell sorting, cryopreservation, antiacinar cytotoxic antibodies, tissue culture, and cell sorting by simple filtration ***(154)***.

Some concern has been raised about the assay used to determine islet viability. The gold standard is the fluorescein diacetate/propidium iodide (FD/PI) membrane integrity technique ***(110,155)***. Preliminary data from our laboratory using Syto-Green and ethidium bromide (SG/EB) suggests that the former method considerably overestimates the extent of islet viability ***(156)***.

Despite efforts to manufacture highly purified and standardized collagenase blends, the heterogeneity of the preparations, the quality and nature of

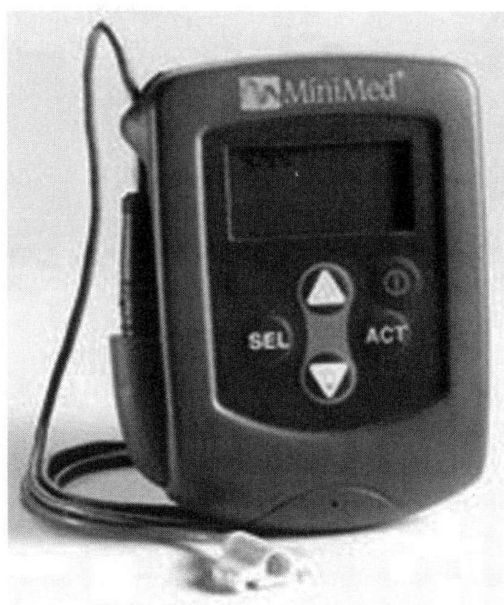

Fig. 6. The Continuous Glucose Monitor System (CGMS) (MiniMed, Sylmar, CA).

donor pancreata, and prolonged cold ischemia times hamper a process that is inherently difficult to control ***(157)***. One solution would be to determine the acinar, ductal, and endocrine elements of the donor pancreas using sophisticated genetic or phenotypic and molecular assays and then prepare an enzyme cocktail incorporating specific recombinant collagenase enzymes for each donor pancreas ***(158,159)***.

Careful patient selection is essential as clinical islet transplantation becomes more widely available. Lability has been difficult to characterize ***(160)***. We have developed a new scoring system, the lability index (LI), as a means to better assist the selection of potential recipients, particularly those with severe metabolic lability, who may have been overlooked by the less reliable mean amplitude glycemic excursion scoring system ***(161)***. The latter, which is based upon seven readings per 24 h for 2 consecutive days, provides an inaccurate analysis of lability. The Continuous Glucose Monitor System (CGMS; MiniMed, Sylmar, CA) has been very effective in monitoring real-time blood glucose trends of highly labile diabetics ***(162)***. This device has helped to document improvements in blood glucose control and predict whether another transplant is required (**Fig. 6**). Metabolic studies have shown that an implant mass of 16,400 IE/kg is necessary to reduce insulin requirements by 1 IU.

3.2. Pancreas Preservation Before Islet Isolation

Although UW solution has proven to be very effective for vascularized pancreas preservation, organs stored in UW solution before islet isolation for even

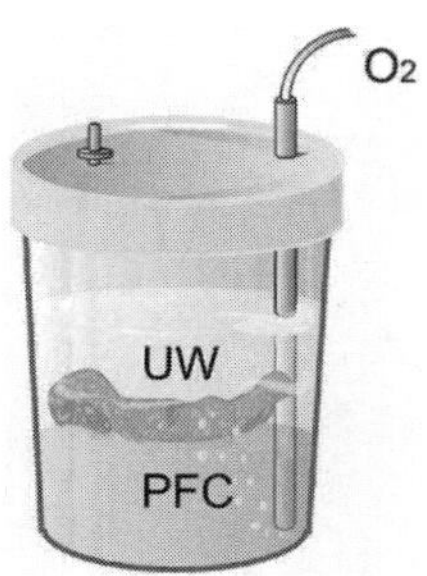

Fig. 7. Two-layer (University of Wisconsin solution/perfluorochemical [UW/PFC]) cold-storage method. The pancreatic graft is on the surface of PFC, covered with UW, and oxygenated during preservation mainly because of direct diffusion of dissolved oxygen in PFC.

short periods has a profoundly negative impact on islet yields and clinical outcomes. In some circumstances it may be more appropriate to defer a cadaveric graft intended for vascularized pancreas transplantation, the rationale being that a pancreas destined for islet transplantation has a more critical CIT (ideally <8 h) than its vascularized counterpart, which can tolerate up to 30 h of cold ischemia ***(163,164)***. We have provided evidence of the detrimental impact of cold ischemia on posttransplant islet function ***(107)***. The ischemic index, which takes into account the CIT for any given islet implant mass, has a positive correlation with insulin secretion.

Refined procurement and preservation techniques would allow better allocation of pancreata among islet-isolation facilities and organ-transplant centers and more efficient use of limited resources. PFC-based preservation (two-layer method [TLM]) supplies oxygen and metabolic substrates to the pancreas during preservation, thereby maintaining cellular integrity and reducing ischemic cell swelling (**Fig. 7**). This method improves metabolic parameters during preservation and optimizes islet recovery (**Fig. 8**) and posttransplant graft function of cold and warm ischemically damaged pancreata without inducing oxidative stress ***(142–147)*** (**Table 2**).

The TLM also improves the viability of vascular endothelium and stabilizes the microcirculation, an effect that can be further augmented by supplementing UW solution with a thromboxane A_2 (TxA_2) synthetase inhibitor such as OKY046 ***(165)***. The immunosuppressive properties of PFCs originally precluded their use as a blood substitute, but animal studies suggest that TLM-preserved pancreata are associated with a reduced incidence of acute rejection when compared to pancreata preserved in UW solution ***(166)***. Thus, the TLM has the potential to maximize the use of donor pancreata that would otherwise be discarded. While the effects of TLM on whole-pancreas transplantation have

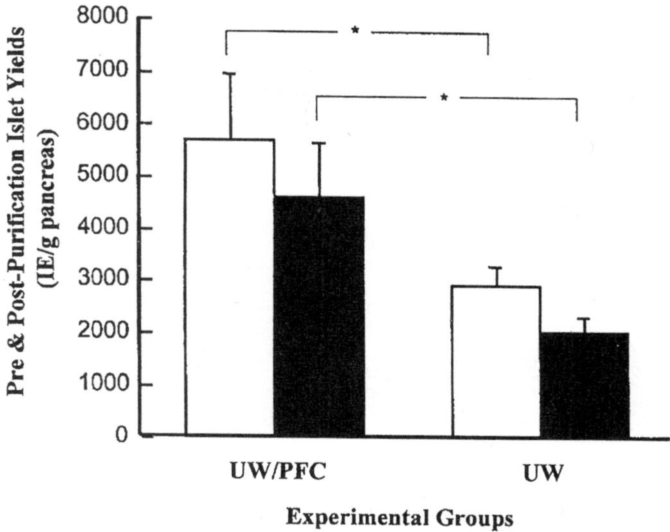

Fig. 8. Prepurification (white) and postpurification (black) islet yields from human pancreases after >10 h of cold storage in UW. Additional preservation by the two-layer method was performed in the UW–PFC group. $*p > 0.05$.

been well documented, little is known about the mechanisms of cold ischemic injury on diminishing islet yield over time. Reliable methods for the detection of ischemically damaged tissue as well as specific markers predictive of successful clinical outcomes are also lacking.

3.3. Strategies to Improve Islet Engraftment

Clinical outcomes are influenced by numerous factors that are known to exist prior to the donor's demise, during procurement and preservation, throughout the isolation and purification process, during culture, and following transplantation ***(66)***. Posttransplant metabolic data suggest that 25–75% of the islets fail to engraft ***(95,96)***. Islets are lost during the early posttransplant phase by a variety of non-immune-related mechanisms, including ischemia, apoptosis, and nonspecific blood-mediated platelet binding and complement activation, a process known as the instant blood-mediated inflammatory reaction (IBMIR) ***(167)***. Ozmen et al. have demonstrated that IBMIR was responsible for both the loss of transplanted islets and portal vein thrombosis ***(168)***. The reaction, which is mediated by exposure to ABO-compatible blood, can be abrogated in an in vitro loop system by blocking the activation of islet-bound tissue factor (TF) with MAbs or inhibiting thrombin activity with Melagatran or its oral prodrug principle, H376/95 (Astra Zeneca, Gothenburg, Sweden).

Table 2
Human Islet Transplantation from Pancreases With Additional Preservation by the Two-Layer Method

Patient	Transplanted islets (IE/kg) of recipient's body weight	Fasting glucose (mmol/L)		C-peptide at 90 min (ng/mL)		Glycosylated hemoglobin (%)		Exogenous isulin use (U/kg/d)	
		Pre-Tx	Post-Tx	Pre-Tx	Post-Tx	Pre-Tx	Post-Tx	Pre-Tx	Post-Tx
1st Tx									
A	7007	17.6	6.4	<0.302	3.80	6.4	5.5	0.67	None
B	6411	8.6	6.2	<0.302	4.59	6.6	5.1	0.57	0.13
C	5086	10.2	5.6	<0.906	2.80	8.9	6.7	0.70	0.53
2nd Tx									
D	5970	8.6	5.8	2.11	3.29	6.5	6.0	0.19	None
E	6310	7.0	5.3	0.87	4.32	6.6	6.0	0.17	None

These studies suggest that inhibition of TF activity before transplantation or clinical protocols incorporating thrombin inhibitors or site-inactivated factor VIIa might prevent IBMIR ***(169)***. Pretreating islets before transplantation with antisensing agents that either block the expression or inhibit the synthesis of TF would also eliminate the adverse effects associated with systemic therapy.

Most centers employ short-term culture (typically 24–48 h) prior to transplantation ***(170)***. It is unknown at this time whether the 10–20% of islets that die during culture would also be lost if they were transplanted immediately following isolation and purification as described in the original Edmonton protocol. Human islets cultured in modified serum-free media (M-SFM) and antioxidant-enriched ITS media have exhibited sustained posttransplant viability and function ***(171)***. Islets cultured in TCM-199 and 95% FCS for 24 h at 37°C, followed by cooling to 24°C for an additional 24 h, has been shown to enhance islet survival in a single-donor–to–single-recipient rat allotransplant model ***(172)***. Because short-term culture eliminates the need for fresh islets, potential recipients are no longer required to live within close proximity of the transplant center. Tissue culture also reduces immunogenicity, improves islet purity, and possibly prevents portal vein thrombosis. Extended islet culture (for days or even months) has the potential to improve clinical outcomes by allowing time to (1) better match the donor to the recipient, (2) precondition the recipient, (3) expand the islet mass in vitro, and (4) manipulate the islets in vitro to improve islet purity, prevent thrombosis, and reduce immunogenicity.

Encouraging strategies in development or early clinical trials include:

1. Therapies with growth factors and other biologics to promote neovascularization and islet growth ***(173,174)***
2. Macrophage sequestration therapy with 15-deoxyspergualin (DSG) to enable the use of unpurified preparations derived from single-donor pancreata ***(175, 176)***
3. Anti-inflammatory treatment directed at neutralizing the effects of pro-inflammatory cytokines, most notably TNF-α, with monoclonal antibodies to improve engraftment of a marginal islet implant mass ***(97)***
4. Low-dose aspirin and other platelet antagonists, low molecular weight heparins, soluble complement receptor-1 antagonists (TP-10) to prevent portal vein thrombosis ***(177)***
5. Antioxidant therapies (nicotinamide with or without verapamil, vitamin D3 analogs, pentoxifylline, lazaroid compounds, and cholesterol-lowering agents) to minimize nonimmunological islet injury ***(178)***
6. Inactivation of major histocompatibility complex (MHC) class II passenger dendritic cells by low-temperature high-oxygen culture, antidentritic cell antibodies, cryopreservation, or ultraviolet irradiation ***(179,180)***

3.4. Single-Donor Islet Transplantation

β-Cell replacement therapy will no doubt replace pancreas transplantation as the definitive treatment for diabetes. The critical shortage of donor pancreata and the inability to recover large numbers of high-quality islets from a single pancreas are major obstacles to the widespread application of clinical islet transplantation. Some clinicians have argued that the ultimate goal should not be insulin independence but rather blood glucose stability ***(181)***. Although this approach would benefit more patients, we strongly believe that most diabetics, particularly those disabled by recurrent episodes of hypoglycemic unawareness and marked metabolic lability, would be reluctant to accept the potential risks of long-term immunosuppressive therapy if they were to have only partial control over their diabetes. While multiple-donor transplants continue to be the norm, single-donor–to–single-recipient transplantation may soon become a reality as better methods of pancreas preservation, improved islet isolation and purification techniques, and innovative strategies designed to promote islet engraftment are developed ***(182)***. Therefore, insulin independence should remain a priority. Autotransplant studies have shown that if ischemic injury and immune reactivity can be circumvented, it is possible to induce and maintain normoglycemia with fewer islets. Several strategies have shown promise in facilitating single-donor islet transplantation limiting non-immune-mediated graft loss and improving islet engraftment, including (1) the taming of endogenous enzyme activity with serine protease inhibitors during the digestion phase, (2) the use of less toxic non-Ficoll gradients, and (3) anti-inflammatory strategies coupled with insulin-sensitizing drugs ***(183,184)***.

3.5. Living-Donor Islet Transplantation

Large animal studies with nonpurified islet grafts suggest that it may be possible to treat multiple recipients from a single pancreas ***(185)***. A review of 111 live-donor segmental pancreas transplants performed at the University of Minnesota initially demonstrated that donors had only a modest increase in procedure-related complications ***(21,22)***. The avoidance of obese donors and high-risk individuals with positive autoantibody serology has largely eliminated this problem ***(41)***. Live donation of a segmental graft specifically for islet transplantation (perhaps by laparoscopic and hand-assisted removal) is an attractive alternative, but the risk of inducing diabetes or creating a pancreatic fistula in an otherwise healthy donor is a major concern ***(186)***.

3.6. Stem Cell Technology, Xenotransplantation, and Gene Therapy

Islet transplantation in its present form would benefit less than 0.5% of type 1 diabetics. It has long been recognized that alternative sources of insulin-producing, glucose-responsive tissue must be found to treat the more than 175 million children and adult diabetics worldwide ***(187)***. "Islet farming" may be one solution. Embryonic stem cells have been transformed into islet-like clusters that reverse diabetes in mice ***(188)***. Human embryonic stem cells have been coaxed to secrete insulin, albeit in low concentrations and without glucose feedback ***(189)***. Human adult stem cells and pancreatic ductal elements have been induced to transdifferentiate into islet-like or insulin-producing cells ***(190)***. Adult stem cells expressing c-kit have induced islet regeneration and reduced hyperglycemia in streptozotocin-induced diabetic mice ***(191)***. A novel proliferating insulin-secreting cell line derived from a neonate with persistent hyperinsulinemic hypoglycemia of infancy (PHHI), also known as nesidioblastosis, has proven to be a useful tool in diabetes-related research. NES2Y β-cells not only lack functional ATP-sensitive K^+ channels, they also exhibit impaired expression of the insulin gene-regulatory protein transcription factor, PDX-1 (or IUF-1). Triple transfection with the genes encoding the two subunits of the K^+ATP channel and PDX-1 appears to restore glucose-responsive insulin secretion in vitro. However, preclinical studies are required to determine if these cells can indeed maintain physiological glucose homeostasis and will not undergo senescence or degenerate into malignant cells over time ***(192)***.

Xenotransplantation has great potential as a means to alleviate the critical shortage of organs, but controversial ethical and epidemiological concerns must be overcome. Pigs are the most favored source of donor tissue because they are in plentiful supply and share a number of physiological and anatomical similarities with humans. Porcine insulin, which differs from human insulin by only one amino acid, was used successfully for decades but has since been replaced with recombinant insulin ***(193)***. The public fear of a porcine endogenous retrovirus (PERV) pandemic has significantly delayed clinical trials. Even though there have been reports that PERV is transcriptionally active and infectious across species in vitro, there is no evidence of viral transmission, clinical infection, or disease in humans with porcine xenografts ***(194)***. Selective breeding, targeted gene deletion (colloquially termed gene knockout), and cloning are possible solutions to this dilemma. Transgenic pigs expressing human complement-regulatory proteins have been developed to overcome hyperacute discordant rejection, but very large doses of cyclophosphamide are required ***(195)***. The role of this phenomenon in xenotransplantation is uncertain because xenograft rejection also occurs in complement-deficient rodent models, suggesting that other mechanisms are also involved ***(196)***. Fetal porcine islet-like cell clusters (ICCs) have reversed diabetes in experimental animals. Although co-transplantation of porcine ICCs and a kidney in human diabetics did not induce insulin independence, porcine C-peptide was detectable in the urine for 200–400 d ***(197)***. Adult porcine islets are very fragile and difficult to isolate, although some researchers have reported some success ***(43,198)***. Korbutt et al. have developed an isolation and culture technique that consistently yields large numbers of functional neonatal porcine islet clusters ***(110)***. Neonatal porcine islets, which have the unique ability to replicate in vitro and in vivo, are more susceptible to hyperacute xenorejection than adult porcine islets. Since the latter expresses very little of the gal α [1,3] gal epitope, microencapsulation of transgenic neonatal pig islet clusters might overcome these barriers ***(199)***. Despite the concerns and problems of xenotransplantation described above, clinical trials using porcine fetal and neonatal ICCs have been undertaken worldwide ***(197,200,201)***.

Conceptually, gene therapy involves treating an organ prior to transplantation by activating or dampening specific genes known to be involved during the early phase of acute graft rejection. The goal is to convince the host immune system to recognize the transplanted organ as self. One major advantage of pretreating the organ before transplantation is the elimination of the recipient's immune response to the viral vector itself when it is administered systemically.

Other promising approaches in β-cell replacement therapy include the generation of a human endocrine pancreatic cell line by transfection with SV40 DNA, induction of islet neogenesis, transformation of hepatocytes to secrete a single-chain insulin analog, expansion of cloned human insulin-producing cell lines, tissue engineering of β-and non-β-cells to secrete insulin, and genetic engineering of intestinal mucosal K-cells to secrete insulin ***(202,203)***. Major challenges thwarting clinical application of these technologies at this time include the inability to both induce physiological glucose-sensing with positive feedback mechanisms and prevent senescence or malignant transformation.

Many technological and biological limitations as well as ethical, political, and regulatory obstacles must be overcome ***(204,205)***. While many of these issues appear to be insurmountable, a large prospective multicenter trial based on a classical randomized control-test paradigm with clearly defined endpoints and rigorous scrutiny of all data would allow these technologies to move closer to clinical reality.

4. Novel Immunosuppressive Strategies in Clinical Islet Transplantation

The ultimate goal of islet transplantation is to reestablish physiological glucose homeostasis with an abundant source of insulin-producing tissue and eliminate the need for immunosuppressive therapy. However, the complexity of the human immune system (and a limited understanding of the mechanisms of autoimmune recurrence in particular), the inability to detect early allograft rejection, and the lack of a preclinical autoimmune model of diabetes are major obstacles ***(64,206)***. Despite overwhelming success in small animal models, the induction of permanent graft function or stable tolerance in large animals, nonhuman primates, and humans have been elusive.

4.1. Graft Accommodation and Minimal Immunosuppression Therapy

Accommodation, or the acceptance of a graft as self, is a well-recognized phenomenon in experimental and clinical organ transplantation. Although the mechanism is not completely understood, it enables the tapering of drug dosages to subtherapeutic levels and, in some cases, the complete withdrawal of all antirejection agents without destabilizing the graft ***(207–211)***. This approach has the potential to significantly reduce the risk of drug-related side effects, lymphoma and other malignancies, graft-vs-host disease (GVHD), and life-threatening nosocomial and opportunistic infections. One of the most effective means of promoting robust tolerance is donor-specific bone marrow transplantation following myeloablation ***(212)***. High-dose whole-body irradiation and powerful chemotherapeutic agents are very effective cytoablative modalities for treating hemopoietic malignancies, but this approach is difficult to justify in islet transplantation. Unlike other transplant recipients whose only hope for survival is a vital organ transplant, the majority of diabetics can be safely managed with insulin ***(7,8)***. However, carefully selected patients with unstable diabetes arguably represent the ideal population to test the efficacy of nonmyeloablative methods and new tolerance protocols as the risk–benefit ratio is clearly in their favor ***(213)***.

Some liver, kidney, and pancreas transplant recipients have been successfully withdrawn from all immunosuppressants for one or more reasons at various times posttransplant ***(207)***. Starzl et al. were able to deliberately wean a small number of patients with liver and kidney grafts off all immunosuppression ***(208)***. This concept of late operational tolerance was further developed in a large study of liver, kidney, pancreas, and intestinal transplants using thymoglobulin induction and tacrolimus monotherapy unless other agents were required to suppress breakthrough rejection ***(209)***. Despite histological evidence of immune activity, about 60% of recipients with surviving grafts after 1 yr were safely weaned to tacrolimus dosing once a week. Tanaka and Kiuchi were also able to successfully withdraw all immunosuppressive agents in more than 60 children who received living-donor liver transplants ***(214)***. Tacrolimus monotherapy was reduced to once a week prior to complete drug withdrawal. Although the mechanism of operational tolerance in these patients has not been defined, it is believed to be a result of the large number of host $CD4^+CD25^+$ regulatory T-cells ***(211)***. It is not known whether this tolerance will remain stable over time. Experimental and clinical studies have shown that there is a risk of accelerated chronic rejection ***(212)***.

4.2. Islet Transplantation in Immunoprivileged Sites

The existence of immunoprivileged sites was recognized very early in the development of organ transplantation when researchers attempted to transplant nonhemopoietic tissues and cells such as thyroid and parathyroid tissue following radical surgery for malignancy and fetal brain tissue or adult adrenal tissue to treat Parkinson's disease *(215)*. The immunoprotective properties of the testis (the most studied site), vitreous humor of the eye, brain, and thymus cannot be explained solely on the basis of a simple physical barrier. Fas-Fas ligand (Fas-FasL) interaction and other antiapoptotic pathways are most likely responsible for this unique feature *(216)*. Islets transplanted in immunoprivileged sites have demonstrated marked prolongation or indefinite survival *(217)*. Islet allografts transplanted into intra-abdominally placed testes, co-transplantation of allogeneic islets and testicular cell aggregates, and co-encapsulation of Sertoli-enriched testicular cell fractions with islet xenografts have afforded some degree of immunological protection *(218,219)*.

4.3. Immunoprotection Through Bioencapsulation

Cell encapsulation technology has enormous clinical potential as a therapeutic modality for the management of a wide range of diseases including diabetes, hemophilia, cancer, and renal failure *(220,221)*. In 1954 Algre et al. demonstrated that cultured cells enveloped by a semi-permeable membrane prevented allograft rejection *(222)*. Ten years later, Chang proposed using artificial microcapsules for the immunoprotection of transplanted cells *(223)*. While bioengineering initially promised to prevent allograft and xenograft rejection by eliminating cell–cell contact and interaction with large molecular weight immuno-globulins, islet graft destruction through toxic cytokine-mediated pathways suggests that complete immunological protection will be a more formidable obstacle if only insulin, nutrients, and metabolic waste products are to diffuse freely across the membrane *(224)*. Several immunoisolation systems have been developed including devices anastomosed to the vascular system as arteriovenous (AV) shunts, diffusion chambers or macrocapsules, and spherical microcapsules *(225)*. Experimental diabetes has been cured in rodents implanted with microencapsulated islets. The intense fibrosis and destruction of the encapsulated tissue induced by contaminants in the alginate carrier or by shed graft antigens has been a frustrating obstacle. Few studies have been able to demonstrate consistent and unequivocal protection against autoimmune recurrence unless combined with immunosuppressants or monoclonal antibodies *(226)*. However, sustained insulin independence has been achieved beyond 9 mo in spontaneously diabetic dogs after intraperitoneal implantation of microencapsulated islet allografts *(227)*. To date, only one patient treated with microencapsulated islets transplanted into the peritoneal space has achieved insulin independence in the absence of immunosuppression ***(228)***. Sun et al. demonstrated the potential of microencapsulated xenografts when cynomologus monkeys with autoimmune diabetes were implanted with adult porcine alginate-encapsulated islets and remained normoglycemic for 803 d without any adjunctive immunosuppression ***(229)***. BALB/c and nonobese diabetic (NOD) mice transplanted with syngeneic and allogeneic islets encapsulated with an inert non-poly-L-lysine-alginate (barium chloride) carrier were rendered normoglycemic beyond 350 d ***(230)***.

4.4. Innovations in Tolerance Induction

T-cell activation and clonal expansion is a complex process that involves engagement of donor antigen with a T-cell receptor (TCR), which consists of the TCR itself and its corresponding CD3 complex, or a non-antigen-specific inductive stimulus (co-stimulator) provided by an antigen-presenting cell (APC) ***(231,232)***. There are two pathways of graft antigen presentation: (1) the direct pathway, where recipient T cells recognize antigens in the context of a major histocompatability complex (MHC) on the surface of donor APCs that are capable of co-stimulatory activity (donor APC dependent), and (2) the indirect pathway, whereby host T cells recognize graft antigen in the form of a peptide in the cleft of the recipient class II molecules, which is then processed and presented by host APCs (host APC dependent). Both pathways are believed to play a role in allograft rejection, although the direct pathway is perhaps the most crucial initially, whereas the indirect pathway is the primary mediator of chronic rejection, particularly in xenograft rejection. The interaction of the TCR complex with the donor antigen activates the first signal (signal 1). Co-stimulation, or signal 2, is provided by the interaction of a myriad of surface molecules and APCs, the most prominent chimeric cell being the dendritic leukocyte ***(233)***. T-cell co-stimulation by molecules on the APC is required for optimal T-cell proliferation (signal 3). Co-stimulation blockade results in functional inactivation (anergy) of the corresponding T cell and triggers apoptosis.

A number of novel immunosuppressive biologics are in preclinical development or early clinical trials ***(234)*** (**Table 3**). The major targets of these agents are (1) cell-surface molecules involved in recipient/donor immune cell interactions (most importantly, the co-stimulatory pathway), (2) signaling pathways involved in T-cell activation, cytokine production, and T-cell proliferation, and (3) trafficking and recruitment of immune cells associated with graft rejection. Some of the most promising agents include (1) campath-1H induction and anti-inflammatory prophylaxis with infliximab ***(97)***, (2) a humanized anti-CD11a MAb (anti-LFA1), (3) a second-generation humanized CTLA4-Ig MAb (LEA29Y) directed against B7.1/B7.2, (4) a humanized CD45 MAb (anti-CD45RB), and (5) a humanized anti-CD52 antibody (anti-CD52).

Table 3
Major Targets of New Agents in Immunosuppression Development

- Interference with cell-surface molecules important in immune cell interactions
- Inhibiting signaling mechanisms
- Inhibiting T-cell proliferation
- Alter trafficking and recruitment of immune cells responsible for rejection

4.5. Intrathymic Induction

The recent discovery by Nomura et al. that the thymus also produces small amounts of insulin has important implications in the pathogenesis and treatment of type 1 diabetes *(235)*. It is believed that the higher levels of thymic pro-insulin expression might promote negative selection (deletion) of autoreactive T lymphocytes. This may explain why NOD mice are protected from primary disease when islets are implanted in the thymus *(236)*. Tolerance is achieved by the deletion of alloreactive cells migrating through the thymus before they encounter donor antigen in the peripheral circulation *(237)*. Intrathymic inoculation of donor antigens such as islets, splenocytes, lymphocytes, and donor-specific MHC peptides has resulted in the long-term survival of rodent islet allografts *(238)*. Intrathymic implantation of bone marrow supplemented with a single dose of ALG has also been shown to induce tolerance in rodents by thymic T-cell-negative selection after donor-specific islet transplantation *(239)*. While small animal studies have confirmed the effectiveness of this approach, clinical application has been limited as a result of age-related thymic atrophy, technical difficulties, and the fact that alternative sites for either positive or negative T-lymphocyte selection have been poorly characterized *(240)*.

4.6. Mixed Hemopoietic Microchimerism

Donor bone marrow infusion following myeloablation has been used to induce high-level microchimerism and tolerance of donor immune cells in recipients with hematological malignancies *(212,241)*. The extent of stable nonresponsiveness depends on the degree of chimeric activity *(242)*. High-dose bone marrow transplantation in the presence of effective immunosuppression significantly reduces human liver rejection rates and enhances graft survival *(243)*. Preliminary trials of bone marrow infusion combined with other solid organ or islet transplants suggest that donor-specific tolerance can be achieved *(244)*. Ricordi et al. demonstrated that donor-specific bone marrow transplantation without myeloablation and temporary immunosuppression resulted in a high level of donor microchimerism and unresponsiveness to islet allografts in rats for more than 6 mo *(245)*.

4.7. Co-Stimulation Blockade

One of the most interesting strategies is co-stimulation blockade with monoclonal antibodies to prevent signal 2 activation at the time of transplantation while leaving signal 1 TCR–antigen engagement unaltered. In 1991 Linsley et al. reported that the fusion protein antigen-4-immunoglobulin (CTA4-Ig) could uncouple second-signal interaction and prevent activation by binding to CD28-B7.1/B7.2 molecules on both cytotoxic T and B cells, respectively ***(246)***. CTLA4-Ig has been shown to prolong allograft and xenograft function in cardiac, renal, small bowel, and lung transplant models in rodents and was more efficacious when combined with donor-specific bone marrow transplantation and/or low-dose immunosuppression ***(229,247)***. CTLA4-Ig administration has enhanced survival of islet allografts and xenografts ***(248,249)***. Co-transplantation of CTLA4-Ig-secreting myoblasts or biolistic delivery of the CTLA4-Ig gene have also been shown to improve islet allograft survival in diabetic mice ***(250)***. Humanized CTLA4-Ig and monkey islet allografts led to suppression of both humoral and cellular immune responses and a prolonged graft-survival rate of 40% ***(251)***. An even more potent CTLA4-Ig, LEA29Y, has been shown in primate islet transplant studies and clinical trials of patients with rheumatoid arthritis and renal transplantation to be safe and effective ***(252,253)***. Murine-skin allograft transplant models treated with either CTLA4-Ig or anti-CD40L alone did not result in long-term engraftment. However, combined co-stimulation blockade with both agents led to dramatic synergistic interaction and long-term survival and function ***(254)***. These inhibitors were also effective in preventing antigen sensitization in murine islet transplantation ***(255)***. This has important implications for clinical islet transplantation, particularly when multiple donors are required to achieve insulin independence. Kirk et al. found that administering anti-CD40L or CTLA4-Ig significantly extended renal graft survival in rhesus monkeys but that co-administration of both agents led to indefinite survival and donor-specific tolerance to secondary skin grafts ***(256)***. We have found that inducible co-stimulator (ICOS) signaling blockade in combination with sirolimus or additional co-stimulatory blockade significantly reduced allospecific T-cell proliferation and effector function and induced operational tolerance of islet allografts ***(257)***.

CD40-CD40L interaction plays a critical role by upregulating T-cell adhesion (B7) molecules and TF expression on the surface of endothelial cells ***(258,259)***. CD40L is expressed on activated $CD4^+$ T cells, stimulated mast cells, basophils, activated platelets, and vascular endothelium of various organs. Blockade of the CD40/CD40 ligand (CD40L) pathway can induce long-term tolerance of renal allografts in monkeys and other nonhuman primates ***(260–261)***. Despite impressive evidence in rodent models and preclinical studies with primates, the phase I trial of a humanized monoclonal antibody directed against

CD40L (anti-CD154) in patients with rheumatoid arthritis was abruptly halted following reports of unexpected thromboembolic complications, including one fatality ***(254)***. Biogen's Hu5C8 MAb has an increased binding capacity for islets, which in turn sets up the scenario for thromboembolism. While thromboembolic complications have been reported previously with other antibodies in humans and monkeys, highly refined humanized preparations have eliminated most of the risk ***(262)***. Kenyon et al. demonstrated that Hu5C8 MAb extended functional islet allograft survival in rhesus monkeys and baboons but also reversed multiple episodes of rejection without any evidence of thromboembolic complications ***(260,261)***. IDEC131 (E6040) (IDEC Pharmaceuticals Corporation, San Diego, CA), which targets a different epitope of Hu5C8, has been used effectively in patients with systemic lupus erythematosus and psoriasis. Anti-CD40 therapy, which targets CD40 directly, has safely extended renal allograft survival in nonhuman primates ***(263)***.

If techniques to induce robust tolerance to alloantigens fail to protect the graft from autoimmune attack, an adjuvant strategy of co-stimulatory blockade or bone marrow conditioning in combination with micro-dose immunosuppression would be a logical approach. Low-dose sirolimus in the absence of glucocorticoids, which are also known to interfere with active tolerance pathways, has a distinct advantage because apoptosis remains unimpaired in activated T cells ***(264)***.

Another effective strategy is the induction of peripheral tolerance with anti-CD3-based diphtheria-conjugated immunotoxin ***(265,266)***. Knechtle et al. reported that renal allografts transplanted into nonhuman primates were able to maintain rejection-free tolerance for more than 4 yr following a 2-wk induction course with diphtheria immunotoxin ***(266)***. The underlying mechanism of this operational tolerance involved the immunotoxin-mediated depletion of circulating and sessile naive and memory T-cell subtypes, while the dual action of DSG blocked the activation of pro-inflammatory cytokines induced by the immunotoxin and promoted indefinite systemic production of T-helper cell (Th2) cytokines.

Calcineurin inhibitors have been the cornerstone of immunosuppression regimens since the introduction of cyclosporine in 1983. However, they have not had a dramatic impact on long-term renal graft outcome as measured by graft half-life ***(267)***. In a side-by-side study of tacrolimus vs cyclosporine, 66% of renal allograft biopsies at 2-yr posttransplant had evidence of chronic transplant nephropathy ***(268)***. Acute rejection and acute nephrotoxicity (especially in cyclosporine-treated patients) at 1 yr posttransplant had a strong correlation with the development of chronic transplant nephropathy. While these agents no doubt provide effective immunosuppression, calcineurin inhibitors also undermine the mechanisms of establishing tolerance. Consequently, there has been much debate about eliminating or reducing the reliance on calcineurin inhibitors. In 1999, Solez et al. reported the first multicenter trial of a calcineurin-inhibitor-sparing regimen in primary renal transplants ***(269)***. Daclizumab, MMF, and steroids were demonstrated to be safe and effective. At 4-mo follow-up, 45% of patients had developed biopsy-proven acute rejection and were treated with corticosteroids and/or a humanized anti-CD3 monoantibody (OKT3-α1-Ala-Ala or OKT3). Patients exhibiting signs of graft failure were treated with calcineurin inhibitors. Even so, 60% of recipients were able to remain off calcineurin inhibitors with excellent renal function, as evidenced by significantly prolonged mean and median times to rejection.

The most promising tolerance protocols use a combination of modalities. Central tolerance through mixed chimerism is based on the intrathymic clonal deletion of alloreactive T cells and the removal of immunoreactive antibodies to the donor graft by implanting donor-specific bone marrow cells in the recipient prior to islet transplantation. This method has been successful with skin allografts in rodents, skin and kidney allografts in pigs, kidney and discordant heart xenografts (pig-to-sheep), and kidney transplants in primates ***(245,270)***. Bone marrow replacement following total body irradiation and anti-CD40L (CD154) antibody therapy induced donor-specific allotolerance in NOD mice without autoimmune recurrence and prolonged islet graft function beyond 100 d ***(271)***. Durham et al. showed that B6 recipients of totally MHC-mismatched BALB/c skin grafts treated with repeated doses of donor bone marrow and anti-CD40L developed durable (>300 d) multilineage hemopoietic chimerism and both indefinite (>300 d) allograft acceptance and donor-specific tolerance to secondary skin grafts without cytoreductive conditioning ***(272)***.

5. Islet Cell Transplantation, Children, and Type 2 Diabetes

Judicious split/mixed or basal/bolus insulin therapies are excellent treatment modalities for the majority of pediatric patients ***(273,274)***. The risks associated with islet transplantation are significantly lower than those associated with pancreas transplantation ***(21,94)***. Because end-organ damage evolves over many years, the trade-off of exchanging frequent blood glucose testing, daily insulin injections, and dietary restrictions for life-long immunosuppression cannot be justified in all children or adolescents at this time ***(275)***. However, deliberately exposing high-risk individuals to the risks of a steroid-free immunosuppression regimen has some merit, especially those experiencing (1) recurrent episodes of unexplained severe hypoglycemia and its life-threatening sequelae, despite optimal medical management ***(7,8)***, (2) the presence of progressive vascular complications (particularly retinopathy and nephropathy), which have the potential of severe disability and premature death in early or mid-adulthood ***(276)***, and (3) concurrent immunosuppressive therapy for a co-morbidity (such as kidney, heart, or liver transplant) that can be safely and effectively treated with a steroid-free regimen ***(277,278)***. Clinical trials are underway in North America and Europe to assess the efficacy of OKT3 in children and adolescents with new-onset type 1 diabetes. We are also assessing the impact of *de novo* islet-alone transplantation in children who are at risk of premature death from severe metabolic lability. In the meantime, insulin therapy will continue to be the method of choice for the majority of type 1 diabetics.

The underlying metabolic defect in type 2 diabetes is the result of insulin resistance from abnormalities in insulin receptor number, function, and postreceptor signaling ***(279)***. β-Cell dysfunction can also coexist in type 2 diabetes and has been demonstrated in small animal models of type 2 diabetes ***(280)***. Chronic liver disease is associated with impaired glucose tolerance and diabetes ***(281)***. Combined islet–liver allografts in patients with cirrhosis and overt type 2 diabetes, which occurs in about 20% of cirrhotic patients, have much greater improvements in insulin requirements, HbA_{1C} levels, and overall metabolic control than one would expect with orthoptic liver transplantation alone ***(282,283)***. Retrospective studies of pancreas transplants performed inadvertently in type 2 diabetics have shown excellent long-term graft function with insulin independence ***(284)***. It is unclear at this time if pancreas transplantation can override the abnormal insulin demand caused by peripheral insulin resistance without β-cell exhaustion, or whether patients with high C-peptide levels inadvertently transplanted represent an atypical subgroup of type 2 diabetics with mutations in the glucokinase gene. Small animal and preliminary clinical studies suggest that 10 times more islets might be required to overcome the effects of peripheral insulin resistance ***(285)***. While islet and pancreas transplantation will continue to dominate the management of type 1 diabetes, prospective randomized trials incorporating metabolic studies would help to define the nature of the disease and whether β-cell replacement therapy has a role in the treatment of type 2 diabetes. Islet transplantation as a treatment option for type 2 diabetes must therefore await the development of other tissue sources.

6. Conclusions

There has been remarkable progress in clinical islet transplantation since the introduction of the Edmonton protocol nearly 5 yr ago. Insulin independence with effective immune prophylaxis can be achieved in more than 83% of recipients at 1 yr posttransplant. Islet transplantation has effectively eliminated glycemic lability and the sequelae of severe hypoglycemia. All of our patients, even those who are not insulin-free, consider the transplant to be worthwhile and beneficial. Emerging worldwide data suggest that positive protective effects on secondary diabetic complications will emerge at 5–10 yr posttransplant. The clinical reality of immunologic tolerance is on the horizon and may very well be first accomplished in the field of islet transplantation. The continuing success of the Edmonton protocol is most encouraging and is only one of many developments in the quest to cure diabetes.

References

1. Gepts, W. (1984) Islet morphology in type I diabetes. *Behring Ins t. Mitt.* **(75)**, 39–41.
2. Atkinson, M. A. and Eisenbarth, G. S.(2001) Type 1 diabetes: new perspectives on disease pathogenesis and treatment. *Lancet* **358(9277)**, 221–229. Erratum in *Lancet* **358(9283)**, 766.
3. Rabinovitch, A. and Suarez-Pinzon, W. L. (2003) Role of cytokines in the pathogenesis of autoimmune diabetes mellitus. *Rev. Endocr. Metab. Disord.* **4(3)**, 291–299.
4. Boyle, J. P., Honeycutt, A. A., Narayan, K. M., et al. (2001) Projection of diabetes burden through 2050: impact of changing demography and disease prevalence in the U.S. *Diabetes Care* **24**, 1936–1940.
5. Tan, M. H. and MacLean, D. R. (1995) Epidemiology of diabetes mellitus in Canada. *Clin. Invest. Med.* **18(4)**, 240–246.
6. Rubin, R. J., Altman, W. M., and Mendelson, D. N. (1994) Health care expenditures for people with diabetes mellitus. *J. Clin. Endocrinol. Metab.* 78(4), 809A–809F.
7. The Diabetes Control and Complications Trial Research Group. (1993) The effect of intensive treatment of diabetes on the development and progression of long-term complications in insulin-dependent diabetes mellitus. *N. Engl. J. Med.* **329 (14)**, 977–986.
8. The Diabetes Control and Complications Trial Research Group. (1997) Hypoglycemia in the Diabetes Control and Complications Trial. The Diabetes Control and Complications Trial Research Group. *Diabetes* **46(2)**, 271–286.
9. Turner, R. C. and Holman, R. R. (1996) The United Kingdom Prospective Diabetes Study. UK Prospective Diabetes Study Group. *Ann. Med.* **28(5)**, 439–444.
10. Chase, H. P., Lockspeiser, T., Peery, B., Shepherd, M., MacKenzie, T., Anderson, J., and Garg, S. K. (2001) The impact of the diabetes control and complications trial and humalog insulin on glycohemoglobin levels and severe hypoglycemia in type 1 diabetes. *Diabetes Care* **24(3)**, 430–434.
11. American Diabetes Association. (2002) Position statement: evidence-based nutrition principles and recommendations for the treatment and prevention of diabetes and related complications. *J. Am. Diet. Assoc.* **102(1)**, 109–118.
12. American Diabetes Association. (2003) Position statement: continuous subcutaneous insulin infusion. *Diabetes Care* **26(Suppl. I)**, S125.
13. Howard, G., O'Leary, D. H., Zaccaro, D., et al. (1996) Insulin sensitivity and atherosclerosis. The Insulin Resistance Atherosclerosis Study (IRAS) Investigators. *Circulation* **93(10)**, 1809–1817.

14. Despres, J. P., Lamarche, B., Mauriege, P., et al. (1996) Hyperinsulinemia as an independent risk factor for ischemic heart disease. *N. Engl. J. Med.* **334(15)**, 952–957.
15. Ryan, E. A. (1998) Pancreas transplants: for whom? *Lancet* **351(9109)**, 1072–1703.
16. Robertson, R. P., Davis, C., Larsen, J., Stratta, R., and Sutherland, D. E. (2003) American Diabetes Association. Pancreas transplantation for patients with type 1 diabetes. *Diabetes Care* **26(Suppl. 1)**, S120.
17. Fioretto, P., Steffes, M. W., Sutherland, D. E., Goetz, F. C., and Mauer, M. (1998) Reversal of lesions of diabetic nephropathy after pancreas transplantation. *N. Engl. J. Med.* **339(2)**, 69–75.
18. Martinenghi, S., Comi, G., Galardi, G., Di Carlo, V., Pozza, G., and Secchi, A. (1997) Amelioration of nerve conduction velocity following simultaneous kidney/pancreas transplantation is due to the glycaemic control provided by the pancreas. *Diabetologia* **40(9)**, 1110–1112.
19. Jukema, J. W., Smets, Y. F., van der Pijl, J. W., et al. (2002) Impact of simultaneous pancreas and kidney transplantation on progression of coronary atherosclerosis in patients with end-stage renal failure due to type 1 diabetes. *Diabetes Care* **25(5)**, 906–911.
20. Kelly, W. D., Lillehi, R. C., Lerkel, F. K., Idezuki, Y., and Goetz, F. C. (1967) Allotransplantation of the pancreas and duodenum along with the kidney in diabetic nephropathy. *Surgery* **61(6)**, 827–837.
21. Sutherland, D. E, Gruessner, R. W., and Gruessner, A. C. (2001) Pancreas transplantation for the treatment of diabetes mellitus. *World J. Surg.* **25**, 487–496.
22. Sutherland, D. E., Gruessner, R. W., Dunn, D. L., et al. (2001) Lessons learned from more than 1,000 pancreas transplants at a single institution. *Ann. Surg.* **233 (4)**, 463–501.
23. Odorico, J. S. and Sollinger H. W. (2002) Technical and immunosuppressive advances in transplantation for insulin-dependent diabetes mellitus. *World J. Surg.* **26(2)**, 94–211.
24. von Mering, J. and Minkowski, O. (1889) Diabetes mellitus after pancreas extirpation. *Archiv. Exp. Path ol. Pharmakol.* **26**, 111.
25. Williams, P. (1894) Notes on diabetes treated with extract and by grafts of sheep's pancreas. *Br. Med. J.* **2**, 1303–1304.
26. Barron, M. (1920) The relation of the islet of Langerhans to diabetes with a special reference to cases of pancreatic lithiasis. *Surg. Gynecol. Obstet.* **31**, 437.
27. Hellerstrôm, C. (1964) A method for the microdissection of intact pancreatic islets of mammals. *Acta Endocrinol.* **45**, 122–132.
28. Younoszai, R., Sorensen, R., and Lindall, A. (1970) Homotransplantation of isolated pancreatic islets. *Diabetes* **19(Suppl. 1)**, 406.
29. Banting, F. G., Best, C. H., Collip, J. B., Campbell, W. R., and Fletcher, A. A. (1922) Pancreatic extracts in the treatment of diabetes mellitus: preliminary report. *Can. Med. Assoc. J.* **12**, 141.
30. Burrow, G. N., Hazlett, B. E., and Phillips, M. J. (1982) A case of diabetes mellitus. *N. Engl. J. Med.* **306**, 340–343.

31. *Nobel Lectures, Physiology or Medicine 1922–1941*, (1965) Elsevier Publishing Company, Amsterdam.
32. Marble, A. (1965) Relation of control of diabetes to vascular sequelae. *Med. Clin. North Am.* **49**, 1137–1145.
33. Starzl, T. E. (1990) The development of clinical renal transplantation. *Am. J. Kidney Dis.* **16(6)**, 548–556.
34. Lacy, P. and Kostianovsky, M. (1967) Method for the isolation of intact islets of Langerhans from the rat pancreas. *Diabetes* **16**, 35–39.
35. Moskalewski, S. (1965) Isolation and culture of the islets of Langerhans of the guinea pig. *Gen. Comp. Endocrinol.* **5**, 342–353.
36. Kemp, C. B., Knight, M. J., Scharp, D. W., Ballinger, W. F., and Lacy, P. E. (1973) Effect of transplantation site on the results of pancreatic islet isografts in diabetic rats. *Diabetologia* **9(6)**, 486–491.
37. White, S. A., James, R. F., Swift, S. M., Kimber, R. M., and Nicholson, M. L. (2001) Human islet cell transplantation—future prospects. *Diabet. Med.* **18(2)**, 78–103.
38. Najarian, J. S., Sutherland, D. E., Matas, A. J., Steffes, M. W., Simmons, R. L., and Goetz, F. C. (1977) Human islet transplantation: a preliminary report. *Transplant. Proc.* **9(1)**, 233–236.
39. Largiader, F., Kolb, E., Binswanger, U., and Illig, R. (1979) Successful allotransplantation of an island of Langerhans. *Schweiz. Med.Wochenschr.* **109(45)**, 1733–1736.
40. Langerhans, P. (1989) Beiträge zur mikroskopischen Anatomie der Bauchspeicheldruse. Inaur disert. Berlin Lange.
41. Lacy, P. (1994) Pancreatic islet cell transplant. *Mt. Sinai J. Med.* **61(1)**, 23–31.
42. Noel, J., Rabinovitch, A., Olson, L., Kyriakides, G., Miller, J., and Mintz, D. H. (1982) A method for large-scale, high-yield isolation of canine pancreatic islets of Langerhans. *Metabolism* **31(2)**, 184–187.
43. Sutherland, D. E., Steffes, M. W., Bauer, G. E., McManus, D., Noe, B. D., and Najarian, J. S. (1974) Isolation of human and porcine islets of Langerhans and islet transplantation in pigs. *J. Surg. Res.* **16(2)**, 102–111.
44. Tzakis, A. G., Ricordi, C., Alejandro R., Zeng, Y., Fung, J. J., Todo, S., Demetris, A. J., Mintz, D. H., and Starzl, T. E. (1990) Pancreatic islet transplantation after upper abdominal exenteration and liver replacement. *Lancet* **336**, 402–405.
45. Ricordi, C., Tzakis, A. G., Carroll, P. B., Zeng, Y. J., Rilo, H. L., Alejandro, R., Shapiro, A., Fung, J. J., Demetris, A. J., Mintz, D. H., et al. (1992) Human islet isolation and allotransplantation in 22 consecutive cases. *Transplantation* **53 (2)**, 407–414.
46. Oberholzer, J., Triponer, F., Mage, R., Andereggen, E., Buhler, L., Cretin, N., Fournier, B., Goumaz, C., Lou, J., Philippe, J., and Morel, P. (2000) Human islet transplantation: lessons from 13 autologous and 13 allogeneic transplantations. *Transplantation* **69(6)**, 1115–1123.
47. Socci, C., Davalli, A. M., Vignali, A., Bertuzzi, F., Maffi, P., Zammarchi, O., Ci Carlo, V., and Pozza, G. (1992) Evidence of in vivo human islet graft func-

tion despite a weak response to in vitro perfusion. *Transplant. Proc.* **24**, 3056–3057.

48. Warnock, G. L., Kneteman, N. M., Ryan, E. A., Rabinovitch, A., and Rajotte, R. V. (1992) Long-term follow-up after transplantation of insulin-producing pancreatic islets ito patients with wild type I (insulin-dependent) diabetes mellitus. *Diabetologia* **35(1)**, 89–95.
49. Pyzdrowski, K. L., Kendall, D. M., Halter, J. B., Nakhleh, R. E., Sutherland, D. E., and Robertson, R. P. (1992) Preserved insulin secretion and insulin independence in recipients of islet autografts. *N. Engl. J. Med.* **327(4)**, 220–226.
50. Sutherland, D. E., Gruessner, R. W., Gores, P. F., Brayman, K., Wahoff, D., and Gruessner, A. (1995) Pancreas transplantation: an update. *Diabetes Metab. Rev.* **11(4)**, 337–363.
51. Farney, A. C., Hering, B. J., Nelson, L., Tanioka, Y., Gilmore, T., Leone, J., Wahoff, D., Najarian, J., Kendall, D., and Sutherland, D.E. (1998) No late failures of intraportal human islet autografts beyond 2 years. *Transplant. Proc.* **30(2)**, 420.
52. Brendel, M. (2001) International Islet Transplant Registry Newsletter No. 9. Volume 8. Number 1.
53. Oberholzer, J., Mathe, Z., Bucher, P., Triponez, F., Bosco, D., Fournier, B., Majno, P., Philippe, J., and Morel, P. (2003) Islet autotransplantation after left pancreatectomy for non-enucleable insulinoma. *Am. J. Transplant.* **3(10)**, 1302–1307.
54. Robertson, R. P., Lanz, K. J., Sutherland, D. E., and Kendall, D. M. (2001) Prevention of diabetes for up to 13 years by autoislet transplantation after pancreatectomy for chronic pancreatitis. *Diabetes* **50(1)**, 47–50.
55. Ricordi, C. and Rastellini, C. (1995) Automated method for pancreatic islet separation, in (Ricordi, C., ed.) *Methods in Islet Implantation.* RG Landes, Austin, TX, p. 433.
56. Yasunami, Y., Ryu, S., and Kamei, T. (1990) FK506 as the sole immunosuppressive agent for prolongation of islet allograft survival in the rat. *Transplantation* **49(4)**, 682–686.
57. Reece-Smith, H., Muller, G., McShane, P., and Morris, P. J. (1983) Combined liver and pancreatic islet transplantation in the rat. *Transplantation* **36(2)**, 230–231.
58. Fukushima, M., Nakai, Y., Taniguchi, A., Imura, H., Nagata, I., and Tokuyama, K. (1993) Insulin sensitivity, insulin secretion, and glucose effectiveness in anorexia nervosa: a minimal model analysis. *Metabolism* **42(9)**, 1164–1168.
59. Warnock, G. L., Kneteman, N. M., Ryan, E. A., et al. (1989) Continued function of pancreatic islets after transplantation in type I diabetes. *Lancet* **2(8662)**, 570–572.
60. Ricordi, C., Gray, D. W., Hering, B. J., et al. (1990) Islet isolation assessment in man and large animals. *Acta Diabetol. Lat.* **27**, 185–195.
61. Ricordi, C., Tzakis, A., Alejandro, R., et al. (1991) Detection of pancreatic islet tissue following islet allotransplantation in man. *Transplantation* **52**, 1079–1080.

62. Scharp, D. W., Lacy, P. E., Santiago, J. V., McCullough, C. S., Weide, L. G., Boyle, P. J., et al. (1991) Results of our first nine intraportal islet allografts in type 1, insulin-dependent diabetic patients. *Transplantation* **51**, 76–85.
63. Rosenberg, L., Wang, R., Paraskevas, S., and Maysinger, D. (1999) Structural and functional changes resulting from islet isolation lead to islet cell death. *Surgery* **126(2)**, 393–398.
64. Kenyon, N. S., Ranuncoli, A., Masetti, M., Chatzipetrou, M., and Ricordi, C. (1998) Islet transplantation: present and future perspectives. *Diabetes Metab. Rev.* **14(4)**, 303–313.
65. Shapiro, A. M., Hao, E., Lakey, J. R., Finegood, D., Rajotte, R V., and Kneteman, N.M. (1998) Diabetogenic synergism in canine islet autografts from cyclosporine and steroids in combination. *Transplant. Proc.* **30(2)**, 527.
66. Hering, B. and Ricordi, C. (1999) Islet transplantation for patients with type 1 diabetes mellitus: results, research priorities and reasons for optimism. *Graft* **2**, 12–27.
67. Luzi, L., Secchi, A., Facchini, F., et al. (1990) Reduction of insulin resistance by combined kidney-pancreas transplantation in type 1 (insulin-dependent) diabetic patients. *Diabetologia* **33(9)**, 549–556.
68. Drachenberg, C. B., Klassen, D. K., Weir, M. R., et al. (1999) Islet cell damage associated with tacrolimus and cyclosporine: morphological features in pancreas allograft biopsies and clinical correlation. *Transplantation* **68(3)**, 396–402.
69. Patane, G., Piro, S., Rabuazzo, A. M., Anello, M., Vigneri, R., and Purrello, F. (2000) Metformin restores insulin secretion altered by chronic exposure to free fatty acids or high glucose: a direct metformin effect on pancreatic beta-cells. Diabetes **49(5)**, 735–740.
70. Ricordi, C., Scharp, D. W., and Lacy, P. E. (1988) Reversal of diabetes in nude mice after transplantation of fresh and 7-day-cultured (24 degrees C) human pancreatic islets. *Transplantation* **45(5)**, 994–996.
71. Lake, S. P., Bassett, P. D., Larkins, A., et al. (1989) Large-scale purification of human islets utilizing discontinuous albumin gradient on IBM 2991 cell separator. *Diabetes* **38**, 143–145.
72. Carlsson, P. O., Palm, F., Andersson, A., and Liss, P. (2001) Markedly decreased oxygen tension in transplanted rat pancreatic islets irrespective of the implanted site. *Diabetes* **50(3)**, 489–495.
73. Ricordi, C., Lacy, P. E., and Scharp, D. W. (1989) Automated islet isolation from human pancreas. *Diabetes* **38**, 140–142.
74. Lakey, J. R., Warnock, G. L., Shapiro, A. M., et al. (1999) Intraductal collagenase delivery into the human pancreas using syringe loading or controlled perfusion. *Cell Transplant.* **8 (3)**, 285–292.
75. Hering, B. J., Bretzel, R. G., Hopt, U. T., et al. (1994) New protocol toward prevention of early human islet allograft failure. *Transplant. Proc.* **26(2)**, 570–571.
76. Bretzel, R. G., Brandhorst, D, Brandhorst, H., et al. (1999) Improved survival of intraportal pancreatic islet cell allografts in patients with type-1 diabetes mellitus by refined peritransplant management. *J. Mol. Med.* **77(1)**, 140–143.

77. Maffi, P., Bertuzzi, F., Guiducci, D., et al. (2001) Pre- and perioperative management influences the clinical outcome of islet transplantation. *Am. J. Transplant.* **1(Suppl. 1)**, 10.
78. Benhamou, P. Y., Oberholzer, J., Toso, C., et al.; GRAGIL Consortium. (2001) Human islet transplantation network for the treatment of Type I diabetes: first data from the Swiss-French GRAGIL consortium (1999–2000). *Diabetologia* **44(7)**, 859–864.
79. Sutherland, D. E., Sibley, R., Xu, X. Z., et al. (1984) Twin-to-twin pancreas transplantation: reversal and reenactment of the pathogenesis of type I diabetes. *Trans. Assoc. Am. Physicians* **97**, 80–87.
80. Feutren, G. and Mihatch, M. J. (1992) Risk factors for cyclosporine-induced nephropathy in patients with autoimmune diseases. International Kidney Biopsy Registry of Cyclosporine in Autoimmune Diseases. *N. Engl. J. Med.* **326(25)**, 1654–1660.
81. Yakimets, W. J., Lakey, J. R., Yatscoff, R. W., et al. (1993) Prolongation of canine pancreatic islet allograft survival with combined rapamycin and cyclosporine therapy at low doses. Rapamycin efficacy is blood level related. *Transplantation* **56(6)**, 1293–1298.
82. Allison, A. C. (2002) Mechanisms of action of mycophenolate mofetil in preventing chronic rejection. *Transplant. Proc.* **34(7)**, 2863–2866.
83. Trofe, J., Buell, J. F., First, M. R., Hanaway, M. J., Beebe, T. M., and Woodle, E. S. (2002) The role of immunosuppression in lymphoma. *Recent Results Cancer Res.* **159**, 55–66.
84. Fishman, J. A. and Rubin, R. H. (1998) Infection in organ-transplant recipients. *N. Engl. J. Med.* **338(24)**, 1741–1751.
85. Gaber, A. O., First, M. R., Tesi, R. J., et al. (1998) Results of the double-blind, randomized, multicenter, phase III clinical trial of thymoglobulin versus Atgam in the treatment of acute graft rejection episodes after renal transplantation. *Transplantation* **66(1)**, 29–37.
86. Sehgal, S. N., Baker, H., and Vezina, C. (1975) Rapamycin (AY-22,989), a new antifungal antibiotic. II. Fermentation, isolation and characterization. *J. Antibiot.* **28(10)**, 727–732.
87. Shapiro, A. M., Gallant, H., Hao, E., et al. (1998) Portal vein immunosuppressant levels and islet graft toxicity. *Transplant. Proc.* **30(2)**, 641.
88. Yakimets, W. J., Lakey, J. R., Yatscoff, R. W., Ket al. (1993) Prolongation of canine pancreatic islet allograft survival with combined rapamycin and cyclosporine therapy at low doses. Rapamycin efficacy is blood level related. *Transplantation* **56(6)**, 1293–1298.
89. Chen, H., Qi, S., Xu, D., et al. (1998) Combined effect of rapamycin and FK 506 in prolongation of small bowel graft survival in the mouse. *Transplant. Proc.* **30(6)**, 2579–2581.
90. McAlister, V. C., Gao, Z., Peltekian, K., Domingues, J., Mahalati, K., and MacDonald, A. S. (2000) Sirolimus-tacrolimus combination immunosuppression. *Lancet* **355(9201)**, 376–377.

91. Vincenti, F., Kirkman, R., Light, S., et al. (1998) Interleukin-2-receptor blockade with daclizumab to prevent acute rejection in renal transplantation. Daclizumab Triple Therapy Study Group. *N. Engl. J. Med.* **338(3)**, 161–165.
92. Kahan, B. D., Rajagopalan, P. R., and Hall, M. (1999) Reduction of the occurrence of acute cellular rejection among renal allograft recipients treated with basiliximab, a chimeric anti-interleukin-2-receptor monoclonal antibody. United States Simulect Renal Study Group. *Transplantation* **67(2)**, 276–284.
93. Halloran, P. F. (1999) T-cell activation pathways: a transplantation perspective. *Transplant. Proc.* **31(1–2)**, 769–771.
94. Shapiro, A. M., Lakey, J. R., Ryan, E. A., et al. (2000) Islet transplantation in seven patients with type 1 diabetes mellitus using a glucocorticoid-free immunosuppressive regimen. *N. Engl. J. Med.* **343(4)**, 230–238.
95. Ryan, E. A., Lakey, J. R., Rajotte, R. V., et al. (2001) Clinical outcomes and insulin secretion after islet transplantation with the Edmonton protocol. *Diabetes* **50(4)**, 710–719.
96. Ryan, E. A., Lakey, J. R., Paty, B. W., et al. (2002) Successful islet transplantation: continued insulin reserve provides long-term glycemic control. *Diabetes* **51(7)**, 2148–2157.
97. Shapiro, A., et al. (2003) Three-year follow-up in clinical islet-alone transplant with the Edmonton protocol, and preliminary impact of infliximab and Campath-1H. *Am. J. Transplant.* **3(Suppl. 5)**, 296.
98. Luzi, L. (1999) Metabolic strategies to predict and improve intrahepatic islet graft function. *J. Mol. Med.* **77(1)**, 49–56.
99. de Mattos, A. M., Olyaei, A. J., and Bennett, W. M. (2000) Nephrotoxicity of immunosuppressive drugs: long-term consequences and challenges for the future. *Am. J. Kidney Dis.* **35(2)**, 333–346.
100. Cryer, P. E., Fisher, J. N., and Shamoon, H. (1994) Hypoglycemia. *Diabetes Care* **17(7)**, 734–755.
101. Dahlquist, G. (1999) Primary and secondary prevention strategies of pre-type 1 diabetes. Potentials and pitfalls. *Diabetes Care* **22 (Suppl. 2)**, B4–B6.
102. http//:www.organandtissue.ca
103. D'Alessndro, M. D., James, H., Southard, J. H., Love, R. B., and Belzer, F. O. (1994) Organ preservation. *Surg. Clin. North Am.* **74(5)**, 1083–1095.
104. Lakey, J. R., Warnock, G. L., Rajotte, R. V., et al. (1996) Variables in organ donors that affect the recovery of human islets of Langerhans. *Transplantation* **61(7)**, 047–1053.
105. Kalayoglu, M., D'Alessandro, A. M., Knechtle, S.J, et al. (1996) Preliminary experience with split liver transplantation. *J. Am. Coll. Surg.* **182(5)**, 381–387.
106. Kneteman, N. M., Lakey, J. R., Kizilisik, T. A., Ao, Z., Warnock, G. L., and Rajotte, R. V. (1994) Cadaver pancreas recovery technique. Impact on islet recovery and in vitro function. *Transplantation* **58(10)**, 1114–1119.
107. Lakey, J. R., Kneteman, N. M., Rajotte, R. V., Wu, D. C., Bigam, D., and Shapiro, A. M. (2002) Effect of core pancreas temperature during cadaveric procurement on human islet isolation and functional viability. *Transplantation* **73(7)**, 1106–1110.

108. Idezuki, Y., Goetz, F. C., and Lillehei, R.C. (1969) Experimental allotransplantation of the preserved pancreas and duodenum. *Surgery* 485–493.
109. Fraga, D. W., Sabek, O., Hathaway, D. K., and Gaber, A. O. (1998) A comparison of media supplement methods for the extended culture of human islet tissue. *Transplantation* **65(8)**, 1060–1066.
110. Korbutt, G. S., Elliot, J. F., Ao, Z., Smith, D. K., Warnock, G. L., and Rajotte, R. V. (1996) Large scale isolation, growth and function of porcine neonatal islet cells. *J. Clin. Invest.* **97**, 2119–2129.
111. Weimar, B., Rauber, K., Brendel, M. D., Bretzel, R. G., and Rau, W. S. (1999) Percutaneous transhepatic catheterization of the portal vein: a combined CT- and fluoroscopy-guided technique. *Cardiovasc. Intervent. Radiol.* **22(4)**, 342–344.
112. Luca, A., D'Amico, G., La Galla, R., Midiri, M., Morabito, A., and Pagliaro, L. (1999) TIPS for prevention of recurrent bleeding in patients with cirrhosis: meta-analysis of randomized clinical trials. *Radiology* **212(2)**, 411–421.
113. Vincenti, F. (2001) Interleukin-2 receptor monoclonal antibodies in renal transplantation: current use and emerging regimens. *Transplant. Proc.* **33(7–8)**, 3169–3171.
114. Halloran, P. F. (2000) Sirolimus and cyclosporin for renal transplantation. *Lancet* **356(9225)**, 179–180.
115. Shapiro, A. M., Geng Hao, E., Lakey, J. R., Finegood, D. T., Rajotte, R. V., and Kneteman, N. M. (2002) Defining optimal immunosuppression for islet transplantation based on reduced diabetogenicity in canine islet autografts. *Transplantation* **74(11)**, 1522–1528.
116. Darenkov, I. A., Marcarelli, M. A., Basadonna, G. P., et al. (1997) Reduced incidence of Epstein-Barr virus-associated posttransplant lymphoproliferative disorder using preemptive antiviral therapy. *Transplantation* **64(6)**, 848–852.
117. Flynn, J. M. and Byrd, J. C. (2000) Campath-1H monoclonal antibody therapy. *Curr. Opin. Oncol.* **12(6)**, 574–581.
118. Kirk, A. D., Hale, D. A., Mannon, R. B., et al. (2003) Results from a human renal allograft tolerance trial evaluating the humanized CD52-specific monoclonal antibody alemtuzumab (CAMPATH-1H).*Transplantation* **76(1)**, 120–129.
119. Tzakis, A. G., Kato, T., Nishida, S., et al. (2002) Campath-1H in intestinal and multivisceral transplantation: preliminary data. *Transplant. Proc.* **34(3)**, 937.
120. Farney, A. C., Xenos, E., Sutherland, D. E., et al. (1993) Inhibition of pancreatic islet beta cell function by tumor necrosis factor is blocked by a soluble tumor necrosis factor receptor. *Transplant. Proc.* **25**, 865–866.
121. Rafael, E., Ryan, E. A., Paty, B. W., et al. (2003) Changes in liver enzymes after clinical islet transplantation. *Transplantation* **76(9)**, 1280–1284.
122. Casey, J. J., Lakey, J. R., Ryan, E. A., et al. (2002) Portal venous pressure changes after sequential clinical islet transplantation. *Transplantation* **74(7)**, 913–915.
123. Shapiro, A. M., Lakey, J. R., Rajotte, R. V., et al. (1995) Portal vein thrombosis after transplantation of partially purified pancreatic islets in a combined human liver/islet allograft. *Transplantation* **59(7)**, 1060–1063.

124. Sacks, D. B., Bruns, D. E., Goldstein, D. E., Maclaren, N. K., McDonald, J. M., and Parrott, M. (2002) Guidelines and recommendations for laboratory analysis in the diagnosis and management of diabetes mellitus. *Clin. Chem.* **48(3)**, 436–472.
125. Braghi, S., Bonifacio, E., Secchi, A., Di Carlo, V., Pozza, G., and Bosi, E. (2000) Modulation of humoral islet autoimmunity by pancreas allotransplantation influences allograft outcome in patients with type 1 diabetes. *Diabetes* **49(2)**, 218–224.
126. Jaeger, C., Allendorfer, J., Hatziagelaki, E., et al. (1997 Persistent GAD 65 antibodies in longstanding IDDM are not associated with residual beta-cell function, neuropathy or HLA-DR status. *Horm. Metab. Res.* **29(10)**, 510–515.
127. Xavier, L., Cunha, M., Goncalves, C., et al. (2003) Hematological remission and long term hematological control of acute myeloblastic leukemia induced and maintained by granulocyte-colony stimulating factor (G-CSF) therapy. *Leuk. Lymphoma* **44(12)**, 2137–2142.
128. Vasquez, E. M. (2000) Sirolimus: a new agent for prevention of renal allograft rejection. *Am. J. Health Syst. Pharm.* **57(5)**, 437–448.
129. Hirshberg, B., Mog, S., Patterson, N., Leconte, J., and Harlan, D. M. (2002) Histopathological study of intrahepatic islets transplanted in the nonhuman primate model using Edmonton protocol immunosuppression. *J. Clin. Endocrinol. Metab.* **87(12)**,5424–5429.
130. Johnson, J. A., Kotovych, M., Ryan, E. A., and Shapiro, A. M. (2004) Reduced fear of hypoglycemia in successful islet transplantation. *Diabetes Care* **27(2)**, 624–625.
131. Paty, B. W., Ryan, E. A., Shapiro, A. M., Lakey, J. R., and Robertson, R. P. (2002) Intrahepatic islet transplantation in type 1 diabetic patients does not restore hypoglycemic hormonal counterregulation or symptom recognition after insulin independence. *Diabetes* **51(12)**, 3428–3434.
132. Hevener, A. L., Bergman, R. N., and Donovan, C. M. (1997) Novel glucosensor for hypoglycemic detection localized to the portal vein. *Diabetes* **46**, 1521–1525.
133. Gupta, V., Wahoff, D. C., Rooney, D. P., et al. (1997) The defective glucagon response from transplanted intrahepatic pancreatic islets during hypoglycemia is transplantation site-determined. *Diabetes* **46**, 28–33.
134. Hevener, A. L., Bergman, R. N., and Donovan, C. M. (2001) Hypoglycemic detection does not occur in the hepatic artery or liver: findings consistent with a portal vein glucosensor locus. *Diabetes* **50**, 399–403.
135. Kneteman, N. M., Lakey, J. R., Wagner, T., and Finegood, D. (1996) The metabolic impact of rapamycin (sirolimus) in chronic canine islet graft recipients. *Transplantation* **61**, 1206–1212.
136. Davalli, A. M., Maffi, P., Socci, C., et al. (2000) Insights from a successful case of intrahepatic islet transplantation into a type 1 diabetic patient. *J. Clin. Endocrinol. Metab.* **85(10)**, 3847–3852.
137. White, S. A., Koppiker, N. P., Burden, A. C., et al. (1998) Insulin deficiency and increased intact and 32/33 split proinsulin secretion following human islet autotransplantation. *Transplant. Proc.* **30(2)**, 627–628.

138. http://www.immunetolerance.org
139. Hering, B. J., Matsumoto, I., Sawada, T., et al. (2002) Impact of two-layer pancreas preservation on islet isolation and transplantation. *Transplantation* **74(12)**, 1813–1816.
140. Herold, K. C., Burton, J. B., Francois, F., Poumian-Ruiz, E., Glandt, M., and Bluestone, J. A. (2003) Activation of human T cells by FcR nonbinding anti-CD3 mAb, hOKT3gamma1(Ala-Ala). *J. Clin. Invest.* **111(3)**, 409–418.
141. Gaber, A. O., Fraga, D. W., Callicutt, C. S., Gerling, I. C., Sabek, O. M., and Kotb, M. Y. (2001) Improved in vivo pancreatic islet function after prolonged in vitro islet culture. *Transplantation* **72(11)**, 1730–1736.
142. Tsujimura, T., Kuroda, Y., Kin, T., et al. (2002) Human islet transplantation from pancreases with prolonged col ischemia using additional preservation by the two-layer (UW solution/perfluorochemical) sold-storage method. *Transplantation* **74(12)**, 1687–1691.
143. Lakey, J. R., Tsujimura, T., Shapiro, A. M., and Kuroda, Y. (2002) Preservation of the human pancreas before islet isolation using a two-layer (UW solution/ perfluorochemical) cold storage method. *Transplantation* **74(12)**, 1809–1811.
144. Ricordi, C., Fraker, C., Szust, J., et al. (2003) Improved human islet isolation outcome from marginal donors following addition of oxygenated perfluorocarbon to the cold-storage solution. *Transplantation* **75**, 1524–1527.
145. Fraker, C. A., Alejandro, R., and Ricordi, C. (2002) Use of oxygenated perfluorocarbon toward making every pancreas count. *Transplantation* **74**, 1811–1813.
146. Matsumoto, S., Rigley, T. H., Qualley, S. A., Kuroda, Y., Reems, J. A., and Stevens, R. B. (2002) Efficacy of the oxygen-charged static two-layer method for short-term pancreaspreservation and islet isolation from nonhuman primate and human pancreata. *Cell Transplant.* **11**, 769–777.
147. Matsumoto, S. and Kuroda, Y. (2002) Perfluorocarbon for organ preservation before transplantation. *Transplantation* **74**, 1804–1809.
148. Markmann, J. F., Deng, S., Desai, N. M., et al. (2003) The use of non-heart-beating donors for isolated pancreatic islet transplantation. *Transplantation* **75(9)**, 1423–1429.
149. Kaufman, D. B., Baker, M. S., Chen, X., Leventhal, J. R., and Stuart, F. P. (2002) Sequential kidney/islet transplantation using prednisone-free immunosuppression. *Am. J. Transplant.* **2**, 674–677.
150. Hering, B., et al. (2003) Successful single donor islet transplantation in type 1 diabetes. *Am. J. Transplant.* **3**, 296.
151. http://spitfire.emmes.com/study/isl/index.html
152. Ricordi, C., Lakey, J. R., and Hering, B. J. (2001) Challenges toward standardization of islet isolation technology. *Transplant. Proc.* **33(1–2)**, 1709.
153. Lakey, J. R. T, Ricordi, D., Hering, B., et al. (2003) Standardization of human islet isolation for a international multicenter transplant trial. *Am. Transplant. Congress* **3(Suppl. 5)**, 297.

154. Salvalaggio, P. R., Deng, S., Ariyan, C. E., et al. (2002) Islet filtration: a simple and rapid new purification procedure that avoids ficoll and improves islet mass and function. *Transplantation* **74(6)**, 877.
155. Kirlew, T. (1999) Viability estimation of islets using fluorescent stains. Cell Transplant Center, Diabetes Research Institute, University of Miami School of Medicine, Miami, FL, pp. 1–6.
156. Bennett, M. J., McGhee-Wilson, D., Shapiro, A. M. J., and Lakey, R. J. T. Variation in human islet viability based on different membrane integrity stains. *Cell Transplant.*, in press.
157. Wolters, G. H., Vos-Scheperkeuter, G. H., Lin, H. C., and van Schilfgaarde, R. (1995) Different roles of class I and class II *Clostridium histolyticum* collagenase in rat pancreatic islet isolation. *Diabetes* **44(2)**, 227–233.
158. Brandhorst, H., Brandhorst, D., Hesse, F., et al. (2003) Successful human islet isolation utilizing recombinant collagenase. *Diabetes* **52(5)**, 1143–1146.
159. Rose, N. L., Palcic, M. M., Helms, L. M., and Lakey, J. R. (2003) Evaluation of Pefabloc as a serine protease inhibitor during human-islet isolation. *Transplantation* **75(4)**, 462–466.
160. Ryan, E. A., Shandro, T., Green, K., et al. (2004) Assessment of the severity of hypoglycemia and glycemic lability in type 1 diabetic subjects undergoing islet transplantation. *Diabetes* **53(4)**, 955–962.
161. Service, F. J., Molnar, G. D., Rosevear, J. W., Ackerman, E., Gatewood, L. C., and Taylor, W. F. (1970) Mean amplitude of glycemic excursions, a measure of diabetic instability. *Diabetes* **19(9)**, 644–655.
162. Bode, B. W., Sabbah, H., and Davidson, P. C. (2001) What's ahead in glucose monitoring? New techniques hold promise for improved ease and accuracy. *Postgrad. Med.* **109(4)**, 41–44, 47–49.
163. Rabkin, J. M., Olyaei, A. J., Orloff, S. L., et al. (1999) Distant processing of pancreas islets for autotransplantation following total pancreatectomy. *Am. J. Surg.* **177(5)**, 423–427.
164. D'Alessandro, A. M., Southard, J. H., Love, R. B., and Belzer, F. O. (1994) Organ preservation. *Surg. Clin. North. Am.* **74(5)**, 1083–1095.
165. Matsumoto, S., Kuroda, Y., Fujita, H., et al. (1996) Extending the margin of safety of preservation period for resuscitation of ischemically damaged pancreas during preservation using the two-layer (University of Wisconsin solution/perfluorochemical) method at 20 degrees C with thromboxane A2 synthesis inhibitor OKY046. *Transplantation* **62(7)**, 879–883.
166. Kuroda, Y., Morita, A., Fujino, Y., Tanioka, Y., Ku, Y., and Saitoh, Y. (1993) Successful extended preservation of ischemically damaged pancreas by the two-layer (University of Wisconsin solution/perfluorochemical) cold storage method. *Transplantation* **56(5)**, 1087–1090.
167. Stadlbauer, V., Schaffellner, S., Iberer, F., et al. (2003) Occurrence of apoptosis during ischemia in porcine pancreas islet cells. *Int. J. Artif. Organs* **26**, 205–210.
168. Ozmen, L., Ekdahl, K. N., Elgue, G., Larsson, R., Korsgren, O., and Nilsson, B. (2002) Inhibition of thrombin abrogates the instant blood-mediated inflamma-

tory reaction triggered by isolated human islets: possible application of the thrombin inhibitor melagatran in clinical islet transplantation. *Diabetes* **51**, 1779–1784.

169. Gustafsson, D., Nystrom, J., Carlsson, S., et al. (2001) The direct thrombin inhibitor Melagatran and its oral prodrug H 376/95: intestinal absorption properties, biochemical and pharmacodynamic effects. *Thromb. Res.* **101**, 171–181.
170. Warnock, G. L., Dabbs, K. D., Cattral, M. S., and Rajotte, R. V. (1994) Improved survival of in vitro cultured canine islet allografts. *Transplantation* **57**, 17–22.
171. Gysemans, C., Van Etten, E., Overbergh, L., et al. (2002) Treatment of autoimmune diabetes recurrence in non-obese diabetic mice by mouse interferon-beta in combination with an analogue of 1alpha,25-dihydroxyvitamin-D3. *Clin. Exp. Immunol.* **128**, 213–220.
172. Jahr, H., Hussmann, B., Eckhardt, T., and Bretzel, R. G. (2002) Successful single donor islet allotransplantation in the streptozotocin diabetes rat model. *Cell Transplant.* **11**, 513–518.
173. Beattie, G. M., Montgomery, A. M., Lopez, A. D., et al. (2002) A novel approach to increase human islet cell mass while preserving beta-cell function. *Diabetes* **51**, 3435–3439.
174. Brand, S. J., Tagerud, S., Lambert, P., et al. (2002) Pharmacological treatment of chronic diabetes by stimulating pancreatic beta-cell regeneration with systemic co-administration of EGF and gastrin. *Pharmacol. Toxicol.* **91**, 414–420.
175. Gores, P. F., Najarian, J. S., Stephanian, E., Lloveras, J. J., Kelley, S. L., and Sutherland, D. E. (1993) Insulin independence in type I diabetes after transplantation of unpurified islets from single donor with 15-deoxyspergualin. *Lancet* **341**, 19–21.
176. Kaufman, D. B., Gores, P. F., Field, M. J., et al. (1994) Effect of 15-deoxyspergualin on immediate function and long-term survival of transplanted islets in murine recipients of a marginal islet mass. *Diabetes* **43**, 778–783.
177. Brandhorst, D., Brandhorst, H., Zwolinski, A., Nahidi, F., and Bretzel, R. G. (2002) High-dosed nicotinamide decreases early graft failure after pig to nude rat intraportal islet transplantation. *Transplantation* **73**, 74–79.
178. Shapiro, A. M., Hao, E., Rajotte, R. V., and Kneteman, N. M. (1996) Impact of Lazaroid U74006F on ischemia and reperfusion injury of islets after transplantation in the rat. *Transplant. Proc.* **28**, 85–86.
179. Papas, K. K., Colton, C. K., Gounarides, J. S., et al. (2001) NMR spectroscopy in beta cell engineering and islet transplantation. *Ann. NY Acad. Sci.* **944**, 96–119.
180. Burridge, P., Lakey, J., and Rajotte, R. (2002) Cryopreservation of human pancreatic islets. *Graft* **5(5)**, 266–273.
181. Waugh, N. (2000) Could fewer islet cells be transplanted in type 1 diabetes? *Br. Med. J.* **321(7275)**, 1534.
182. Shapiro, J., Ryan, E., Warnock, G. L., et al. (2001) Could fewer islet cells be transplanted in type 1 diabetes? Insulin independence should be dominant force in islet transplantation. *Br. Med. J.* **322(7290)**, 861.

183. Lakey, J. R., Helms, L. M., Kin, T., et al. (2001) Serine-protease inhibition during islet isolation increases islet yield from human pancreases with prolonged ischemia. *Transplantation* **72(4)**, 565–570.
184. Huang, G. C., Zhao, M., Jones, P., et al. (2004) The development of new density gradient media for purifying human islets and islet-quality assessments. *Transplantation* **77(1)**, 143–145.
185. Payne, W. D., Sutherland, D.E, Matas, A. J., Gorecki, P., and Najarian, J. S. (1979) DL-Ethionine treatment of adult pancreatic donors. Amelioration of diabetes in multiple recipients with tissue from a single donor. *Ann. Surg.* **189 (2)**, 248–256.
186. Gruessner, R. W., Kendall, D. M., Drangstveit, M. B., Gruessner, A. C., and Sutherland, D. E. (1997) Simultaneous pancreas-kidney transplantation from live donors. *Ann. Surg.* **226(4)**, 471–480.
187. http://www.who.int/hpr/gs.fs.diabetes.shtml
188. Soria, B., Roche, E., Berna, G., et al. (2000) Insulin-secreting cells derived from embryonic stem cells normalize glycemia in streptozotocin-induced diabetic mice. *Diabetes* **49**, 157–162.
189. Lumelsky, N., Blondel, O., Laeng, P., Velasco, I., Ravin, R., and McKay, R. (2001) Differentiation of embryonic stem cells to insulin-secreting structures similar to pancreatic islets. *Science* **292(5520)**, 1389–1394. Erratum in *Science* **293(5529)**, 428.
190. Ulrich, A. B., Schmied, B. M., Standop, J., Schneider, M. B., and Pour, P. M. (2002) Pancreatic cell lines: a review. *Pancreas* **24(2)**, 111–120.
191. Hess, D., Li, L., Martin, M., et al. (2003) Bone marrow-derived stem cells initiate pancreatic regeneration. *Nat. Biotechnol.* **21**, 763–770.
192. Macfarlane, W. M., O'Brien, R. E., Barnes, P. D., et al. (2000) Sulfonylurea receptor 1 and Kir6.2 expression in the novel human insulin-secreting cell line NES2Y. *Diabetes* **49(6)**, 953–960.
193. Hannon, J. P., Bossone, C. A., and Wade, C. E. (1990) Normal physiological values for conscious pigs used in biomedical research. *Lab. Anim. Sci.* **40(3)**, 293–298.
194. van der Laan, L. J., Lockey, C., Griffeth, B. C., et al. (2000) Infection by porcine endogenous retrovirus after islet xenotransplantation in SCID mice. *Nature* **407 (6800)**, 90–94.
195. Cowan, P. J., Shinkel, T. A., Aminian, A., et al. (1998) High-level co-expression of complement regulators on vascular endothelium in transgenic mice: CD55 and CD59 provide greater protection from human complement-mediated injury than CD59 alone. *Xenotransplantation* **5**, 184–190.
196. Karlsson-Parra, A., Ridderstad A., Wallgren, A. C., Moller E., Ljunggren, H. G., and Korsgren, O. (1996) Xenograft rejection of porcine islet-like cell clusters in normal and natural killer cell-depleted mice. *Transplantation* **61(9)**, 1313–1320.
197. Groth, C. G., Korsgren, O., Tibell, A., et al. (1994) Transplantation of porcine fetal pancreas to diabetic patients. *Lancet* **344**, 1402–1404.

198. O'Neil, J. J., Stegemann, J. P., Nicholson, D. T., Gagnon, K. A., Solomon, B. A., and Mullon, C. J. (2001) The isolation and function of porcine islets from market weight pigs. *Cell Transplant.* **10(3)**, 235–246.
199. Rayat, G. R., Rajotte, R. V., Elliott, J. F., and Korbutt, G. S. (1998) Expression of Gal alpha(1,3)gal on neonatal porcine islet beta-cells and susceptibility to human antibody/complement lysis. *Diabetes* **47(9)**, 1406–1411.
200. Birmingham, K. (2002) Skepticism surrounds diabetes xenograft experiment. *Nat. Med.* **8(10)**, 1047.
201. Valdes, R. (2002) Xenotransplantation trials. *Lancet* **359(9325)**, 2281.
202. Lee, H. C., Kim, S. J., Kim, K. S., Shin, H. C., and Yoon, J. W. (2000) Remission in models of type 1 diabetes by gene therapy using a single-chain insulin analogue. *Nature* **408(6811)**, 483–488.
203. Cheung, A. T., Dayanandan, B., Lewis, J. T., et al. (2000) Glucose-dependent insulin release from genetically engineered K cells. *Science* **290(5498)**, 1959–1962.
204. Orive, G., Hernandez, R. M., Gascon, A. R., Igartua, M., and Pedraz, J. L. (2003) Controversies over stem cell research. *Trends Biotechnol.* **21(3)**, 109–112.
205. Chapman, L. E. (2003) Xenotransplantation: public health risks — patient vs. society in an emerging field. *Curr. Top. Microbiol. Immunol.* **278**, 23–45.
206. Boitard, C., Timsit, J., Larger, E., Sempe, P., and Bach, J. F. (1993) Pathogenesis of IDDM: immune regulation and induction of immune tolerance in the NOD mouse. *Autoimmunity* **15 (Suppl.)**, 12–13.
207. Mazariegos, G. V., Reyes, J., Marino, I., Flynn, B., Fung, J. J., and Starzl, T. E. (1997) Risks and benefits of weaning immunosuppression in liver transplant recipients: long-term follow-up. *Transplant. Proc.* **29**, 1174–1177.
208. Starzl, T. E., Murase, N., Abu-Elmagd, K., et al. (2003) Tolerogenic immunosuppression for organ transplantation. *Lancet* **361**, 1502–1510.
209. Wood, K. J. and Sakaguchi, S. (2003) Regulatory T cells in transplantation tolerance. *Nat. Rev. Immunol.* 3, 199–210.
210. Sakaguchi, S. (2003) Control of immune responses by naturally arising CD4+ regulatory T cells that express toll-like receptors. *J. Exp. Med.* **197**, 397–401.
211. Buhler, L. H., Spitzer, T. R., Sykes, M., et al. (2002) Induction of kidney allograft tolerance after transient lymphohematopoietic chimerism in patients with multiple myeloma and end-stage renal disease. *Transplantation* **74**, 1405–1409.
212. Buhler, L. H., Spitzer, T. R., Sykes, M., et al. (2002) Induction of kidney allograft tolerance after transient lymphohematopoietic chimerism in patients with multiple myeloma and end-stage renal disease. *Transplantation* **74**, 1405–1409.
213. Shapiro, A. M., Nanji, S. A., and Lakey, J. R. (2003) Clinical islet transplant: current and future directions towards tolerance. *Immunol. Rev.* **196**, 219–236.
214. Tanaka, K. and Kiuchi, T. (2002) Living-donor liver transplantation in the new decade: perspective from the twentieth to the twenty-first century. *J. Hepatobiliary Pancreat. Surg.* **9(2)**, 218–222.
215. Madrazo, I., Leon, V., Torres, C., et al. (1988) Transplantation of fetal substantia nigra and adrenal medulla to the caudate nucleus in two patients with Parkinson's disease. *N. Engl. J. Med.* **318(1)**, 51.

216. Takeda, Y., Gotoh, M., Dono, K., et al. Protection of islet allografts transplanted together with Fas ligand expressing testicular allografts. *Diabetologia* 1998 **41**, 315–321.
217. Levy, M. M., Ketchum, R. J., Tomaszewski, J. E., Naji, A., Barker, C. F., and Brayman, K. L. (2002) Intrathymic islet transplantation in the canine: I. Histological and functional evidence of autologous intrathymic islet engraftment and survival in pancreatectomized recipients. *Transplantation* **73(6),** 842–852.
218. Korbutt, G. S., Elliott, J. F., and Rajotte, R. V. (1997) Cotransplantation of allogeneic islets with allogeneic testicular cell aggregates allows long-term graft survival without systemic immunosuppression. *Diabetes* **46**, 317–322.
219. Yang, H. and Wright, J. R., Jr. (1999) Co-encapsulation of Sertoli enriched testicular cell fractions further prolongs fish-to-mouse islet xenograft survival. *Transplantation* **67**, 815–820.
220. Xu, W., Liu, L., and Charles, I. G. (2002) Microencapsulated iNOS-expressing cells cause tumor suppression in mice. *FASEB J.* **16**, 213–215.
221. Prakash, S. and Chang, T. M. S. (1996) Microencapsulated genetically engineered live *E. coli* DH5 cells administered orally to maintain normal plasma urea level in uremic rats. *Nat. Med.* **2**, 883–887.
222. Algre, G. H., Weaver, J. M., and Prehn, R. T. (1954) Growth of cells in vivo in diffusion chambers. I Survival of homografts in immunized mice. *J. Natl. Cancer Inst.* **15**, 493–507.
223. Chang, T. M. S. (1964) Semipermeable microcapsules. *Science* **146**, 524–525.
224. Orive, G., Hernandez, R. M., Gascon, A. R., et al. (2003) Cell encapsulation: promise and progress. *Nat. Med.* **9**, 104–107.
225. Lanza, R. P. and Chick W. L. (1997) Transplantation of pancreatic islets. *Ann. NY Acad. Sci.* **831**, 323–331.
226. Calafiore, R., Basta, G., Luca, G., et al. (2003) Grafts of microencapsulated pancreatic islet cells for the therapy of diabetes mellitus in nonimmunosuppressed animals. *Biotechnol. Appl. Biochem.* [Epub ahead of print.]
227. Soon-Shiong, P., Feldman, E., Nelson, R., et al. (1992) Successful reversal of spontaneous diabetes in dogs by intraperitoneal microencapsulated islets. *Transplantation* **54**, 769–774.
228. Soon-Shiong, P., Heintz, R. E., Merideth, N., et al. (1994) Insulin independence in a type 1 diabetic patient after encapsulated islet transplantation. *Lancet* **343**, 950–951.
229. Sun, W., Wang, Q., Zhang, L., et al. (2003) Blockade of CD40 pathway enhances the induction of immune tolerance by immature dendritic cells genetically modified to express cytotoxic T lymphocyte antigen 4 immunoglobulin. *Transplantation* **76(9)**, 1351–1359.
230. Duvivier-Kali, V. F., Omer, A., Parent, R. J., O'Neil, J. J., and Weir, G. C. (2001) Complete protection of islets against allorejection and autoimmunity by a simple barium-alginate membrane. *Diabetes* **50(8)**, 1698–1705.
231. Delves, P. J. and Roitt I. M. (2000) The immune system. First of two parts. *N. Engl. J. Med.* **343(1)**, 108–117.

232. Delves, P. J. and Roitt I. M. (2000) The immune system. Second of two parts. *N. Engl. J. Med.* **343(2)**, 37–49.
233. Coyle, A. J. and Gutierrez-Ramos, J. C. (2001) The expanding B7 superfamily: increasing complexity in costimulatory signals regulating T cell function. *Nat. Immunol.* **2**, 203–209.
234. Vincenti, F. (2002) What's in the pipeline? New immunosuppressive drugs in transplantation. *Am. J. Transplant.* **2(10)**, 898–903.
235. Nomura, Y., Mullen, Y., and Stein, E. (1993) Syngeneic islets transplanted into the thymus of newborn mice prevent diabetes and reduce insulitis in the NOD mouse. *Transplant. Proc.* **25**, 963–964.
236. Pugliese, A. (2002) Peripheral antigen-expressing cells and autoimmunity. *Endocrinol. Metab. Clin. North Am.* **31(2)**, 411–430, viii.
237. Remuzzi, G., Perico, N., Carpenter, C. B., and Sayegh, M. H. (1995) The thymic way to transplantation tolerance. *J. Am. Soc. Nephrol.* **5(9)**, 1639–1646.
238. Chowdhury, N. C., Saborio, D. V., Garrovillo, M., et al. (1998) Comparative studies of specific acquired systemic tolerance induced by intrathymic inoculation of a single synthetic Wistar-Furth (RT1U) allo-MHC class I (RT1.AU) peptide or WAG (RT1U)-derived class I peptide. *Transplantation* **66**, 1059–1066.
239. Posselt, A. M., Odorico, J. S., Barker, C. F., and Naji, A. (1992) Promotion of pancreatic islet allograft survival by intrathymic transplantation of bone marrow. *Diabetes* **41**, 771–775.
240. Ali, A., Garrovillo, M., Jin, M. X., Hardy, M. A., and Oluwole, S. F. (2000) Major histocompatibility complex class I peptide-pulsed host dendritic cells induce antigen-specific acquired thymic tolerance to islet cells. *Transplantation* **69(2)**, 221–226.
241. Starzl, T. E., Demetris, A. J., Murase, N., Thomson, A. W., Trucco, M., and Ricordi, C. (1998) Transplantation tolerance, microchimerism, and the two-way paradigm. *Theor. Med. Bioeth.* **19(5)**, 441–455.
242. Wekerle, T., Blaha, P., Koporc, Z., Bigenzahn, S., Pusch, M., and Muehlbacher, F. (2003) Mechanisms of tolerance induction through the transplantation of donor hematopoietic stem cells: central versus peripheral tolerance. *Transplantation* **75(9 Suppl.)**, 21S–25S.
243. Ricordi, C., Karatzas, T., Nery J., Webb, M., Selvaggi, G., Fernandez, L., Khan, F. A., Ruiz, P., Schiff, E., Olson, L., Fernandez, H., Bean, J., Esquenazi, V., Miller, J., and Tzakis, A. G. (1997) High-dose donor bone marrow infusions to enhance allograft survival: the effect of timing. *Transplantation* **63(1)**, 7–11.
244. Li, H., Inverardi, L., Molano, R. D., Pileggi, A., and Ricordi, C. (2003) Nonlethal conditioning for the induction of allogeneic chimerism and tolerance to islet allografts. *Transplantation* **75(7)**, 966–970.
245. Ricordi, C., Murase, N., Rastellini, C., Behboo, R., Demetris, A. J., and Starzl, T. E. (1996) Indefinite survival of rat islet allografts following infusion of donor bone marrow without cytoablation. *Cell Transplant.* **5(1)**, 53–55.

246. Linsley, P. S., Wallace, P. M., Johnson, J., et al. (1992) Immunosuppression in vivo by a soluble form of the CTLA-4 T cell activation molecule. *Science* **257**, 792–795.
247. Jordan, S. C., Matsumara Y., Zuo, X. J., Marchevsky, A., Linsley, P., and Matloff, J. (1996) Donor-specific transfusions enhance the immunosuppressive effects of single-dose cyclosporine A and CTLA4-Ig but do not result in long-term graft acceptance in a histoincompatible model of rat lung allograft rejection. *Transplant. Immunol.* **4**, 33–37.
248. Roy-Chaudhury, P., Nickerson, P. W., Manfro, R. C., Zheng, X. X., Steiger, J., Li, Y. S., and Strom, T. B. (1997) CTLA4Ig attenuates accelerated rejection (presensitization) in the mouse islet allograft model. *Transplantation* **64**, 172–175.
249. Lenschow, D. J., Zeng, Y., Thistlethwaite, J. R., et al. (1992) Long-term survival of xenogeneic pancreatic islet grafts induced by CTLA4lg. *Science* **257**, 789–792.
250. Gainer, A. L., Suarez-Pinzon, W. L., Min W. P., et al. (1998) Improved survival of biolistically transfected mouse islet allografts expressing CTLA4-Ig or soluble Fas ligand. *Transplantation* **66**, 194–199.
251. Levisetti, M. G., Padrid, P. A., Szot, G. L., et al. (1997) Immunosuppressive effects of human CTLA4Ig in a non-human primate model of allogeneic pancreatic islet transplantation. *J. Immunol.* **159**, 5187–5191.
252. Adams, A. B., Shirasugi, N., Durham, M. M., et al. (2002) Calcineurin inhibitor-free CD28 blockade-based protocol protects allogeneic islets in nonhuman primates. *Diabetes* **51**, 265–270.
253. Moreland, L. W., Alten, R., Van den Bosch, F., et al. (2002) Costimulatory blockade in patients with rheumatoid arthritis: a pilot, dose-finding, double-blind, placebo-controlled clinical trial evaluating CTLA-4Ig and LEA29Y eighty-five days after the first infusion. *Arthritis Rheum.* **46**, 1470–1479.
254. Larsen, C. P., Elwood, E. T., Alexander, D. Z., et al. (1996) Long-term acceptance of skin and cardiac allografts after blocking CD40 and CD28 pathways. *Nature* **381**, 434–438.
255. Zheng, X. X., Markees, T. G., Hancock, W. W., et al. (1999) CTLA4 Signals are required to optimally induce allograft tolerance with combined donor-specific transfusion and anti-CD154 monoclonal antibody treatment. *J. Immunol.* **162**, 4983–4990.
256. Kirk, A. D., Harlan, D. M., Armstrong, N. N., et al. (1997) CTLA4-Ig and anti-CD40 ligand prevent renal allograft rejection in primates. *Proc. Natl. Acad. Sci. USA* **94**, 8789–8794.
257. Nanji, S. A., Hancock, W. W., Anderson, C. C., Zhu, L. F., Kneteman, N. M., and Shapiro, A. M. (2003) Combination therapy with anti-ICOS and cyclosporine enhances cardiac but not islet allograft survival. *Transplant. Proc.* **35(7)**, 2477–2478.
258. Yang, Y. and Wilson, J. M. (1996) CD40 ligand-dependent T cell activation. requirement of B7-CD28 signaling through CD40. *Science* **273**, 1862–1864.

259. Grewal, I. S., Foellmer, H. G., Grewal, K. D., et al. (1996) Requirement for CD40 ligand in costimulation induction, T cell activation, and experimental allergic encephalomyelitis. *Science* **273**, 1864–1867.
260. Kenyon, N. S., Chatzipetrou, M., Masetti, M., et al. (1999) Long-term survival and function of intrahepatic islet allotrafts in rheses monkeys treated with humanized anti-CD154. *Proc. Natl. Acad. Sci. USA* **96(14)**, 8132–8137.
261. Kenyon, N. S., Fernandez, L. A., Lehmann, R., et al. (1999) along-term survival and function of intrahepatic islet allografts in baboons treated with humanized anti-CD154. *Diabetes* **48(7)**, 1473–1481.
262. Kawai, T., Andrews, D., Colvin, R. B., Sachs, D. H., and Cosimi, A. B. (2000) Thromboembolic complications after treatment with monoclonal antibody against CD40 ligand. *Nat. Med.* **6(2)**, 114.
263. Pearson, T. C., Trambley, J., Odom, K., Aet al. (2002) Anti-CD40 therapy extends renal allograft survival in rhesus macaques. *Transplantation* **74**, 933–940.
264. Li, Y., Li, X. C., Zheng, X. X., Wells, A. D., Turka, L. A., and Strom, T. B. (1999) Blocking both signal 1 and signal 2 of T-cell activation prevents apoptosis of alloreactive T cells and induction of peripheral allograft tolerance. *Nat. Med.* **5**, 1298–1302.
265. Asiedu, C. K., Dong, S. S., Lobashevsky, A., Jenkins, S. M., and Thomas, J. M. (2003) Tolerance induced by anti-CD3 immunotoxin plus 15-deoxyspergualin associates with donor-specific indirect pathway unresponsiveness. *Cell Immunol.* **223(2)**, 103–112.
266. Knechtle, S. J. (2001) Treatment with immunotoxin. *Philos. Trans. R. Soc. Lond. B Biol. Sci.* **356(1409)**, 681–689. Knechtle, S. J., Hamawy, M. M., Hu, H., Fechner, J. H., Jr., Cho, C. S. (2001) Tolerance and near-tolerance strategies in monkeys and their application to human renal transplantation. *Immunol. Rev.* **183**, 205–213.
267. Vincenti, F. (1999) Daclizumab: novel biologic immunoprophylaxis for prevention of acute rejection in renal transplantation. *Transplant. Proc.* **31(6)**, 2206–2207.
268. Spitzer, T. R., Delmonico, F., Tolkoff-Rubin, N., et al. (1999) Combined histocompatibility leukocyte antigen-matched donor bone marrow and renal transplantation for multiple myeloma with end stage renal disease: the induction of allograft tolerance through mixed lymphohematopoietic chimerism. *Transplantation* **68**, 480–484.
269. Solez, K., Vincenti, F., and Filo, R. S. (1998) Histopathologic findings from 2-year protocol biopsies from a U.S. multicenter kidney transplant trial comparing tacrolimus versus cyclosporine: a report of the FK506 Kidney Transplant Study Group. *Transplantation* **66(12)**, 1736–1740.
270. Jin, Y., Zhang, Q., Hao, J., Gao, X., Guo, Y., and Xie, S. (2003) Simultaneous administration of a low-dose mixture of donor bone marrow cells and splenocytes plus adenovirus containing the CTLA4Ig gene result in stable mixed chimerism and long-term survival of cardiac allograft in rats. *Immunology* **110(2)**, 275–286.

271. Seung, E., Iwakoshi, N., Woda, B. A., et al. (2000) Allogeneic hematopoietic chimerism in mice treated with sublethal myeloablation and anti-CD154 antibody: absence of graft-versus-host disease, induction of skin allograft tolerance, and prevention of recurrent autoimmunity in islet-allografted NOD/Lt mice. *Blood* **95**, 2175–2182.
272. Durham, M. M., Bingaman, A. W., Adams, A. B., et al. (2000) Cutting edge: administration of anti-CD40 ligand and donor bone marrow leads to hemopoietic chimerism and donor-specific tolerance without cytoreductive conditioning. *J. Immunol.* **165(1)**, 1–4.
273. Dunger, D. B. (2002) Use of continuous glucose monitoring to investigate nocturnal hypoglycaemia prevalence in relation to insulin regimen and exercise. *Diabetes* **51(Suppl. 2)**, A2.
274. Amin, R., Ross, K., Acerini, C. L., Edge, J. A., Warner, J., and Dunger, D. B. (2003) Hypoglycemia prevalence in prepubertal children with type 1 diabetes on standard insulin regimen: use of continuous glucose monitoring system. *Diabetes Care* **26(3)**, 662–667.
275. Hathout, E., Lakey, J., and Shapiro, J. (2003) Islet transplant: an option for childhood diabetes? *Arch. Dis. Child.* **88(7)**, 591–594.
276. Edge, J. A., Hawkins, M. M., Winter, D. L., and Dunger, D. B. (2001) The risk and outcome of cerebral oedema developing during diabetic ketoacidosis. *Arch. Dis. Child.* **85**, 16–22.
277. Wallot, M. A., Mathot, M., Janssen, M., et al. (2002) Long-term survival and late graft loss in pediatric liver transplant recipients—a 15-year single-center experience. *Liver Transplant.* **8**, 615–622.
278. Gjertson, D. W. and Cecka, J. M. (2001) Determinants of long-term survival of pediatric kidney grafts reported to the United Network for Organ Sharing kidney transplant registry. *Pediatr. Transplant.* **5**, 5–15.
279. Goldstein, B. J. (2003) Insulin resistance: from benign to type 2 diabetes mellitus. *Rev. Cardiovasc. Med.* **4(Suppl. 6)**, S3–S10.
280. Polonsky, K. S. (1995) Lilly Lecture 1994. The beta-cell in diabetes: from molecular genetics to clinical research. *Diabetes* **44(6)**, 705–717.
281. Petrides, A. S. and DeFronzo R. A. (1989) Glucose metabolism in cirrhosis: a review with some perspectives for the future. *Diabetes Metab. Rev.* **5(8)**, 691–709.
282. Ricordi, C., Alejandro, R., Angelico, M. C., et al. (1997) Human islet allografts in patients with type 2 diabetes undergoing liver transplantation. *Transplantation* **63(3)**, 473–475.
283. Angelico, M. C., Alejandro, R., Nery, J., et al. (1999) Transplantation of islets of Langerhans in patients with insulin-requiring diabetes mellitus undergoing orthotopic liver transplantation—the Miami experience. *J. Mol. Med.* **77(1)**, 144–147.
284. Sasaki, T. M., Gray, R. S., Ratner, R. E., et al. (1998) Successful long-term kidney-pancreas transplants in diabetic patients with high C-peptide levels. *Transplantation* **65(11)**, 1510–1512.
285. Ricordi, C., Angelico, M. C., Alejandro, R., et al. (1997) Liver-islet transplantation in type 2 diabetes. *Transplant. Proc.* **29(4),** 2240.

4

Current Status of Lung Transplantation

Allan R. Glanville

Summary

Lung transplantation has come of age with the development of a critical mass of experienced clinicians who are committed to pooling their knowledge to solve the clinical problems that continue to confound the benefits individual patients may enjoy from these life-saving procedures. Adequately powered clinical trials are in progress to assist decision making regarding the role of newer immunosuppressive agents. Therapeutic drug monitoring has become critical to minimizing preventable complications such as renal dysfunction with calcineurin inhibitors. Fibroproliferation inhibitors are used more widely to ameliorate the abnormal healing response to allodependent or alloindependent injury, the latter perhaps related to underrecognized gastroesophageal reflux disease for which fundoplication is now proposed as an effective preventative measure. Cumulative damage to the graft from low-grade rejection is now appreciated as a potential cause of graft loss perhaps via an insidious small vessel vasculitis causing bronchiolar ischemic injury. Clearly, despite some progress, substantive challenges remain.

Key Words: Lung transplantation; broncholitis obliterans; rejection; therapeutic monitoring.

1. Introduction

The last 20 yr have been both exciting and fulfilling for those privileged to be involved in this rapidly changing modality of care. Patients for whom no other therapy offered a realistic chance of ongoing survival and quality of life at last had hope. During these years the science of lung transplantation evolved from an experimental procedure to an investigative procedure to an accepted mainstream therapy for patients with life-threatening pulmonary diseases ***(1–5)***. Similarly, living lobar pulmonary transplantation, first performed in 1993, has now achieved a position as a legitimate therapy, particularly where lung transplantation using a cadaveric donor is not available in a timely fashion ***(6,7)***.

From: *Methods in Molecular Biology, vol. 333: Transplantation Immunology: Methods and Protocols*
Edited by: P. Hornick and M. Rose © Humana Press Inc., Totowa, NJ

International guidelines for the referral of patients for the consideration of listing for lung transplantation have been promulgated, debated, and revised ***(8,9)***. The consensus achieved by the working groups involved with the production of these documents has not only set a benchmark for international collaboration in the field of solid organ transplantation, but also typifies the willingness of the medical community to identify and solve key problem areas in this new field. As a result of this type of collaboration, adequately powered multicenter trials of new immunosuppressive agents are building on earlier single-center studies ***(10)*** to identify superior drug combinations for the prevention of rejection and obliterative bronchiolitis (OB) ***(11)***. Similar trials using rapamycin derivative (RAD; everolimus; Novartis Pharmaceuticals Corporation, East Hanover, NJ) are investigating effective therapies for established bronchiolitis obliterans syndrome (BOS), and a new position paper has been developed to assist in the diagnosis of BOS ***(12,13)***. Experiences gained in lung transplantation have provided new insights into other orphan diseases, such as primary pulmonary hypertension (PPH) ***(14–17)***, α_1-antitrypsin deficiency (AATD) ***(18)***, and pulmonary lymphangioleiomyomatosis ***(19)***. Viable alternatives to lung transplantation have been developed for certain patients, including PPH ***(20)***, postthromboembolic pulmonary hypertension ***(21)***, and, most importantly for emphysema, where the role of lung-volume-reduction surgery is under review ***(22)***. Diagnostic bronchoscopic techniques such as transbronchial lung biopsy ***(23)*** and interventional techniques such as laser therapy ***(24)***, balloon dilatation, and stent placement have undergone major advances as a direct result of the need to examine the allograft for rejection and infection ***(25)*** and to manage the sequelae of bronchial anastomotic strictures ***(26–29)***. These techniques have been transferred to the management of patients with conditions including lung cancer, posttuberculosis stricture, and tracheo-esophageal fistula ***(30)***.

The development of isolated lung transplantation, coupled with the early high perioperative mortality rates reported for heart–lung transplantation (HLT), led to a reduction in the yearly rate of HLT from a plateau of about 220 procedures per annum in 1988–1995 to only 71 procedures in 2002 ***(31)***. For the 2973 patients in the International Society for Heart and Lung Transplantation (ISHLT) Registry database up to 2002, 1-yr survival was 62% and 5-yr survival was 41%. However, while the overall $T_{1/2}$ was only 2.8 yr, the conditional $T_{1/2}$ (i.e., for 1-yr survivors) was 8.3 yr. In contrast, 1-yr survival for HLT at St Vincent's (Sydney, Australia) has been 81% overall and 93% during the last decade ($n = 42$). For experienced units with higher-than-average 1-yr survival, this is still an excellent operation with a substantial number of patients now in the 15- to 20-yr survival group ***(32)***. Predominant indications remain congenital heart disease (CHD) (32%), PPH (24%), cystic fibrosis (CF) (15%), chronic obstructive pulmonary disease (COPD) (6%), AATD (2%), and idiopathic pulmonary fibrosis (IPF) (3%). Retransplantation accounts for 2%. Arguments still exist regarding the equity of performing this triple organ transplant where separation of the donor bloc might service two or even three individuals, but in truth, few surgeons have achieved substantive experience with the nuances of this procedure, and this alone biases toward the performance of separate heart- and lung-only transplants. Moreover, where the heart transplant team is involved with the discussion regarding organ allocation, there are often cardiac patients who seem to have a more pressing need than the potential HLT recipient. As a result, the majority of units now routinely service all indications other than CHD with the lung-only procedures ***(5)***.

For lung-only transplants, an activity plateau of about 1650 procedures per annum was reached during 1996–2002. The numbers of bilateral sequential single lung transplants (BSSLT) have slowly risen during this time to account for just over half of the procedures performed per year. It is of interest that although the 1-yr survival figures for single lung transplant (SLT) ($n = 8581$) and BSSLT ($n = 6686$) are superior to HLT at 73 and 75% with $T_{1/2}$ of 3.9 and 5.3 yr, respectively, the 5-yr figures are equivalent for SLT but superior for BSSLT at 43% and 51%, with conditional $T_{1/2}$ (conditional on 1-yr survival) of 6.2 and 8.3 yr, respectively. St Vincent's has a 90% survival at 1 yr for BSSLT ($n = 275$) and 80% for SLT ($n = 140$), with 5-yr survivals of 65 and 57%, respectively.

Indications for SLT remain COPD (53%), IPF (24%), and AATD (9%). In comparison, CF (31%) comprises the largest group for BSSLT, followed by COPD (23%), AATD (10%), IPF (10%), and PPH (8%). Differences in organ-allocation systems throughout the world are associated with regional differences in mortality rates on the waiting list. The equity of duration of time waiting versus medical urgency as a criterion for priority of transplantation remains questionable. IPF and CF have the highest mortality rates on the waiting list ***(33)***. Late referral compounds this problem, particularly for patients with IPF ***(34)***.

Some 46% of all lung transplant recipients are in the age range of 50–64 yr, with 50% of procedures during 1997–2003 performed in this age group. Similarly, the mean donor age rose from 24 yr in 1989 to 34 yr in 2002. The number of pediatric recipients (<10 yr) has been static at 35 per year during this time, emphasizing the fact that no pediatric program can have the benefits that accrue from the experiences gained in a high-volume transplant unit. Registry data confirm lower survival rates for units performing fewer than nine lung transplants per year ***(35)***. Coupling adult and pediatric units in adjacent facilities may allow sharing of expertise, better outcomes, and increasing rates of pediatric transplants if a cooperative approach is utilized.

2. Long-Term Outcomes

2.1. Survival

The causes of death after lung transplantation vary with the time posttransplant; to provide ease of grouping of like causes it is useful to divide the time after lung transplantation into operative, perioperative (within 30 d of transplant), early (defined as within the first postoperative year), medium term (1–3yr), and late (beyond 3 yr). To add some complexity to this analysis, it is important to acknowledge that causes of death are still evolving, representing the dynamic nature of developments in the field over the last 10 yr. Although some units have reached maturation, many have become defunct. Only a few have taken up the challenge anew. In fact only 44 of 126 centers that have performed HLT are still active compared with 91 of 161 SLT centers and 91 of 148 bilateral lung transplant centers ***(35)***.

Thirty-day mortality, not surprisingly, is predominantly dependent on surgical factors, factors related to donors, organ harvesting, ex vivo preservation, and early high-dose immunosuppression. In order of prevalence, causes of death include nonspecific graft failure (NSGF) (31%), noncytomegalovirus (non-CMV) infection (24%), technical factors (8%), cardiac causes (12%), acute rejection (5%), OB (0.5%), and CMV infection (0.1%). Primary graft failure carried a mortality rate of 63% in one series ***(36)***.

1. Early deaths (31 d to 1 yr) are largely the result of non-CMV infections (39%), and NSGF (18%), followed by OB (6%), cardiac (4%), posttransplant lymphoproliferative disease (PTLD) (3%), CMV (4%), technical (3%), malignancy (2%), and acute rejection (2%).
2. Medium term (1–3 yr), the pendulum has swung toward OB, which accounts for 29% of deaths. Other major causes include non-CMV infections (39%) and NSGF (16%). Minor causes include malignancy (5%), cardiac (3%), PTLD (2%), acute rejection (2%), CMV (2%), and technical (1%).
3. Late deaths (beyond 3 yr) are dominated by OB (32%), non-CMV infection (20%), and NSGF (17%). Malignancy accounts for 7%, with other minor causes including cardiac (4%), PTLD (2%), acute rejection (1%), and CMV (1%).

It is perhaps disappointing that NSGF accounts for so many deaths, as it suggests that an in-depth analysis of etiology has not been made, nor has postmortem information been available. It is likely the effects of ischemia-reperfusion injury account for the majority of cases ***(37)***. Few centers have routinely reported postmortem data, but this final assessment is strongly recommended ***(38)***. One center that has analyzed postmortem data found an especially high rate of pulmonary thromboembolism in ventilated patients ***(39)***. Although acute rejection does not account for a significant proportion of deaths, these data do not include an assessment of the relationship between therapy for rejection and resulting infection. This potential relationship is perhaps even more important in the nexus between OB and infectious death. The major trend, however, is the dominance of OB as the cause of death for long-term survivors, with an increasing frequency of malignancy as a late cause of death. It is important to emphasize that the cause of death is not confirmed by postmortem examination in the majority of these, and therefore the diagnosis of OB as the cause is usually based on the presence of BOS ***(13)***. This can only result in an overestimate of the real incidence of OB as a factor. Significant OB is always associated with a loss of lung function.

Data from 1995 to 2002 identify the major risks for 1-yr survival as retransplantation with an odds ratio (OR) of 2.42, diagnosis of sarcoidosis (OR 2.2), use of intravenous inotropes (OR 2.26), diagnosis of PPH (OR 2.24), transplantation from a ventilator (OR 2.21), donor diagnosis of diabetes mellitus (DM) (OR 1.95), diagnosis of AATD (OR 1.67), recipient diagnosis of malignancy (OR 1.61), diagnosis of IPF (OR 1.60), and CMV mismatch of donor (seropositive) and recipient (seronegative) (OR 1.32).

Both linear and quadratic analysis identify risk factors as increasing age (OR 1.0 at 51) ($p < 0.0001$), reduced center volume (OR 1.0 at 20 transplants/yr) ($p < 0.0001$), and increasing pulmonary vascular resistance (OR 1.0 at 3) ($p < 0.02$), as well as a combination of increasing donor age with increasing ischemic time ($p = 0.03$). Factors not associated with an increased risk of 1-yr survival include recipient factors such as pCO_2, chronic steroid use, transfusions, and recent infection requiring intravenous drug therapy; donor factors such as clinical infection, history of hypertension, and history of cancer; and transplant factors such as procedure type, ABO compatibility, human leukocyte antigen (HLA) mismatch, year of transplant, and height ratio of donor and recipient.

Recipient age (30–50 yr OR 1.0 with 65 yr OR 2.0) and donor age (55 yr OR 1.5) remain important factors for 5-yr survival, as do transplantation from a ventilator (OR 2.24), retransplantation (OR 1.98), donor infection within 2 wk of transplant needing intravenous therapy (OR 1.36), diagnosis of IPF (OR 1.07), and HLA mismatch (OR 1.07/mismatch). Of interest, donor weight of less than 70 kg is protective ($p = 0.02$), as is recipient pulmonary vascular resistance less than 3 wood units ($p = 0.002$).

Factors not associated with increased risk of 5-yr survival include recipient factors such as hospitalized status, chronic steroid use, transfusions, history of malignancy, panel reactive antibody positivity, gender, forced vital capacity (FVC), forced expiratory volume in 1 s (FEV_1), height, and weight, whereas donor factors not associated include gender, clinical infection, history of hypertension, history of cancer, history of diabetes, and height. Transplant factors include procedure type and ABO compatibility.

2.2. Morbidity

2.2.1. Overview

Given the depressing list of potential complications that have been recorded after lung transplantation, it is encouraging that most are infrequent or, at least, well-known and predictable sequelae of immunosuppression for which there are now preventative strategies. Hypertension is the most prevalent serious complication, occurring in 50% of recipients at 1 yr and 86.4% at 5 yr; renal dysfunction occurs in 25.8 and 38.4%, respectively, with 1.9 and 3.4% requiring dialysis. Hyperlipidemia occurs in 16.3 and 45.5% and diabetes mellitus in 20.1 and 29.4%. These four complications are all predominantly related to immunosuppressive therapy with calcineurin inhibitors and corticosteroids superimposed on pretransplant risk factors related to underlying disease states. Recent data suggest that changes in monitoring techniques hold promise in ameliorating renal dysfunction ***(40–42)***, but these techniques have not yet been embraced by the broader lung transplant community, although an international trial is about to commence.

2.2.2. Surgical Complications

Despite recent improvements in perioperative mortality rates, morbidity related to wound dehiscence remains an important cause of prolonged impatient stay. Common causes include wound infection with common bacterial pathogens, particularly multiresistant *Staphylococcus aureus* (MRSA), but even fastidious organisms such as *Mycoplasma hominis* are reported to cause wound breakdown and should be considered where wound swabs show pus cells but no organisms on Gram stain ***(43)***. Culture takes 5–8 d, so plates should not be discarded early in this situation. Preliminary evidence also implicates *Chlamydia pneumoniae* as a potential contributor to early postoperative mortality from airway dehiscence and inflammatory airway disease, but confirmation of diagnosis requires more sophisticated tools such as polymerase chain reaction (PCR) of bronchoalveolar fluid because most laboratories are not able to culture wild strains ***(44)***. Empiric prophylactic antibiotic therapy with macrolides with or without a tetracycline may eradicate this organism if treatment is sufficiently prolonged (>6 wk).

An inevitable consequence of bilateral thoracosternotomy performed for bilateral lung transplantation is cutaneous paresthesia and commonly dysesthesia related to surgical section of cutaneous nerves. Return of sensation is variable, and it is prudent to warn patients of the likely alterations in chest wall and nipple sensation at the time of acquiring informed consent. Postoperative arrhythmias are predominantly atrial in origin and probably no more frequent than with other forms of thoracic surgery ***(45)***. Most patients cope well with the rate disturbance, but the risk of embolic phenomena makes it worth considering prophylaxis and/or early electroconversion. Pharmacological therapy with amiodarone is often effective, but the potential risks of acute and chronic pulmonary toxicity should be kept in mind, particularly if pulmonary infiltrates develop ***(46)***. Fungal anatomical infection may present with exsaguinating hemoptysis due to erosion into a pulmonary artery. Preventative strategies include the use of prophylactic inhaled amphotericin in the perioperative period ***(47)***. Inherent in the risk profile of thoracic surgery is the risk of operative ischemic events, perhaps related to inadvertent hypotension and hypoperfusion secondary to uncontrolled bleeding. Pulmonary vein thrombosis has been reported with an increased frequency in lung transplantation but may be successfully managed by early intervention ***(48,49)***. The use of cardiopulmonary bypass, however, does not necessarily prevent these events and adds a significant risk of cognitive dysfunction, which may persist in the long term ***(50)***. Atrial anastomotic thrombus, which may be detected by transeosophageal echocardiography, adds another potential embolic risk of neurological deficit.

One surgical complication that may respond to medical therapy is the development of significant gastroparesis with secondary gastroesophageal reflux disease (GERD) resulting from either section, traction, or thermal trauma to vagal efferents ***(51)***. Therapy with dietary advice, elevation of the head of the bed, prokinetic agents, acid suppression, and newer anti-reflux therapies such as proton pump inhibitors may ameliorate symptoms. It is often the passage of time, however, that affords resolution of simple traction or thermal injuries. Abdominal weight loss is important in this group to further reduce the risk of aspiration. Silent nocturnal aspiration of gastric contents is now recognized as a potential risk factor for the development of BOS ***(52–54)***. The mechanism may be complex, involving the interaction of a competent immune response to epithelial injury followed by the development of an autonomous propagation of the response to alloepithelial antigens ***(55)***. Surgical attempts at cure using fundoplication should be undertaken before permanent airway damage ensues ***(56–58)***. Phrenic nerve palsy, whether by inadvertent intraoperative section, thermal trauma, or traction may delay weaning from assisted ventilation and pose ongoing problems with breathing while recumbent, particularly at the time of bronchoscopy.

2.2.3. Iatrogenic Complications

Bronchoscopy with transbronchial biopsy (TBBx) carries an appreciable iatrogenic risk for patients undergoing lung transplantation. In services where a policy of allograft surveillance with TBBx is followed, the majority of patients will undergo at least six procedures in the first postoperative year. The total risk for an individual patient, therefore, is the unit risk per procedure multiplied by the number of procedures. Complications of TBBx in lung transplant recipients include pneumothorax (1–3%), pulmonary hemorrhage (10–15%), postprocedure fever (5–7%), need for assisted ventilation (0.1–0.5%), arrhythmia (2%), upper airway obstruction requiring intervention (10%). and cardiorespiratory arrest and death (~0.01%) ***(59)***. The putative benefit rests in the hope that early therapeutic intervention resulting from the diagnostic procedure might prevent development of permanent allograft dysfunction.

Interventional bronchoscopy for the management of airway anastomotic breakdown or stricture by its very nature has a much higher risk profile. Torrential bleeding from granulation tissue, airway rupture, creation of a false passage, misplacement of a stent, migration of a stent, and late stent occlusion from granulation tissue or inspissated secretions are all recognized complications. Nevertheless, excellent individual results can be obtained with long-term good-quality survival, but group results are inferior to those seen in patients who do not need airway intervention ***(28)***.

Other common but potentially risky procedures include insertion of central venous access devices, particularly Swan-Ganz catheters ***(60–62)*** and large-bore indwelling vascular catheters for dialysis, pleural drainage tubes, and urinary catheters. Death from perforation of the jugular vein leading to hemothorax and hypotension, air embolism ***(63)***, undiagnosed tension pneumothorax, lacerations of intercostals arteries, splenic puncture, and direct myocardial transfixion have all been recorded ***(64,65)***.

In addition to morbidity related to immunosuppressive agents, three relatively common idiosyncratic adverse drug reactions seem to have a predilection for transplant patients. Ciprofloxacin-associated Achilles tendon disease is characterized by pain, gait disturbance, swelling, and occasionally rupture and is reported to occur frequently in lung transplant recipients ***(66)***. It does not appear to be a dose-related phenomenon. Nor is it related to postoperative steroid dose, age, or underlying disease process. Aminoglycoside ototoxicity is a potential complication worth considering in addition to renal toxicity and may occur even with inhaled therapy. Risks are even more difficult to assess in the ventilated patient. Formal audiological testing at the time of transplant assessment is particularly useful in patients with CF to identify patients at high risk. Statin-related acute and chronic rhabdomyolysis may be a devastating complication with profound global weakness, myoglobinuria, and renal failure or may present simply with subtle fatiguability ***(67)***. Triazole antifungal agents alter calcineurin metabolism so that catastrophic levels of muscle breakdown may ensue in patients taking statins. Pravastatin is reported to have the lowest rate of this effect at low and intermediate dosages.

2.2.4. Generic Complications of Immunosuppression

Opportunistic infections are perhaps the most frequent cause of morbidity and direct mortality following lung transplantation. Common agents include CMV ***(68,69)***, MRSA, other herpesviruses, including Epstein–Barr virus (EBV), varicella-zoster, and human herpesvirus 8 ***(70)***, typical and atypical mycobacteria ***(71)***, *Pneumocystis carinii*, *Aspergillus fumigatus*, *Nocardia* species, *Burkholderia cepacia* ***(72)***, and *Pseudomonas aeruginosa*. Concerns regarding multiresistant agents such as vancomycin-resistant *Enterococcus* (VRE) affect all who work in this area.

PTLD is found more commonly after lung transplantation than other forms of solid organ transplantation, which may reflect the bulk of lymphoid tissue transplanted with the pulmonary allograft, the tendency for young lung transplant recipients to be EBV-naïve, or simply use of a higher level of immunosuppression after lung transplantation ***(73,74)***. EBV mismatch, where an EBV-naïve recipient receives an EBV-positive graft is reported to carry such a high incidence (30–50%) ***(75)*** of PTLD that serious questions have been raised regarding the utility of transplant for EBV-naïve recipients because PTLD is often fatal. Not all units have found this association, however, or such a high mortality rate ***(76)***. One recent report outlines a strategy to reduce the incidence of PTLD to an acceptable, almost negligible level by avoiding cytolytic therapy using low-level immunosuppression and lifelong antiviral therapy in the high-risk group of EBV-mismatched recipients ***(77)***. The specific role of antiviral therapy is debatable. However, once PTLD is diagnosed, most units advise reduction of the ambient level of immune suppression guided by serial monitoring of EBV viral load kinetics. Indeed, this latter strategy can be used prospectively to determine a threshold for preemptive therapy akin to strategies used for CMV ***(78–81)***. PTLD represents 53% of posttransplant malignancy occurring in the first postoperative year but only 17% by the fifth year posttransplant. Conversely, cutaneous malignancy assumes a more important role as time passes posttransplant. At 1 yr it causes 15% of malignancy, but by 5 yr 56% of cases ***(35)***. In particular, cutaneous squamous cell carcinoma (SCC) in the immunosuppressed lung transplant recipient has a predilection for metastatic spread, thereby causing significant morbidity in this group. While exhortations to practice sun-safe behavior are frequently made to this group, it is more likely that the rate of SCC reflects solar damage that occurred 10–20 yr previously. Regular and frequent dermatological review is nevertheless important to detect early SCC at a stage where interventional management may be efficacious to avoid disfiguring surgery and fatal metastatic spread. The issues of female genital health and especially the risk of genital tract neoplasm related to human papillomavirus infection have received scant attention in the literature to date.

Our recent review records a higher rate of cervical intraepithelial neoplasia (CIN; grades 1–3) after lung transplantation ***(82)***. Frequent surveillance PAP smears are needed to detect early recurrence after therapeutic endeavors. Extensive surgery may be required for vulval intraepithelial neoplasia (VIN). Routine surveillance mammography or indeed self-examination for the early detection of breast carcinoma after lung transplantation has not been proven to have advantageous cost–benefit ratio, but logic dictates that benefits might accrue to individual patients who have higher risk profiles.

Lung cancer may occur in the transplanted lung, but more reports have dealt with the problem of lung cancer in either the explanted lung or the remaining native lung ***(83,84)***. Depending on the underlying disease process, it may be very difficult to detect a small primary neoplasm, and where patients spend a protracted time on the waiting list, it is wise to perform review thoracic computed tomography scans on a 6-mo basis to detect early lesions. The cost efficiency of this strategy is such that only 1 case per 100 lung transplants needs to be detected to provide a favorable cost-utility ratio. There are no prospective data on the potential role or cost-efficiency ratio for the use of positron emission tomography (PET) scans in this group. Careful review of chest radiography performed on the night of the transplant is of course invaluable to detect larger lesions (>1 cm), but chest x-ray is neither sensitive nor specific, and the decision to defer lung transplantation is difficult in this situation. The risk of proceeding needs to be weighed against the likelihood that a particular lesion is malignant and will not be cured by resection.

2.2.5. Multifactorial Complications

Coronary artery disease (CAD) rarely causes death after lung transplantation, but transplant-related CAD after HLT occurs frequently in conjunction with OB, suggesting that both may be forms of chronic allograft rejection. Transplant-related CAD is often difficult to appreciate on standard coronary angiography, which underestimates the severity and extent of pathology due to the diffuse and concentric nature of intimal changes ***(85)***. Intravascular ultrasound is the procedure of choice. Hypertension (HT) is the most frequent complication after lung transplantation. Therapy with calcineurin inhibitors, corticosteroids, renal dysfunction, obesity, and underlying disease states combine to produce an incidence of HT of 50% at 1 yr and 86.4% at 5 yr. HT is often refractory to therapy with conventional agents but may respond to angiotensin-converting enzyme (ACE) receptor antagonists, which fortunately have a lower rate of troublesome cough and angioedema than ACE inhibitors *per se*.

Oral health is not always appreciated as a *sine qua non* of optimum success after lung transplantation, but recent studies demonstrate improvements in quality of life and outcome measures with attention to oral health issues. Severe gingival hyperplasia related to cyclosporine therapy may require conversion to alternative agents.

Libido may be depressed or enhanced after lung transplantation. Alterations in body image, postoperative chest pain, side effects of medications—especially corticosteroids—and changes in the dynamics of longstanding relationships related to shifts in the need for care/caregiving may all impact negatively on the desire to maintain a sexual relationship. Conversely, the freedoms that accrue with the liberation from the shackles of oxygen therapy, improvements in exercise tolerance, and a general feeling of health all conspire in the opposite direction. It may be commented that the desire to procreate often transcends common sense in healthy young transplant recipients. A considered individualized approach is advised as the preferred method for discussing these issues, after which optimum perinatal care is required for both mother and child ***(86)***. Fortunately, outcomes are often more positive than anticipated.

2.2.6. Corticosteroids

Although the ramifications of corticosteroid therapy are legion and well known, it is puzzling that more attempts to individualize therapy based on solid pharmacokinetic data are not made. It is as if the oldest and most frequently prescribed immunosuppressive in the pharmacopeia is somehow blighted by the curse of familiarity, and hence our patients pay a heavy penalty of unwanted and largely preventable side effects. A move towards routine performance of area under the curve (AUC) monitoring for prednisolone therapy may assist in the rational utilization of this most dangerous medication ***(87)***.

Subtle alterations in bone mineral density occur promptly after lung transplantation, and the greatest damage is done during the first 6 mo ***(88,89)***. Steroids combine with calcineurin inhibitors to promote rapid bone loss during this time and preemptive strategies to prevent this trend should be part of routine management ***(90,91)***. The risk of osteoporosis (OP) after lung transplantation should not be underestimated. OP is a mortality risk factor in some series, and the reduction of quality of life and rehabilitation potential associated with pathological fracture resulting from OP is well recognized ***(92)***.

Proximal myopathy related to steroid therapy seriously hinders rehabilitation as well and may be so severe as to prevent independent walking and resumption of activities of daily living. Relative inactivity due to proximal myopathy forms part of a vicious cycle leading to further deconditioning and loss of function ***(93,94)***. In addition to the direct effects of steroid therapy, posttransplant myopathy is a complex end result of pretransplant deconditioning ***(95)***, the preexisting disease state ***(96)***, and cyclosporine effects ***(97, 98)***. The success or failure of lung transplantation as a discipline ultimately depends on the functionality of the survivors, so it behooves all working in the area to act aggressively in the interests of optimum patient care to minimize the incidence of these catastrophic complications. In one sense, lung transplantation is perhaps the key for true pulmonary rehabilitation for selected patients ***(99)***.

Cutaneous fragility remains problematic even on low-dose steroid therapy and is a great source of concern to many older patients. Seemingly minor trauma often results in significant skin tears requiring surgery, with or without skin grafting to repair the defect. The risk of secondary infection further compounds the impact of this all-too-frequent complication. In the younger age group, by comparison, acne is the usual problem, and while it may be controlled by topical therapies, it is the passage of time that more often provides resolution. Again, the distress of what we see as a relatively minor complication cannot be underestimated. Quality of life may be significantly impaired because of alterations in personal image. Acne may therefore require more aggressive systemic therapy in selected patients.

DM occurs *de novo* posttransplant in 15–20% of patients. Patients with CF and patients on tacrolimus are at the highest risk, but onset is often related to augmented immunosuppression, with high-dose corticosteroids given for rejection. In addition to the usual risks of ketoacidosis and therapy-related hypoglycemia, DM may be associated with accelerated microvascular disease and thereby contribute to overall vasculopathy in the transplant recipient. Dietary management is important to help maintain optimal body mass index (BMI) and a balanced nutritional intake ***(100–102)***. Many transplant recipients blame their overeating on their steroid therapy, and for this reason alone, attempts to minimize steroid dosage are justifiable. Hyperlipidemia is, of course, exacerbated by dietary indiscretion, poor diabetic control, and excessive alcohol intake. Calcineurin inhibitors and rapamycin, in particular, all contribute to the difficulty of normalizing lipids after transplant.

Posterior subcapsular cataract formation is the ocular hallmark of steroid therapy after lung transplantation and is so frequent that it is good policy to incorporate a yearly eye examination schedule ***(103)***. Fortunately, lens extraction is now performed as a minor procedure, and thus, the burden of diminished visual activity in this group may be reduced. The accelerated nature of cataract formation in this group mandates expediting ophthalmic surgery to maximize quality of life. Avascular necrosis of the femoral head presents with pain and a limp. Bone scan findings are typical, and treatment of choice is total hip replacement for severe cases. Perhaps 5% of patients are so afflicted, but age and previous treatment are cofactors in assessing relative risk.

Obstructive sleep apnea syndrome (OSAS) is an important but little appreciated cause of morbidity after lung transplantation ***(104)***. Whereas lung transplantation cures OSAS in the immediate postoperative period, a number of subjects develop OSAS rapidly thereafter. Lung transplantation behaves as an accelerated model for development of OSAS. Pulmonary denervation *per se* does not cause sleep disturbance ***(105,106)***. Potential mechanisms include localized fat deposition in and around the upper airway and steroid-induced myopathy of the genioglossus. Weight gain is both a cause and consequence of OSAS in this group. Other sequelae include sleep fragmentation, hypertension, cardiac dysfunction, and a tendency to desaturate during fiberoptic bronchoscopy. The latter may be managed by therapeutic or, indeed, prophylactic insertion of a nasopharyngeal tube ***(107)***.

2.2.7. Calcineurin Inhibitors

The relative roles of the principal calcineurin inhibitors, cyclosporine and tacrolimus, in the generation of HT, hyperlipidemia, DM, and oral health issues have already been discussed. HT, particularly in the younger patient, is implicated in the potentially fatal complication of cerebral neurotoxicity manifest by major motor epilepsy and, on occasion, status epilepticus ***(108)***. Blood pressure control is essential for satisfactory short-term management. Other forms of neurotoxicity include tremor, an exaggerated physiological tremor that may be ameliorated by the use of a small dose of β-blocker, and peripheral neuropathy, which may respond to dose reduction if detected early. Delirium may be seen as an idiosyncratic response in new transplant recipients with initial drug exposure. Hypomagnesemia and hypokalemia are thought to be contributory factors ***(108)***. High-dose steroids alone may cause a similar response.

Hirsutism may seem a small price to pay for adequate immunosuppression, but insofar as it impacts negatively on self-esteem and thereby limits social interaction, it can defeat the aim of lung transplantation to return functional patients to real-world situations ***(109)***. Therefore, a proactive strategy is needed to provide patients so afflicted access to optimal therapies to manage this problem. Nephrotoxicity was and is the major complication that requires ongoing consideration ***(110)***. Some 38.4% of lung transplant recipients have significant renal dysfunction by 5 yr posttransplant ***(35)***. This rate alone calls for an urgent reappraisal of current immunosuppressive strategies. The technology and pharmacological knowledge already exist to allow more sophisticated use of current drugs, and for the sake of renal preservation we must forgo outmoded approaches and embrace a new strategy ***(111)***. Every nephron is important, and the minor inconvenience of performing AUC monitoring or a limited sampling strategy is eminently worth the investment of time and cost if superior outcomes can be achieved.

3. Bronchiolitis Obliterans Syndrome

Other authors will discuss the issues regarding BOS, but it would be remiss in this summary of the status of lung transplantation not to provide some further commentary. It is important when discussing BOS to clearly differentiate it from the diagnosis of OB, which is a pathological description ***(112–114)***. The two conditions are not mutually exclusive, however, and most but not all patients with OB will have BOS and vice versa. A distinct number with BOS will have other diagnoses, such as undetected invasive fungal infection, necrotizing bronchiolitis, chondromalacia, native lung volume hyperinflation syndrome, mycobacterial infection, *Chlamydia* infection, or PTLD. The value of postmortem studies as a teaching tool in this regard should not be discounted. The logical corollaries are (1) that all attempts to achieve a firm tissue diagnosis should reasonably be made within a suitable risk–benefit framework and (2) that empiric augmented immunosuppression carries a mortality risk for a percentage of patients with BOS ***(115)***. One year after lung transplantation the rate of BOS is 9.4%. By 5 yr it rises to 34.4%. These are conservative estimates in that they are based on self-reporting of rates determined from 1- and 5-yr survivors, not all of whom will have had regular lung function testing assessed for this complication. Furthermore, there is a well-recognized trend for units to underreport complications. Does BOS always connote OB? Certainly, the recognition of "reversible" BOS and the recently reported impact of therapy with azithromycin ***(116)*** as well as surgical therapy for GERD ***(52)*** point to an alloindependent mechanism associated with airflow limitation in the absence of bronchiolar obliteration. The paucity of careful postmortem studies correlating physiological with pathological findings limits observations in this area; nevertheless, it is likely significant OB is associated with severe airflow limitation, and once a terminal bronchiole is lost, the effect is permanent no matter the etiology. Hence, recurrent injury leads irrevocably to a cumulative situation of airway loss, which may be conceptualized as the progressive loss of the cross-sectional area of all the terminal bronchioles summed together. Notwithstanding the damage done to the whole respiratory epithelium, as posttransplant allograft epithelial injury is widespread, it is the impact on the terminal bronchioles that is so devastating from a functional perspective. It is these guardians of the acinus that stand as the last barrier in and out of the gas-exchange unit. Indeed, there is no effective collateral ventilation beyond this level that can be accessed breath by breath.

The paradigm of graft injury and defective repair with an exuberant fibroproliferative response has been the basis of much research in this area. Recent careful pathological work from the Cambridge group has identified a reduction in the number and patency of the tiny vessels that comprise the microvasculature surrounding the terminal bronchioles in patients who developed

OB ***(117)***. Perhaps rejection-associated microvasculitis is the root cause of most OB and the resultant ischemic injury the reason that repair is so inefficient. Bronchial vessels strangely have been ignored in the focus of rejection determined by TBBx, largely because the pulmonary vessels are so accessible to biopsy and so visible in the section. Most centers that report according to the ISHLT grading of pulmonary vasculature (A grade) and bronchial mucosa (B grade) will have detected the close correlation of A and B grades, so it is not difficult to assume that the missing link in the equation is the direct allodependent damage of the bronchial microvasculature, which would lead to mucosal loss. Whether epithelial injury occurs independent of microvascular injury is a moot point in true rejection but may explain the ability of alloindependent epithelial injury (such as GERD) to heal effectively. Microvascular ischemia may well be the true limiting factor after all. Ischemia itself likely leads to amplification of the inflammatory response by cytokine release with activation of resident dendritic cells, and upregulation of epithelial HLA expression to augmented airway epithelial damage.

Several studies have linked the finding of acute pulmonary allograft rejection with the subsequent development of BOS, but none has then analyzed the positive predictive value of the diagnosis of BOS for the confirmation of OB postmortem in sufficient numbers to allow meaningful analysis ***(118–122)***. The possibility that treatment of BOS confounds the natural history should not be excluded from any proper discussion in this area. Perhaps a more useful signal for the development of (possibly) BOS or (certainly) OB will be the severity and persistence of lymphocytic bronchiolitis on transbronchial lung biopsy ***(28)***. It seems strange that the focus for so long in this area has been on the parenchyma rather than the airway.

Approaches to the management of BOS have been described in this volume and elsewhere ***(123,124)***. Early-recognition signals ***(125)*** are needed to allow institution of therapies at a stage where maximum preservation of lung function can be achieved. Every terminal bronchiole is important and, once lost to fibrosis, will never be recovered. A suitable metaphor for the effect of OB is to consider the total cross-sectional area of the 30,000 terminal bronchioles summed together as the area of a clock face. As the area of a single terminal bronchiole is lost to fibrosis, just over a second passes. Initially, there is no clinical evidence of disease because the lung has such a great functional reserve. By 6 o'clock the loss of 50% of the cross-sectional area is now appreciable, physiologically and symptomatically. Much irreversible damage has already been done, and it is here that the majority of interventional studies have usually commenced management! It is no wonder that the rate of effectiveness is so small. Proven effective treatments can only be established by properly powered multicenter trials that are not biased to a negative result by the time of entry to the study. We need the best evidence as soon as it can collected to guide management in this area, which is so critical to the long-term viability of individual patients and to lung transplantation *per se*. Similarly, in the scientific domain, research should focus on vascular and epithelial injury patterns ***(126)*** and the fibroproliferative response of the human lung fibroblast ***(127,128)*** with or without epithelial interactions ***(129)***. This information will then allow a rational choice of therapies for individual patients. Ultimately, the goal remains prevention, which hopefully will make early detection and therapy redundant.

4. Future Trends

The future of lung transplantation looks secure as a vigorous and determined global scientific approach is now being taken to identify and solve the major problems that bedevil the chance of an optimum outcome for the individual patient. Positive trends to guide forward planning and development include the development of consensus documents from the international community in the areas of listing of candidates, donor selection and management, primary graft dysfunction, the diagnosis and grading of acute and chronic pulmonary allograft rejection, and the description and grading of pulmonary allograft dysfunction ***(8,13,113,114,130)***. The revised grading of the pulmonary allograft dysfunction document includes a more sensitive descriptor of small airway dysfunction with the aim of identifying BOS at an earlier stage, which may be more amenable to reversal with interventional therapy, or at least to allow stabilization with maximal preservation of pulmonary functional reserve ***(131)***. Publication of the results of trials designed to prevent and manage BOS is awaited with great interest. Whether positive or not, the proper template now exists to examine these questions in a scientifically rigorous manner. The recognition of the precious nature of donor resources has led rightly to the reevaluation of evidence describing acceptable criteria for pulmonary organ utilization ***(130)***. Recommendations from the ISHLT position paper are yet to be tested widely in the crucible of clinical practice, but a patent willingness exists to implement them based on the experiences of a handful of *avant garde* units ***(132,133)***. Knowledge gained from the study of patients with orphan diseases referred for transplantation has led to the development of therapeutic alternatives for pulmonary hypertension and emphysema with further refinements of listing criteria ensuing. It is likely that organ-allocation strategies will continue to reflect the dynamics of the local transplant community, with major differences existing between countries and indeed within some larger countries. It is to be hoped that inequities of organ allocation thus accruing can be solved ultimately by a system that takes cognizance of differing rates of urgency between disease states and rates of decline. Only thus can we, as a global community, hope to minimize the phenomenon of death on the waiting list *(33)*.

5. Summary and Conclusions

1. Alternatives to lung transplantation: The focus on lung failure generated by the transplant community has led to new initiatives and understandings of alternative therapies for specific conditions. Lung transplantation remains the optimal therapy for selected patients.
2. Expanding the donor envelope: Traditional conservative concepts of the optimal donor are being superceded by a reasoned, outcome-based approach, with acceptable results taking into account the opportunity cost of not using a suboptimal donor for a potential recipient.
3. Expanding the recipient envelope: The concept of whom to exclude from transplant has been superceded by the approach of whom to include within an acceptable risk–benefit ratio individualized to a specific patient.
4. Sophisticated drug monitoring: High rates of renal dysfunction mandate the use of more sophisticated techniques such as AUC monitoring and limited sampling strategies targeted to reflect this.
5. Individualized immunosuppressive therapy: The availability of techniques to examine in vitro the response of individual patient's tissues to immunosuppressive agents lends itself to high level information regarding likely response in vivo.
6. Multicenter trials: The template now exists to help answer the important questions. Initial studies are underway.
7. Risk factor management: This remains essential for optimal outcomes.
8. Side effect prophylaxis: The price of freedom is eternal vigilance.
9. OB: the last challenge: As in Arthurian legend, OB is the once and future challenge and its conquest the holy grail of lung transplantation.

Acknowledgment

The author continues to acknowledge with much gratitude the privilege of being involved with the lung transplant community over the last 21 yr and in particular the experiences and lessons learned from exposure to this remarkable patient group.

References

1. Reitz, B. A., Wallwork, J. L., Hunt, S. A., et al. (1982) Heart-lung transplantation: successful therapy for patients with pulmonary vascular disease. *N. Engl. J. Med.* **306**, 557–564.
2. Harringer, W. and Haverich, A. (2002) Heart and heart-lung transplantation: standards and improvements. *World J. Surg.* **26**, 218–225.
3. Spratt, P., Glanville, A. R., MacDonald, P., Farnsworth, A., Bryant, D., Keogh, A., and Chang, V. P. (1990) Heart/lung transplantation in Australia: early results of the St Vincent's program. *Transplant. Proc.* **22**, 2142–2142.

4. Whyte, R. I., Robbins, R. C., Altinger, J., et al. (1999) Heart-lung transplantation for primary pulmonary hypertension. *Ann. Thorac. Surg.* **67**, 937–942.
5. Barlow, C. W., Robbins, R. C., Moon, M. R., Akindipe, O., Theodore, J., and Reitz, B. A. (2000) Heart-lung versus double-lung transplantation for suppurative lung disease. *J. Thorac. Cardiovasc. Surg.* **119**, 466–476.
6. Cohen, R. G. S. (2001) Living donor lung transplantation. *World J. Surg.* **25**, 244–250.
7. Starnes, V. A., Bowdish, M. E., Woo, M. S., et al. (2004) A decade of living lobar lung transplantation: recipient outcomes. *J. Thorac. Cardiovasc. Surg.* **127**, 114–122.
8. Maurer, J. R., Frost, A. E., Estenne, M., Higenbottam, T., and Glanville, A. R. (1998) International guidelines for the selection of lung transplant candidates. The International Society for Heart and Lung Transplantation, the American Thoracic Society, the American Society of Transplant Physicians, the European Respiratory Society. *Transplantation* **66**, 951–956.
9. Glanville, A. R. and Estenne, M. (2003) Indications, patient selection and timing of referral for lung transplantation. *Eur. Respir. J.* **22**, 845–852.
10. Griffith, B., Bando, K., Hardesty, R., et al. (1994) A prospective randomized trial of FK506 versus cyclosporine after human pulmonary transplantation. *Transplantation* **57**, 848–851.
11. Corris, P., Glanville, A., McNeil, K., et al. (2001) One year analysis of an ongoing international radomised study of mycophenolate mofetil (MMF) vs azathioprine (AZA) in lung transplantation. *J. Heart Lung Transplant.* **20**, 208.
12. Estenne, M. and Hertz, M. I. (2002) Bronchiolitis obliterans after human lung transplantation. *Am. J. Respir. Crit. Care Med.* **166**, 440–444.
13. Estenne, M., Maurer, J. R., Boehler, A., et al. (2002) Bronchiolitis obliterans syndrome 2001: an update of the diagnostic criteria. *J. Heart Lung Transplant.* **21**, 297–310.
14. Rubin, L. J. (1997) Primary pulmonary hypertension. *N. Engl. J. Med.* **336**, 111–117.
15. Fouty, B. and Rodman, D. M. (1999) Pulmonary vascular gene transfer: Prospects for successful therapy of pulmonary hypertension. *Am. J. Respir. Cell Mol. Biol.* **21**, 555–557.
16. D'Alonzo, G. E., Barst, R. J., Ayres, S. M., et al. (1991) Survival in patients with primary pulmonary hypertension. Results from a national prospective registry. *Ann. Intern. Med.* **115**, 343–349.
17. Glanville, A. R., Burke, C. M., Theodore, J., and Robin, E. D. (1987) Primary pulmonary hypertension. Length of survival in patients referred for heart-lung transplantation. *Chest* **91**, 675–681.
18. Janus, E. B. J. (1990) Alpha-1-antitrypsin deficiency and emphysema: new horizons in treatment. *Aust. NZ J. Med.* **20**, 755–757.
19. Taylor, J., Ryu, J., Colby, T., and Raffin, T. (1990) Lymphangioleiomatosis. *N. Engl. J. Med.* **323**, 1254–1260.
20. Conte, J. V., Gaine, S. P., Orens, J. B., Harris, T., and Rubin, L. J. (1998) The influence of continuous intravenous prostcyclin therapy for primary pulmonary

hypertension on the timing and outcome of transplantation. *J. Heart Lung Transplant.* **17**, 679–685.

21. Archibald, C. J., Auger, W. R., Fedullo, P. F., et al. (1999) Long-term outcome after pulmonary thromboendarterectomy. *Am. J. Respir. Crit. Care Med.* **160**, 523–528.
22. Meyers, B. F. and Patterson, G. A. (2001) Lung transplantation versus lung volume reduction as surgical therapy for emphysema. *World J. Surg.* **255**, 238–243.
23. Higenbottam, T., Stewart, S., Penketh, A., and Wallwork, J. (1988) Transbronchial lung biopsy for the diagnosis of rejection in heart-lung transplant patients. *Transplantation* **46**, 532–539.
24. Hertz, M. I., Harmon, K. R., Knighton, D. R., et al. (1991) Combined laser phototherapy and growth factor treatment of bronchial obstruction after lung transplantation. *Chest* **100**, 1717–1719.
25. Sibley, R. K., Berry, G. J., Tazelaar, H. D., et al. (1993) The role of transbronchial biopsies in the management of lung transplant recipients. *J. Heart Lung Transplant.* **12**, 308–324.
26. Chhajed, P. N. M., Malouf, M., Tamm, M., Spratt, P., and Glanville, A. R. (2001) Interventional bronchoscopy for the management of airway complications following lung transplantation. *Chest* **120**, 1894–1899.
27. Chhajed, P. N. M., Tamm, M., and Glanville, A. R. (2001) Early experience with nitinol (ultraflex) stents for the management of benign airway lesions. *Am. J. Respir. Crit. Care Med.* **163**, A700.
28. Aboyoun, C. L., Tamm, M., M. Chhajed, P. N., et al. (2001) Diagnostic value of follow-up transbronchial lung biopsy after lung rejection. *Am. J. Respir. Crit. Care Med.* **164**, 460–463.
29. Schafers, H- J., Haydock, D. A., and Cooper, J. D. (1991) The prevalence and management of bronchial anamostic complications in lung transplantation. *J. Thorac. Cardiovasc. Surg.* **101**, 1044–1052.
30. Chhajed, P. N., Malouf, M., and Glanville, A. R. (2001) Bronchoscopic dilation in the management of benign (non-transplant) tracheobronchial stenosis. *Intern. Med. J.* **31**, 512–516.
31. Trulock, E. P., Edwards, L. B., Taylor, D. O., et al. (2004) The Registry of the International Society for Heart and Lung Transplantation: twenty-first official adult heart transplant report—2004. *J. Heart Lung Transplant.* **23**, 804–815.
32. Stoica, S. C., McNeil, K. D., Perreas, K., et al. (2001) Heart-lung transplantation for Eisenmenger syndrome: early and long-term results. *Ann. Thorac. Surg.* **72**, 1887–1891.
33. De Meester, J., Smits, J. M., Persijn, G. G., and Haverich, A. (2001) Listing for lung transplantation: life expectancy and transplant effect, stratified by type of end-stage lung disease, the Eurotransplant experience. *J. Heart Lung Transplant.* **20**, 518–524.
34. Lok, S. (1999) Interstitial lung disease clinics for the management of idiopathic pulmonary fibrosis: a potential advantage to patients. *J. Heart Lung Transplant.* **18**, 884–890.

35. Hosenpud, J. D., Bennet, L. E., Keck, B. M., Boucek, M. M., and Novick, R. J. (2001) The registry of the International Society for Heart and Lung Transplantation: eighteenth official report—2001. *J. Heart Lung Transplant.* **20**, 805–815.
36. Christie, J. D., Sager, J. S., Kimmel, S. E., et al. (2005) Impact of primary graft failure on outcomes following lung transplantation. *Chest* **127**, 161–165.
37. de Perrot, M., Liu, M., Waddell, T. K., and Keshavjee, S. (2003) Ischemia-reperfusion-induced lung injury. *Am. J. Respir. Crit. Care Med.* **167**, 490–511.
38. Husain, A. N., Siddiqui, M. T., Reddy, V. B., Yeldandi, V., Montoya, A., and Garrity, E. R. (1996) Post-mortem findings in lung transplant recipients. *Mod. Pathol.* **9**, 752–761.
39. Burns, K. E. and Iacono, A. T. (2004) Pulmonary embolism on post-mortem examination: an under-recognized complication in lung-transplant recipients? *Transplantation* **77**, 692–628.
40. Henry, M. (1999) Cyclosporine and tacrolimus (FK506): a comparison of efficacy and safety profiles. *Clin. Transplant.* **13**, 209–220.
41. Glanville, A. R., Morton, J. M., Aboyoun, C. L., Plit, M. L., and Malouf, M. A. (2004) Cyclosporine C2 monitoring improves renal dysfunction after lung transplantation. *J. Heart Lung Transplant.* **23**, 1170–1174.
42. Modry, D. L., Oyer, P. E., Jamieson, S. W., et al. (1985) Cyclosporine in heart and heart-lung transplantation. *Can. J. Surg.* **28**, 274–280, 282.
43. Hopkins, P. M., Winlaw, D. S., Chhajed, P. N., et al. (2002) *Mycoplasma hominis* infection in heart and lung transplantation. *J. Heart Lung Transplant.* **21**, 1225–1229.
44. Glanville, A. G., Gencay, M., Tamm, M., et al. (2005) *Chlamydia pneumoniae* infection after lung transplantation. *J. Heart Lung Transplant.* **24**, 131–136.
45. Hoffman, T. M., Rhodes, L. A., Wieand, T. S., Spray, T. L., and Bridges, N. D. (2001) Arrhythmias after pediatric lung transplantation. *Pediatr. Transplant.* **5**, 349–352.
46. Ashrafian, H. and Davey, P. (2001) Is amiodarone an underrecognized cause of acute respiratory failure in the ICU? *Chest* **120**, 275–282.
47. Reichenspurner, H., Gamberg, P., Nitschke, M., et al. (1997) Significant reduction in the number of fungal infections after lung-, heart-lung, and heart transplantation using aerosolized amphotericin B prophylaxis. *Transplant. Proc.* **29**, 627–628.
48. Nagahiro, I., Horton, M., Wilson, M., Bennetts, J., Spratt, P., and Glanville, A. R. (2003) Pulmonary vein thrombosis treated successfully by thrombectomy after bilateral sequential lung transplantation: report of a case. *Surg. Today* **33**, 282–284.
49. Leibowitz, D. W., Smith, C. R., Michler, R. E., et al. (1994) Incidence of pulmonary vein complications after lung transplantation: a prospective transesophageal echocardiographic study. *J. Am. Coll. Cardiol.* **24**, 671–675.
50. van Dijk, D., Keizer, A. M., Diephuis, J. C., Durand, C., Vos, L. J., and Hijman, R. (2000) Neurocognitive dysfunction after coronary artery bypass surgery: a systematic review [see comments]. *J. Thorac. Cardiovasc. Surg.* **120**, 632–639.

51. Reid, K. R., McKenzie, F. N., Menkis, A. H., et al. (1990) Importance of chronic aspiration in recipients of heart-lung transplants. *Lancet* **336**, 206–208.
52. Hadjiliadis, D., Duane Davis, R., Steele, M. P., et al. (2003) Gastroesophageal reflux disease in lung transplant recipients. *Clin. Transplant.* **17**, 363–368.
53. Hoeskstra, H. J., Hawkins, K., de Boer, W. J., Rottier, K., and van der Bij, W. (2001) Gastrointestinal complications in lung transplant survivors that require surgical intervention. *Br. J. Surg.* **88**, 433–438.
54. Yiannopoulos, A., Shafazand, S., Ziedalski, T. et al. (2004) Gastric pacing for severe gastroparesis in a heart-lung transplant recipient. *J. Heart Lung Transplant.* **23**, 371–374.
55. Palmer, S. M., Burch, L. H., Trindade, A. J., et al. (2005) Innate immunity influences long-term outcomes after human lung transplant. *Am. J. Respir. Crit. Care Med.* **171**, 780–785.
56. Hadjiliadis, D., Davis, R. D., and Palmer, S. M. (2002) Is transplant operation important in determining post transplant risk of brochiolitis obliterans syndrome in lung transplant recipients? *Chest* **122**, 1168–1175.
57. Lau, C. L., Palmer, S. M., Howell, D. N., et al. (2002) Laparoscopic antireflux surgery in the lung transplant population. *Surg. Endosc.* **16**, 1674–1678.
58. O'Halloran, E. K., Reynolds, J. D., Lau, C. L., et al. (2004) Laparoscopic Nissen fundoplication for treating reflux in lung transplant recipients. *J. Gastrointest. Surg.* **8**, 132–137.
59. Chhajed, P. N., Aboyoun, C. L., Malouf, M. A., Hopkins, P.M., Plit, M. L., and Glanville, A. R. (2003) Risk factors and management of bleeding associated with transbronchial lung biopsy in lung transplant recipients. *J. Heart Lung Transplant.* **22**, 195–197.
60. Robin, E. D. (1985) The cult of the Swan-Granz catheter. Overuse and abuse of pulmonary flow catheters. *Ann. Intern. Med.* **103**, 445–449.
61. Robin, E. D. (1987) Death by pulmonary artery flow-directed catheter: time for a moratorium? *Chest* **92**, 727–731.
62. Robin, E. D. (1988) Defenders of the pulmonary artery catheter. *Chest* **93**, 1059–1066.
63. Muth, C. S. (2000) Gas embolism. *N. Engl. J. Med.* **342**, 476–482.
64. Kleinfeld, G. (1980) Iatrogenic splenic trauma. *JAMA* **244**, 1784.
65. Hesselink, D. A., Van Der Klooster, J. M., Bac, E. H., Scheffer, M. G., and Brouwers J. W. (2001) Cardiac tamponade secondary to chest tube placement. *Eur. J. Emerg. Med.* **8**, 237–239.
66. Chhajed, P. N., Plit, M., Hopkins, P., Malouf, M., and Glanville, A. R. (2002) Achilles tendon disease in lung transplant recipients: association with ciproflaxcin. *Eur. Respir. J.* **19**, 469–471.
67. Malouf, M. A., Bicknell, M., and Glanville, A. R. (1997) Rhabdomyolysis after lung transplantation. *Aust. NZ J. Med.* **27**, 186.
68. Duncan, A. J., Dummer, J. S., Paradis, I., et al. (1991) Cytomegalovirus infection and survival in lung transplant recipients. *J. Heart Lung Transplant.* **10**, 638–646.

69. Burke, C. M., Glanville, A. R., Macoviak, J. A., et al. (1986) The spectrum of cytomegalovirus infection following human heart-lung transplantation. *J. Heart Transplant.* **5**, 267–272.
70. Ho, M. (1998) Human herpesvirus 8—let the transplantation physician beware. *N. Engl. J. Med.* **339**, 1391–1392.
71. Malouf, M. A. and Glanville, A. R. (1999) The spectrum of mycobacterial infection after lung transplantation. *Am. J. Respir. Crit. Care Med.* **160**, 1611–1616.
72. Aris, R. M., Gillingan, P. H., Neuringer, I. P., Gott, K. K., Rea, J., and Yankaskas, J. R. (1997) The effects of panresistant bacteria in cystic fibrosis patients on lung transplant outcome. *Am. J. Respir. Crit. Care Med.* **155**, 1699–1704.
73. Yousem, S. A., Randhawa, P., Locker, J., et al. (1989) Posttransplant lymphoproliferative disorders in heart-lung transplant recipients. *Hum. Pathol.* **20**, 361–369.
74. Swerdlow, A. J., Higgins, C. D., Hunt, B. J., et al. (2000) Risk of lymphoid neoplasia after cardiothoracic transplantation. *Transplantation* **69**, 897–904.
75. Aris, R. M., Maia, D. M., Neuringer, I. P., et al. (1996) Post-transplantation lymphoproliferative disorder in the Epstein-Barr virus-naïve lung transplant recipient. *Am. J. Respir. Crit. Care Med.* **154**, 1712–1717.
76. Reams, B. D., McAdams, H. P., Howell, D. N., Steele, M. P., Davis, R. D., and Palmer, S. M. (2003) Post transplant lymphoproliferative disorder: incidence, presentation, and response to treatment in lung transplant recipients. *Chest* **124**, 1242–1249.
77. Malouf, M. A., Chhajed, P. N., Hopkins, P., Plit, M., Turner, J., and Glanville, A. R. (2002) Antiviral prophylaxis reduces the incidence of lymphoproliferative disease in lung transplant recipients. *J. Heart Lung Transplant.* **21**, 547–554.
78. Verschuuren, E. A., Stevens, S., Pronk, I., et al. (2001) Frequent monitoring of Epstein-Barr virus DNA load in unfractionised whole blood is essential for early detection of post-transplant lymphoproliferative disease in lung transplant patients. *J. Heart Lung Transplant.* **20**, 199–200.
79. Verschuuren, E., van der Bij, W., de Boer, W., Timens, W., Middeldorp, J., and The, T. H. (2003) Quantitive Epstein-Barr virus (EBV) serology in lung transplant recipients with primary EBV infection and/or post-transplant lymphoproliferative disease. *J. Med. Virol.* **69**, 258–266.
80. Guiver, M., Fox, A. J., Mutton, K., Mogulkoc, N., and Egan, J. (2001) Evaluation of CMV viral load using TaqMan CMV quantitive PCR and comparison with CMV antigenemia in heart and lung transplant recipients. *Transplantation* **71**, 1609–1615.
81. Michaelides, A., Facey, D., Spelman, D., Wesselingh, S., and Kostimbos, T. (2003) HCMV DNA detection and quantitation in the plasma and PBL of lung transplant recipients: COBAS Amplicor HCMV monitor test versus in-house quantitative HCMV PCR. *J. Clin. Virol.* **28**, 111–120.
82. Malouf, M. A., Hopkins, P. M., Singleton, L., Chhajed, P. N., Plit, M. L., and Glanville, A. R. (2002) Female sexual health issues after lung transplantation:the importance of screening. *Am. J. Respir. Crit. Care Med.* **165**, A391.

83. Abrahams, N. A., Meziane, M., Ramalingam, P., Mehta, A., DeCamp, M., and Farver, C. F. (2004) Incidence of primary neoplasms in explanted lungs: long-term follow-up from 214 lung transplant patients. *Transplant. Proc.* **36**, 2808–2811.
84. Stagner, L. D., Allenspach, L. L., Hogan, K. K., Willcock, L. C., Higgins, R. S., and Chan, K. M. (2001) Bronchogenic carcinoma in lung transplant recipients. *J. Heart Lung Transplant.* **20**, 908–911.
85. Glanville, A. R., Baldwin, J. C., Hunt, S. A., and Theodore, J. (1990) Long-term cardiopulmonary function after human heart-lung transplantation. *Aust. NZ J. Med.* **20**, 208–214.
86. Armenti, V. T., Radomski, J. S., Moritz, M. J., Philips, L. Z., McGrory, C. H., and Coscia, L. A. (2000) Report from the National Transplantation Pregnancy Registry (NTPR): outcomes of pregnancy after transplantation. *Clin. Transplant.* 123–134.
87. Morton, J. M., Mcwhinney, B., Hickman, P. E., and Potter, J. M. (2001) Therapeutic drug monitoring (TDM) of predinsolone in lung transplantation. *J. Heart Lung Transplant.* **20**, 192.
88. Henderson, K., Eisman, J., Keogh, A., et al. (2001) Protective effect of short-term calcitriol or cyclical etidronate on bone loss after cardiac or lung transplantation. *J. Bone Miner. Res* .**16**, 565–571.
89. Sambrook, P., Henderson, N. K., Keogh, A., et al. (2000) Effect of calcitriol on bone loss after cardiac or lung transplantation. *J. Bone Miner. Res.* **15**, 1818–1824.
90. Aris, R. M., Lester, G. E., Renner, J. B., et al. (2000) Efficacy of pamidronate for osteoporosis in patients with cystic fibrosis following lung transplantation. *Am. J. Respir. Crit. Care Med.* **162**, 941–946.
91. Spira, A., Gutierrez, C., Chaparro, C., Hutcheon, M. A., and Chan, C. K. (2000) Osteoporosis and lung transplantation: a prospective study. *Chest* **117**, 476–481.
92. Shane, E., Papadopoulos, A., Staron, R., et al. (1999) Bone loss and fracture after lung transplantation. *Transplantation* **68**, 220–227.
93. Epstein, F. H. (2000) Exercise limitation in health and disease. *N. Engl. J. Med.* **343**, 632–641.
94. Morrison, W. L. Gibson, J. N., Scrimgeour, C., and Rennie, M. J. (1988) Muscle wasting in emphysema. *Clin. Sci. (Colch.)* **75**, 415–420.
95. Williams, T. J., Patterson, G. A., McClean, P. A., Zamel, N., and Maurer, J. R. (1992) Maximal exercise testing in single and double lung transplant recipients. *Am. Rev. Respir. Dis.* **145**, 101–105.
96. Otulana, B., Higenbottam, T. and Wallwork, J. (1992) Causes of exercise limitation after heart-lung transplantation. *J. Heart Lung Transplant.* **11**, S244–251.
97. Evans, A., Al-Himyary, A., Hrovat, M., et al. (1997) Abnormal skeletal muscle oxidative capacity after lung transplantation by ^{31}P-MRS. *Am. J. Respir. Crit. Care Med.* **155**, 615–621.
98. Wang, X. N., Williams, T. J., McKenna, M. J., et al. (1999) Skeletal muscle oxidative capacity, fiber type, and metabolites after lung transplantation. *Am. J. Respir. Crit. Care Med.* **160**, 57–63.

99. Resnikoff, P. M. and Ries, A. L. (1998) Pulmonary rehabilitation for chronic lung disease. *J. Heart Lung Transplant.* **17**, 643–650.
100. Schwebel, C., Pin, I., Barnoud, D., et al. (2000) Prevalence and consequences of nutritional depletion in lung transplant candidates. *Eur. Respir. J.* **16**, 1050–1055.
101. Snell, G. I., Bennetts, K., Bartolo, J., et al. (1998) Body mass index as a predictor of survival in adults with cystic fibrosis referred for lung transplant candidates. *J. Heart Lung Transplant.* **17**, 1097–1103.
102. Madill, J., Maurer, J. R., and de Hoyos, A. (1993) A comparison of preoperative and postoperative nutritional states of lung transplant recipients. *Transplantation* **56**, 347–350.
103. Ng, P., McCluskey, P., McCaughan, G., et al. (1998) Ocular complications of heart, lung, and liver transplantation. *Br. J. Ophthalmol.* **82**, 423–428.
104. Malouf, M. A., Chhajed, P. N., Jankelson, D., Aboyoun, C., Grunstein, R., and Glanville, A. R. (2001) Prevalence of sleep disordered breathing after lung transplantation. *J. Heart Lung Transplant.* **20**, 225.
105. Shea, S. A., Horner, R. L., Banner, N. R., et al. (1988) The effect of human heart-lung transplantation upon breathing at rest and during sleep. *Respir. Physiol.* **72**, 131–149.
106. Sanders, M. H., Costantino, J. P., Owens, G. R., et al. (1989) Breathing during wakefulness and sleep after human heart-lung transplantation. *Am. Rev. Respir. Dis.* **140**, 45–51.
107. Chhajed, P. N., Aboyoun, C., Malouf, M., et al. (2002) Management of acute hypoxaemia during flexible bronchoscopy with insertion of a nasopharyngeal tube in lung transplant recipients. *Chest* **121**, 1350–1354.
108. Goldstein, L. S., Haug, M. T., 3rd, Perl, J., 2,et al. (1998) Central nervous system complications after lung transplantation. *J. Heart Lung Transplant.* **17**, 185–191.
109. Cohen, L., Littlefield, C., Kelly, P., Maurer, J., and Abbey, S. (1998) Predictors of quality of life and adjustment after lung transplantation. *Chest* **113**, 633–644.
110. Imoto, E. M., Glanville, A. R., Baldwin, J. C., and Theodore, J. (1987) Kidney function in heart-lung transplant recipients: the effect of low-dosage cyclosporine therapy. *J. Heart Transplant.* **6**, 204–213.
111. Dumont, R. J., Partovi, N., Levy, R. D., Fradet, G., and Ensom, M. H. (2001) A limited sampling strategy for cyclosporine area under the curve monitoring in lung transplant recipients. *J. Heart Lung Transplant.* **20**, 897–900.
112. Burke, C. M., Theodore, J., Dawkins, K. D., et al. (1984) Post-transplant obliterative broncholitis and other late lung sequelae in human heart-lung transplantation. *Chest* **86**, 824–829.
113. Berry, G. J., Brunt, E. M., Chamberlain, D., et al. (1990) A working formulation for the standardization of nomenclature in the diagnosis of heart and lung rejection: Lung Rejection Study Group. The International Society for Heart Transplantation. *J. Heart Transplant.* **9**, 593–601.
114. Yousem, S. A., Berry, G. J., Cagle, P. T., et al. (1996) Revision of the 1990 working formulation for the classification of pulmonary allograft rejection: Lung Rejection Study Group. *J. Heart Lung Transplant.* **15**, 1–15.

115. Glanville, A. R., Baldwin, J. C., Burke, C. M., Theodore, J., and Robin, E. D. (1987) Obliterative bronchiolitis after heart-lung transplantation: apparent arrest by augmented immunosuppression. *Ann. Intern. Med.* **107**, 300–304.
116. Gerhadt, S. G., McDyer, J. F., Girgis, R. E., Conte, J. V., Yang, S. C.,and Orens, J. B, (2003) Maintenance azithromycin therapy for broncholitis obliterans syndrome: results of a pilot study. *Am. J. Respir. Crit. Care Med.* **168**, 121–125.
117. Luckraz, H., Goddard, M., McNeil, K., et al. (2004) Microvascular changes in small airways predispose to obliterative bronchiolitis after lung transplantation. *J. Heart Lung Transplant.* **23**, 527–531.
118. Keller, C. A., Cagle, P. T., Brown, R. W., Noon, G., and Frost, A. E. (1995) Bronchiolitis obliterans in recipients of single, double, and heart-lung transplantation. *Chest* **107**, 973–980.
119. Girgis, R. E., Tu, I., Berry, G. J., et al. (1996) Risk factors for the development of obliterative bronchiolitis after lung transplantation. *J. Heart Lung Transplant.* **15**, 1200–1208.
120. Heng, D., Sharples, L. D., McNeil, K., Stewart, S., Wreghitt, T., and Wallwork, J. (1998) Bronchiolitis obliterans syndrome: incidence, natural history, prognosis, and risk factors. *J. Heart Lung Transplant.* **17**, 1255–1263.
121. Sharples, L. D., Tamm, M., McNeil, K., Higenbottam, T. W., Stewart, S., and Wallwork, J. (1996) Development of bronchiolitis obliterans syndrome in recipients of heart-lung transplantation—early risk factors. *Transplantation* **61**, 560–566.
122. Husain, A. N., Siddiqui, M. T., Holmes, E. W., et al. (1999) Analysis of risk factors for the development of bronchiolitis obliterans syndrome. *Am. J. Respir. Crit. Care Med.* **159**, 829–833.
123. Trulock, E. P. (1997) Lung transplantation. *Am. J. Respir. Crit. Care Med.* **155**, 789–818.
124. Glanville, A. R. (2000) Current and prospective treatments of obliterative bronchiolitis. *Curr. Opin. Organ Transplant.* **5**, 396–401.
125. Reynaud-Gaubert, M., Thomas, P., Badier, M., Cau, P., Giudicelli, R., and Fuentes, P. (2000) Early detection of airway involvement in obliterative bronchiolitis after lung transplantation. Functional and bronchoalveolar lavage cell findings. *Am. J. Respir. Crit. Care Med.* **161**, 1924–1929.
126. Zheng, L., Orsida, B. E., Ward, C., et al. (1999) Airway vascular changes in lung allograft recipients. *J. Heart Lung Transplant.* **18**, 231–238.
127. Jonosono, M., Fang, K., Keith, F., et al. (1999) Measurement of fibroblast proliferative activity in bronchoalveolar lavage fluid in the analysis of obliterative bronchiolitis among lung transplant recipients. *J. Heart Lung Transplant.* **18**, 972–985.
128. Tamm, M., Roth, M., Malouf, M., et al. (2001) Primary fibroblast cell cultures from transbronchial biopsies of lung transplant recipients. *Transplantation* **71**, 337–339.
129. Hostettler, K. E., Roth, M., Burgess, J. K., et al. (2004) Cyclosporine A mediates fibroproliferation through epithelial cells. *Transplantation* **77**, 1886–1893.

130. Orens, J. B., Boehler, A., de Perrot, M., et al. (2003) A review of lung transplant donor acceptability criteria. *J. Heart Lung Transplant.* **22**, 1183–1200.
131. Estenne, M. Maurer, J. R., Boehler, A., et al. (2001) Bronchiolitis obliterans syndrome 2001: an update of the diagnostic criteria. *J. Heart Lung Transplant.*, **21**, 297–310.
132. Gabbay, E., Williams, T. J., Griffiths, A. P., et al. (1999) Maximising the utilization of donor organs offered for lung transplantation. *Am. J. Respir. Crit. Care Med.* **160**, 265–271.
133. Bhorade, S. M., Vigneswaran, W., McCabe, M. A., and Garrity, E. R. (2000) Liberalization of donor criteria may expand the donor pool without adverse consequence in lung transplantation. *J. Heart Lung Transplant.* **19**, 1199–1204.

5

Chronic Rejection in the Heart

Philip Hornick and Marlene Rose

Summary

The dramatic improvements in 1-yr survival following cardiac transplantation have not been matched by similar improvements in long-term graft survival. Long-term survival of allografted hearts is limited by a progressive fibroproliferative disease, resulting in intimal thickening and occlusion of the grafted coronary vessels. This disease, variously known as accelerated transplant coronary artery disease or cardiac graft vasculopathy, is also known as chronic rejection. The histology and clinical sequelae are briefly described. The disease can be thought of as a model for nontransplant atherosclerosis, postangioplasty restenosis, and vein graft atherosclerosis. There is compelling evidence that it is driven by alloantigen-dependent mechanisms. The evolution of the disease consists of three phases, an antibody-mediated phase, a cell-mediated phase, and a phase of tissue remodeling that is dependent on cytokines and growth factors. Experimental studies show that adoptive transfer of immunglobulin can transfer features of intimal hyperplasia to transplanted arteries in immunodeficient recipients. Damage to donor endothelium is likely to be an important initiating factor in this disease because it exposes a thrombogenic subendothelial matrix. Whether T cells of antibody are most important in damaging the endothelium is currently the subject of much research. Although T cells are sometimes present in atherosclerotic lesions, an association with acute rejection has never been consistently shown.

Key Words: Rejection; graft vasculopathy; intimal hyperplasia; smooth muscle cells; endothelium; antibodies.

1. Introduction

Despite improvements in the short-term success rate of clinical organ transplantation during recent years, the rate of long-term graft attrition has remained constant *(1–3)*. The progressive improvement in short-term patient and graft survival since the inception of organ transplantation is principally because of better immunosuppressive management of acute rejection episodes, improved

From: *Methods in Molecular Biology, vol. 333: Transplantation Immunology: Methods and Protocols*
Edited by: P. Hornick and M. Rose © Humana Press Inc., Totowa, NJ

diagnosis and treatment of infectious complications, more effective organ preservation, and improved donor selection. However, the acquisition of increasingly detailed knowledge of the immunobiology of rejection and more effective methods of immunosuppression have both failed to prolong the long-term functional survival of organ allografts as a result of chronic rejection. In this regard transplantation has not yet lived up to its potential as a long-term treatment for a lifetime disease.

Chronic rejection may be defined as the progressive functional deterioration of transplanted tissue occurring months or years after engraftment. It is associated with vascular obliteration and other structural changes that lead gradually to organ fibrosis ***(2,4–6)***. The half-life of cadaveric renal transplants after the first year has elapsed has remained constant at 6–7 yr ***(1–3,7,8)***.

Cardiac transplants exhibit graft arteriosclerosis, which produces a progressive luminal narrowing and obstruction in 40–45% of recipients at 5 yr following transplantation ***(9–12)*** and remains the leading cause of death after the first year has elapsed. The incidence of this vasculopathy has been cited as between 15 and 20% of patients per year ***(9,11)***.

Chronic rejection of the cardiac allograft is manifest by the development of transplant-associated coronary artery disease (TxCAD) and was first described in humans by Bieber et al. ***(13)***. It is similar to the type of proliferative vascular lesions observed in renal allografts with chronic vascular rejection ***(14,15)***. Its morphological characteristics differ from conventional coronary artery disease, although in its most advanced form it may resemble conventional non-transplant-associated atheroma ***(11)***. It can therefore act as a model for atherosclerosis in nontransplanted hearts, postangioplasty restenosis, and vein graft atherosclerosis. In recipients with TxCAD in the implanted donor allograft, the epicardial vessels can be palpated as firm and cord-like, often bulging onto the epicardial surface. Grossly, the cut surface of an epicardial vessel affected with TxCAD will contain orange or yellow gummous material ***(16)***. Although the term TxCAD invokes similarities with nontransplant atherosclerosis, conventional atherosclerotic lesions are focal, involve proximal bifurcations of the coronary vasculature, and are eccentric in their distribution ***(17)***. The lesions frequently contain calcium and disrupt the internal elastic lamina ***(17)***. Finally, even in patients with familial hyperlipidemia, the conventional atherosclerotic lesions develop over many years ***(18)***. TxCAD, however, tends to affect the epicardial arteries as well as the proximal parts of the intramyocardial arteries in a diffuse fashion, and less extensive changes have been described in coronary veins ***(19)***. The process involves the great arteries and venous structures up to but not beyond the transplant suture line (the division between donor and native tissue). In the early stages of the disease there is a diffuse, concentric intimal proliferation with preservation of the internal elastic lamina. The main components of the intimal thickening are smooth muscle cells and endothelial cells (ECs), as well as cellular infiltrates consisting predominantly of fibroblasts, dendritic cells (DCs), macrophages, and T lymphocytes (CD4 and CD8) ***(16,20,21)***. Lipid-containing foam cells and later cholesterol clefts appear in a segmental fashion with eventual replacement of lesions very similar to those encountered in atherosclerotic plaques with occasional necrosis and secondary thrombosis. These late atheromatous lesions tend to be segmental, the internal elastic lamina is intact until only very late in the disease process, when it can be disrupted, and calcium deposition is occasional ***(11,16)***. Such lesions are almost always superimposed on the diffuse type of the disease and possibly represent a later stage or a different form of the disease ***(22)***. Some authors have described this as a superimposed "naturally occurring atherosclerosis"***(23)***. The media of the affected arteries is usually normal or thin. Some patients develop extensive necrotising arteritis with destruction of all layers including the media and internal elastic lamina ***(20)***. TxCAD is exclusively limited to the allograft, and its progression is more rapid in comparison to conventional atheroma ***(9,11,24–26)***. Distal vessels are the earliest to occlude, presumably because of their smaller luminal area ***(19)***. TxCAD has been observed as early as 3 mo posttransplantation ***(16)***.

The clinical manifestations of TxCAD result from perfusion failure and ischemia and include myocardial infarcts, arrhythmias, mitral regurgitation secondary to ischemia, heart failure, and sudden death ***(27)***. Angina pectoris, the classical sign of myocardial ischemia, is usually absent in the denervated cardiac allograft ***(28,29)***.

The primary method by which TxCAD is diagnosed is by surveillance coronary angiography, with many centers performing this on at least an annual basis, with some performing routine postdischarge angiography in order to obtain baseline comparative information. It is also pertinent to note that current financial constraints have impinged on this practice, with some UK centers abandoning routine angiography altogether. Although coronary angiography is quite specific for nontransplant coronary atheromatous disease, it appears that it underestimates the presence of TxCAD due to its circumferential and diffuse nature, as well as the involvement of intramyocardial branches ***(30)***. The advent of intravascular ultrasound and its application to the assessment of TxCAD can show intimal thickening developing in the epicardial coronary arteries of cardiac allografts even in the face of a normal-appearing angiogram ***(31–35)***.

The difficulty in the accurate assessment of TxCAD is further compounded the absence of effective therapy. Prevention remains the primary goal, which continues to be elusive despite advances in immunosuppression. The incidence of TxCAD does not appear to have been affected since the introduction of cyclosporine alone or in combination with or without azathioprine and/or steroids ***(10,30,36–39)***, nor is TxCAD generally responsive to antilymphocyte antibody treatment ***(40)***, and in an animal model of transplantation FK506 has not been shown to affect the development of TxCAD ***(41)***.

Invasive therapeutic options for focal nontransplant coronary atherosclerosis include coronary artery bypass grafting (CABG) and coronary angioplasty and ultimately heart retransplantation. Apart from anecdotal reports, CABG is generally not attempted due to the diffuse nature of TxCAD. Angioplasty is attempted more frequently because of the less invasive nature of this therapeutic modality and is reserved for the small numbers with higher-grade lesions superimposed on the generalized process ***(42)***. Ultimate improvement in prognosis is likely to be hampered by the rapidity of this diffuse and progressive process. The only definitive therapy for TxCAD is retransplantation ***(27)***. This raises obvious philosophical issues as well as concern as to whether patients who receive retransplants actually have an overall worse prognosis compared to first-time recipients ***(43)***.

2. Mechanisms of Chronic Allograft Rejection, Antigen- and Non-Antigen-Dependent Events in Chronic Rejection

Although the designation of rejection implies a central role for immunological mechanisms in the histopathological changes responsible for TxCAD, the protracted time course allows the additional influence of other factors that are nonimmune in origin. Chronic rejection is undoubtedly a multifactorial disease. The vascular tissue bears characteristic changes of diffuse concentric intimal hyperplasia leading to progressive and obliterative vasculopathy. These changes may thus be regarded as the end result of immune and nonimmune interactions with the coronary vasculature, which also include responsive adaptations including tissue remodeling as part of a response to injury and tissue repair mechanisms in much the way Ross described in the context of conventional atheroma ***(50)***.

3. Non-Antigen-Dependent Events in Chronic Cardiac Allograft Rejection

Non-antigen-dependent factors thought to be important in the development of TxCAD are (1) those pertinent to the recipient, including the conventional risk factors for atherogenesis, namely, age, sex, obesity, hyperlipidemia, hypertension, smoking, and diabetes, as well as (2) pretransplant diagnosis, (3) donor age and sex, (4) immunosuppressive agents and protocols, (5) nonimmune endothelial injury (donor ischemic time and reperfusion injury), and (6) cytomegalovirus (CMV) infection (reviewed in **ref. *51***). In the main, the available data from major transplant centres are variable and somewhat conflicting (e.g., **refs.**

27,30,37,38,52–57; reviewed in **ref. *51***). The variability of such data is most likely the result of the limitations of the studies concerned as well as the fact that these studies are retrospective, include small patient numbers, and utilize coronary angiography for the detection of TxCAD. The most consistently described relationship is that between hyperlipidemia and TxCAD. The observation of a posttransplant lipid disorder is in part related to the fact that a high proportion of recipients suffer from this condition pretransplant and it was responsible for their preoperative diagnosis of ischemic cardiomyopathy. However, it appears most likely that obesity and the immunosuppressive agents prednisone and cyclosporine play a significant predisposing role in the development of posttransplant hyperlipidemia.

4. Alloantigen-Dependent Events in Chronic Rejection

Despite the foregoing, a consensus exists that TxCAD is primarily immune or alloantigen mediated. Any explanation for the pathogenesis of TxCAD must explain the preferential involvement of the engrafted vessels with sparing of the host's native arteries. This suggests that some factors pertaining selectively to the allograft vasculature rather than some nonspecific consequence of the transplanted state must underlie the pathogenesis of TxCAD. An acquired dyslipidemia or acquired CMV infection alone would not account for selective involvement of the grafted vessels. Immunological mechanisms could explain arteriosclerosis in the engrafted arteries and veins with sparing of the native vessels as well as the rapid progression of TxCAD in comparison to conventional atherogenesis. The histopathological distinction with conventional atheroma suggests a different pathogenesis until at least late in the disease process. Non-antigen-dependent processes, e.g., dyslipidemias, may exacerbate the early immune-mediated injury and may play a more important role with prolonged allograft residence. In this regard, antigen-independent processes such as ischemia or other types of injury to the endothelium around the time of transplantation may also contribute to this process.

5. Experimental Evidence for an Immune Basis for TxCAD

Lurie et al. showed in a deliberately mismatched rat heart transplant model that almost all of the animals developed a proliferative vascular lesion within 20 d ***(58)***. In a rabbit heterotopic heart transplant model, animals receiving high-cholesterol diets and those receiving a normal diet developed proliferative vascular lesions in the allograft to the same degree; however, fatty proliferative lesions developed only in the cholesterol-treated animals ***(59)***. These data would suggest that the proliferative lesion itself is independent of the lipid milieu, but when hyperlipidemia is present, this appears to affect the makeup of the vascular lesion.

A number of experimental approaches have provided more tangible evidence for the involvement of alloantigen-specific immune mechanisms in chronic rejection. Pretransplant immunization with donor splenocytes accelerated the rate of development and progression of TxCAD compared with nonimmunized recipients in a rat cardiac transplant model ***(60)***. Manipulations aimed at induction of donor-antigen unresponsiveness, such as pretransplant intrathymic inoculation of donor cells in combination with recipient lymphocyte ablation, resulted in a significant decrease in the extent and degree of TxCAD ***(61)***. The receptor-ligand pairs CD28-B7 and CD40-gp39 are essential for the initiation and amplification of T-cell-dependent immune responses ***(62,63)***. Larsen et al. ***(64)*** have shown that by blocking CD40 and CD28 costimulatory pathways, T-cell clonal expansion in vitro and in vivo promotes long-term survival of fully allogeneic skin grafts and inhibits the development of TxCAD.

The evolution of chronic rejection in general and of the vascular lesions in particular has been conceptualized as consisting of three phases, an antibody-mediated phase, a cell-mediated phase, and a phase of tissue remodeling that is largely dependent on cytokines and growth factors ***(65,66)***.

Chronic rejection has long been considered an antibody-mediated phenomenon because anti-human leukocyte antigen (HLA) immunoglobulins, complement, and antiendothelial antibodies have been found in areas of vessel wall necrosis and intimal thickening ***(67)***, although it has also been suggested that this may be the result of altered vascular permeability ***(68)***. Recent studies in severe combined immune-deficient mice have shown that passive transfer of antidonor antibody causes TxCAD in long-standing cardiac allografts ***(69)***. The best established example of a contribution of humoral immunity to vascular complications of transplantation is hyperacute rejection, where preformed natural antibodies directed against determinants on the surface of the allogeneic ECs elicit an immediate complement-mediated injury that leads to acute thrombosis and immediate failure of the allograft ***(70)***. The generation of major histocompatibility complex (MHC)-derived or EC antibodies following engraftment might lead to a similar but less dramatic process on an ongoing basis. Sublytic injury of vascular cells by complement might promote the release of growth factors that could contribute to a fibroproliferative rather than a desquamative or necrotic process ***(71)***. In the 1970s Minick and Murphy demonstrated that antigen–antibody complexes can potentiate atherosclerosis as well as its development in cholesterol-fed rabbits ***(72)***. Shed alloantigen combining with host antibodies could furnish one source of antigen–antibody complexes. In the human the importance of anti-HLA and antiendothelial antibodies in the development of chronic rejection has been suggested by a number of groups ***(73–76)***. The precise significance of the initial wave of antibody deposition remains unknown, especially as such alloantibody formation is often associated with cell-mediated rejection. In small-animal models of transplantation, the progression of vascular lesions is often associated with a decline or disappearance of detectable antidonor antibody titers.

A clearer perspective on the relative contribution of the cells involved in alloantigen-mediated damage was shown by Shi et al. *(77)*. In a mouse model of TxCAD in which carotid arteries were transplanted across multiple histocompatibility barriers into seven mutant strains with immunological defects, an acquired immune response with the participation of $CD4^+$ (helper) T cells, antibody, and macrophages was essential to the development of the concentric neointimal proliferation and luminal narrowing characteristic of TxCAD. $CD8^+$ (cytotoxic) T cells and natural killer cells were not involved in the process. Arteries allografted into mice deficient in both T-cell receptors and antibody showed almost no neointimal proliferation, whereas those grafted into mice deficient only in helper T cells, antibody, or macrophages developed small neointimas. These small neointimas and the large neointimas of control animals contained a similar number of inflammatory cells; however, smooth muscle cell number and collagen deposition were diminished in the small neointimas. The reduction in neointimal size in arteries allografted into mice deficient in helper T cells, antibody, or macrophages may be accounted for by a decrease in smooth muscle cell migration or proliferation.

Despite the differences between TxCAD and conventional atherosclerosis, hypotheses regarding the pathogenesis of atherosclerosis may be qualitatively applicable to the transplantation scenario, with the differences being more quantitative. In this regard, Ross's response-to-injury model is particularly attractive *(50,78,79)*. This hypothesis states that the primary process is injury to ECs, which then leads to subsequent vascular damage. If the injury produces EC death and denudation, then the loss of local prostacyclin (PGI_2) production combined with the exposure of the thrombogenic subendothelial collagen matrix would lead to platelet aggregation and release of platelet factors such as platelet-derived growth factor (PDGF), which is a potent smooth muscle cell mitogen *(17)*. Replacement of individually detached ECs by neighbouring ECs can result in a more subtle nondenuding form of injury *(80,81)*. Although this type of injury may not have any morphological manifestations, it may result in increased permeability of the endothelial barrier, allowing constituents of plasma access to the subendothelial layers and increased uptake of plasma constituents (e.g., immunoglobulin) by the endothelium itself, or stimulate EC production of growth factors such as PDGF *(17)*. Modifications to the endothelium such as those mentioned may occur when ECs are injured in a sublethal manner that does not result in replacement or morphological changes. In the case of TxCAD, it could be that one or more of the various forms of endothelial injury described results from an immune response directed against allogeneic vascular endothelium, resulting in an atherosclerotic vascular response.

6. Acute Rejection and TxCAD

Because acute rejection episodes constitute one of the most frequent causes of profound tissue damage in the early posttransplant period, it is likely that they are among the most powerful events to initiate chronic rejection. Alloantigen-independent events factors such as prolonged ischemia, surgical manipulation, reperfusion injury, and lipid-mediated tissue injury may enhance antigen-dependent events either through upregulation of alloantigens and cell adhesion molecules or at the level of increased production of mediators common to various pathways of tissue injury. As indicated previously, there is compelling experimental evidence suggesting that chronic rejection is primarily allo-antigen driven and that immune mechanisms resulting in acute cardiac allograft rejection also contribute to the pathogenesis of TxCAD. However, in clinical cardiac transplantation the association between acute rejection and TxCAD remains controversial. Studies that have attempted to clarify the relationship between acute rejection and TxCAD have produced conflicting results. Whereas a positive correlation was found in some studies *(27,55,82–84)*, others have been unable to confirm a direct correlation of TxCAD with biopsy-diagnosed rejection, incidence, or severity *(30,35,55,85–87)*. Limitations to these studies include the fact that they are all retrospective and include small patient numbers, the use of varying grades of severity of biopsy-proven clinical rejection, and, in most cases, angiographic detection of coronary arterial abnormalities. Furthermore, prophylactic and maintenance immunosuppressive regimes vary among patients within each study and between studies. Acute rejection that merits treatment varies according to the immunosuppressive policy of the particular transplant center, and accordingly some series focus on International Society for Heart and Lung Transplantation (ISHLT) grade 3A *(88)* or above as being clinically significant. The policy at Harefield Hospital (United Kingdom) of minimizing the long-term use of steroids in maintenance immunosuppression has led to the view that mild diffuse disease (ISHLT 1B) should be treated with a brief course of intravenous steroids. This center and others *(87)* therefore regard grade 1B as clinically significant, particularly because recurrent mild episodes may insidiously damage vascular endothelium. In a study by Winters et al. *(38)*, the number of previous clinically treated (moderate or severe) rejection episodes only weakly correlated with percent luminal narrowing demonstrated by digitized video-image analysis. However, if the total number of rejection episodes was analyzed (including even minimal rejection that normally would not be treated), the difference in percent luminal narrowing between patients having fewer versus those having more rejection episodes became highly significant. As acute cellular rejection diminishes dramatically over time ***(19)***, the practice of most centers is to reduce the dose of all immunosuppressive agents over the first year after transplantation in order to reduce toxic side effects. Although this may be quite reasonable for the prevention of acute cellular rejection, it may not be the correct approach for TxCAD. Moreover, mild subclinical cellular rejection episodes may still substantially contribute to TxCAD development and/or progression. Finally, TxCAD in all of these studies is considered as being either present or absent. However, stratification on the basis of time when TxCAD developed may help to apportion both immunological and nonimmunological risk factors more appropriately.

References

1. Paul, L. and Benediktsson, H. (1993) Chronic transplant rejection, magnitude of the problem and pathogenetic mechanisms. *Transplant Rev.* **7**, 96–113.
2. Hayry, P., Isoniemi, H., Yilmaz, S., Mennander, A., Lemstrom, K., Raisanen-Sokolowski, A., et al. (1993) Chronic allograft rejection. *Immunol. Rev.* **134**, 33–81.
3. Tilney, N., Schmid, C., Azuma, H., and Heemann, U. (1994) Transplantation immunology: an introduction. *Transplant. Immunol.* **2**, 99–102.
4. Azuma, H., and Tilney, N. (1994) Chronic graft rejection. *Curr. Opin. Immunol.* **6**, 770–776.
5. Adams, H., Russell, M., Hancock, W., Sayegh, M., Wyner, L., and Karnovsky, M. (1993) Chronic rejection in experimental cardiac transplantation: studies in the Lewis-F344 model. *Immunol. Rev.* **143**, 5–19.
6. Ewel, C. and Foegh, M. (1993) Chronic graft rejection: accelerated transplant arteriosclerosis. *Immunol. Rev.* **134**, 21–31.
7. Schweitzer, E., Matas, A., Gillingham, K., et al. (1991) Causes of renal allograft loss. *Ann. Surg.* **214**, 679–688.
8. Cook, D. (1987) Long term survival of kidney allografts, in (Terasaki, P., ed.) *Clinical Transplants*, Los Angeles, UCLA Tissue Typing Laboratory.
9. Uretsky, B., Murali, S., Reddy, P., Rabin, B., Lee, A., Bartley, P., et al. (1987) Development of coronary artery disease in cardiac transplant patients receiving immunosuppressive therapy with cyclosporin and prednisolone. *Circulation* **76**, 827–833.
10. Gao, S., Schroeder, J., Alderman, E., Hunt, S., Valantine, H., Wiederhold, V., et al. (1989) Prevalence of accelerated coronary artery disease in heart transplant survivors, comparison of cyclosporin and azathioprine regimens. *Circulation* **80 (Suppl. III)**, 100–105.
11. Billingham, M. (1987) Cardiac transplant atherosclerosis. *Transplant. Proc.* **19 (Suppl. 5)**,19–25.
12. Billingham, M. (1989) Graft coronary disease: the lesions and the patients. *Transplant. Proc.* **21**, 3665–3666.

13. Bieber, C., Stinson, E., Shumway, N., Payne, R., and Kosek, J. (1970) Cardiac transplantation in man, VII, Cardiac allograft pathology. *Circulation* **41**, 753–779.
14. Porter, K., Thomson, W., Owen, K., Kenyon, J., Mowbray, J., and Peart, W. (1963) Obliterative vascular changes in four human kidney homotransplants. *Br. Med. J.* **II**, 639–645.
15. Busch G, Galvanek E, and Reynolds E. (1971) Human renal allografts. *Hum Pathol* **2**, 253–298.
16. Billingham, M. (1997) Graft coronary disease: old and new dimensions. *Cardiovasc. Pathol.* **6**, 95–101.
17. Ross, R. (1986) Factors influencing atherogenesis, in (Hurst, J., ed.) *The Heart* New York, McGraw-Hill, pp. 801–815.
18. Gotto, A. and Farmer, J. (1988) Risk factors for coronary artery disease, in (Braunwald, E., ed.) *Heart Disease* Philadelphia, WB Saunders Inc., pp. 1153–1190.
19. Hosenpud, J., Shipley, J., and Wagner, C. (1992) Cardiac allograft vasculopathy, Current concepts, recent developments and future directions. *J Heart Lung Transplant.* **11**, 9–23.
20. Hruban, R., Beschorner, W., Baumgartner, W., Austine, S., Ren, H., and Reitz, B. (1990) Accelerated arteriosclerosis in heart transplant recipients is associated with a T-lymphocyte-mediated endothelialitis. *Am. J. Pathol.* **137**, 871.
21. Usy, C. and Rose, A. (1983) Cardiac transplantation, aspects of the pathology. *Pathol. Annu.* **17**, 147.
22. Yacoub, M. and Rose, M. (1993) Accelerated coronary sclerosis, in (Rose, M. and Yacoub, M., eds.) *Immunology of Heart and Lung Transplantation*, London, Edward Arnold, pp. 289–299.
23. Pucci, A., Forbes, C., and Billingham, M. (1990) Pathologic features in long term cardiac allografts. *J. Heart Transplant.* **9**, 339–345.
24. Gao, A., Alderman, E., Schroeder, J., Silverman, .J, and Hunt, S. (1988) Accelerated coronary vascular disease in the heart transplant patient, coronary arteriographic findings. *J. Am. Coll. Cardiol.* **12**, 334–340.
25. Hess, J., Hastillo, A., Mohanakumar, T., Cowley, M., Vetrovac, G., Szentpetery, S., et al. (1983) Accelerated atherosclerosis in cardiac transplantation, role of cytotoxic B-cell antibodies and hyperlipidaemia. *Circulation* **68(Suppl. 2)**, 94–101.
26. Zerbe, T., Uretsky, B., Kormos, R., Armitage, J., Wolyn, T., Groffith, B., et al. (1992) Graft atherosclerosis: effects of cellular rejection and human lymphocyte antigen. *J. Heart Lung Transplant.* **11**, S104–110.
27. Gao, S., Schroeder, J., Hunt, S., and Stinson, E. (1988) Retransplantation for severe accelerated coronary artery disease in heart transplant recipients. *Am. J. Cardiol.* **62**,.876.
28. Stark, R., McGinn, A., and Wilson, R. (1991) Chest pain in cardiac transplant recipients, evidence of sensory reinnervation after cardiac transplantation. *N. Engl. J. Med.* **234**, 1791–1794.
29. Vora, K., Hosenpud, J., Ray, J., et al. (1991) Angina pectoris in a cardiac allograft recipient. *Clin. Transplant.* **5**, 20–22.

30. Gao, S., Schroeder, J., Alderman, E., Hunt, S., Siverman, J., Wiederhold, V., et al. (1987) Clinical and laboratory correlates of accelerated coronary artery disease in the cardiac transplant patient. *Circulation* **76**, 56–61.
31. Schroeder, J., Gao, S., Hunt, S., and Stinson, E. (1992) Accelerated graft coronary artery disease: diagnosis and prevention. *J. Heart Lung Transplant.* **11(Suppl.)**, 258–265.
32. St. Goar, F., Pinto, F., Alderman, E., et al. (1992) Intracoronary ultrasound in cardiac transplant recipients. In vivo evidence of "angiographically silent" intimal thickening. *Circulation* **85**, 979–987.
33. Ventura, H., Ramee, S., Jain, A., et al. (1992) Coronary artery imaging with intravascular ultrasound in patients following cardiac transplantation. *Transplantation* **53**, 216–219.
34. Rickenbacher, P., Pinto, F., Chenzbraun, A., et al. (1992) Incidence and severity of transplant artery disease early and up to 15 years after transplantation as detected by intravascular ultrasound. *J. Am. Coll. Cardiol.* **25**, 171–177.
35. Rickenbacher, P., Kemna, M., Pinto, F., Hunt, S., Alderman, E., Schroeder, J., et al. (1996) Coronary artery intimal thickening in the transplanted heart. *Transplantation* **61**, 46–53.
36. Kirkman, R., Strom, T., Weir, M., and Tilney, N. (1982) Late mortality and morbidity in recipients of long-term allografts. *Transplantation* **34**, 347–351.
37. Olivari, M., Homans, D., Wilson, R., Kubo, S., and Ring, W. (1989) Coronary artery disease in cardiac transplant patients receiving triple-drug immunosuppressive therapy. *Circulation* **80(Suppl.)**, 111–115.
38. Winters, G., Kendall, T., and Radio, S. (1990) Post-transplant obesity and hyperlipidaemia, major predictors of severity of coronary arteriopathy in failed human allografts. *J. Heart Transplant.* **9**, 364.
39. Hess, M., Hastillo, A., Thompson, J., et al. (1987) Lipid mediators in organ transplantation: does cyclosporin accelerate coronary atherosclerosis? *Transplant Proc.* **19(Suppl. 5)**, 71–73.
40. Paul, L. and Fellstrom, B. (1992) Chronic vascular rejection of the heart and the kidney, have rational treatment options emerged? *Transplantation* **53**, 1169–1179.
41. Arai, S., Okada, M., Morimoto, T., Hisamochi, K., Senoo, Y., and Teramoto, S. (1991) The impact of FK506 on graft coronary disease and graft infiltrating lymphocyte subsets following rat heart transplantation, comparison with cyclosporin A [abstract]. *J. Heart Lung Transplant.* **10**, 175.
42. Vetrovec, G., Cowley, M., Newton, C., et al. (1988) Applications of percutaneous transluminal angioplasty in cardiac transplantation. Preliminary results in five patients. *Circulation* **78(Suppl. III)**, 83–86.
43. Karwande, S., Ensley, R., and Renlund, D. (1992) Cardiac retransplantation: a viable option? *Ann. Thorac. Surg.* **54**, 840–844.
44. Jamieson, S., Oyer, P., and Baldwin, J. (1984) Heart transplantation for end-stage ischemic heart disease, The Stanford experience. *Heart Transplant* **3**, 224–227.
45. Kaye, M. (1993) The registry of the international society for heart and lung transplantation, Tenth official report—1993. *J. Heart Lung Transplant.* **12**, 541–548.

46. Sarris, G., Moore, K., and Schroeder, J. (1994) Cardiac transplantation: the Stanford experience in the cyclosporin era. *J. Thorac. Cardiovasc. Surg.* **108**, 240.
47. Hosenpud, J. (1996) The Registry of the International Society for Heart and Lung Transplantation: Thirteenth Official Report. *J. Heart Lung Transplant.* **15**, 655.
48. Evans, R., Orians, C., and Ascher, N. (1992) The potential supply of organ donors: an assessment of the efficacy of organ procurement efforts in the United States. *JAMA* **267**, 239.
49. Baumgartner, W., Augustine, S., and Borkon, A. (1987) Present experience in cardiac transplantation. *Ann. Thorac. Surg.* **6**, 585.
50. Ross, R. (1993) The pathogenesis of atherosclerosis, a perspective for the 1990s. *Nature* **362**, 801–809.
51. Johnson, M. (1993) Transplant coronary disease, non-immunologic risk factors. *J. Heart Lung Transplant.* **11(Suppl.)**, 124–132.
52. Pahl, E., Fricker, F., Armitage, J., et al. (1990) Coronary arteriosclerosis in pediatric heart transplant survivors, limitation of long-term survival. *J. Pediatr.* **116**, 177–183.
53. Eich, D., Thompson, J., Daijin, K., et al. (1991) Hypercholesterolaemia in long-term survivors of heart transplantation, an early marker of accelerated coronary artery disease. *J. Heart Lung Transplant.* **10**, 45–49.
54. Sharples, L., Caine, N., Mullins, P., et al. (1991) Risk factor analysis for the major hazards following heart transplantation—rejection, infection, and coronary occlusive disease. *Transplantation* **52**, 244.
55. Gao, S., Schroeder, J., Hunt, S., Valantine, H., Hill, I,, and Stinson, E. (1993) Influence of graft rejection on incidence of accelerated graft coronary artery disease: a new approach to analysis. *J. Heart Lung Transplant.* **12**, 1029.
56. McDonald, K., Rector, T., Braulin, E., Kubo, S., and Olivari, M. (1989) Association of coronary artery disease in cardiac transplant recipients with cytomegalovirus infection. *Am. J. Cardiol.* **64**, 359.
57. Barbir, M., Kushwaha, S., Hunt, B., Macken, A., Thomson, G., Mitchell, A., et al. (1992) Lipoprotein (a) and accelerated coronary artery disease in cardiac transplant patients. *Lancet* **340**, 1500–1502.
58. Lurie, K., Billingham, M., Jamieson, S., Harrison, D., and Reitz, B. (1981) Pathogenesis and prevention of graft arteriosclerosis in an experimental heart transplant model. *Transplantation* **31**, 41–47.
59. Alonso, D., Starek, P., and Minick, C. (1977) Studies on the pathogenesis of atheroarteriosclerosis induced in rabbit cardiac allografts by synergy of graft rejection and hypercholesterolaemia. *Am. J. Pathol.* **87**, 265–292.
60. Cramer, D., Chapman, F., Wu, G., Harnaha, J., Quian, S., and Makowka, L. (1990) Cardiac transplantation in the rat. II. Alteration of the severity of donor graft arteriosclerosis by modulation of the host immune response. *Transplantation* **50**, 554–558.
61. Shin, Y., Adams, D., Wyner, L., Akalin, E., Sayegh, M., and Karnovsky, M. (1995) Intrathymic tolerance in the Lewis-to-F344 chronic cardiac allograft rejection model. *Transplantation* **59**, 1647–1653.

62. Bluestone, J. (1995) New perspectives of CD28-B7-mediated costimulation. *Immunity* **2**, 555–559.
63. Banchereau, J., et al. (1994) The CD40 antigen and its ligand. *Ann. Rev. Immunol.* **12**, 881–922.
64. Larsen, C., Elwood, E., Alexander, D., Ritchie, S., Hendrix, R., Tucker-Burden, C., et al. (1996) Long-term acceptance of skin and cardiac allografts after blocking CD40 and CD28 pathways. *Nature* **381**, 434–438.
65. Fellstom, B., Larsson, E., and Tufveson, G. (1989) Strategies in chronic rejection of transplanted organs: a current view on pathogenesis, diagnosis and treatment. *Transplant Proc.* **21**, 1435–1439.
66. Foegh, M. (1990) Chronic rejection-graft arteriosclerosis. *Transplant. Proc.* **22**, 119–122.
67. Taylor, D., Ibrahim, H., Tolman, D., and Hess, M. (1991) Accelerated coronary arteriosclerosis in cardiac transplantation. *Transplant. Rev.* **5**, 165–174.
68. Higgy, N., Davidoff, A., Grothman, G., Hollenberg, M., Benediktsson, H., and Paul, L. (1991) Platelet derived growth factor–receptor expression in rat heart allografts. *J. Heart Lung Transplant.* **10**, 5135–5141.
69. Russell, P., Chase, C., Winn, H., and Colvin, R. (1994) Coronary atherosclerosis in transplanted rat heart. II. The importance of humoral immunity. *J. Immunol.* **152**, 389–398.
70. Dalmasso, A., Vercellotti, G., Fischel, R., Bolman, R., Bach, F., and Platt, J. (1992) Mechanisms of complement activation in the hyperacute rejection of porcine organs transplanted into primate recipients. ***Am. J. Pathol.*** **140**, 1157–1166.
71. Benzaquen, L., Nicholson-Weller, A., and Halperin, J. (1994) Terminal complement proteins C5b-9 release fibroblast growth factor and platelet derived growth factor from endothelial cells. *J. Exp. Med.* **179**, 985–992.
72. Minick, C. and Murphy, G. (1973) Experimental induction of arteriosclerosis by the synergy of allergic injury to arteries and lipid-rich diet. II. Effect of repeatedly injected foreign protein in rabbits fed a lipid-rich cholesterol-poor diet. *Am. J. Pathol.* **73**, 265–300.
73. Dunn, M., Crisp, S., Rose, M., Taylor, P., and Yacoub, M. (1992) Anti-endothelial antibodies and coronary artery disease after cardiac transplantation. *Lancet* **339**, 1566–1570.
74. Crisp, S., Dunn, M., Rose, M., Taylor, P., and Yacoub, M. (1994) Anti-endothelial antibodies after heart transplantation, The accelerating factor in transplant associated coronary artery disease. *J. Heart Lung Transplant.* **13**, 81–92.
75. Suciu-Foca, N., Reed, E., Marboe, C., Harris, P., Yu, P., Sun, Y., et al. (1991) The role of anti-HLA antibodies in heart transplantation. *Transplantation* **51**, 716–724.
76. Reed, E., Hong, B., Ho, E., Harris, P., Weinberger, J., and Suciu-Foca ,N. (1996) Monitoring of soluble HLA alloantigens and anti-HLA antibodies identifies heart allograft recipients at risk of transplant-associated coronary artery disease. *Transplantation* **61**, 566–572.

77. Shi, C., Lee, W., He, Q., Zhang, D., Fletcher, Jr., D., Newell, J., et al. (1996) Immunologic basis of transplant-associated arteriosclerosis. *Proc. Natl. Acad. Sci. USA* **93(9)**, 4051–4056.
78. Ross, R. and Glomset, J. (1976) The pathogenesis of atherosclerosis. *N. Engl. J. Med.* **295**, 369–420.
79. Ross, R. (1986) The pathogenesis of atherosclerosis, an update. *N. Engl. J. Med.* **314**, 488–500.
80. Reidy, M. and Schwartz, S. (1981) Endothelial injury and regeneration. III. Time course of intimal changes after small defined injury to rat aortic endothelium. *Lab. Invest.* **44**, 301–308.
81. Reidy, M. and Schwartz, S. (1983) Endothelial injury and regeneration. IV. Endotoxin, a non-denuding injury to aortic endothelium. *Lab. Invest.* **48**, 24–34.
82. Narrod, J., Kormos, R., Armitage, J., Hardesty, R., Ladowski, J., and Griffith B. (1989) Acute rejection and coronary artery disease in long-term survivors of heart transplantation. *J. Heart Transplant.* **5**, 418–421.
83. Radnovancevic, B, Poindexter, S, Birovljev, S, et al. (1990) Risk factors for development of accelerated coronary artery disease in cardiac transplant patients. *Eur. J. Cardiothorac. Surg.* **4**, 309.
84. Schutz, A., Kemkes, B., Kugler, C., et al. (1990) The influence of rejection episodes on the development of accelerated coronary artery disease after heart transplantation. *Eur. J. Cardiothorac. Surg.* **4**, 309.
85. Ratkovec, R., Wray, R., Renlund, D., et al. (1990) Influence of corticosteroid-free maintenance immunosuppression on allograft coronary disease: a new approach to analysis. *J. Thora.c Cardiovasc. Surg.* **100**, 6.
86. Stovin, P., Sharples, P., Hutter, J., Wallwork, J., and English, T. (1991) Some prognostic factors of the development of transplant-related coronary artery disease in human cardiac allografts. *J. Heart Lung Transplant.* **1**, 38–44.
87. Stovin, P., Sharples, L., Schofield, P., Cary, N., Mullins, P., English, T., et al. (1993) Lack of association between endomyocardial evidence of rejection in the first six months and the later development of transplant coronary artery disease. *J. Heart Lung Transplant.* **12**, 110–116.

6

Direct and Indirect Allorecognition

Philip Hornick

Summary

The design and effectiveness of strategies to promote long-term graft acceptance requires a fundamental understanding of the mechanisms underlying acute and chronic rejection. This chapter discusses the two pathways of allorecognition—direct and indirect—and suggests that the direct pathway plays a major role in the early weeks after transplantation and that the indirect pathway may contribute to the process of chronic rejection. The results of in vitro and in vivo experimental models are discussed, together with clinical data.

Key Words: Direct allorecognition; indirect allorecognition; chronic rejection; acute rejection.

1. Introduction

One of the most striking features of the T-cell response provoked by major histocompatibility complex (MHC)-incompatible cells is its vigor. This is reflected by the mixed leukocyte reaction (MLR) in vitro *(1)* and in vivo by the rejection of solid organ transplants and graft-vs-host disease in recipients of allogeneic bone marrow transplants. Indeed, it was the very strength of the alloresponse that led to the discovery of MHC molecules and their products, which were first designated "transplantation antigens." The strength of this response is accounted for by the uniquely high precursor frequency of T cells with specificity for allogeneic MHC molecules. This feature of the alloresponse was first detected by Skinner and Marbrook *(2)* and Fischer-Lindahl and Wilson *(3)* for class I-reactive T cells.

Direct allorecognition is defined as the recognition by recipient T cells of the intact MHC alloantigens displayed at the surface of donor (dendritic) cells carried within the graft. No other cells intervene in this initial step of the direct pathway.

From: *Methods in Molecular Biology, vol. 333: Transplantation Immunology: Methods and Protocols*
Edited by: P. Hornick and M. Rose © Humana Press Inc., Totowa, NJ

Any discussion pertaining to the direct recognition of allogeneic cells needs initially to focus on two fundamental issues: (1) the high precursor frequency of alloreactive T cells that recognize allogeneic MHC molecules and (2) the fact that the rules of self-MHC restriction are apparently disregarded in the direct binding of the T-cell receptor (TCR) to the allogeneic MHC molecules.

T-cell precursor frequencies of $1{:}10^3$–10^4 have frequently been recorded against foreign MHC molecules compared with $1{:}10^5$ or less for nominal, antigen-specific, self-MHC restricted T cells. It appears that recognition of nominal antigen in the context of self-MHC molecules and the recognition of alloantigen is not by two distinct T-cell populations, but rather by an overlapping population. T-cell clones have been generated that recognize nominal antigen in a self-MHC restricted fashion and cross-react on allogeneic cells ***(4,5)***. It has further been shown that approximately half of the cells involved in generating an alloresponse have been primed previously to nominal antigen ***(6)***. The precise nature of the ligand recognized by the alloreactive T cells still remains unclear. There are two main hypotheses, which make very different assumptions about the nature of the ligand bound by the alloreactive T cells. The multiple binary complex hypothesis was proposed by Matzinger and Bevan in 1977 ***(7)***. This hypothesis proposes that the antigen-binding grooves of the MHC molecules expressed on normal cells are occupied with an extreme diversity of peptides derived from the processing of serum and cellular proteins, presented with class I or class II MHC molecules. Alloreactive T cells are specific for individual complexes of MHC and peptide, as are nominal antigen-specific T cells. As a consequence, a single allogeneic MHC molecule will be able to stimulate a large number of different T-cell clones, each with a distinct peptide, MHC specificity, and hence account for the high precursor frequency.

The second hypothesis, proposed by Bevan, is referred to as the high-determinant-density hypothesis ***(8)***. It proposes that the attention of the alloreactive T cell's receptor is focused on the exposed residues of the allogeneic MHC molecule that differ from the responder, whether the antigen-binding site of the molecule is occupied or not. If the specificity of the alloreactive T cell is for the allogeneic MHC molecule itself, then in theory all foreign MHC molecules of any given isotype (e.g., human leukocyte antigen [HLA]-DR) displayed by the allogeneic stimulator cell could act as ligands for the alloreactive responder T cell. The implication of this hypothesis becomes obvious when the total number of MHC molecules, i.e., ligand density, is compared to the ligand density available to an antigen-specific T cell. This issue has been addressed by Harding and Unanue ***(9)***. Following the internalization, processing, and presentation of an antigen by a class II-expressing antigen-expressing cell (APC), it is probable that only a small fraction, probably <1%, of class II molecules will be occupied with the particular peptide for which the T cell is specific. It follows that there may be a 100-fold higher number of ligands or determinant density per cell available for the alloreactive T cell than is available to an antigen-specific T cell. The corollary of this is that cells of lower affinity than is required for an antigen-specific response may be called into the alloreactive repertoire such that T cells with low and medium as well as high affinity for the allo-MHC molecule could lead to the generation of a high precursor frequency.

In order to understand fully the phenomenon of direct allorecognition, this now needs to be accommodated within the framework of a T-cell repertoire that has been positively selected to recognize peptide in the context of self-MHC.

At face value the foregoing discussion appears to break the rules of self-MHC restriction, but the two hypotheses to account for the high precursor frequency of alloreactive T cells can be accommodated within the context of self-MHC restriction. This is easiest to envisage where responder and stimulator MHC molecules are similar, sharing conserved sequences in the exposed TCR-contacting surface of the molecule. Differences in the peptide-binding groove allow binding and display of different sets of peptides ***(10)***. The alloresponse is thus directed to the multiplicity of different peptides bound by the MHC molecule. When the exposed surfaces of the responder and stimulator MHC molecules are substantially different, the alternative, high-determinant-density hypothesis may provide a better explanation for the observed strength of the alloresponse. In order to reconcile this with self-MHC restriction, it only needs to be suggested that a small fraction of T cells whose receptors were selected for self-MHC recognition cross-react, by chance, with a foreign MHC structure. Given the bias that appears to exist in TCR genes for MHC recognition ***(11)***, this is likely to occur in structurally dissimilar responder, stimulator combinations with sufficient frequency to account for the numbers of alloreactive T cells identified by limiting dilution analysis.

It has long been assumed that the in vitro MLR correlates with acute transplant rejection. Until recently it had not been shown that T cells with exclusive direct allospecificity can effect acute rejection. Pietra et al. ***(12)*** reconstituted severe combined immunodeficiency mice (SCID) with syngeneic $CD4^+$ T cells. This led to rejection of MHC class II-expressing heart grafts, but not MHC class II-deficient grafts. Moreover, they were also able to show that SCID mice, also MHC class II deficient, rejected allogeneic grafts when reconstituted with $CD4^+$ T cells. Because these mice had no $CD8^+$ cells and no MHC class II-expressing APCs, direct cytotoxic and indirect allorecognition would not have occurred. Thus, $CD4^+$ cells were both necessary and sufficient to mediate allograft rejection.

2. Observations of Direct Pathway Hyporesponsiveness

In vitro primed donor-specific direct pathway alloreactive T-helper (Th) cells have been found to induce acute graft rejection when adoptively transferred into irradiated recipients that had been transplanted with an allogeneic kidney. Rejection occurred only in the presence of donor genotype dendritic cells (DCs) ***(13)***. However, in animals bearing an established graft, the renal parenchymal cells were unable to reactivate the alloreactive T cells. These results indicate that while direct alloreactive T cells play a dominant role in acute rejection, in the absence of donor DCs, T-cell hyporesponsiveness can occur.

Direct alloreactive T cells are primed in the spleen and draining lymph nodes following the migration and maturation of donor DCs ***(14)***. Effector functions are carried out by $CD8^+$ cytotoxic T lymphocytes (CTLs) within the graft without necessarily further input from Th or DCs. While cytokines secreted by Th cells will facilitate the initial stages of clonal expansion of the $CD8^+$ compartment, thus amplifying the rejection response, thereafter $CD8^+$ cells are likely to be autonomous in their activity ***(15)***. Th cells can initiate antibody production at sites distant from the allograft by allospecific B cells. Delayed-type hypersensitivity (DTH) responses may be orchestrated by Th cells that have infiltrated the graft having left the recipient lymphoid tissue. Here, primed or memory antigen-specific $CD4^+$ cells may be activated by immature donor DCs that still persist within the graft. Such activation has been demonstrated in vitro ***(16)***, and memory T-cell activation by antigen-loaded, immature tissue DCs may be one mechanism by which secondary antigen-specific responses are initiated very quickly ***(17)***. It would thus appear that for the allograft, MHC-expressing, immature DCs within the graft may play an important role as immunogenic targets for activated $CD4^+$ cells. The eventual replacement of donor DCs by recipient interstitial DCs ***(18)*** and the apparent paucity of cells capable of stimulating direct allorecognition left within the graft and their potential for inducing anergy is likely to account for the hyporesponsiveness of direct pathway T cells in the experimental systems thus far examined.

3. Clinical Correlates of Donor-Specific Hyporesponsiveness

In recipients receiving immunosuppression, episodes of acute rejection become less frequent and less destructive with the passage of time following transplantation, while the progression of chronic rejection remains unaffected ***(19)***.

Limiting dilution techniques specific for the direct pathway have been utilized to estimate recipient, antidonor Th and CTL frequencies in patients who have chronic rejection. Following preliminary investigations by Deacock and Lechler ***(20)***, Mason et al., utilizing a range of B-lymphoblastoid cell lines expressing donor DR antigens have been able to show donor-specific hyporesponsiveness in some patients with chronic renal failure ***(21)***. Such findings are important because they indicate that for humans as for rodents, the prolonged residence of an allograft can induce donor-specific hyporesponsiveness in T cells with direct allospecificity. These findings also suggest that chronic rejection can progress despite such hyporesponsiveness.

Chronic rejection is under the influence of alloantigen-dependent and non-alloantigen-dependent factors. The importance of HLA matching, acute graft rejection, rapid progression in allogeneic as compared to syngeneic grafts, as well as more tangible experimental evidence *(22–24)*, points to a determining role for alloantigen-dependent processes. Direct allorecognition is likely to be an important event in the initiation of chronic rejection in that the clinical picture in the early posttransplant period is dominated by tissue damage caused by episodes of acute rejection. However, chronic rejection may occur in the absence of previous episodes of acute rejection *(25)*, and the observation of direct pathway hyporesponsiveness following graft residence and depletion of donor DCs mitigates against this pathway being a driving force in the progression of chronic rejection.

4. Indirect Allorecognition

Tangible evidence for a second route of allorecognition was provided by retransplantation experiments in a rat model. Lechler and Batchelor observed that MHC-incompatible kidney allografts depleted of indigenous passenger leukocytes (by "parking" kidneys in enhanced hosts) were permanently accepted without immunosuppression in certain donor/recipient combinations, but in others suffered rejection *(26)*. This second route for the recognition of allogeneic MHC is known as the indirect pathway, whereby allogeneic MHC molecules and/or other donor alloantigens are processed and presented by recipient APCs. This is the normal mechanism of T-cell stimulation by nominal antigens, i.e., as processed peptides associated with self (recipient)-MHC class II molecules. Alloantigens shed from a graft will in general be treated as exogenous antigens by recipient APCs, leading to a dominance of Th cells recognizing allopeptides bound to MHC self class II molecules. The observations made thus far indicate that T cells sensitized by the direct pathway might initially dominate the rejection process occurring in nonimmune recipients, but that T cells sensitized by indirect allorecognition might contribute substantially to continuing long-term or chronic graft damage after the allograft has lost its DC population *(26)* and direct alloreactive T cells have been rendered hyporesponsive.

5. Evidence for Indirect Allorecognition in Small Mammalian Models

In a murine system, Benichou et al. *(27)* showed that T cells collected from mice that had been sensitized by allogeneic splenocyte infusion or skin grafting proliferated to synthetic peptides derived from the polymorphic regions of

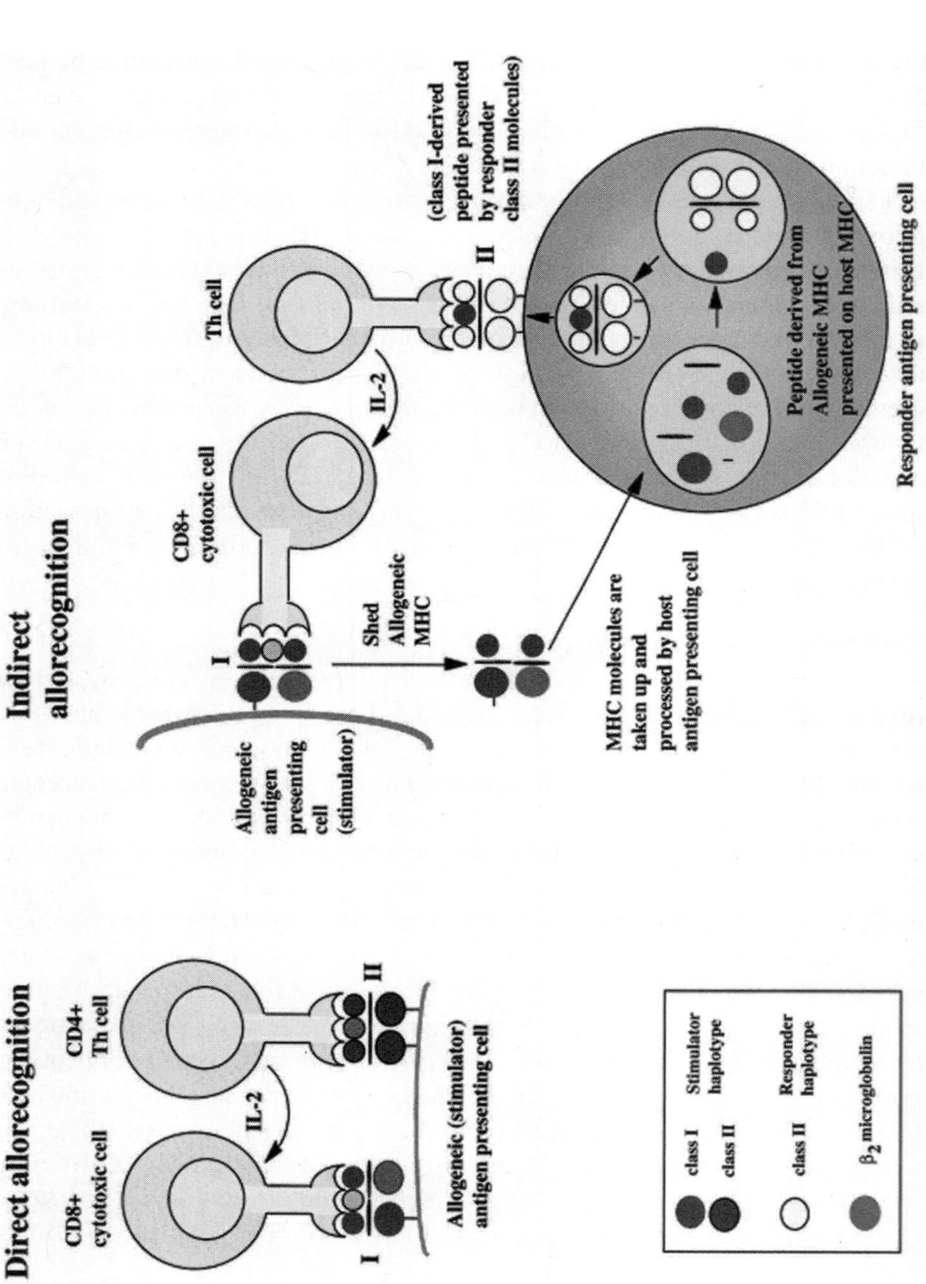

Direct allorecognition

CD8+
cytotoxic cell

CD4+
Th cell

IL-2

I

II

Allogeneic (stimulator)
antigen presenting cell

Indirect allorecognition

Allogeneic
antigen
presenting
cell
(stimulator)

I

CD8+
cytotoxic cell

Th cell

Shed
Allogeneic
MHC

IL-2

II

(class I-derived
peptide presented
by responder
class II molecules)

MHC molecules are
taken up and
processed by host
antigen presenting cell

Peptide derived from
Allogeneic MHC
presented on host MHC

Responder antigen presenting cell

class I
class II
Stimulator
haplotype

class II
Responder
haplotype

β_2 microglobulin

the α and β chains of the allogeneic class II MHC molecule presented by host APCs.

Peptide immunization of allogeneic MHC antigens has been shown to hasten the rate of graft rejection for skin and kidney allografts ***(28, 29)***. Perhaps the most compelling evidence showing that an indirect response could initiate allograft rejection was generated once MHC class II-deficient knockout mice were generated by targeted gene disruption ***(30)***. Since grafts from these mice were unable to stimulate a direct $CD4^+$ T-cell response, rapid rejection of their graft in a $CD4^+$-dependent manner suggested that indirect T-cell stimulation could lead to graft rejection ***(31)***. Further importance of indirect alloresponses is suggested by the downregulation of T-cell responses following thymic administration of allogeneic MHC-derived peptides leading to prolonged survival of subsequent renal allografts. Such peptides could not have affected the direct pathway, which suggests that indirect presentation is critical to the rejection process ***(32)***. These data also imply dominance over the direct pathway.

6. Evidence for Indirect Allorecognition In Vitro

Evidence that processing and presentation of MHC-derived peptides occurs physiologically has been provided by Chicz et al. ***(33)***, who eluted peptides from HLA-DR1 molecules derived from naturally processed self MHC polypeptides from either the invariant chain or HLA-A2. This suggests that processing and presentation of such peptides is a common event in vivo.

Both MHC class I ***(34)*** and class II ***(35)*** allogeneic peptides may be presented in the context of self-MHC class II. It is probable that the precise cellular origins of donor antigens will be of little significance, as donor antigens are processed and presented by recipient APCs, the important factor being the quantity of donor antigen available. Class I MHC antigens are likely to be of greater importance than class II antigens, being more common in the long-term life span of the allograft ***(36)***, at least in the absence of acute rejection episodes **(37)**. With the knowledge that crosstalk between the endogenous and exogenous pathways can take place, presentation of exogenous antigens by self-MHC class I molecules may also occur. The actual physiological significance

---

Fig. 1. *(opposite page)* Direct allorecognition involves the recognition by T cells of the polymorphism of the C alloantigens displayed at the surface of donor dendritic cells. No other cells intervene in this initial step of the direct pathway. Indirect allorecognition involves the recognition of donor alloantigens (primarily allogeneic MHC molecules) in the same way as for any nominal protein antigen, i.e., as processed peptides associated with self (recipient)-MHC class II molecules. Following activation of indirect T-helper cells, allospecific effector cells may be stimulated in the same localized environment.

of this in graft rejection is questionable. One view is that CD8+ cells sensitized by peptides presented in the context of recipient MHC class I molecules will not find such a determinant expressed by donor cells except in cases where donor and recipient MHC class I molecules are matched *(38)*. IL-2 secreting CTL **(39)** may, however, potentially react with such self-restricted peptides and thus provide the cytokines necessary (in addition to cytokines generated from indirect HTL) for driving directly sensitized CTL, B-cell, and DTH responses against the graft and not by their own actual interaction with the donor and hence lysis of donor cells.

7. Evidence of the Indirect Pathway in Humans

The frequency of T cells engaged in the indirect recognition of synthetic DR1 peptides in an in vitro culture system was found to be about 100-fold lower than that of T cells participating in direct recognition of native HLA-DR antigen *(40)*. Such data, however, do not necessarily imply dominance of direct pathway mechanisms, as there is the potential for the generation of a multiplicity of epitopes derived from MHC molecules. The strength of the indirect response would therefore be the sum total of all indirect frequencies estimated for each epitope. It thus becomes clear that a failure to demonstrate an indirect alloreactive frequency might reflect the sensitivity of the assay system and the methodology utilized *(41)*. This conceptually challenges the precept that direct allorecognition dominates the rejection process in its early stages just because high precursor frequencies are produced in vitro.

Recent data derived in the context of acute rejection in recipients of heart grafts and utilizing synthetic peptides corresponding to the hypervariable regions of the mismatched donor HLA-DR antigens have indicated an association between acute rejection and activation of the indirect pathway *(42)*. Frasca et al. raised T-cell clones from an HLA-A2-negative patient whose A2-positive kidney failed as a result of chronic rejection. The clones responded in a self-restricted manner to a single peptide of HLA-A2 *(43)*.

The relative contribution of alloantibody in the rejection process is not well understood. In the context of chronic rejection, humoral mechanisms have long been thought to make important contributions. Taylor et al. *(44)* and Russell et al. *(45)* indicate in the rat the importance of humoral immune mechanisms in the development of chronic rejection. In humans, recent evidence indicates their potential importance in chronic rejection *(46,47)*. Because the alloantibodies formed during chronic rejection react with donor cells and often exhibit antidonor specificity, this process is likely to be mediated by Th cells recognizing donor MHC-derived peptides and bound to host MHC molecules. Donor alloantigens released from the injured graft may provide soluble MHC molecules, which produce antigens for indirect allorecognition. Such processes may expose the graft to the continuous attack of allopeptide-reactive Th cells, which can mediate rejection long after the donor APCs have migrated from the graft and provide help to B cells to produce antidonor HLA antibodies ***(48)***. Anti-HLA antibodies can bind soluble HLA antigens, forming immune complexes that are internalized by APCs via Fc receptors. This again would result in efficient processing of alloantigens and stimulation of allopeptide reactive Th cells ***(49,50)***. It is possible that sublytic injury of vascular cells by complement may promote the release of growth factors that could contribute to a fibroproliferative rather than a desquamative or frankly necrotic process ***(51)***. B-cell antibody production thus must involve T cells with indirect allospecificity.

References

1. Bach, F., Bach, M., and Sondel, P. (1976) Differential function of major histocompatibility complex antigens in T lymphocyte activation. *Nature* **259**, 273–281.
2. Skinner, M. and Marbrook J. (1976) An estimation of the frequency of frequency of precursor cells which generate cytotoxic lymphocytes. *J. Exp. Med.* **143**, 1562–1567.
3. Fischer-Lindahl, K. and Wilson, D. (1976) *J. Exp. Med.* **145**, 500–507.
4. Hunig, T. and Bevan, M. (1980) Self-H2 antigens influence the specificity of alloreactive cells. *J. Exp. Med.* **151**, 1288–1298.
5. Lombardi, G., Sidhu, S., Batchelor, J., and Lechler, R. (1989) Allorecognition of DR1 by T cells from a DR/Dw13 responder mimics self-restricted recognition of endogenous peptides. *Proc. Natl. Acad. Sci.* **86**, 4190–4194.
6. Lombardi, G., Sidhu, S., Daly, M., Batchelor, J., Makgoba, W., and Lechler, R. (1990) Are primary alloresponses truly primary? *Int. Immunol.* **2**, 9–13.
7. Matzinger, P. and Bevan, M. (1977) Why do so many lymphocytes respond to major histocompatibility antigens? *Cell. Immunol.* **29**, 1–5.
8. Bevan, M. (1984) High determinant density may explain the phenomenon of alloreactivity. *Immunol. Today* **5**, 128-–130.
9. Harding, C. and Unanue, E. (1990) Quantitation of antigen-presenting cell MHC class II/peptide complexes necessary for T cell stimulation. *Nature* **346**, 574.
10. Lechler, R., Lombardi, G., Batchelor, J., Reinsmoen, N., and Bach, F. (1990) The molecular basis of alloreactivity. *Immunol. Today* **11**, 83–88.
11. Merkenschlager, M., Graf, D., Lovatt, M., Bommhardt, U., Zamoyska, R., and Fisher, A. (1997) How many thymocytes audition for selection? *J. Exp. Med.* **186**, 1149–1158.
12. Pietra, B., Wiseman, A., Bolwerk, A., Rizeq, M., and Gill, R. (2000) CD4 T cell-mediated cardiac allograft rejection requires donor but not host MHC class II. *J. Clin. Invest.* **106**, 1003–1010.
13. Braun, M., McCormack, A., Webb, G., and Batchelor, J. (1993) Mediation of acute but not chronic rejection of the MHC incompatible rat kidney grafts by alloreactive CD4 T cells activated by the direct pathway of sensitisation. *Transplantation* **55**, 177–182.

14. Austyn, J. and Larsen, C. (1990) Migration patterns of dendritic leucocytes. Implications for transplantation. *Transplantation* **49**, 1–7.
15. Harding, F. and Allison, J. (1993) CD28-B7 interactions allow the induction of CD8+ cytotoxic T lymphocytes in the absence of exogenous help. *J. Exp. Med.* **176**, 519–529.
16. Dai, R., Grammar, S., and Streilein, J. (1993) Fresh and cultured Langerhans cells display differential capacities to activate hapten-specific T cells. *J. Immunol.* **150**, 59–66.
17. Streilein, J., Grammar, S., Yoshikawa, T., Demidem, A., and Vermeer, M. (1990) Functional dichotomy between Langerhans cells that present antigen to naive and to memory/effector T lymphocytes. *Immunol. Rev.* **117**, 159–183.
18. Milton, A., Spencer, S., and Fabre, J. (1986) The effects of cyclosporin A on the induction of donor class I and class II MHC antigens in heart and kidney allografts in the rat. *Transplantation* **42**, 337.
19. Hosenpud, J., Shipley, J., and Wagner, C. (1992) Cardiac allograft vasculopathy, Current concepts, recent developments and future directions. *J. Heart Lung Transplant.* **11**, 9–23.
20. Deacock, S. J. and Lechler, R. L. (1992) Positive correlation of T cell sensitization with frequencies of alloreactive T helper cells in chronic renal failure patients. *Transplantation* **54**, 338–343.
21. Mason, P., Robinson, C., and Lechler, R. (1996) Detection of donor-specific hyporesponsiveness following late failure of human renal allografts. *Kidney Int.* **50**, 1019–1025.
22. Cramer, D., Chapman, F., Wu, G., Harnaha, J., Quian, S., and Makowka, L. (1990) Cardiac transplantation in the rat. II. Alteration of the severity of donor graft arteriosclerosis by modulation of the host immune response. *Transplantation* **50**, 554–558.
23. Shin, Y., Adams, D., Wyner, L., Akalin, E., Sayegh, M., and Karnovsky, M. (1995) Intrathymic tolerance in the Lewis-to-F344 chronic cardiac allograft rejection model. *Transplantation* **59**, 1647–1653.
24. Cramer, D., Qian, S., Harnaha, J., et al. (1989) Cardiac transplantation in the rat, I. The effect of histocompatibility differences on graft atherosclerosis. *Transplantation* **47**, 414–419.
25. Isoniemi, H., Nurminen, M., Tikkanen, M., et al. (1994) Risk factors predicting chronic rejection of renal allografts. *Transplantation* **57**, 68–72.
26. Lechler, R. and Batchelor, J. (1982) Restoration of immunogenicity to passenger cell- depleted kidney allografts by the addition of donor strain dendritic cells. *J. Exp. Med.* **155**, 31–41.
27. Benichou, G., Takizawa, A., Olson, A., McMillan, M., and Sercarz, E. (1992) Donor major histocompatibility complex (MHC) peptides are presented by recipient MHC molecules during graft rejection. *J. Exp. Med.* **175**, 305–308.
28. Fangmann, J., Dalchau, R., and Fabre, J. (1992) Rejection of skin allografts by indirect allorecognition of donor class I major histocompatibility complex peptides. *J. Exp. Med.* **175**, 1521–1529.

29. Benham, A., Sawyer, G., and Fabre, J. (1995) Indirect T cell recognition of donor antigens contributes to the rejection of vascularized kidney allografts. *Transplantation* **59**, 1028–1032.
30. Grusby, M., Johnson, R., Papaioannou, V., and Glimcher, L. (1991) Depletion of CD4 T cells in major histocompatibility complex class II-deficient mice. *Science* **253**, 1417–1420.
31. Auchinloss, H. J., Lee, R., Shea, S., Markowitz, J., Grusby, M., and Glimcher, L. (1993) The role of 'indirect' recognition in initiating rejection of skin grafts from major histocompatibility complex class II-deficient mice. *Proc. Natl. Acad. Sci. USA* **90**, 3373–3377.
32. Sayegh, M., Perico, N., Gallon, L., Imberti, O., Hancock, W., Remuzzi, G., et al. (1994) Mechanisms of acquired thymic unresponsiveness to renal allografts. *Transplantation* **58**, 125–132.
33. Chicz, R., Urban, R., Lane, W., Gorga, S., Stern, L., Vignali, D., et al. (1992) Predominant naturally processed peptides bound to HLA-DR1 are derived from MHC relayed molecules and are heterogeneous in size. *Nature* **358**, 764–768.
34. Essaket, S. and Fabron, J. (1990) Co-recognition of HLA-A1 and HLA DPw3 by a human CD4+ alloreactive T cell clone. *J. Exp. Med.* **172**, 387–390.
35. de Koster, H., Anderson, D., Termijtelen, A. (1990) T cells sensitized to synthetic HLA-DR3 peptide give evidence of continuous presentation of denatured HLA-DR3 molecoles by HLA-DP. *J. Exp. Med.* **169**, 1191–1196.
36. Hart, D. and Fabre, J. (1979) Quantitative studies on the tissue distribution of Ia and SD antigens in the DA and Lewis rat strains. *Transplantation* **27**, 110.
37. Milton, A., Spencer, S., and Fabre, J. (1986) Massive induction of donor type class I and class II MHC antigens in rejecting cardiac allografts in the rat. *J. Exp. Med.* **161**, 98.
38. Auchinloss, H. J. and Sutan, H. (1996) Antigen processing and presentation in transplantation. *Curr. Opin. Immunol.* **8**, 681–687.
39. Joos, J., Zanker, B., Wagnar, H., and Kabelitz, D. (1988) Quantitative assessment of interleukin-2-producing alloreactive human T cells by limiting dilution analysis. *J. Immunol. Methods* **112**, 85.
40. Liu, Z., Sun, Y., Xi, Y., Maffai, A., Reed, E., Harri,s P., et al. (1993) Contribution of direct and indirect allorecognition pathways to T cell alloreactivity. *J. Exp. Med.* **177**, 1643–1650.
41. Van Besouw, N., Vaessen, L., Daane, C., Jutte, N., Balk, A., Claas, F., et al. (1996) Peripheral monitoring of direct and indirect alloantigen presentation pathways in clinical heart transplant recipients. *Transplantation* **61**, 165–167.
42. Liu, Z., Coloval, A., Tugulea, S., Reed, E., Fisher, P., Mancini, D., et al. (1996) Indirect recognition of donor HLA-DR peptides in organ allograft rejection. *J. Clin. Invest.* **98**, 1150–1157.
43. Frasca, L., Amendola, A., Hornick, P., Uren, J., Marelliberg, F., Lechler, R., et al. (1998) The role of donor and recipient antigen presenting cells in priming and maintaining T cells with indirect specificity. *Transplantation* **66**, 1238–1243.

44. Taylor, D., Ibrahim, H., Tolman, D., and Hess, M. (1991) Accelerated coronary arteriosclerosis in cardiac transplantation. *Transplant. Rev.* **5**, 165–174.
45. Russell, P., Chase, C., Winn, H., and Colvin, R. (1994) Coronary atherosclerosis in transplanted rat heart. II. The importance of humoral immunity. *J. Immunol.* **152**, 389–398.
46. Dunn, M. J., Crisp, S. J., Rose, M. L., Taylor, P. M., Yacoub, M. H. (1992) Anti-endothelial antibodies and coronary artery disease after cardiac transplantation. *Lancet.* **339**, 1566–1570.
47. Reed, E. F., Hong, B., Ho, E., Harris, P. E., Weinberger, J., Suciu-Foca, N. (1996) Monitoring of soluble HLA alloantigens and anti-HLA antibodies identifies heart allograft recipients at risk of transplant-associated coronary artery disease. *Transplantation.* **61**, 566–572.
48. Bradley, J., Mowat, A. M., and Bolton, E. (1992) Processed MHC class I alloantigen as the stimulus for CD4+ T-cell dependent antibody-mediated graft rejection. *Immunol. Today* **13(11)**, 434–438.
49. Simitsek, P., Campbell, D., Lanzavecchia, A., Fairweather, N., and Watts, C. (1995) Modulation of antigen processing by bound antibodies can boost or suppress class II major histocompatibility complex presentation of different T cell determinants. *J. Exp. Med.* **181**, 1957.
50. Sallusto, F. and Lanzavecchia, A. (1994) Efficient presentation of soluble antigen by cultured human dendritic cells is maintained by granulocyte/macrophage colony-stimulating factor plus interleukin 4 and down regulated by tumour necrosis factor alpha. *J. Exp. Med.* **179**, 1109.
51. Benzaquen, L., Nicholson-Weller, A., and Halperin, J. (1994) Terminal complement proteins C5b-9 release fibroblast growth factor and platelet derived growth factor from endothelial cells. *J. Exp. Med.* **179**, 985–992.

7

HLA Typing and Its Influence on Organ Transplantation

Stephen Sheldon and Kay Poulton

Summary

Human leukocyte antigen (HLA) molecules are expressed on almost all nucleated cells, and they are the major molecules that initiate graft rejection. There are three classical loci at HLA class I: HLA-A, -B, and -Cw, and five loci at class II: HLA-DR, -DQ, -DP, -DM, and -DO. The system is highly polymorphic, there being many alleles at each individual locus. Three methods for HLA typing are described in this chapter, including serological methods and the molecular techniques of sequence-specific priming (SSP) and sequence-specific oligonucleotide probing (SSOP). The influence of HLA matching on solid organ and bone marrow transplantation is also described. HLA matching has had the greatest clinical impact in kidney and bone marrow transplantation, where efforts are made to match at the HLA-A, -B, and -DR loci. In heart and lung transplantation, although studies have shown it would be an advantage to match especially at the DR locus, practical considerations (ischemic times, availability of donors, clinical need of recipients) make this less of a consideration. Corneal grafts are not usually influenced by HLA matching, unless being transplanted into a vascularized (or inflamed) bed.

Key Words: HLA molecules; crossmatching; tissue-typing; serology.

1. Introduction

Human leukocyte antigen (HLA) molecules are expressed on the surface of virtually all nucleated cells and play a pivotal role in the fundamental necessity of the immune system to distinguish self from non-self. HLA antigens are the vehicles used to present peptides on the cell surface. Non-self determinants presented by HLA can instigate an appropriate immune response through HLA/T-cell-receptor interaction. In humans, the genes that code for the HLA antigens are located on the short arm of chromosome 6 (6p21.3) within a region termed the major histocompatibility complex (MHC).

From: *Methods in Molecular Biology, vol. 333: Transplantation Immunology: Methods and Protocols*
Edited by: P. Hornick and M. Rose © Humana Press Inc., Totowa, NJ

The evolution of this complex of HLA genes within the MHC has been driven by the need of the immune system to effectively identify and respond to pathogens. The HLA system has responded to the evolutionary pressure generated by the ability of pathogens to constantly mutate, by itself becoming highly polymorphic within populations. This strategy increases the chances of at least a portion of a population being capable of effectively presenting and responding to new pathogens as they appear. If HLA polymorphisms are lacking within a population, a new pathogen has a greater potential to wipe that population out. The high level of polymorphism found within the HLA gene pool may well be central to the efficiency of the immune system in dealing with infection, but this has proved to be a major problem within the field of transplantation. In the artificial situation of transplantation, HLA molecules function as histocompatibility antigens.

Because each individual inherits sets of several highly polymorphic HLA genes from both father and mother, the chance of two nonsibling individuals having an identical HLA phenotype is small. Because HLA antigens act as the markers that serve to communicate the identity of self or non-self within the immune system, any transplanted HLA disparity may act as the stimulus for an immune response. In the case of an HLA-mismatched allograft, the response is to initiate a cellular- and/or antibody-mediated rejection of the graft. Such a response can be instigated by passenger antigen-presenting cells (APCs) of donor origin, which can persist for some time posttransplant. This pathway is referred to as direct allorecognition and is unique to transplantation. If recipient APCs activate a rejection process, this is referred to as indirect allorecognition, this mechanism being comparable to the host's natural response to an infection.

The field of histocompatibility and immunogenetics has therefore evolved mainly through the need to identify and catalog the genetic polymorphisms within the HLA system in order to quantify the levels of disparity between donors and recipients.

2. Early History

The origins of HLA typing as we know it today stem from observations made by hematologists in the 1930s, who observed leukoagglutinating antibodies in patients with leukopenia. In the late 1950s, workers including Jean Dausset, Rose Payne, and Jon van Rood observed leukoagglutinins in serum, which were attributed to the patients having been exposed to alloantigens through transfusions or pregnancy ***(1–3)***. The reaction patterns displayed by the different antibodies identified against random cell panels revealed clusters of antisera with similar specificities. Individual research groups were therefore able to use these antibodies as reagents to phenotype individuals for the different specificities identified. The analogy with the genetically determined mice histocompatibility antigens described by Snell at the Jackson Laboratories and Gorer in England in the 1950s *(4,5)* was soon recognized, as was the impact that the study of these gene products could have in understanding the processes of allograft rejection.

As the number of investigators increased, collaboration was needed to develop a standardized nomenclature and typing methods. In 1964, the first International Workshop was convened in Durham, North Carolina. HLA antigens were categorized according to their structural and functional similarities into class I and class II. Since 1964, there have been 14 International Workshops, during which time three HLA class I (HLA-A, -B, and -Cw) and five HLA class II (HLA-DR, -DQ, -DP, -DM, and -DO) loci have been identified and comprehensively studied. More than 1800 polymorphisms have now been defined, with more continuing to be identified *(6)*.

3. Typing Methods

3.1. Serology

The earliest methods used to define HLA polymorphisms were entirely based on serological techniques. The complement-dependent lymphocytotoxicity (CDC) assay was developed in the 1964 by Terasaki and McClelland to dramatically reduce the volume of precious typing reagents required to define an individual phenotype *(7)*. The CDC assay requires only 1 mL of typing reagent per test and 1 mL of target cells at a concentration of 2–4 × 10^6/mL. Cells and sera are mixed under oil to avoid evaporation in sloping-sided wells of a Terasaki tray. After 30 min, rabbit serum is added as a source of complement (4–5 mL) and the assay is incubated for a further 60 min. If a well contains an antibody with specificity to HLA molecules expressed on the cells' surface, the binding of that antibody will activate the rabbit complement. The lytic action of the activated complement results in cell death. The reactions are then fixed, stained, and read through the underside of the Terasaki tray using an inverted microscope. Cell death is recorded as a positive reaction, and the pattern of these reactions is interpreted to assign an HLA phenotype.

Screening individuals who have been previously exposed to non-self HLA antigens can identify HLA-typing reagents. The most productive source of high-titer monospecific HLA-typing reagents is multiparous women. During pregnancy, women may produce HLA-specific antibodies after immunological exposure to non-self paternal HLA antigens expressed by the fetus *(3)*. Serum from these women can be screened against a panel of cells of previously defined phenotype. The pattern of positive reactions can therefore be analyzed to determine the specificity or specificities of any detected antibodies. These well-characterized sera can subsequently be used as typing reagents. Patients who have had transfusions or a previous transplant with some degree of HLA mismatch may also develop HLA-specific antibodies, although these patients are more likely to develop antibodies directed against multiple HLA antigens. If this is the case, a serum becomes less useful as a typing reagent.

The target cells used in the CDC assay are usually peripheral blood lymphocytes (PBLs), which can be isolated from anticoagulated whole blood by density gradient centrifugation. As an alternative source, lymphocytes can also be flushed from the spleen or lymph nodes of cadaveric donors. Other cell-preparation techniques available include negative selection of PBLs by lysis of red cells and nonlymphocyte leukocytes with monoclonal antibodies (MAbs; e.g., LymphoKwik, One Lambda Inc). Antibody-coated magnetizable microbeads can also be used (e.g., Dynabeads, Dynal Ltd, or Fluorobeads, One Lambda Inc). These bind to specific cell populations and are then isolated using a strong magnet. These later methods allow class II-expressing B cells to be isolated independently as a target cell for class II (HLA-DR and -DQ) typing *(8)*.

The costs with respect to time and human resources required to screen, identify, and control the quality of alloantisera for use as CDC typing reagents has driven most HLA-typing laboratories to use class I and class II monoclonal antibody typing trays, which are now commercially available. Because the supply of MAbs provided is in theory unlimited and the avidity of the antibodies can be adjusted, this CDC method provides an added advantage in that the target cell can be added to both the MAb and complement in a one-step assay without reducing sensitivity. This simplifies the protocol and reduces the total incubation time required to just 1 h.

Although serology-based techniques allowed scientists to first identify the polymorphic nature of the HLA system, the advent of molecular biology has allowed us to radically improve the level of polymorphic definition that can be achieved.

3.2. HLA Typing by Molecular Methods

Our understanding of the HLA system was dramatically improved when it became possible to define HLA specificities by genetic analysis. The very earliest techniques involved probing Southern blots of genomic DNA digested using restriction enzymes, yielding a variety of banding patterns, which were crudely related to HLA class II alleles. As more sequence data became available and DNA-based technologies progressed, it became possible to identify HLA alleles present by testing specifically for individual alleles.

By the early 1990s, two diverse DNA-based HLA-typing systems were established and embraced by the HLA community. Both of these methods utilize the polymerase chain reaction (PCR) to produce multiple copies of the HLA genes, focusing predominantly on exons 2, 3, and 4. These exons encode the peptide-binding grooves of the HLA molecules, where most of the base changes are located, giving each allele its unique sequence. One of these methods involved specific amplification of HLA alleles using PCR-sequence-specific priming (SSP) ***(9)***. The second technique involved locus-specific amplification of HLA genes and resolution of specific alleles present by probing the PCR-amplified DNA using PCR-sequence-specific oligonucleotide probes (SSOP) ***(10,11)***. These methods have proved so efficient and adaptable that they are still widely used today in some form.

3.2.1. PCR-SSP

When HLA typing using SSP, multiple simultaneous tests are performed on a single sample. Each test looks for the presence or absence of one polymorphism using PCR primers specific only for that sequence. The system relies on the lack of 5' to 3' exonuclease activity of *Taq* DNA polymerase, used in the PCR reaction. Using this enzyme, PCR amplification only occurs if alleles with sequences identical to those of the PCR primers used are present in the sample to be tested. Specificity of the PCR amplification is conferred by the base at the 3' end of each primer, where an exact match is required in order to allow the synthesis of a new strand of DNA.

It is necessary to run multiple simultaneous SSP reactions in order to obtain an HLA typing. Typically, at least 96 reactions are required to define HLA-A, -B, and -DRB1 alleles present at the lowest resolution. As a control against amplification failure, which could give a false-negative result, primers that amplify a highly conserved gene (often human growth hormone) are included in each reaction. These internal control primers amplify a band that is easily distinguished from specific amplification by size, using conventional agarose gel electrophoresis stained with ethidium bromide under ultraviolet light **(Fig. 1)**. In some cases, primers do not amplify specific alleles but amplify allele groups, and specificity is defined by looking at combinations of positive and negative results. Results are interpreted by comparing these reaction patterns either manually or with the aid of a computerized software package designed specifically for each test.

The major advantage of this system is that it is the quickest method of obtaining a full HLA typing using molecular methods widely available at the moment. From receipt of sample to interpretation of the gel image, a complete HLA typing by DNA-based methods takes approx 3.5 h. It is possible that this technology may be replaced in future by real-time PCR methodologies (e.g., TaqMan, Applied Biosystems Inc.), which will remove the need to analyze PCR product using gel electrophoresis, but at the time of going to press these technologies were not readily available in most laboratories. As the most rapid of the DNA-based technologies available, PCR-SSP is still the technology of choice for most centers performing HLA typing of cadaveric donors for transplantation. As a

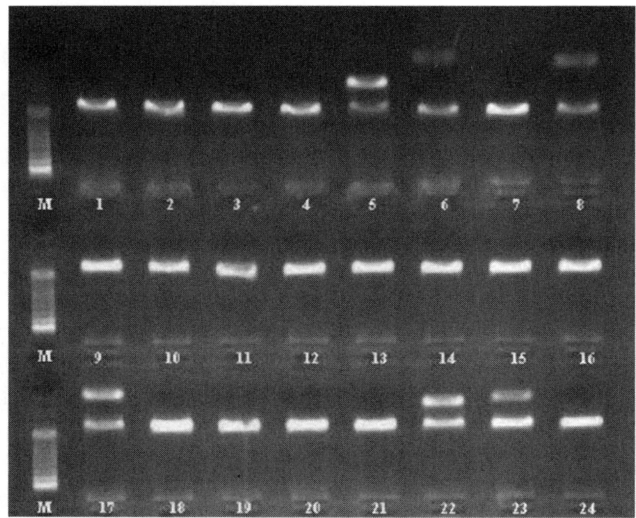

Fig. 1. HLA-DRB1 typing by PCR-SSP (low resolution).The presence of specific amplification bands in lanes 5, 6, and 17 indicates the presence of HLA-DRB1*03, and a positive reaction in lane 8 indicates the presence of DRB1*04. The specific amplification in lane 22 indicates the presence of DRB3* alleles, which are in linkage with DRB1*03 alleles. Lane 23 shows the presence of DRB4* alleles, in linkage with DRB1*04. M = size marker to identify size of amplified products (bp)

result, this technique has been heavily exploited commercially, and a number of manufacturers now market comprehensive PCR-SSP HLA-typing reagents (Dynal Biotech, One Lambda, Protrans, and Biotest, among others)

One disadvantage of PCR-SSP is that it remains a comparatively expensive technique, consuming relatively large quantities of primers and DNA polymerase and using relatively large amounts of DNA. For HLA typing of multiple samples, it could also be regarded as a rather time-consuming procedure. The 3.5 h it takes to process a sample is not reduced dramatically by processing multiple samples, and the ability to process samples simultaneously is limited by resources such as the number of thermal cyclers available at any one time. A far more suitable system for HLA typing of multiple samples is based on the alternative technology established again in the early 1990s: SSOP.

3.2.2. SSOP

This is also a PCR-based system, relying on amplification not of specific alleles as in PCR-SSP, but of exons in the HLA genes containing the hypervariable regions that confer allele specificity. Multiple Southern blots of the amplified PCR product are prepared on nylon membranes, which are then hybridized against a series of labeled SSO probes directed against specific base changes that bind to regions of complementarity. Excess or nonspecifically bound probes are removed after hybridization using stringent washing procedures with either tetramethylammonium chloride or sodium saline citrate. SSO probes remain bound after stringent washing procedures only when the sequence of the probes is an exact match to that of an HLA allele present in the sample. Bound probe is detected, usually using enhanced chemiluminescence-based techniques, and the HLA type of the individual is interpreted by comparing patterns of positive and negative reactions ***(12)***.

One obvious advantage of PCR-SSOP is that this system is best suited for typing large numbers of samples simultaneously. When compared with HLA typing by PCR-SSP, little additional expenditure is required to process 96 samples compared with processing a single sample in terms of thermal cyclers, technician time, and reagents. This approach to HLA typing is also the most economical in terms of the amount of DNA required because only one PCR amplification is required per sample. This makes PCR-SSOP the method of choice for research studies, where it is essential to conserve sample whenever possible.

Over the years, the PCR-SSOP system has been subject to various technological modifications used to improve the efficiency or the safety of the methodology used in routine practice. For example, the most efficient labeling of the oligonucleotide probes was originally achieved using radioactive labels (^{32}P). In time, this was superceded by substituting biotin-labeled probes, followed by an enhanced chemiluminescence detection system. Robotic workstations and automated (real-time) development systems have replaced laborious manual pipetting and interpretation of autoradiographs, reducing the potential for introducing human error into the system. A modification of the SSOP is used successfully in the form of reverse slot blot assays produced commercially for HLA typing ***(13)***. An overview of this method is summarized in **Fig. 2**.

4. HLA Nomenclature

As would be expected in this fast-growing field, nomenclature for both existing and novel alleles is strictly regulated by the WHO Nomenclature Committee for factors of the HLA system. Regular updates documenting the details of newly identified HLA alleles are published in *Tissue Antigens*, but the official repository for HLA sequences is the IMGT/HLA sequence database, which can be accessed at www.ebi.ac.uk/imgt/hla. In July 2005 this database contained sequences for 1325 class I alleles and 763 class II alleles. The database is updated at 3-mo intervals.

Over time, major revisions of HLA nomenclature have been necessary to accommodate the increasing number of HLA alleles identified. The most recent

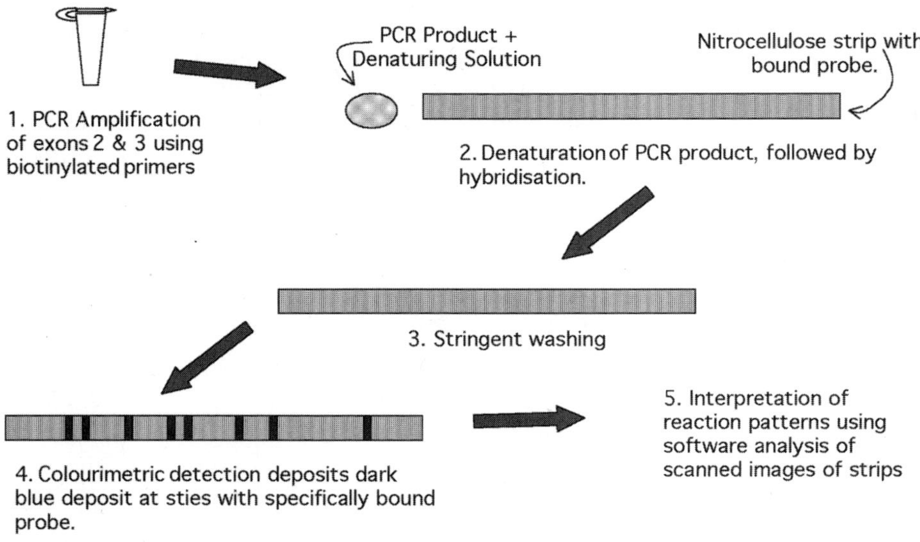
PCR Product +
Denaturing Solution
Nitrocellulose strip with
bound probe.
1. PCR Amplification
of exons 2 & 3 using
biotinylated primers
2. Denaturation of PCR product, followed by
hybridisation.
3. Stringent washing
4. Colourimetric detection deposits dark
blue deposit at sties with specifically bound
probe.
5. Interpretation of
reaction patterns using
software analysis of
scanned images of strips
Reli SSO HLA Typing Strips (Dynal, UK),
LiPA Strips (Innogenetics)

Fig. 2. The principle of sequence-specific oligonucleotide probing (SSOP) has been used in the manufacture of reverse slot blot strips for HLA typing. PCR, polymerase chain reaction; HLA, human leukocyte antigen.

major revision was published in July 2002 *(6)*. A guide to the current nomenclature for HLA antigens and alleles is summarized in **Table 1**. HLA alleles described in publications printed before July 2002 may have changed their nomenclature, and it is advisable to refer to **ref. *6*** for clarity.

5. Influence of HLA Matching

5.1. Solid Organ Transplantation

We shall see that the influence of HLA matching in solid organ transplants depends on which organ is being considered for transplant. The degree of HLA matching deemed suitable or necessary by individual transplant communities is very much country- and center-specific. In general, the degree of HLA mismatch for a particular transplant is the number of broad antigen specificities (as defined by serological nomenclature) mismatched at the HLA-A, -B, and -DR loci, in that order. A totally HLA-mismatched transplant is therefore referred to as a 2:2:2, whereas a 0:0:0 transplant would indicate that no broad antigens were mismatched at any of the three loci.

Table 1
Reference Guide to HLA Nomenclature

Nomenclature	Interpretation	
HLA-A	Indentification of HLA locus	
HLA-A24	Serologically defined HLA antigen	
HLA-A*	Asterisk denotes HLA alleles defined by analysis of DNA	
HLA-A*24	2-digit resolution	Denotes the allele group (corresponds where possible to the serological group; often termed "low resolution"
HLA-A*2402	4-digit resolution	Sequence variation between alleles results in amino acid substitutions (Coding variation, or nonsynonymous changes)
HLA-A*240201	6-digit resolution	Noncoding variation; sequence changes are synonymous, do not result in amino acid substitution
HLA-A*24020102	8-digit resolution	Sequence variation occurs within introns, or 5'/3' extremities of the gene
HLA-A*24020102L	Alphabetical suffice	Letters (see below) may be used as a suffix to describe the biological expression of the encoded molecule A Aberrant expression C Molecule present in the cytoplasm only L Low levels of expression N Null allele (not expressed) S Secreted molecule present only as soluble form

HLA, human leukocyte antigen.

5.1.1. Kidney Transplantation

The surgical event of kidney transplantation has been developed to the point of becoming a relatively routine procedure. As a result, technical failure rates are very low, and the major barrier to successful transplantation is preventing and/or managing graft-rejection processes.

The immediate concern is the risk of early antibody-mediated rejection, often referred to as hyperacute rejection. This can be prevented by ensuring that both donor and recipient are ABO blood group compatible, which eliminates the potential thrombotic effect of naturally occurring anti-ABO isoagglutinins.

Early antibody-mediated rejection owing to preformed HLA-specific antibodies is also a risk factor ***(14)***. Recipients need to be screened pretransplant for the presence or development of HLA-specific antibodies. If sensitization to any HLA specificities is identified, these can be highlighted as "unacceptable antigens" and avoided as mismatches with any potential donor. A prospective CDC crossmatch is also used to identify transplants with potential for hyperacute rejection. More recently protocols involving flow cytometry have been introduced to provide a more sensitive method of crossmatching if required.

In kidney transplantation it is widely accepted that the avoidance of HLA mismatches improves actuarial graft survival and reduces the incidence of acute rejection and sensitization to mismatched specificities. Evidence-based single- and multicenter studies can demonstrate an incremental increase in actuarial graft survival over time as the number of HLA mismatches is reduced ***(15–18)***. Opelz et al. ***(15)*** showed that graft survival was 17% lower for 2:2:2 mismatched transplants than 0:0:0 10 yr after transplant. The strongest impact is accepted as being due to HLA-DR mismatching, followed by HLA-B and finally HLA-A. Beyond 10 yr, the influence on graft survival of the three loci was found to be equivalent and additive.

The sharing of kidneys between centers can dramatically minimize HLA mismatches within transplant programs. The benefit of allocation of kidneys on the basis of HLA specificity matching is still debated, however ***(19)***, given that multidrug, high-dose immunosuppressive regimens can minimize the influence of poorly HLA-matched transplants. The counterargument for shipping organs to improve matching, however, arises from the inevitable extension of cold ischemia times incurred in doing so ***(20)***, which is itself a well-documented risk factor. The potential for longer waiting times for patients with less common HLA phenotypes (such as those belonging to ethnic minorities) also exists.

There is a balance, therefore, between making efforts to minimize HLA mismatches or to rely on more aggressive immunosuppressive regimens to counteract the influence of increased HLA disparity. The payback for the latter protocol is increased susceptibility to posttransplant complications including infection and cancers.

The policies used in different parts of the world for the allocation of kidneys tend to be influenced to a great extent by the geographic constraints of organ sharing. Where localized alliances can be used to exchange organs to improve the degree of matching, it has been demonstrated that the cold ischemic time need not be significantly increased ***(21)***. The time implications generated by shipping organs over vast distances across the United States, however, has resulted in legislation requiring kidneys to be shared only when there are no HLA-A, -B, or -DR (0:0:0) mismatches. Beyond this, kidneys are transplanted locally using other criteria. In Eurotransplant, kidneys are shared whenever possible to minimize HLA mismatches. The United Kingdom has developed a system whereby sharing of kidneys occurs for 0:0:0, 1:0:0, 0:1:0, and 1:1:0 mismatched transplants. If only poorer HLA matches can be identified, kidneys are transplanted locally, with priority recommended to recipients with minimum mismatch at HLA-DR. Where a tie exists, other factors are considered. The factors used highlight the transplantability of an individual as predicted by the commonality of their HLA type in combination with their level of preexisting sensitization to other HLA specificities. In addition, factors such as donor–recipient age disparity and transport times where excessive cold ischemia time is predicted are also weighted into the allocation decision (www.uktrans plant.org.uk).

In the long run, one further advantage of minimizing HLA mismatches that is often overlooked is the effect that this has of limiting the potential for a recipient to become sensitized to multiple non-self HLA epitopes. Following a poorly matched kidney transplant, a patient can become highly sensitized, developing antibodies reactive with more than 50% of the donor population. In this situation it becomes much more difficult to find a cross-match-negative donor should these patients subsequently require a second transplant. Highly sensitized patients may remain relisted for many years before a suitable donor can be found, if at all. Opelz et al. *(15)*, using multicenter analysis, also demonstrated that the influence of HLA mismatches when transplanting sensitized patients was even stronger. The difference between graft survival at 5 yr for these patients is 30% less for recipients with six mismatches when compared to those with no mismatches. Such evidence-based practice should be recognized by transplant centers and used to develop allocation policies to make the best use of the precious but limited supply of donor kidneys.

5.1.2. Heart Transplantation

Alternatives to heart transplantation such as the use of angiotensin-converting enzyme inhibitors *(22)* are noticeably reducing the number of patients being listed for heart transplantation. This may be compounded in the future by the use of implantable ventricular assist devices, which are currently under development. Heart transplant activity is currently on the decline and may well continue to decrease *(23)*. Given the highly polymorphic nature of the HLA system, shorter waiting lists only exacerbate the difficulty of finding a well-matched recipient for an individual heart. In contrast to kidney transplantation, much more consideration is required in terms of size matching the donor and recipient. Once this, together with ABO blood group compatibility, age matching, and perhaps Cytomegalovirus (CMV) compatibility has been taken into account, selecting suitable HLA-matched recipients from a small waiting list is extremely limiting and may not even be possible in some instances. Given the clinical urgency to transplant patients who are listed, the addition of a further selection tier allowing HLA compatibility to be considered has not been supported. In addition, the relatively short cold ischemia time permissible for hearts (ideally <3 h with a 6-h upper limit) prevents long-distance shipping of the organ from being a viable option in the pursuit of better matching. Even when a patient with identified HLA-specific antibodies requires a prospective crossmatch, the limited time available can exclude donors where sample transportation time to the laboratory is too excessive. In this respect the field of kidney transplantation has big advantages.

The influence of HLA in the allocation of donor hearts is, therefore, on the whole overridden by these other risk factors. If a center has two potential recipients with equal clinical suitability, there is evidence to support using HLA mismatch, with particular emphasis on HLA-DR, as a supplement to the selection process ***(24–27)***. The level of HLA matching achieved in kidney transplantation will never be reached in heart transplantation. However, by not considering the level of HLA mismatching within the recipient selection process, who knows what golden opportunities may be being overlooked.

5.1.3. Lung Transplantation

The influence of HLA in lung transplantation is open to debate. As with heart transplantation, and for much the same reasons, donated lungs are allocated on the whole without consideration of HLA compatibility. Only when a potential recipient has been found to be sensitized to predefined HLA specificities is the donor HLA type used to determine suitability. As a result, HLA-mismatch data collected for heart and lung transplants record few cases in which little or no mismatch exists. With time, more cases where few HLA mismatches exist are gradually added. This, however, is a slow process, and the bias of data collected toward transplants with few matches has been a major obstacle to comparative analysis. The poorer outcome of lung transplants compared to hearts is indicative of additional risk factors that help to mask other influences such as HLA.

More recently, as databases have expanded, publications have indicated that HLA mismatches have an influence on acute rejection ***(28)*** as well as on the development of bronchiolitis obliterans syndrome, one of the most significant posttransplant obstacles to long-term graft function ***(29)***. Yet again, HLA-DR mismatch is commonly recognized as having the greatest influence ***(30,31)***.

5.1.4. Liver Transplantation

The influence of HLA compatibility in liver transplantation has not yet been clearly determined. A dualistic effect of HLA matching, first reported by the Pittsburgh group in the late 1980s, postulates that the potential benefit of a liver transplant having reduced allogenicity through HLA matching is masked as a result of the graft being more subject to recurrent disease. Donaldson et al.

(32) examined this theory in the early 1990s in a study of 466 liver transplants. This study concluded that full class I matching in liver transplantation may have an adverse effect, but that some matching may be desirable.

Subsequent studies have found contradictory evidence, leaving unclear the influence of HLA matching in liver transplantation. There is one constant finding, however, that influences other than HLA compatibility are also involved in determining graft outcome.

The unusual divergence from the expected with liver allografts is further extended by them apparently being much more tolerant to ABO blood group incompatibilities that other solid organ transplants. Even positive HLA-specific crossmatches have been reported as being tolerated in some cases. Both of these scenarios are still on the whole identified as strong risk factors.

5.1.5. Corneal Transplantation

Each year, more than 2000 people in the United Kingdom have their sight restored following corneal transplantation. In the United States, this figure is more than 40,000. Less than 10% of primary grafts undergo immune rejection despite no routine HLA matching and with immunosuppressive protocols limited to the topical application of corticosteroids. This success is indicative of the eye being an immunologically privileged site. The avascularity of successful corneal allografts is the traditional explanation for this phenomenon, but other mechanisms have now been recognized in sustaining this process. Suppression of inflammatory resources in the eye has thought to have arisen through evolutionary pressures to protect vision *(33)*. The expression of Fas ligand (CD95L) in the eye acts to induce apoptosis of infiltrating inflammatory cells, whereas T-helper-cell-1 responses are actively suppressed. The fact that no passenger donor APCs are transplanted with the allograft, as in other solid organ transplants, means that the potential for direct allorecognition is eliminated. This is also thought to be a protective factor.

Graft rejection does, however, occur if the graft bed becomes vascularized. In cases where a regraft is required, HLA matching, or the avoidance of HLA mismatches identified from the primary graft is required *(34)*. As in all solid organ transplantation, any reexposure to mismatched HLA antigens in a second graft that have provided the target for a primary sensitization event is a contraindication to transplant.

5.2. Hematopoietic Stem Cell Transplantation

Hematopoietic stem cell transplantation (HSCT) is used to restore impaired bone marrow and is most commonly used to treat acute and chronic leukemias, myeloma, or aplastic anemia. In some cases HSCT may be used to resolve a congenital metabolic disorder, such as an enzyme deficiency. Autologous HSCTs may be carried out by stimulating an individual to produce a large number of stem cells, which can then be harvested, stored, and returned to the donor after intensive chemotherapy. This technique allows the delivery of more extensive chemotherapy, knowing that the patient's immune system can be restored safely after treatment. There is no need for HLA matching for autologous HSCT.

Allogeneic HSCT refers to transplantation where the donor is a second individual. It is in these instances where HLA matching is of prime importance. In HSCT, the recipient's bone marrow is ablated and replaced by the donor's hematopoietic stem cells. The donor's stem cells migrate to the recipient's marrow cavity, where they seed and produce a new, healthy immune system. It is essential that the HLA match of the donor be as close as possible to that of the recipient, and it should be matched not only for HLA-A, -B, and -DR, but also for HLA-C, -DQ, and, if possible, -DP *(35)*. Otherwise, as the donor marrow engrafts, the circulating donor leukocytes may identify the recipient as foreign and produce an immune response directly against the recipient. This phenomenon, graft-vs-host disease (GVHD), may affect skin, gut, and liver, among other organs. GVHD ranges in severity from mild (skin involvement) to life threatening (multiple organs affected).

It is interesting that where the donor is a monozygotic twin of the recipient, there is an increased risk of leukemia returning posttransplant (relapse), compared with cases where the donor is an HLA-identical sibling. There is clearly a compromise with matching, therefore, where there is an advantage for the donor to have a slightly different genetic background. This facilitates the elimination of any residual leukemic cells within the recipient's marrow by the leukocytes of the newly seeded graft. This phenomenon, the graft-vs-leukemia (GVL) effect, is associated with increased overall survival.

In matching for HSCT, we aim to achieve a balance between the GVL effect and GVHD. The best overall survival rates are obtained when the donor is an HLA-identical sibling. Unfortunately, this is an option for only approx 25% of patients. The remaining 75% of patients in need of donor stem cells must rely on finding a suitably matched unrelated donor from one of the many donor registries worldwide. The biggest limitation on HSCT is the availability of adequately matched unrelated donors. The probability of finding a suitably matched donor is directly related to the population frequency of the HLA alleles present in the recipient.

In 1999 a special report recommended that typing of HLA alleles should be at allele group resolution (two digits) *(36)*. This has now been recognized as inadequate, and accreditation bodies such as the European Federation for Immunogenetics recommend that donors and recipients be matched for all loci at the allele level (four digits), where possible, with priority given to matching for class II alleles. Using this approach, survival rates for patients receiving transplants from unrelated donors are not significantly different from those where the donor is an HLA-identical sibling ***(37)***. Some centers have extended matching by including additional markers within the MHC in an attempt to extend the matching of HLA haplotypes ***(38)***.

Petersdorf et al. ***(39)*** suggested that in unrelated donation, a single mismatch at the allele level (four digits) at either HLA-A, -B, -Cw, -DRB1, or -DQB1 does not significantly increase the risk of graft failure, whereas a single mismatch at the allele-group level (two digits) does. This introduces the concept that it may be possible to "trade off" acceptable mismatches in unrelated donors in favor of other desirable characteristics of a donor, such as matching for CMV serostatus, donor age, and donor gender ***(40)***.

6. The Future

There is overwhelming clinical support for transplantation as the treatment of choice for end-stage organ failure. As a result, this is a quickly expanding field both clinically and academically. Technical advances in developing molecular methodologies for high-resolution HLA typing are always in progress. The most promising of these methods are the Luminex and Microarray technologies, both of which use the underlying principals of PCR-SSOP described earlier.

Clinically, it is quite possible that the near future will see an expansion in the use of single-cell populations in transplantation. This approach, utilizing pancreatic islets and neural cells, has already been pioneered at some specialist centers. Scientific manipulation of embryonic stem cells may also hold the key to future advances. Until such advances materialize or developments in immunosuppressive therapies allow grafts to be protected with no known side effects, there will always be a need for HLA matching.

References

1. Dausset, J. (1958) Iso-leuco anticorps. *Acta Haematol.* **20**, 156–166.
2. Van Rood, J. J. and Van Leeuwen, A. (1963) Leucocyte grouping. A method and its applications. *J. Clin. Invest.* **42**, 1382–1390.
3. Payne, R., Trip, M., Weigle, J., Bodmer, W., and Bodmer, J. (1964) A new leukocyte iso-antigen system in man. *Cold Spring Harbour Symp.* **29**, 285–295.
4. Snell, G. D. (1948) Methods for the study of histocompatibility genes. *J. Genet.* **49**, 87–108.
5. Gorer, P. A. (1937) The genetic and antigenic basis for tumor transplantation. *J. Pathol. Bacteriol.* **44**, 691–697.
6. Marsh, S. G. E., Albert, E. D., Bodmer, W. F., et al. (2002) Nomenclature for factors of the HLA system 2002. *Tissue Antigens* **60**, 407–464.
7. Terasaki, P. I. and McClelland, J. D. (1964) Microdroplet assay of human cytotoxins. *Nature* **204**, 998–1000.

8. Vartdal, F., Gaudernack, G., Funderud, S., et al. (1986) HLA class I and II typing using cells positively selected from blood by immunomagnetic isolation—a fast and reliable technique. *Tissue Antigens* **28**, 301–312.
9. Olerup, O. and Zetterquist, H. (1993) HLA-DR typing by PCR amplification with sequence-specific primers (PCR-SSP) in 2 hours; an alternative to serological DR typing in clinical practice including donor recipient matching in cadaveric transplantation. *Tissue Antigens* **39**, 225–235.
10. Bignon, J. D., Fernandez-Vina, M. A., Cheneau, M. L., et al. (1997) HLA DNA class II typing by PCR-SSOP: 12th International Histocompatibility Workshop experience, in *HLA Genetic Diversity of HLA Functional and Medical Implication*, Proceedings of the 12th International Histocompatibility Workshop, Vol. 1 (Charron, D. ed.), EDK Press, Paris, pp. 21–25.
11. Kennedy, L. J., Poulton, K. V., Thomson, W., et al. (1997) HLA class I DNA typing using sequence specific oligonucleotide probes (SSOP), in *HLA Genetic Diversity of HLA Functional and Medical Implication*, Proceedings of the 12th International Histocompatibility Workshop, Vol. 1 (Charron, D., ed.), EDK Press, Paris, pp. 216–225.
12. Cao, K., Chopek, M., and Fernandez-Vina, M. A. (1999) High and intermediate resolution DNA typing systems for class I HLA-A, B, C genes by hybridisation with sequence specific oligonucleotide probes (SSOP). *Rev, Immunogenet.* **1**, 177–208.
13. Buyse, I., Decorte, R., Baens, M., et al. (1993) Rapid DNA typing of class II HLA antigens using the polymerase chain reaction and reverse dot blot hybridisation. *Tissue Antigens* **41**, 1–14.
14. Patel, R. and Terasaki, P. I. (1969) Significance of the positive crossmatch test in kidney transplantation. *N. Engl. J. Med.* **280(14)**, 735–739.
15. Opelz, G., Wujciak, T., Dohler, B., Scherer, S., and Mytilineos, J. (1999) HLA compatibility and organ transplant survival. *Rev. Immunogenet.* **1**, 334–342.
16. Dyer, P. A., Johnson, R. W., Martin, S., et al. (1989) Evidence that matching for HLA antigens significantly increases transplant survival in 1001 renal transplants performed in the northwest region of England. *Transplantation* **48(1)**, 131–135.
17. Festenstein, H., Doyle, P., and Holmes, J. (1986) Long-term follow-up in London Transplant Group recipients of cadaver renal allografts. The influence of HLA matching on transplant outcome. *N. Engl. J. Med.* **314(1)**, 7–14.
18. Ayoub, G. and Terasaki, P. (1982) HLA-DR matching in multicenter, single-typing laboratory data. *Transplantation* **33(5)**, 515–517.
19. Starzl, T. E., Eliasziw, M., Gjertson, D. J., et al. (1997) HLA and cross-reactive group matching for cadaveric kidney allocation. *Transplantation* **64**, 983–991.
20. Mange, K. C., Cherikh, W. S., Maghirang, J., and Bloom, R. D. (2001) A comparison of the survival of shipped and locally transplanted cadaveric renal allografts. *N. Engl. J. Med.*. **34** ,1237–1242.
21. Oniscu, G. C., Plant, W., Pocock, P., and Forsythe, J. L. (2002) Scotland-Northern Ireland Alliance in conjunction with UK Transplant, United Kingdom. Does a

kidney-sharing alliance have to sacrifice cold ischemic time for better HLA matching? *Transplantation* **73**, 1647–1652.
22. Eichhorn, E. J. (2001) Prognosis determination in heart failure. *Am. J. Med.* **110 (Suppl. 7A)**, 14s–36s.
23. Large, S. R.(2002) Is there a crisis in cardiac transplantation? *Lancet* **359**, 803–803.
24. Sheldon, S., Yonan, N. A., Aziz, T. N., et al. (1999) The influence of histocompatibility on graft rejection and graft survival within a single centre population of heart transplant recipients. *Transplantation* **68**, 515–519.
25. Smith, J. D., Rose, M. L., Pomerance, A., Burke, M., and Yacoub, M. H. (1995) Reduction of cellular rejection and increase in longer-term survival after heart transplantation after HLA-DR matching. *Lancet* **346(8986)**, 1318–1322.
26. Opelz, G. and Wujciak, T. (1994) The influence of HLA compatibility on graft survival after heart transplantation. *N. Engl. J. Med.* **330(12)**, 816–819.
27. Kerman, R. H., Van-Buren, C. T., Lewis, R. M., Frazier, O. H., Cooley, D., and Kahan, B. D. (1988) The impact of HLA A, B, and DR blood transfusions and immune responder status on cardiac allograft recipients treated with cyclosporine. *Transplantation* **45(2)**, 333–337.
28. Schulman, L. L., Weinberg, A. D., McGregor, C., Galantowicz, M. E., Suciu-Foca, N. M., and Itescu, S. (1998) Mismatches at the HLA-DR and HLA-B loci are risk factors for acute rejection after lung transplantation. *Am. J. Respir. Crit. Care Med.* **157**, 1833–1837.
29. Schulman, L. L., Weinberg, A. D., McGregor, C., Suciu-Foca, N. M., and Itescu, S. (2001) Influence of donor and recipient HLA locus mismatching on the development of obliterative bronchiolitis after lung transplantation. *Am. J. Respir. Crit. Care Med.* **163**, 437–442.
30. van den Berg, J. W., Hepkema, B. G., Geertsma, A., et al. (2001) Long-term outcome of lung transplantation is predicted by the number of HLA-DR mismatches. *Transplantation* **71(3)**, 368–373.
31. Chalermskulrat, W., Neuringer, I. P., Schmitz, J. L., et al. (2003) Human leukocyte antigen mismatches predispose to the severity of bronchiolitis obliterans syndrome after lung transplantation. *Chest* **123(6)**, 1825–1831.
32. Donaldson, P., Underhill, J., Doherty, D., et al. (1993) Influence of human leukocyte antigen matching on liver allograft survival and rejection: "the dualistic effect." *Hepatology* **17**, 1008–1015.
33. Niederkorn, J. Y. (2002) Immune privilege in the anterior chamber of the eye. *Crit. Rev. Immunol.* **22**, 13–46.
34. Bartels, M. C., Doxiadis, I. N., Colen, T. P., and Beekhuis, W. H. (2003) Long-term outcome in high-risk corneal transplantation and the influence of HLA-A and HLA-B matching. *Cornea* **22**, 552–556.
35. Charron D. (2003) Immunogenomics of hematopoietic stem cell transplantation. *Transfus. Clin. Biol.* **10**, 156–158.
36. Hurley, C. K., Wade, J. A., Oudshoorn, M., et al, on behalf of the Quality Assurance and Donor Registries Working Groups of the World Marrow Donor Asso-

ciation. (1999) A special report: histocompatibility testing guidelines for haematopoietic stem cell transplantation using volunteer donors. *Hum. Immunol.* **60**, 347–360.

37. Mickelson, E. M., Petersdorf, E., Anasetti, C., Martin, P., and Hansen. J. A. (1998) HLA matching in haematopoietic cell transplantation, in *HLA 1998* (Gjertson, D. W. and Terasaki, P. L., eds.), American Society for Histocompatibility and Immunogenetics, Lenexa, KS, pp. 47–56.
38. Gaudieri, S., Longman-Jacobson, N., Tay, G. K., and Dawkins, R. L. (2001) Sequence analysis of the MHC class I region reveals the basis of the genomic matching technique. *Hum. Immunol.* **62(3)**, 279–285.
39. Petersdorf, E. W., Hansen, J. A., Martin, P. J., et al. (2001) Major histocompatibility complex class I alleles and antigens in haematopoietic cell transplantation. *N. Engl. J. Med.* **345**, 1794–1800.
40. Kollman, C., Howe, C. W. S., Anasetti, C., et al. (2001) Donor characteristics as risk factors after transplantation of bone marrow from unrelated donors: the effect of donor age. *Blood* **97(7)**, 2043–2051.

8

Strategies for Gene Transfer to Solid Organs

Viral Vectors

Charlotte Lawson

Summary

A major complication associated with transplantation of solid organs is immunological rejection, which is currently controlled pharmacologically with immunosuppressive drugs, which must be administered indefinitely and may have harmful side effects. Gene transfer to donor organs or recipient immune cells prior to transplantation could limit their use. The effects of transfer of candidate genes in experimental models of allograft rejection is outlined in this chapter, followed by a description of the features of an ideal gene-therapy vector. Finally, a brief overview of viral vector systems used commonly for gene transfer is presented.

Key Words: Gene therapy; transplantation; viral vectors; retrovirus; adenovirus; adeno-associated virus; herpes simplex virus.

1. Introduction

Solid organ grafting remains the only cure for several end-stage diseases. A major complication associated with transplantation is immunological rejection of organs, which is currently controlled by systemic administration of immunosuppressive drugs indefinitely. This can lead to opportunistic infections and drug-specific toxicity. One of the major challenges in transplant immunology today is to overcome the need for such long-term regimes. Ex vivo gene transfer to donor organs or recipient immune cells prior to transplantation is an attractive approach.

2. Genes To Be Delivered to Solid Organ Grafts

Although at this time no gene-therapy trials are registered in either the United States (www4.od.nih.gov/oba/Rdna.htm) or the United Kingdom (www.doh.

From: *Methods in Molecular Biology, vol. 333: Transplantation Immunology: Methods and Protocols*
Edited by: P. Hornick and M. Rose © Humana Press Inc., Totowa, NJ

gov.uk/genetics/gtac) addressing the complications of solid organ transplantation, gene-transfer strategies have been employed in several animal models of allotransplantation using a number of different approaches. These therapies fall broadly into three categories: induction of immune tolerance, reduction of inflammatory responses, and prevention of ischemia/reperfusion (I/R) injury.

2.1. Induction of Immune Tolerance

A recent review ***(1)*** has described some of the strategies for the induction of immune tolerance of allografts by co-stimulatory blockade or molecular chimerism. Transfer of genes encoding soluble co-stimulatory molecules such as cytotoxic T-lymphocyte antigen-4-Ig or CD40-Ig can prolong survival of renal ***(2)***, islet ***(3)***, hepatic ***(4)***, or cardiac ***(5,6)*** allografts in rodent models.

Donor-specific hyporesponsiveness has been achieved by transfer of autologous hematopoietic stem cells genetically modified to express donor-specific major histocompatibility complex (MHC) genes (molecular chimerism) in several rodent and large-animal allotransplantation models. This prolongs survival of renal and skin allografts ***(7–9)*** and can induce long-term T-cell tolerance ***(9)***.

2.2. Cytokine Gene Transfer

Cytokines play a critical role in modulating inflammation and cellular infiltration in transplanted organs. Proinflammatory and T-helper-type cytokines such as tumor necrosis factor, interferon (IFN)-γ, interleukin (IL)-8, IL-12, and IL-18 are upregulated during cold ischemia and are associated with poor outcome. It has been hypothesized, therefore, that overexpression of potent anti-inflammatory cytokines such as IL-10 and IL-4 in graft tissue could limit ongoing inflammation and prevent further injury ***(10)***. Gene transfer of human ***(10)***, mouse ***(11)***, or viral (derived from Epstein-Barr virus *BCRFI* open reading frame [ORF] ***[12]***) IL-10 in animal models of lung transplantation has been shown to prolong early graft function and reduce bronchial obliteration, while gene transfer of human ***(13)*** or viral ***(14,15)*** IL-10 has also been shown to prolong cardiac allograft survival. Gene transfer of IL-13, another anti-inflammatory cytokine, prior to allotransplantation modestly improved graft survival ***(16)***. Intracoronory transfer of transforming growth factor-β gene to donor hearts was also beneficial ***(14)***. In contrast, administration of autologous dendritic cells engineered to express IL-4 prior to transplantation led to enhanced pro-inflammatory gene expression and accelerated organ rejection of murine cardiac allografts ***(17)***.

2.3. Modulation of Ischemia/Reperfusion Injury

Nonallospecific processes also have an important role in graft survival, not least of which are inflammatory responses and I/R injury to donor organs at time of transplantation. Several studies have examined the possibility of reducing the impact of this damage by transduction of potentially cytoprotective genes. Transduction of rat hearts with heat-shock proteins-70 and -72 or IL-1 receptor antagonist using inactivated hemagglutinating virus of Japan prior to heterotopic transplantation has been shown to reduce I/R injury ***(18–20)***, whereas in a model of liver transplantation, gene transfer of copper–zinc superoxide dismutase led to indefinite graft survival and reduction in necrosis ***(21, 22)***. Catalase and hemoxygenase-1 can also protect against I/R injury ***(21–27)***.

2.4. Inhibition of Vasculopathy

Vasculopathy is a well-described feature of chronic rejection of solid organ allografts comprising formation of an extensive neointima within grafted vessels. The lesion is similar in many respects to the lesion seen after restenosis injury with proliferation of smooth muscle cells, recruitment of inflammatory and hematopoietic cells, platelet aggregation, and thrombus formation. Several studies have shown that overexpression of genes that negatively regulate cellular proliferation in vitro can reduce neointima formation in vivo in animal models of restenosis injury ***(28)***. Overexpression of the cyclin-dependent kinase inhibitor $p27^{kip1}$ ***(29)*** or a fusion protein of $p27^{kip1}$ and $p16^{Ink4}$ ***(30)*** attenuated smooth muscle cell proliferation and neointima formation in a balloon-injured porcine artery model. Inhibition of transcriptional activity of the transcription factor E2F by expression of a constitutively active form of Rb, a negative regulator of cell-cycle regulation ***(31)***, or Rb2 ***(32)*** or Rb-E2F fusion protein ***(33)*** has also all been shown to be effective in limiting neointima formation. The transfer of similar genes to allografts could prolong graft function beyond current expectations.

2.5. RNA Interference

An exciting possibility for the future is the inhibition of genes that may promote allo-immune reactions (e.g., co-stimulatory molecules, adhesion molecules, cytokines, or their receptors). Delivery of antisense oligodeoxynucleotides to intercellular adhesion molecule-1, using nonviral methods, to allografts at the time of implantation has been described and has been shown improve graft survival ***(34–36)***. The efficacy of such approaches may be improved with the development of techniques for RNA interference. This is a conserved process that involves the silencing of specific genes with double-stranded RNA ***(37,38)***. Short double-stranded RNA oligonucleotides (small interfering RNA [siRNA]) have been shown to "knock down" specific genes in vitro ***(39–41)***, whereas adenovirus vectors encoding the sequence required to produce complementary strands of siRNA attached via a linker can infect cells, leading to gene silencing of targeted genes in vitro ***(42)*** and in vivo **(43)**. Recently, gene silencing of Fas has been achieved in vivo, leading to significant amelioration of fulminant hepatitis ***(44)***.

3. General Considerations for Gene Transfer

Although there are some examples of efficient transfer of naked DNA into cells and tissues, introduction of genetic material into most sites requires the use of a vector to efficiently deliver the DNA to cells. The ideal gene-therapy vector has several properties, which are outlined here. Current research into the development of vectors for gene therapy can be divided into viral and nonviral vector-mediated gene delivery. The relative advantages and disadvantages of both delivery methods are discussed in the next chapter.

1. *Efficient delivery of DNA*: In general, naked DNA is very inefficiently taken up by cells, so there has been much effort to improve gene delivery using either modified viruses (viral vectors; *see* below) or refining nonviral delivery by targeting to cell-surface proteins (discussed in the following chapter).
2. *Safety*: Vectors must not be pathogenic or toxic to patients. Although nonviral delivery systems are considered to be a relatively safe method of gene transfer, there are several safety concerns with viral vectors. One concern is that recombination events could occur in vivo between endogenous viral elements and transduced viral vectors, leading to the formation of potentially pathogenic replication-competent virus. Second, although the integration of introduced genetic material into the host cell genome is desirable, since it leads to longer term expression of the transgene, it carries with it the risk of insertional mutagenesis and activation of oncogenes. Introduction of plasmid DNA (either naked or packaged) is not without risk, however. A recent study has shown that bacterial lipopolysaccharide (LPS) contamination is an obligatory contaminant of plasmid DNA purified from bacteria by standard laboratory procedures and cannot be completely removed from plasmid preparations. Thus, introduction of plasmid DNA could have pathological consequences, triggering LPS-mediated toxicity in vivo ***(45)***. In addition, selectable markers derived from bacterial genomes, which may be incorporated into vectors for ex vivo propagation, could be antigenic if they enter the hematopoietic cell lineage. It is possible for protein to be expressed, which could be presented in MHC class I and cause CD8 T-cell immune responses (i.e., genetic immunization could occur). This could be detrimental to the patient ***(46)***.
3. *Specificity*: It is important to avoid unpredictable side effects because of the ectopic expression of the transgene in normal tissues (in the context of transplantation these are recipient tissues).
4. *Regulation*: This is a highly desirable property, allowing for activation of a transgene when needed, maintenance of transgene expression within a therapeutic window, and the possibility of silencing if necessary. There has been some success in vitro and in animal models using antibiotic-responsive promoters (e.g., TetON) ***(47)*** or use of a hypoxia switch ***(48–50)***, which may be of particular use in the transplant setting.

5. *Delivery of any gene, whatever size or function*: In theory, there is no limit to the size of DNA that can be delivered by nonviral methods of gene transfer. On the other hand, there is often a limit to the amount of foreign DNA that can be inserted into viral vectors depending on the size of the wild-type viral genome and the number of viral genes deleted because inserts much larger than the endogenous DNA that has been removed will not be efficiently packaged by viral structural proteins.
6. *High-level and long-term expression*: DNA delivered by nonviral methods can be rapidly removed from cells by lysosomal degradation. There are many strategies to overcome this (*see* Chapter 9). Viral transfer of DNA is more efficient than nonviral transfer, and viruses have evolved strategies to avoid degradation within the host cell. However, immunogenicity of viral genes, necessary for transduction of target cells, may limit the duration of transgene expression.
7. *Cost-effectiveness*: Vectors should be inexpensive to produce in large quantities. The production of sufficient quantities of viruses for gene-therapy applications often requires complex purification procedures and quality-control measures. On the other hand, vectors for nonviral transfer of DNA take less time to prepare, do not require such stringent quality control assays before use, and have less batch-to-batch variation in potency.

4. Viral Vectors

The viral life cycle has evolved to efficiently transfer genetic material into host cells (infection) followed by expression of viral proteins and assembly of new viral particles (replication). Gene-therapy vectors have been developed that take advantage of the viral life cycle with a modified genome carrying a therapeutic gene cassette in place of the viral genome. Transduction is defined as the abortive (nonreplicative) infection introducing functional genetic information expressed from recombinant vectors in target cells.

The viral genome comprises genes required for replication and infection as well as *cis*-acting regulatory sequences. In order to improve safety and prevent reconstitution into productive viral particles by recombination events, where possible most viral genes and regulatory sequences are removed during construction of viral vector plasmids. It has been found that viral genes can be expressed in *trans* on separate plasmids in “helper” or “packaging” cells to ensure stability and limit remobilization ***(51)***. Packaging cells are engineered eukaryotic cells that express viral proteins needed for propagation of vectors. This is generally achieved by permanent transfection of plasmids encoding viral proteins into cultured cell lines. Packaging cell lines typically express the viral proteins required to package the vectors but lack a packaging signal. In contrast, viral vector plasmids typically lack some or all of the genes required for propagation, but they will have a packaging signal and other virally encoded essential regulatory sequences, as well as a strong constitutive promoter (sometimes endogenous to the original virus or from other viruses, e.g., cytomegalovirus [CMV] early promoter) and polyadenylation signals. They may also contain sequences required for efficient propagation of the vector in bacteria and a multicloning site for cloning of insert DNA. To further minimize replication-competent virus production, these genes may be encoded on more than one separate plasmid. Shuttle vectors or gutless vectors encoding only the gene of interest together with a strong promoter and polyadenylation sequences and essential viral packaging signals have also been employed in different viral delivery systems. Helper viruses are not often used because of the likelihood that a replication-competent virus could be generated through high-frequency recombination *(52)* **(Fig. 1)**.

Several different virus families have been exploited for gene therapy-applications owing to the efficiency of infection and cell tropism **(Table 1)**. A brief overview of viral vector systems used commonly for gene transfer is given here.

5. Retroviruses

Retroviruses are RNA viruses that replicate through an integrated DNA intermediate (*see* **ref.** ***53*** for full description). Retroviral particles encapsulate two copies of the full-length viral RNA, each copy containing the full genetic information needed for virus replication, including the *gag* (group-specific antigen), *pro* (protease), *pol* (polymerase), and *env* (envelope) genes. Retroviruses can be classified into simple and complex retroviruses. Complex viruses encode the essential viral genes above as well as several accessory genes. Further classification divides retroviruses into oncoretroviruses (mostly simple retroviruses, e.g., murine leukemia virus [MLV]), lentiviruses (complex retroviruses, e.g., human immunodeficiency virus-1 [HIV-1]), and spumaviruses (complex retroviruses, e.g., human foamy virus). Currently all three types are being exploited as gene-therapy tools. (For recent reviews *see* **refs.** ***52***, ***54***, and ***55***.)

Fig. 1. *(opposite page)* Strategy for viral vector production. (**A**) Typical viral genome with essential viral genes, regulatory sequences, and packaging signal. In order to produce replication deficient viral vectors, the genetic material is separated onto (**B**) plasmid encoding viral packaging signal and minimum viral regulatory sequences, and (**C**) helper plasmids encoding essential viral genes required for viral replication and packaging. (**D**) Production of packaging cell line by transfection of helper plasmids. (**E**) Production of producer cell line by transfection of packaging cell line with viral vector plasmid. (**F**) Isolation and purification of virus particles from producer cell culture supernatants (e.g., retrovirus vectors) or lysates (e.g., Ad5 vectors). (**G**) Infection of target cells with viral vectors and (**H**) expression of protein of interest in target cells (can be secreted, cell surface, or intracellular protein or could be siRNA to inhibit expression of endogenous protein).

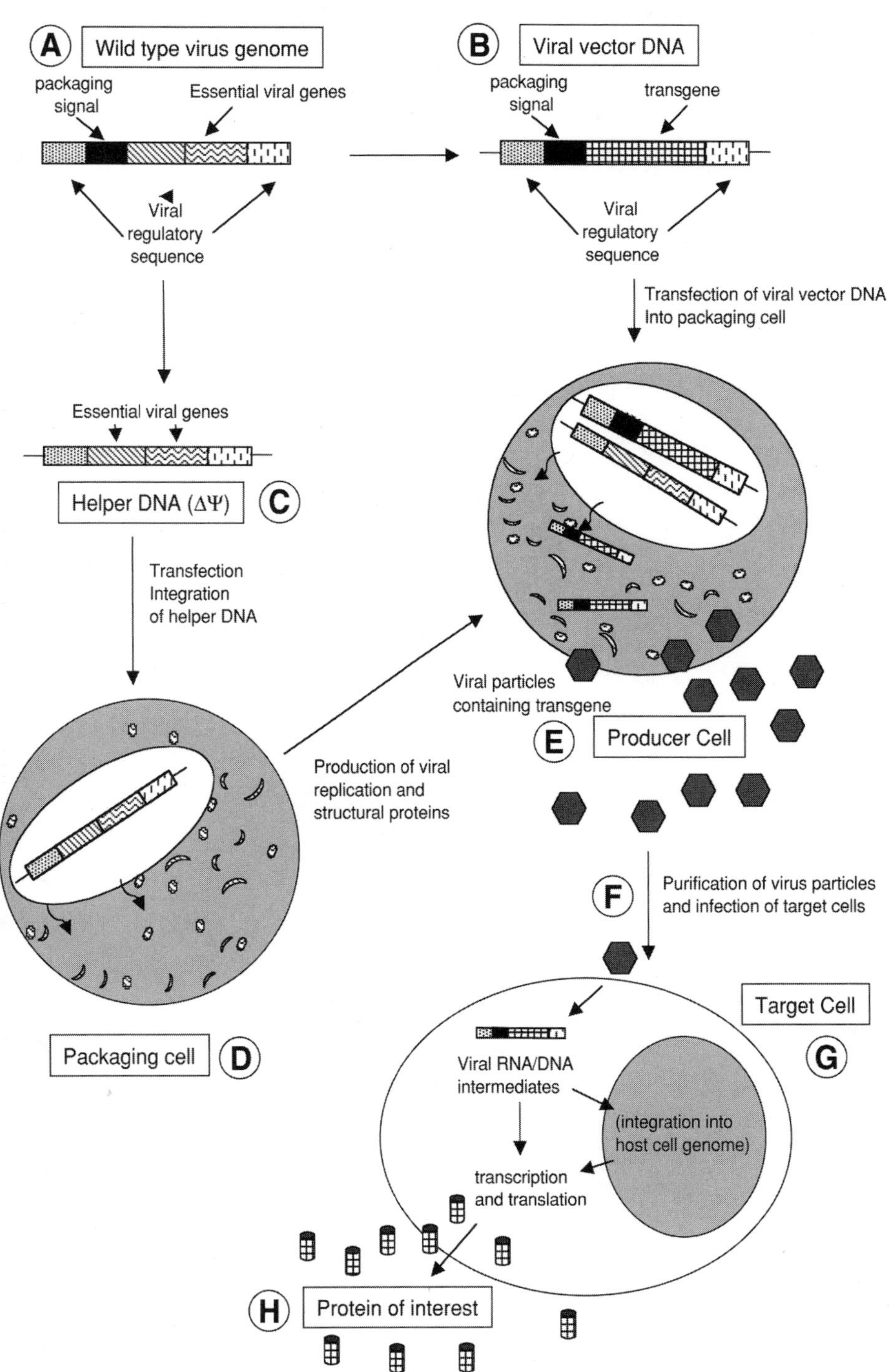
A
Wild type virus genome
packaging signal
Essential viral genes
Viral regulatory sequence
B
Viral vector DNA
packaging signal
transgene
Viral regulatory sequence
Transfection of viral vector DNA Into packaging cell
Essential viral genes
Helper DNA (ΔΨ)
C
Transfection Integration of helper DNA
Production of viral replication and structural proteins
Viral particles containing transgene
E
Producer Cell
Packaging cell
D
F
Purification of virus particles and infection of target cells
Target Cell
G
Viral RNA/DNA intermediates
(integration into host cell genome)
transcription and translation
H
Protein of interest

Table 1
Characteristics of Commonly Used Viral Vectors

	Characteristics	Advantages/future potential	Drawbacks
Oncoretrovirus	Single-stranded RNA simple retrovirus	Relatively high titers (10^8–10^7 cfu/mL) Broad cell tropism Viral genome integration leading to long-term expression of transgene transgene No toxic effects on infected cells Up to 10 kb can be inserted	Risk of insertional mutagenesis Possibility of formation of replication-competent retrovirus by homologous recombination with HERVs Degradation of virus particles by complement Only infect dividing cells
Lentivirus	Single-stranded RNA complex retrovirus	Can infect nondividing cells Expanded cell tropism by pseudotyping Stable gene expression due to integration of viral genome Relatively high titres (10^6–10^7 cfu/mL) Up to 10 kb can be inserted	Possible serum convesion to HIV-1 (current generation vectors) Insertional mutagenesis Presence of tat and rev regulatory proteins may cause immune response Possible recombination with HERVs leading to replication-competent virus
Foamy vius	Complex retrovirus with some simularities to herpes simplex virus life cycle	Stable gene expression due to viral genome integration Innocuous to natural hosts in vivo, although cytopathic to cells in culture Humans are "dead-end hosts" Resistant to complement-mediated lysis Can be pseudotyped Relatively high titers (10^6–10^7 cfu/mL) Up to 14 kb can be inserted	Risk of insertional mutagenesis Recombination with HERVs Serum conversion to human foamy virus (not shown to be pathogenic to humans accidentally infected)

Adenovirs (Ad)	Nonenveloped virus with linear double-standed DNA genome	Very high titers (10^{12} pfu/mL) High levels of gene expression (transient) Can infect nondividing cells Up to 7 kb can be inserted (can be greater if more of Ad genome is detected)	Inflammatory and cytotoxic host immune responses Preformed neutralizing antibodies to Ad particles Not suitable for long-term expression of gene since no integration into host cell genome Complicated vector genome
Adeno-associated virus (AAV)	Small nonenveloped single-stranded DNA genome Belongs to Parvoviridae family	Wide cell tropism Infection of nondividing cells High titers (10^{10} cfu/mL) Possibility of latent infection and integration into host cell genome Up to 4 kb can be inserted Nonpathogenic, nontoxic	Difficult to purify Helper virus (Ad or HSV) may be required for propagation Preformed neutralizing antibodies to AAV Integration into host cell genome is not directed in AAV vectors and could result in insertional mutagenesis
Herpes simplex virus (HSV)	Large enveloped double-stranded DNA virus 152 kb genome Wild-type HSV is highly pathogenic	Titres in the range (10^4–10^8 cfu/mL) Up to 30 kb can be inserted (including multiple genes) No integration into host cell genome Long-term episomal expression of transgene in neuronal cells Cytopathic effects in cancer cell	Inflammatory and toxic reactions in patients Complicated genome and propagation

HERV, human endogenous retrovirus.

5.1. Oncoretroviruses

To date, several registered gene-therapy trials using retroviral transfer have used vectors based on MLV, an amphotropic (able to infect human cells) oncoretrovirus. Oncoretroviruses have a relatively simple genome, which can be easily rearranged to generate replication-defective recombinant viral vectors. In general, they retain retroviral long-terminal repeat sequences, a minimal packaging signal, and the gene of interest. Recombinant replication-defective particles are produced after transfection of oncoretroviral vectors (e.g., pMFG ***[56]***, pBAbe series ***[57]***) into a suitable eukaryotic packaging cell line (e.g., Omega E; GP+E; GP EnvAm12 ***[57–59]***). One disadvantage is that these vectors require dividing cells to be taken up and integrated into the host cell genome for long-term expression of the transgene. Therefore, their usefulness may be limited in clinical applications in which nondividing cells are the targets for gene therapy ***(60)***.

5.2. Lentiviruses

There has been some progress in the development of vectors based on lentiviruses, in particular HIV-1. The lentiviruses have a more complex genome than oncoretroviruses and therefore a more complex replication cycle. Lentiviruses are able to infect nondividing and terminally differentiated cell types, which is a major advantage over oncoretrovirus vectors for gene-therapy applications ***(60)***. The development of lentivirus vectors and packaging cell lines has been more difficult than that of oncoretrovirus vector-delivery systems. Early vectors based on HIV were nearly intact viral genomes with the *env* gene deleted and substituted in *trans*. This enabled the vectors to target CD4-expressing cells efficiently, but targeting to other cells was limited, and viral titers were low. Substitution of the amphotropic MLV envelope glycoprotein broadened the cell-type specificity of these vectors ***(61)***, while vesicular stomatitis virus-G-protein (VSV-G) improved vector titer and greater stability of virus particles ***(62)***. This is known as pseudotyping. Literally, a pseudotyped virus is one in which one or more of the structural proteins of each virus particle are not encoded by the genetic material carried by the virus. However, in the gene-transfer field a pseudotyped virus is one in which the outer shell (the use of envelope glycoproteins from an enveloped virus or the capsid proteins from a nonenveloped virus) originates from a virus that differs from the source of the genome and replication apparatus (for review *see* **ref. *63***).

A second approach was to delete almost all of the viral genome, leaving only a few essential *cis*-acting sequences and providing viral proteins in *trans*. Early attempts relied on co-transfection of viral vectors with helper DNA plasmid constructs. However, this strategy resulted in low titers and increased the risk for generation of recombinant replication-competent virus. The newest vectors (e.g., VSV-G pseudotyped HIV-1 vectors) can be produced with relatively high titers *(64–66)*. They are able to infect cell cycle-arrested cells in culture as well as retinal, muscle, and hepatic cells in vivo with stable expression for several months *(64,67–69)*.

There are now many lentiviral vectors are based on HIV-1 in part because of the huge amount of research into HIV-1 biology. However, owing to concerns over safety, vectors have also been developed from other lentiviruses, which are less pathogenic to humans, including HIV-2 and simian immunodeficiency virus, as well as from feline lentivirus (feline immunodeficiency virus). Chimeric lentivirus vector systems have also been developed. Pseudotyping with VSV-G combined with strong promoters such as CMV promoter has been used to improve cell tropism and transgene expression *(55)*.

5.3. Spumaviruses

Spumaviruses or foamy viruses (FVs) are so named because of the cytopathic foam effect they induce in culture. They are complex retroviruses encoding three accessory genes designated bel1, bel2, and bel3 *(70,71)*. They are innocuous in their natural hosts, which are mainly primates, although nonprimate FVs have been identified *(72)*, and appear to be absent in humans. There have been some cases of accidental infection in humans, but they appear to be apathogenic *(73)*, and there have been no reports of horizontal transmission, suggesting that humans may represent dead-end hosts *(74)*. They persist indefinitely in their hosts, even in the presence of antibodies directed against FV proteins *(75)*. There is a striking similarity between the replication cycles of FV and hepatitis B virus *(76)*.

FVs are highly lytic in culture and have a large cellular tropism *(77)*. FV vectors have been developed that contain only the minimal viral sequences necessary for efficient gene transfer. This vector has been shown to transduce human hematopoietic $CD34^+$ cells and human mesenchymal stem cells in vitro using a four-plasmid packaging cell system *(78)*. Because of the lack of endogenous human FV, the apathogenicity after accidental infection, lack of horizontal transmission, ability to infect nondividing cells, and wide cell tropism, FVs are a promising prospect for future gene-therapy applications.

6. Adenoviruses

Adenoviruses (Ads) are nonenveloped viruses with a linear double-stranded DNA genome. There are 50 distinct serotypes in humans. They are associated with the common cold and can cause respiratory, intestinal, and eye infections in humans *(79,80)*. Ads have been widely used for gene transfer because they have a broad host range and can infect proliferating or nondividing cells. Infection with Ad vectors lead to transient gene expression because the Ad genome does not integrate into the host cell genome.

The genome is functionally divided into early (E) and late (L) regions based on the time of transcription of each gene after infection, with inverted terminal repeats (ITRs) at either end ***(80–82)***. Ad enters the host cell via specific cell-surface receptors, including the well-described coxsackievirus and Ad receptor ***(83)***. It is internalized rapidly via receptor-mediated endocytosis, facilitated via receptors including integrins αvβ3 and αvβ5 ***(84)***.

Many types of Ad vectors have been developed, including replication-competent and replication-defective vectors, mostly based on serotype 2 (Ad2) or serotype 5 (Ad5). The first generation of Ad vectors were E1- and E3-deleted. The second generation includes E1-, E3-, and E4- or E2-deleted vectors based on Ad5. E1-deleted Ad5 vectors are replication defective, but they can be grown in specific cell lines transformed with Ad E1, e.g., human embryonic kidney 293 cells ***(85)***, to supply E1 in *trans*. Deletions of up to 3.2 kb can be made in the E1 region. The nonessential E3 region has also been deleted to accommodate larger inserts. The left-hand ITR and packaging signals from the left-hand 300 bp of the genome are required for replication in 293 cells ***(86)***.

First-generation Ad vectors were only transiently expressed due to a strong immune response elicited by the viral proteins. The use of immunosuppressive drugs could be used to extend transgene expression in the eye ***(87)***, lungs ***(88)***, and in a model of cardiac transplantation ***(89)***.

Second-generation Ad vectors have overcome Ad immunogenicity to some extent by introduction of a mutation in the Ad E2a gene ***(90–92)*** or deletion in E4 ***(93)***. However, these modifications did not mediate significant prolongation of transgene expression compared to first-generation Ad vectors ***(94)***.

A gutted (or gutless) Ad vector has been developed with all of the viral genes deleted in order to reduce immunogenicity. It contains only the ITR required for replication and 5'-*cis*-acting Ad encapsulation signals necessary for packaging ***(95–100)***. However, this vector is difficult to produce, requiring the use of helper virus to provide all the viral proteins in *trans* ***(80)***.

7. Adeno-Associated Virus

Adeno-associated virus (AAV) is a small nonenveloped, single-stranded DNA virus belonging to the parvoviridae group (for review, *see* **ref. *101***). There are two ORFs encoding for nonstructural proteins (Rep) and capsid proteins (Cap). ITR sequences at each end of the genome have been identified as the only *cis*-acting elements required for replication, packaging, and integration of AAV. Thus, AAV vectors can be generated by removal of ORFs with the gene of interest, between the two ITRs, giving AAV vectors a packaging capacity of 4.1–4.9 kb ***(102)***.

Between 50 and 90% of the population is seropositive for AAV. There is no conclusive evidence of any association of AAV with pathology at this time. Six

AAV serotypes have been identified in primates. Serotype 2 has been isolated from humans and extensively studied. Heparin sulfate proteoglycan, fibroblast growth factor-R1, and αvβ5 have been identified as primary and co-receptors for AAV ***(80)***.

AAV is dependent on the presence of a helper virus for propagation, usually Ad or herpesvirus ***(103,104)***. Some genotoxic agents may also induce AAV to replicate ***(105–107)***. In the absence of help, AAV integrates into human chromosome 19 at a particular locus on q13.3qter and establishes latency. After co-infection with the helper virus, the AAV genome is rescued, replicated, and encapsidated into progeny viruses ***(108–110)***.

AAV vectors have been produced by co-transfection of the AAV plasmid together with AAV helper plasmid containing the *Rep* and *Cap* genes into a human cell line (e.g., **ref.** ***293***). Early vectors required infection with helper Ad, but this has been eliminated by co-transfection of plasmids encoding Ad E2A, E4orf6, and VA RNA transcription units ***(80)***, eliminating the possibility of infection of the host with replication-competent helper Ad and subsequent adverse immune responses.

Site-specific integration of latent AAV into human chromosome 19q13.3-qter has generated much interest. However, this process requires AAV Rep proteins, which are not present in AAV vectors, although transgene expression has been reported for months and up to several years in some in vivo models ***(111–116)***, possibly owing to the presence of long-lived double-stranded episomal rAAV genomes ***(117–120)*** or random integration into the host cell genome ***(96,121–125)***.

AAV vectors have been used to deliver transgenes to proliferating and quiescent cells of various species in vitro and in vivo, including muscle, liver, lung central nervous system, eye, and heart ***(111,112,114,121,126–129)***. One difficulty that has been encountered is a variation in transduction efficiency between different cell types.

One advantage of using AAV vectors has been the apparent lack of induction of cellular immune responses, possibly because of the fact that the only genes expressed are the viral capsid and the transgene or the poor transduction of antigen-presenting cells. Lack of immunogenicity may account for the prolonged expression of transgenes in vivo. There is limited activation of the innate immune system and chemokine production, but to a lesser extent than for Ad ***(130)***. Humoral responses to AAV have been detected in animal models, and the presence of neutralizing antibodies greatly reduces the success of vector re-administration ***(131,132)***. Up to 32% of human subjects could have preformed neutralizing antibodies to AAV-2 ***(133)***, which could limit the usefulness of AAV for gene-therapy applications ***(80)***.

8. Herpes Simplex Virus-1

Herpes simplex virus-1 (HSV-1) is a relatively large enveloped double-stranded DNA virus with a 152-kb genome, encoding at least 89 proteins with well-characterized disease pathology ***(134,135)***. Wild-type HSV-1 is a highly pathogenic virus, infecting mucosal epithelial tissue with subsequent lysis of the infected cells. The virus infects sensory neurons and is transported to the nucleus of the neuron. The virus then enters either a lytic or a latent state, both of which are attractive to exploit for gene-therapy applications ***(136–139)***. The lytic cycle of HSV-1 has been exploited for cancer therapy with attenuated replication-competent HSV-1 ***(140–142)***. In the latent state, viral DNA remains extrachromasomal, with only latency-associated transcripts being transcribed. This process is poorly understood but is attractive to gene therapists.

Given the relatively large size of HSV-1, the major benefit of utilizing replication-defective HSV-1 rather than other viral transfection systems is the ability to insert large and/or multiple foreign genes into these vectors. Also, HSV-1 has a relatively large cell tropism, and the genome remains extrachromasomal, minimizing risks of insertional mutagenesis.

HSV-1 genes have been classified as essential or nonessential, depending on their requirement for viral replication in cell culture. However, even genes classified as nonessential are important for HSV-1 replication, and so HSV-1 mutants have been categorized as either helper virus dependent or independent. The helper virus-dependent viruses are also termed amplicons and consist minimally of packaging sequences and an origin of viral DNA replication ***(143,144)***. Helper virus-independent viruses (replication defective) have deletions in one or more essential genes (e.g., deletion of immediate early genes *a 4*, *a 22*, and *a 27*) ***(145)*** and can be grown in packaging cell lines that express the essential gene(s) to provide the gene product in *trans*.

It is possible to insert up to 12 kb of new genetic material into a replication-defective HSV-1 vector by deletion of essential genes (immediate early genes) as well as nonessential genes. In one such vector, genes encoding IL-2, granulocyte-macrophage–colony-stimulating factor, B7.1, and LacZ or IFN-γ were inserted as separate transcriptional units and simultaneously expressed in vitro in primary melanoma cells for up to 1 wk ***(146)*** or L929 tumors ***(147)***. HSV-1 replication-defective vectors are therefore an attractive tool in the transplant setting because genes to induce tolerance, limit I/R injury, and dampen inflammatory responses could all be combined into one vector for delivery.

9. Summary

Gene transfer to donor organs remains an exciting possibility for the future in that it could overcome the need for lifelong immunosuppression of recipients and allow the implantation of allogeneic or xenogeneic organs without adverse consequences. At this time there are no registered trials for human gene therapy to prolong allograft survival, but several research groups are focusing on prolongation of allograft function using gene-transfer technology. Most of these studies have used viral methods of gene transfer, which, as outlined above, provide an effective route of administration, although concerns about safety, immunogenicity, and longevity of expression of transgenes may limit the use of current generations of viral vectors in human transplantation gene-therapy trials. However, many gene-therapy trials using viral vectors have been approved and have shown minimal harmful side effects in other areas of medicine, and research continues to improve vector safety and efficiency.

Acknowledgments

CL is supported by a British Heart Foundation Intermediate Fellowship and grants from the Harefield Research Foundation and Royal Brompton and Harefield NHS Trust Clinical Research Committee.

References

1. Bagley, J. and Iacomini, J. (2003) Gene therapy progress and prospects: gene therapy in organ transplantation. *Gene Ther.* **10**, 605–611.
2. Tomasoni, S., Azzollini, N., Casiraghi, F., Capogrossi, M. C., Remuzzi, G., and Benigni, A. (2000) CTLA4Ig gene transfer prolongs survival and induces donor-specific tolerance in a rat renal allograft. *J. Am. Soc. Nephrol.* **11**, 747–752.
3. Takehara, M., Murakami, M., Inobe, M., et al. (2001) Long-term acceptance of allografts by in vivo gene transfer of regulatable adenovirus vector containing CTLA4IgG and loxP. *Hum. Gene Ther.* **12**, 415–426.
4. Nomura, M., Yamashita, K., Murakami, M., et al. (2002) Induction of donor-specific tolerance by adenovirus-mediated CD40Ig gene therapy in rat liver transplantation. *Transplantation* **73**, 1403–1410.
5. Matsuno, Y., Iwata, H., Yoshikawa, S., et al. (2002) Suppression of graft coronary arteriosclerosis by gene gun-mediated CTLA4-Ig gene transfer. *Transplant. Proc.* **34**, 2619–2621.
6. Guillot, C., Guillonneau, C., Mathieu, P., et al. (2002) Prolonged blockade of CD40-CD40 ligand interactions by gene transfer of CD40Ig results in long-term heart allograft survival and donor-specific hyporesponsiveness, but does not prevent chronic rejection. *J. Immunol.* **168**, 1600–1609.
7. Heim, D. A., Hanazono, Y., Giri, N., et al. (2000) Introduction of a xenogeneic gene via hematopoietic stem cells leads to specific tolerance in a rhesus monkey model. *Mol. Ther.* **1**, 533–544.
8. Sonntag, K. C., Emery, D. W., Yasumoto, A., et al. (2001) Tolerance to solid organ transplants through transfer of MHC class II genes. *J. Clin. Invest.* **107**, 65–71.
9. Bagley, J., Tian, C., Sachs, D. H., and Iacomini, J. (2002) Induction of T-cell tolerance to an MHC class I alloantigen by gene therapy. *Blood* **99**, 4394–4399.

10. de Perrot, M., Fischer, S., Liu, M., et al. (2003) Impact of human interleukin-10 on vector-induced inflammation and early graft function in rat lung transplantation. *Am. J. Respir. Cell Mol. Biol.* **28**, 616–625.
11. Shoji, F., Yonemitsu, Y., Okano, S., et al. (2003) Airway-directed gene transfer of interleukin-10 using recombinant Sendai virus effectively prevents post-transplant fibrous airway obliteration in mice. *Gene Ther.* **10**, 213–218.
12. Itano, H., Mora, B. N., Zhang, W., et al. (2001) Lipid-mediated ex vivo gene transfer of viral interleukin 10 in rat lung allotransplantation. *J. Thorac. Cardiovasc. Surg.* **122**, 29–38.
13. Hong, Y. S., Laks, H., Cui, G., Chong, T. ,and Sen, L. (2002) Localized immunosuppression in the cardiac allograft induced by a new liposome-mediated IL-10 gene therapy. *J. Heart Lung Transplant.* **21**, 1188–1200.
14. Brauner, R., Nonoyama, M., Laks, H., et al. (1997) Intracoronary adenovirus-mediated transfer of immunosuppressive cytokine genes prolongs allograft survival. *J. Thorac. Cardiovasc. Surg.* **114**, 923–933.
15. DeBruyne, L. A., Li, K., Chan, S. Y., Qin, L., Bishop, D. K., and Bromberg, J. S. (1998) Lipid-mediated gene transfer of viral IL-10 prolongs vascularized cardiac allograft survival by inhibiting donor-specific cellular and humoral immune responses. *Gene Ther.* **5**, 1079–1087.
16. Ke, B., Shen, X. D., Zhai, Y., et al. (2002) Heme oxygenase 1 mediates the immunomodulatory and antiapoptotic effects of interleukin 13 gene therapy in vivo and in vitro. *Hum. Gene Ther.* **13**, 1845–1857.
17. Kaneko, K., Wang, Z., Kim, S. H., Morelli, A. E., Robbins, P. D., and Thomson, A. W. (2003) Dendritic cells genetically engineered to express IL-4 exhibit enhanced IL-12p70 production in response to CD40 ligation and accelerate organ allograft rejection. *Gene Ther.* **10**, 143–152.
18. Suzuki, K., Murtuza, B., Sammut, I. A., et al. (2002) Heat shock protein 72 enhances manganese superoxide dismutase activity during myocardial ischemia-reperfusion injury, associated with mitochondrial protection and apoptosis reduction. *Circulation* **106**, I270–1276.
19. Suzuki, K., Murtuza, B., Smolenski, R. T., et al. (2001) Overexpression of interleukin-1 receptor antagonist provides cardioprotection against ischemia-reperfusion injury associated with reduction in apoptosis. *Circulation* **104(12 Suppl 1)**, I308–I313.
20. Jayakumar, J., Suzuki, K., Sammut, I. A., et al. (2001) Heat shock protein 70 gene transfection protects mitochondrial and ventricular function against ischemia-reperfusion injury. *Circulation* **104**, I303–307.
21. Lehmann, T. G., Wheeler, M. D., Schoonhoven, R., Bunzendahl, H., Samulski, R. J.,and Thurman, R. G. (2000) Delivery of Cu/Zn-superoxide dismutase genes with a viral vector minimizes liver injury and improves survival after liver transplantation in the rat. *Transplantation* **69**, 1051–1057.
22. Lehmann, T. G., Wheeler, M. D., Schwabe, R. F., et al. (2000) Gene delivery of Cu/Zn-superoxide dismutase improves graft function after transplantation of fatty livers in the rat. *Hepatology* **32**, 1255–1264.

23. Zhu, H. L., Stewart, A. S., Taylor, M. D., Vijayasarathy, C., Gardner, T. J. ,and Sweeney, H. L. (2000) Blocking free radical production via adenoviral gene transfer decreases cardiac ischemia-reperfusion injury. *Mol. Ther.* **2**, 470–475.
24. Kato, H., Amersi, F., Buelow, R., et al. (2001) Heme oxygenase-1 overexpression protects rat livers from ischemia/reperfusion injury with extended cold preservation. *Am. J. Transplant.* **1**, 121–128.
25. Coito, A. J., Buelow, R., Shen, X. D., et al. (2002) Heme oxygenase-1 gene transfer inhibits inducible nitric oxide synthase expression and protects genetically fat Zucker rat livers from ischemia-reperfusion injury. *Transplantation* **74**, 96–102.
26. Ke, B., Shen, X. D., Melinek, J., et al. (2001) Heme oxygenase-1 gene therapy: a novel immunomodulatory approach in liver allograft recipients? *Transplant. Proc.* **33**, 581–582.
27. Ke, B., Buelow, R., Shen, X. D., et al. (2002) Heme oxygenase 1 gene transfer prevents CD95/Fas ligand-mediated apoptosis and improves liver allograft survival via carbon monoxide signaling pathway. *Hum. Gene Ther.* **13**, 1189–1199.
28. Crook, M. F. and Akyurek, L. M. (2003) Gene transfer strategies to inhibit neointima formation. *Trends Cardiovasc. Med.* **13**, 102–106.
29. Tanner, F. C., Boehm, M., Akyurek, L. M., et al. (2000) Differential effects of the cyclin-dependent kinase inhibitors p27(Kip1), p21(Cip1), and p16(Ink4) on vascular smooth muscle cell proliferation. *Circulation* **101**, 2022–2025.
30. Tsui, L. V., Camrud, A., Mondesire, J., et al. (2001) p27-p16 fusion gene inhibits angioplasty-induced neointimal hyperplasia and coronary artery occlusion. *Circ. Res.* **89**, 323–328.
31. Chang, M. W., Barr, E., Lu, M. M., Barton, K., and Leiden, J. M. (1995). Adenovirus-mediated over-expression of the cyclin/cyclin-dependent kinase inhibitor, p21 inhibits vascular smooth muscle cell proliferation and neointima formation in the rat carotid artery model of balloon angioplasty. *J. Clin. Invest.* **96**, 2260–2268.
32. Claudio, P. P., Fratta, L., Farina, F., et al. (1999) Adenoviral RB2/p130 gene transfer inhibits smooth muscle cell proliferation and prevents restenosis after angioplasty. *Circ. Res.* **85**, 1032–1039.
33. Wills, K. N., Mano, T., Avanzini, J. B., et al. (2001) Tissue-specific expression of an anti-proliferative hybrid transgene from the human smooth muscle alpha-actin promoter suppresses smooth muscle cell proliferation and neointima formation. *Gene Ther.* **8**, 1847–1854.
34. Poston, R. S., Mann, M. J., Hoyt, E. G., Ennen, M., Dzau, V. J., and Robbins, R. C. (1999) Antisense oligodeoxynucleotides prevent acute cardiac allograft rejection via a novel, nontoxic, highly efficient transfection method. *Transplantation* **68**, 825–832.
35. Feeley, B. T., Poston, R. S., Park, A. K., et al. (2000) Optimization of ex vivo pressure mediated delivery of antisense oligodeoxynucleotides to ICAM-1 reduces reperfusion injury in rat cardiac allografts. *Transplantation* **69**, 1067–1074.
36. Toda, K., Kayano, K., Karimova, A., et al. (2000) Antisense intercellular adhesion molecule-1 (ICAM-1) oligodeoxyribonucleotide delivered during organ preserva-

tion inhibits posttransplant ICAM-1 expression and reduces primary lung isograft failure. *Circ. Res.* **86**, 166–174.

37. Fire, A., Xu, S., Montgomery, M. K., Kostas, S. A., Driver, S. E. and Mello, C. C. (1998) Potent and specific genetic interference by double-stranded RNA in *Caenorhabditis elegans*. *Nature* **391**, 806–811.
38. Tuschl, T., Zamore, P. D., Lehmann, R., Bartel, D. P., and Sharp, P. A. (1999) Targeted mRNA degradation by double-stranded RNA in vitro. *Genes Dev.* **13**, 3191–3197.
39. Elbashir, S. M., Harborth, J., Lendeckel, W., Yalcin, A., Weber, K., and Tuschl, T. (2001) Duplexes of 21-nucleotide RNAs mediate RNA interference in cultured mammalian cells. *Nature* **411**, 494–498.
40. Paddison, P. J., Caudy, A. A., Bernstein, E., Hannon, G. J., and Conklin, D. S. (2002) Short hairpin RNAs (shRNAs) induce sequence-specific silencing in mammalian cells. *Genes Dev.* **16**, 948–958.
41. Paddison, P. J., Caudy, A. A. and Hannon, G. J. (2002) Stable suppression of gene expression by RNAi in mammalian cells. *Proc. Natl. Acad. Sci. USA* **99**, 1443–1448.
42. Shen, C., Buck, A. K., Liu, X., Winkler, M. and Reske, S. N. (2003) Gene silencing by adenovirus-delivered siRNA. *FEBS Lett.* **539**, 111–114.
43. Xia, H., Mao, Q., Paulson, H. L., and Davidson, B. L. (2002) siRNA-mediated gene silencing in vitro and in vivo. *Nat. Biotechnol.* **20**, 1006–1010.
44. Song, E., Lee, S. K., Wang, J., et al. (2003) RNA interference targeting Fas protects mice from fulminant hepatitis. *Nat. Med.* **9**, 347–351.
45. Gordillo, G. M., Xia, D., Mullins, A. N., Bergese, S. D., and Orosz, C. G. (1999) Gene therapy in transplantation: pathological consequences of unavoidable plasmid contamination with lipopolysaccharide. *Transplant. Immunol.* **7**, 83–94.
46. Riddell, S. R., Elliott, M., Lewinsohn, D. A., et al. (1996) T-cell mediated rejection of gene-modified HIV-specific cytotoxic T lymphocytes in HIV-infected patients. *Nat. Med.* **2**, 216–223.
47. Apparailly, F., Millet, V., Noel, D., Jacquet, C., Sany, J. and Jorgensen, C. (2002) Tetracycline-inducible interleukin-10 gene transfer mediated by an adeno-associated virus: application to experimental arthritis. *Hum. Gene Ther.* **13**, 1179–1188.
48. Tang, Y., Schmitt-Ott, K., Qian, K., Kagiyama, S., and Phillips, M. I. (2002) Vigilant vectors: adeno-associated virus with a biosensor to switch on amplified therapeutic genes in specific tissues in life-threatening diseases. *Methods* **28**, 259–266.
49. Modlich, U., Pugh, C. W., and Bicknell, R. (2000) Increasing endothelial cell specific expression by the use of heterologous hypoxic and cytokine-inducible enhancers. *Gene Ther.* **7**, 896–902.
50. Hernandez-Alcoceba, R., Pihalja, M., Qian, D., and Clarke, M. F. (2002) New oncolytic adenoviruses with hypoxia- and estrogen receptor-regulated replication. *Hum. Gene Ther.* **13**, 1737–1750.
51. Kay, M. A., Glorioso, J. C., and Naldini, L. (2001) Viral vectors for gene therapy: the art of turning infectious agents into vehicles of therapeutics. *Nat. Med.* **7**, 33–40.

52. Hu, W. S. and Pathak, V. K. (2000) Design of retroviral vectors and helper cells for gene therapy. *Pharmacol. Rev.* **52**, 493–511.
53. Coffin, J. M., Hughes, S. H., and Varmus, H. E. (1997) *Retroviruses* (Coffin, J. M., Hughes, S. H., and Varmus, H. E., eds.), Cold Spring Harbor Laboratory Press, New York.
54. Brenner, S. and Malech, H. L. (2003) Current developments in the design of onco-retrovirus and lentivirus vector systems for hematopoietic cell gene therapy. *Biochim. Biophys. Acta* **1640**, 1–24.
55. Buchschacher, G. L., Jr. and Wong-Staal, F. (2001) Approaches to gene therapy for human immunodeficiency virus infection. *Hum. Gene Ther.* **12**, 1013–1019.
56. Riviere, I., Brose, K., and Mulligan, R. C. (1995). Effects of retroviral vector design on expression of human adenosine deaminase in murine bone marrow transplant recipients engrafted with genetically modified cells. *Proc. Natl. Acad. Sci. USA* **92**, 6733–6737.
57. Morgenstern, J. P. and Land, H. (1990) Advanced mammalian gene transfer: high titre retroviral vectors with multiple drug selection markers and a complementary helper-free packaging cell line. *Nucleic Acids Res.* **18**, 3587–3596.
58. Markowitz, D. G., Goff, S. P., and Bank, A. (1988). Safe and efficient ecotropic and amphotropic packaging lines for use in gene transfer experiments. *Trans. Assoc. Am. Physicians* **101**, 212–218.
59. Markowitz, D., Goff, S., and Bank, A. (1988). A safe packaging line for gene transfer: separating viral genes on two different plasmids. *J. Virol.* **62**, 1120–1124.
60. Lewis, P. F. and Emerman, M. (1994). Passage through mitosis is required for oncoretroviruses but not for the human immunodeficiency virus. *J. Virol.* **68**, 510–516.
61. Page, K. A., Landau, N. R., and Littman, D. R. (1990). Construction and use of a human immunodeficiency virus vector for analysis of virus infectivity. *J. Virol.* **64**, 5270–5276.
62. Yee, J. K., Miyanohara, A., LaPorte, P., Bouic, K., Burns, J. C., and Friedmann, T. (1994). A general method for the generation of high-titer, pantropic retroviral vectors: highly efficient infection of primary hepatocytes. *Proc. Natl. Acad. Sci. USA* **91**, 9564–9568.
63. Sanders, D. A. (2002) No false start for novel pseudotyped vectors. *Curr. Opin. Biotechnol.* **13**, 437–442.
64. Naldini, L., Blomer, U., Gage, F. H., Trono, D., and Verma, I. M. (1996) Efficient transfer, integration, and sustained long-term expression of the transgene in adult rat brains injected with a lentiviral vector. *Proc. Natl. Acad. Sci. USA* **93**, 11,382–11,388.
65. Naldini, L., Blomer, U., Gallay, P., et al. (1996) In vivo gene delivery and stable transduction of nondividing cells by a lentiviral vector. *Science* **272**, 263–267.
66. Blomer, U., Naldini, L., Kafri, T., Trono, D., Verma, I. M. and Gage, F. H. (1997) Highly efficient and sustained gene transfer in adult neurons with a lentivirus vector. *J. Virol.* **71**, 6641–6649.

67. Miyoshi, H., Takahashi, M., Gage, F. H., and Verma, I. M. (1997) Stable and efficient gene transfer into the retina using an HIV-based lentiviral vector. *Proc. Natl. Acad. Sci. USA* **94**, 10,319–10,323.
68. Kafri, T., Blomer, U., Peterson, D. A., Gage, F. H., and Verma, I. M. (1997) Sustained expression of genes delivered directly into liver and muscle by lentiviral vectors. *Nat. Genet.* **17**, 314–317.
69. Kafri, T., van Praag, H., Ouyang, L., Gage, F. H., and Verma, I. M. (1999) A packaging cell line for lentivirus vectors. *J. Virol.* **73**, 576–584.
70. Vogt. (1997) Retroviral virions and genomes, in *Retroviruses* (Coffin, J. M., Hughes, S. H., and Varmus, H. E., eds.), Cold Spring Harbor Press, New York, pp. 27–69.
71. Rethwilm, A., Darai, G., Rosen, A., Maurer, B., and Flugel, R. M. (1987) Molecular cloning of the genome of human spumaretrovirus. *Gene* **59**, 19–28.
72. Lecellier, C. H. and Saib, A. (2000) Foamy viruses: between retroviruses and pararetroviruses. *Virology* **271**, 1–8.
73. Heneine, W., Switzer, W. M., Sandstrom, P., et al. (1998) Identification of a human population infected with simian foamy viruses. *Nat. Med.* **4**, 403–407.
74. Callahan, M. E., Switzer, W. M., Matthews, A. L., et al. (1999) Persistent zoonotic infection of a human with simian foamy virus in the absence of an intact orf-2 accessory gene. *J. Virol.* **73**, 9619–9624.
75. Linial, M. (2000) Why aren't foamy viruses pathogenic? *Trends Microbiol.* **8**, 284–289.
76. Seeger, C. and Mason, W. S. (1996) DNA replication in eukaryotic cells, in *DNA Replication in Eukaryotic Cells* (de Pamphilis, M., ed.), Cold Spring Harbor Laboratory Press, New York, pp. 815–831
77. Hill, C. L., Bieniasz, P. D., and McClure, M. O. (1999) Properties of human foamy virus relevant to its development as a vector for gene therapy. *J. Gen. Virol.* **80(Pt 8)**, 2003–2009.
78. Trobridge, G., Josephson, N., Vassilopoulos, G., Mac, J., and Russell, D. W. (2002) Improved foamy virus vectors with minimal viral sequences. *Mol. Ther.* **6**, 321–328.
79. Rowe, W. P., Huebner, R. J., Gilmore, L. K., Parrott, R. H., and Ward, T. G. (1953) Isolation of a cytopathogenic agent from human adenoids undergoing spontaneous degeneration in tissue culture. *Proc. Soc. Exp. Biol. Med.* **84**, 570–573.
80. Lai, C. M., Lai, Y. K. and Rakoczy, P. E. (2002) Adenovirus and adeno-associated virus vectors. *DNA Cell Biol.* **21**, 895–913.
81. Ginsberg, H. S. (1984) *The Adenoviruses*, Plenum Press, New York.
82. Ginsberg, H. S., Lundholm-Beauchamp, U., Horswood, R. L., et al. (1989) Role of early region 3 (E3) in pathogenesis of adenovirus disease. *Proc. Natl. Acad. Sci. USA* **86**, 3823–3827.
83. Bergelson, J. M., Cunningham, J. A., Droguett, G., et al. (1997) Isolation of a common receptor for Coxsackie B viruses and adenoviruses 2 and 5. *Science* **275**, 1320–1323.

84. Wickham, T. J., Mathias, P., Cheresh, D. A., and Nemerow, G. R. (1993). Integrins alpha v beta 3 and alpha v beta 5 promote adenovirus internalization but not virus attachment. *Cell* **73**, 309–319.
85. Graham, F. L., Smiley, J., Russell, W. C., and Nairn, R. (1977) Characteristics of a human cell line transformed by DNA from human adenovirus type 5. *J. Gen. Virol.* **36**, 59–74.
86. Hearing, P., Samulski, R. J., Wishart, W. L., and Shenk, T. (1987). Identification of a repeated sequence element required for efficient encapsidation of the adenovirus type 5 chromosome. *J. Virol.* **61**, 2555–2558.
87. Shen, W. Y., Lai, M. C., Beilby, J., et al. (2001) Combined effect of cyclosporine and sirolimus on improving the longevity of recombinant adenovirus-mediated transgene expression in the retina. *Arch. Ophthalmol.* **119**, 1033–1043.
88. Cassivi, S. D., Liu, M., Boehler, A., et al. (1999) Transgene expression after adenovirus-mediated retransfection of rat lungs is increased and prolonged by transplant immunosuppression. *J. Thorac. Cardiovasc. Surg.* **117**, 1–7.
89. Yap, J., O'Brien, T., Tazelaar, H. D., and McGregor, C. G. (1997) Immunosuppression prolongs adenoviral mediated transgene expression in cardiac allograft transplantation. *Cardiovasc. Res.* **35**, 529–535.
90. Engelhardt, J. F., Litzky, L., and Wilson, J. M. (1994). Prolonged transgene expression in cotton rat lung with recombinant adenoviruses defective in E2a. *Hum. Gene Ther.* **5**, 1217–1229.
91. Engelhardt, J. F., Ye, X., Doranz, B., and Wilson, J. M. (1994). Ablation of E2A in recombinant adenoviruses improves transgene persistence and decreases inflammatory response in mouse liver. *Proc. Natl. Acad. Sci. USA* **91**, 6196–6200.
92. Yang, Y., Nunes, F. A., Berencsi, K., Gonczol, E., Engelhardt, J. F., and Wilson, J. M. (1994). Inactivation of E2a in recombinant adenoviruses improves the prospect for gene therapy in cystic fibrosis. *Nat. Genet.* **7**, 362–369.
93. Qian, H. S., Channon, K., Neplioueva, V., et al. (2001) Improved adenoviral vector for vascular gene therapy : beneficial effects on vascular function and inflammation. *Circ. Res.* **88**, 911–917.
94. Wen, S., Schneider, D. B., Driscoll, R. M., Vassalli, G., Sassani, A. B., and Dichek, D. A. (2000) Second-generation adenoviral vectors do not prevent rapid loss of transgene expression and vector DNA from the arterial wall. *Arterioscler. Thromb. Vasc. Biol.* **20**, 1452–1458.
95. Fisher, K. J., Choi, H., Burda, J., Chen, S. J., and Wilson, J. M. (1996) Recombinant adenovirus deleted of all viral genes for gene therapy of cystic fibrosis. *Virology* **217**, 11–22.
96. Fisher, K. J., Jooss, K., Alston, J., et al. (1997) Recombinant adeno-associated virus for muscle directed gene therapy. *Nat. Med.* **3**, 306–312.
97. Kochanek, S., Clemens, P. R., Mitani, K., Chen, H. H., Chan, S., and Caskey, C. T. (1996) A new adenoviral vector: Replacement of all viral coding sequences with 28 kb of DNA independently expressing both full-length dystrophin and beta-galactosidase. *Proc. Natl. Acad. Sci. USA* **93**, 5731–5736.

98. Kumar-Singh, R. and Chamberlain, J. S. (1996) Encapsidated adenovirus minichromosomes allow delivery and expression of a 14 kb dystrophin cDNA to muscle cells. *Hum. Mol. Genet.* **5**, 913–921.
99. Kumar-Singh, R. and Farber, D. B. (1998) Encapsidated adenovirus mini-chromosome-mediated delivery of genes to the retina: application to the rescue of photoreceptor degeneration. *Hum. Mol. Genet.* **7**, 1893–1900.
100. Kumar-Singh, R., Yamashita, C. K., Tran, K., and Farber, D. B. (2000) Construction of encapsidated (gutted) adenovirus minichromosomes and their application to rescue of photoreceptor degeneration. *Methods Enzymol.* **316**, 724–743.
101. Berns, K. I. and Giraud, C. (1996) Biology of adeno-associated virus, in *Adeno-Associated Virus (AAV) Vectors in GeneTherapy* (Berns, K. I. and Giraud, C., eds.), Springer Verlag, Berlin, pp. 1–24.
102. Dong, J. Y., Fan, P. D., and Frizzell, R. A. (1996) Quantitative analysis of the packaging capacity of recombinant adeno-associated virus. *Hum. Gene Ther.* **7**, 2101–2112.
103. Casto, B. C., Atchison, R. W., and Hammon, W. M. (1967) Studies on the relationship between adeno-associated virus type I (AAV-1) and adenoviruses. I. Replication of AAV-1 in certain cell cultures and its effect on helper adenovirus. *Virology* **32**, 52–59.
104. Buller, R. M., Janik, J. E., Sebring, E. D.,and Rose, J. A. (1981) Herpes simplex virus types 1 and 2 completely help adenovirus-associated virus replication. *J. Virol.* **40**, 241–247.
105. Yalkinoglu, A. O., Heilbronn, R., Burkle, A., Schlehofer, J. R., and zur Hausen, H. (1988) DNA amplification of adeno-associated virus as a response to cellular genotoxic stress. *Cancer Re.s.* **48**, 3123–3129.
106. Yalkinoglu, A. O., Zentgraf, H., and Hubscher, U. (1991) Origin of adeno-associated virus DNA replication is a target of carcinogen-inducible DNA amplification. *J. Virol.* **65**, 3175–3184.
107. Sanlioglu, S., Duan, D., and Engelhardt, J. F. (1999) Two independent molecular pathways for recombinant adeno-associated virus genome conversion occur after UV-C and E4orf6 augmentation of transduction. *Hum. Gene Ther.* **10**, 591–602.
108. Kotin, R. M., Siniscalco, M., Samulski, R. J., et al. (1990) Site-specific integration by adeno-associated virus. *Proc. Natl. Acad. Sci. USA* **87**, 2211–2215.
109. Kotin, R. M., Linden, R. M., and Berns, K. I. (1992) Characterization of a preferred site on human chromosome 19q for integration of adeno-associated virus DNA by non-homologous recombination. *EMBO J.* **11**, 5071–5078.
110. Samulski, R. J., Zhu, X., Xiao, X., et al. (1991) Targeted integration of adeno-associated virus (AAV) into human chromosome 19. *EMBO J.* **10**, 3941–3950.
111. Flotte, T. R., Afione, S. A., Conrad, C., et al. (1993) Stable in vivo expression of the cystic fibrosis transmembrane conductance regulator with an adeno-associated virus vector. *Proc. Natl. Acad. Sci. USA* **90**, 10,613–10,617.
112. Kaplitt, M. G., Leone, P., Samulski, R. J., et al. (1994) Long-term gene expression and phenotypic correction using adeno-associated virus vectors in the mammalian brain. *Nat. Genet.* **8**, 148–154.

113. McCown, T. J., Xiao, X., Li, J., Breese, G. R., and Samulski, R. J. (1996) Differential and persistent expression patterns of CNS gene transfer by an adeno-associated virus (AAV) vector. *Brain Res.* **713**, 99–107.
114. Snyder, R. O., Spratt, S. K., Lagarde, C., et al. (1997) Efficient and stable adeno-associated virus-mediated transduction in the skeletal muscle of adult immunocompetent mice. *Hum. Gene Ther.* **8**, 1891–1900.
115. Lalwani, A. K., Walsh, B. J., Carvalho, G. J., Muzyczka, N., and Mhatre, A. N. (1998) Expression of adeno-associated virus integrated transgene within the mammalian vestibular organs. *Am. J. Otol.* **19**, 390–395.
116. Schimmenti, S., Boesen, J., Claassen, E. A., Valerio, D., and Einerhand, M. P. (1998) Long-term genetic modification of rhesus monkey hematopoietic cells following transplantation of adenoassociated virus vector-transduced CD34+ cells. *Hum. Gene Ther.* **9**, 2727–2734.
117. Duan, D., Yue, Y., Yan, Z., McCray, P. B., Jr., and Engelhardt, J. F. (1998) Polarity influences the efficiency of recombinant adenoassociated virus infection in differentiated airway epithelia. *Hum. Gene Ther.* **9**, 2761–2776.
118. Malik, A. K., Monahan, P. E., Allen, D. L., Chen, B. G., Samulski, R. J. and Kurachi, K. (2000) Kinetics of recombinant adeno-associated virus-mediated gene transfer. *J. Virol.* **74**, 3555–3565.
119. Nakai, H., Storm, T. A., and Kay, M. A. (2000) Recruitment of single-stranded recombinant adeno-associated virus vector genomes and intermolecular recombination are responsible for stable transduction of liver in vivo. *J. Virol.* **74**, 9451–9463.
120. Nakai, H., Yant, S. R., Storm, T. A., Fuess, S., Meuse, L., and Kay, M. A. (2001) Extrachromosomal recombinant adeno-associated virus vector genomes are primarily responsible for stable liver transduction in vivo. *J. Virol.* **75**, 6969–6976.
121. Xiao, X., Li, J., and Samulski, R. J. (1996) Efficient long-term gene transfer into muscle tissue of immunocompetent mice by adeno-associated virus vector. *J. Virol.* **70**, 8098–8108.
122. Miao, C. H., Snyder, R. O., Schowalter, D. B., et al. (1998) The kinetics of rAAV integration in the liver. *Nat. Genet.* **19**, 13–15.
123. Miao, C. H., Nakai, H., Thompson, A. R., et al. (2000) Nonrandom transduction of recombinant adeno-associated virus vectors in mouse hepatocytes in vivo: cell cycling does not influence hepatocyte transduction. *J. Virol.* **74**, 3793–3803.
124. Nakai, H., Iwaki, Y., Kay, M. A., and Couto, L. B. (1999) Isolation of recombinant adeno-associated virus vector-cellular DNA junctions from mouse liver. *J. Virol.* **73**, 5438–5447.
125. Wu, P., Phillips, M. I., Bui, J., and Terwilliger, E. F. (1998) Adeno-associated virus vector-mediated transgene integration into neurons and other nondividing cell targets. *J. Virol.* **72**, 5919–5926.
126. Kaplitt, M. G., Xiao, X., Samulski, R. J., et al. (1996) Long-term gene transfer in porcine myocardium after coronary infusion of an adeno-associated virus vector. *Ann. Thorac. Surg.* **62**, 1669–1676.

127. Ali, R. R., Reichel, M. B., Thrasher, A. J., et al. (1996) Gene transfer into the mouse retina mediated by an adeno-associated viral vector. *Hum. Mol. Genet.* **5**, 591–594.
128. Ponnazhagan, S., Mukherjee, P., Wang, X. S., et al. (1997) Adeno-associated virus type 2-mediated transduction in primary human bone marrow-derived CD34+ hematopoietic progenitor cells: donor variation and correlation of transgene expression with cellular differentiation. *J. Virol.* **71**, 8262–8267.
129. Rolling, F., Shen, W. Y., Tabarias, H., et al. (1999) Evaluation of adeno-associated virus-mediated gene transfer into the rat retina by clinical fluorescence photography. *Hum. Gene Ther.* **10**, 641–648.
130. Zaiss, A. K., Liu, Q., Bowen, G. P., Wong, N. C., Bartlett, J. S., and Muruve, D. A. (2002) Differential activation of innate immune responses by adenovirus and adeno-associated virus vectors. *J. Virol.* **76**, 4580–4590.
131. Xiao, W., Chirmule, N., Berta, S. C., McCullough, B., Gao, G., and Wilson, J. M. (1999) Gene therapy vectors based on adeno-associated virus type 1. *J. Virol.* **73**, 3994–4003.
132. Chirmule, N., Xiao, W., Truneh, A., et al. (2000) Humoral immunity to adeno-associated virus type 2 vectors following administration to murine and nonhuman primate muscle. *J. Virol.* **74**, 2420–2425.
133. Chirmule, N., Propert, K., Magosin, S., Qian, Y., Qian, R., and Wilson, J. (1999) Immune responses to adenovirus and adeno-associated virus in humans. *Gene Ther.* **6**, 1574–1583.
134. Roizman, B. and Sears, A. E. (1996) Human herpes viruses and their replication, in *Fundamental Virology,* 3rd ed.. (Fields, B. N., Knipe, D. M., Howley, P. M., Chanock, R. M., and Melnick, J. L., eds.), Lippincott-Raven, Philadelphia, pp. 2231–2296.
135. Advani, S. J., Weichselbaum, R. R., Whitley, R. J., and Roizman, B. (2002) Friendly fire: redirecting herpes simplex virus-1 for therapeutic applications. *Clin. Microbiol. Infect.* **8**, 551–563.
136. Burton, E. A., Bai, Q., Goins, W. F., and Glorioso, J. C. (2001) Targeting gene expression using HSV vectors. *Adv. Drug Deliv. Rev.* **53**, 155–170.
137. Burton, E. A., Wechuck, J. B., Wendell, S. K., Goins, W. F., Fink, D. J., and Glorioso, J. C. (2001) Multiple applications for replication-defective herpes simplex virus vectors. *Stem Cells* **19**, 358–377.
138. Burton, E. A., Bai, Q., Goins, W. F., and Glorioso, J. C. (2002) Replication-defective genomic herpes simplex vectors: design and production. *Curr. Opin. Biotechnol.* **13**, 424–428.
139. Burton, E. A., Fink, D. J., and Glorioso, J. C. (2002) Gene delivery using herpes simplex virus vectors. *DNA Cell. Biol.* **21**, 915–936.
140. Martuza, R. L., Malick, A., Markert, J. M., Ruffner, K. L., and Coen, D. M. (1991) Experimental therapy of human glioma by means of a genetically engineered virus mutant. *Science* **252**, 854–856.
141. Mineta, T., Rabkin, S. D., and Martuza, R. L. (1994) Treatment of malignant gliomas using ganciclovir-hypersensitive, ribonucleotide reductase-deficient herpes simplex viral mutant. *Cancer Res.* **54**, 3963–3966.

142. Pyles, R. B., Warnick, R. E., Chalk, C. L., Szanti, B. E., and Parysek, L. M. (1997) A novel multiply-mutated HSV-1 strain for the treatment of human brain tumors. *Hum. Gene Ther.* **8**, 533–544.
143. Frenkel, N., Singer, O., and Kwong, A. D. (1994) Minireview: the herpes simplex virus amplicon—a versatile defective virus vector. *Gene Ther.* **1(Suppl 1)**, S40–S46.
144. Fraefel, C., Jacoby, D. R., and Breakefield, X. O. (2000) Herpes simplex virus type 1-based amplicon vector systems. *Adv. Virus Res.* **55**, 425–451.
145. Krisky, D. M., Wolfe, D., Goins, W. F., et al. (1998) Deletion of multiple immediate-early genes from herpes simplex virus reduces cytotoxicity and permits long-term gene expression in neurons. *Gene Ther.* **5**, 1593–1603.
146. Krisky, D. M., Marconi, P. C., Oligino, T. J., et al. (1998) Development of herpes simplex virus replication-defective multigene vectors for combination gene therapy applications. *Gene Ther.* **5**, 1517–1530.
147. Moriuchi, S., Oligino, T., Krisky, D., et al. (1998) Enhanced tumor cell killing in the presence of ganciclovir by herpes simplex virus type 1 vector-directed coexpression of human tumor necrosis factor-alpha and herpes simplex virus thymidine kinase. *Cancer Res.* **58**, 5731–5737.

9

Nonviral Vectors

Louise Collins

Summary

Gene therapy holds great promise for treating a variety of human diseases and conditions. The field of gene therapy has advanced rapidly in the last decade. However, a major limiting factor remains the lack of a suitable vector for gene delivery. Although viruses are currently the most commonly researched vector, because of continuing safety concerns research has broadened to developing nonviral alternatives.

Nonviral vectors fall into several categories. They can be physical methods, which provide relatively crude delivery approaches, such as direct cell injection, or chemical delivery vehicles. Chemical vectors almost always include a polycation component to assist the passage of DNA to the cell's nucleus.

The passage of the transgene through the cell to the nucleus is hampered by many obstacles. Approaches to overcome these, both intracellularly and extracellularly, in order to maximize gene expression are currently under investigation.

Nonviral vectors offer a safe and versatile alternative to their viral counterparts. Although still in their infancy, the different nonviral approaches under development hold great potential for many clinical applications.

Key Words: Nonviral; gene therapy; vector.

1. Introduction

Viral vectors have been successfully developed to produce relatively long-term, high-level transfection efficiencies to a wide variety of cells, both replicating and postmitotic. However, they are still far from the perfect vector. Nonviral gene-delivery vehicles have received increasing focus in recent years because they offer substantial safety advantages over viral vectors. The predominant concern with viral gene delivery is that of insertional activation within the host genome, leading to oncogenic or tumor-suppressor activation. Concerns have been highlighted, first following the death of a teenager from

From: *Methods in Molecular Biology, vol. 333: Transplantation Immunology: Methods and Protocols*
Edited by: P. Hornick and M. Rose © Humana Press Inc., Totowa, NJ

Table 1
Advantages and Disadvantages of Viral and Nonviral DNA Vectors

Viral vectors	Nonviral vectors
Advantages	*Advantages*
High transfection efficiency	No viral components
Long term gene expression through integration of transgene (retrovirus, AAV)	Low or no immunogenicity
Intrinsic properties for intracellular trafficking	No limit to DNA insert size
	Cell specificity possible with targeted ligands
	Relatively simple preparation procedures
	Standardized homogenous, stable reagents
	Scale up possible
Disadvantages	*Disadvantages*
Replication competent virus formation by homologous recombination	Low transfection efficiency
Oncogenic activation following integration	Transient gene expression–episomal expression
Helper virus carryover (AAV)	Intracellular barrier–may require additional agents
Immunogenicity	Cellular toxicity with some vectors (PEI,liposomes)
Viral protein overload	Inflammation due to unmethylated CpG DNA sequences
Limited cell tropism	
Time consuming preparation	
Batch to batch variation	

AAV, adeno-associated virus; PEI, polyethyleneimine.

adverse immune responses to adenoviral treatment for a liver enzyme deficiency *(1)* and, more recently, in reports of two boys developing leukemia after being treated for severe combined immunodeficiency with retroviruses *(2)*.

It is with this concern, as well as other well-documented disadvantages, illustrated in **Table 1**, that research into nonviral alternatives has advanced with such speed in recent years. Nonviral vectors must achieve by design what viruses have evolved to do naturally, mimicking the advantageous components for rapid transport and efficient expression of foreign DNA within a host cell, but including none of the associated limitations. For transplantation applications they offer a nonimmunogenic alternative for delivery of genes to the graft or to the host immune system in an otherwise immunologically overloaded environment.

Many different approaches to nonviral vector design have been documented. These use both physical and chemical methods, but as yet there is not one single system that can be effectively applied in every gene-therapy situation.

Although publications involving nonviral vectors for immunoregulatory gene delivery to a specific transplantation target are few, there is significant progress in gene delivery to targeted cells or transplantable tissues. Additionally, ex vivo gene delivery has shown great potential with many nonviral gene-delivery systems. Relevant research is discussed here, in reference to the appropriate vectors.

2. Physical Methods

The need for a vector at all is questionable because delivery can be crudely, but effectively, achieved by direct administration of naked plasmid DNA to the target tissue or cell (reviewed in **ref.** *3*). Direct injection to skeletal muscle tissue results in transient gene expression, which indicates its promise as a vaccination procedure ***(4)***. Direct delivery of donor major histocompatibility complex class I antigen to skeletal muscle has been shown to modify allograft response in a transplantation model ***(5)***. Efficient levels of transfection have also been achieved with direct injection into the liver ***(6)***, myocardium ***(7,8)***, skin ***(9)***, as well as brain ***(10,11)*** and solid tumors ***(12)***.

The development of intravascular plasmid delivery has markedly increased the interest in the field of naked DNA gene therapy. Vascular delivery may be systemic or regional, in which DNA is introduced directly into vessels that supply a specific tissue, improving cell access ***(13)***. Intravascular or direct injection of immunomodulatory genes in donor grafts is an attractive alternative to current systemic immunosuppression treatments. Delivery of the functionally immunosuppressive cytokine transforming growth factor-β1 to murine cardiac transplant models by direct DNA injection was shown to significantly prolong graft survival ***(7)***.

Untargeted systemic injection of naked DNA into whole animals results in low-level, short-term, and wide tissue distribution of gene expression ***(14)***. However, increasing hydrodynamic pressure by rapid delivery of a large DNA volume results in a substantial increase in transgene expression, almost exclusively located in the liver following systemic administration ***(15)***. More importantly, hydrodynamic gene delivery can be applied to localized delivery for specific organs including the liver (unpublished data) and kidney ***(16)***.

Other physical methods for DNA delivery include particle bombardment using DNA-coated gold beads ***(17,18)*** and ultrasound methods to temporarily disrupt membranes ***(19)***. Most important in recent years, however, has been the development of electroporation technology. This is a technique routinely used in the laboratory for making transient pores in cell membranes ***(20)***. Refinement of pulse conditions to reduce cell toxicity, and the development of equipment that enables in vivo use, have renewed interest in it for gene-therapy applications ***(21,22)***.

The advantage of these physical methods, apart from the lack of viral components, is their obvious simplicity. However, physical methods are generally harsh and unphysiological in their nature of cell entry. A fine balance is required to keep cell stress to a minimum but, at the same time, achieve sufficient membrane disruption to allow the DNA in.

3. Chemical Methods

There are many different nonviral gene delivery vehicles that make use of the properties of chemicals and proteins to assist cell entry. Nearly all successful nonviral DNA-delivery systems contain some form of polycation. The charge enables binding to plasmid DNA resulting in condensation, as well as electrostatic binding to anionic cell surface groups such as proteoglycans *(23)*.

3.1. Liposomes

Liposomal gene delivery, or Lipoplex, was the first purely nonviral system to reach clinical trials through the pioneering work of Felgner and colleagues in 1987 *(24)*. They developed a cationic lipid that forms small (average diameter 100 nm) unilamellar liposomes under optimal conditions *(25)*. The surface of these liposomes is positively charged and thus readily attracted to the negative phosphate backbone of DNA, spontaneously forming lipid/DNA complexes in which the DNA is protected from intracellular degradation *(26)*. Internalization is thought to occur via both coated pit and noncoated endocytosis pathways, depending on the positive charge of the liposome and the size of the complexes, resulting in efficient cell transfection *(27)*.

Since the initial design, many effective variations have been reported, some of which are shown in **Fig. 1**. Several of these are available commercially (reviewed in **ref.** *28*). A cationic lipid generally consists of four different functional domains: a positively charged head group (usually a single or multiple amine-derived group), a spacer of varying lengths, a linker bond, and a hydrophobic anchor. The relationship between structure and efficiency of gene delivery has been an area of intense research *(29)*.

Most of the cationic lipid preparations used for cell transfection have constituted a cationic amphiphile together with a neutral "helper" lipid, such as dioleoylphosphatidylethanolamine or cholesterol. The helper lipid is required for stabilization and has been shown to improve transfection significantly *(30)*. It is also thought to play a role in membrane disruption, enhancing passage of DNA through the cell, although the precise mechanism remains unclear *(31)*.

The success of lipoplex delivery is widespread. Reports of efficient cationic lipid-mediated delivery of DNA and RNA both in vitro and in vivo have been extensively published, providing transient and stable transfectants to a wide range of tissues and organs in many animal species. Several transplant models

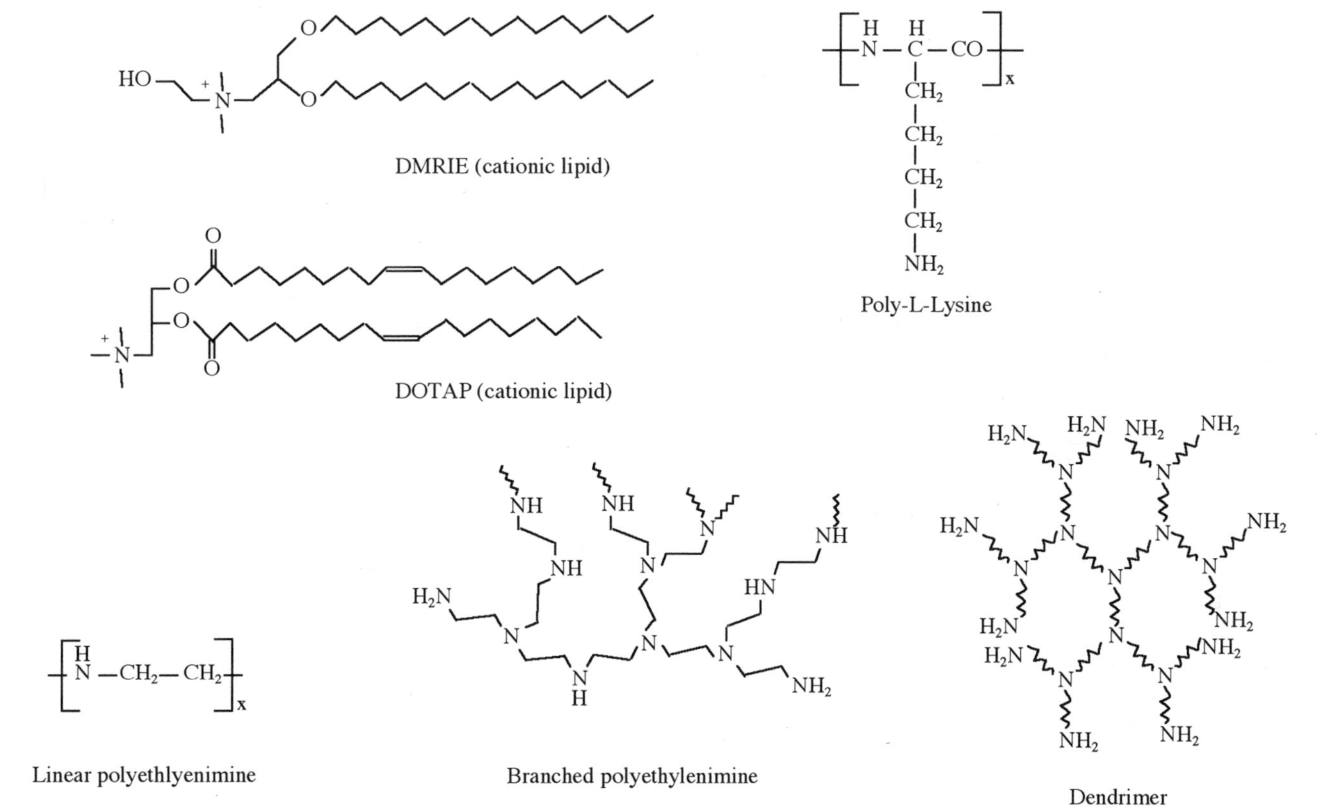

Fig. 1. Structures of commonly used chemical nonviral vectors. DMRIE, 1,2-dimyriotyloxypropyl-3-dimethyl-hydroxy ethyl ammonium bromide; DOTAP, dioleoyltrimethylamino propane.

have used liposomal delivery methods. Viral interleukin (IL)-10 has been delivered using lipid-mediated gene transfer to both rat lung *(32)* and murine cardiac *(33)* allografts and has shown enhanced graft survival by inhibiting donor-specific cellular and humoral immune responses.

Intravenous injection of lipid–DNA complexes produces increased levels of gene expression compared to naked DNA alone *(34)*, with accumulation in the lung endothelium *(35)*. However, because of the high positive charge, complexes aggregate with serum proteins *(36)* and potentially with other body fluids **(37)**, leading to problems in vivo. Some cell toxicity has been reported *(38)*. It has been shown to be possible to lengthen the circulation time, shield the cationic charges, and divert the lipoplexes to other organs by incorporating a hydrophilic polymer, polyethylene glycol (PEG) *(39,40)*. This can occur with or without added tissue selectivity by including natural targeting ligands such as transferrin *(41)*, folate *(42)*, asialofetuin *(43)*, or antibodies *(44)*. Transferrin-enhanced lipids have been shown to successfully deliver viral IL-10 to corneal endothelium, suppressing corneal allograft rejection *(44)*.

The inclusion of additional features to enhance liposomal DNA delivery have consisted of polylysine *(45,46)* or membrane-permeabilizing agents *(27)*. In a similar way, liposomes have been shown to enhance other nonviral vector systems, such as the arginine-glycine-aspartate (RGD)-peptide integrin targeting vector *(47–49)*, and also to improve transfection with some viruses, including adenoviruses *(50)* and the hemaglutinating virus of Japan *(51)*.

3.2. Receptor-Mediated Gene Transfer With Polylysine-Based Polymers

Receptor-mediated gene transfer takes advantage of the ability of receptors on the cell surface to bind and internalize a ligand, enabling increased cell-target specificity. Targeting ligands can be natural or recombinant proteins, synthetic peptides, vitamins, carbohydrates, or specific antibodies.

The fundamental components of a receptor-mediated gene-delivery system (*see* **Fig. 2**) are the ligand that binds effectively and specifically to a cell surface receptor and the DNA-binding moiety, usually a polycation, that is conjugated or synthesized with the ligand, and which electrostatically binds and condenses the plasmid DNA.

The DNA-binding moiety serves as the link, binding the DNA to the targeting ligand, and in addition it compresses the helical structure of the plasmid and condenses it into a small, tightly packed molecule. Most of the DNA-condensing agents are polycations, although other high-affinity binding molecules have also been used, including the DNA-intercalating agents bisacridine *(52)* and Hoechst 33258 *(53)*, sequence-specific DNA-binding proteins, such as the DNA-binding domain of the yeast GAL4 transcription factor *(54)*, or naturally

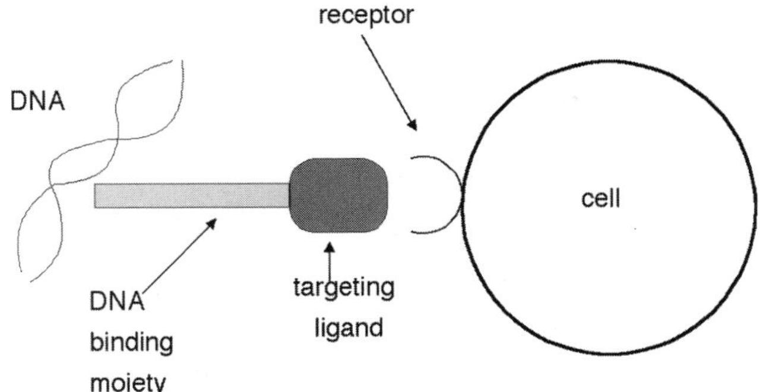

Fig. 2. Basic components of a receptor-mediated gene-delivery system.

occurring DNA-binding proteins, such as spermine ***(55)***, histones ***(56)***, and protamines ***(57)***.

Undoubtedly the most effective and extensively researched DNA-binding moiety to date is the naturally occurring, biodegradable peptide poly(L-lysine). It has been shown to be a highly effective condensing agent ***(58,59)***. As part of several different polyplex vector systems, it has been shown to shield the DNA effectively from degradation by cell nucleases ***(46,60)***. It has also been suggested that polylysine may possess nuclear trafficking properties, further enhancing gene delivery. The length and type of positively charged amino acids have been reported to influence DNA condensation and ultimately the size and stability of the resulting DNA–ligand complexes in solution ***(59,61)***.

The ligand is the most important component of the receptor-mediated gene-delivery vehicle. Lysine chains of high molecular weight have been shown to mediate gene delivery effectively alone. However, polylysine is most effective when linked with a targeting ligand. The ligand provides the specificity of the system by the initial contact with the cell surface and subsequent internalization. Three categories have been used to date: whole naturally occurring proteins (such as asialorosomucoid, transferrin, or insulin), structural motifs of receptor-binding affinity from natural ligands (galactose residues or RGD peptide), or antibodies against an epitope on the extracellular portion of the receptor (e.g., polymeric immunoglobulin receptor).

Table 2 illustrates the wide range of targeting ligands and antibodies that have been investigated as DNA vectors, together with the polycations utilized and their intended cellular targets. It is apparent that many of these targeted systems have huge potential in the transplantation gene-therapy field. Many are targeted to organs such as liver and lung as well as to specific cell types such as endothelium and vascular smooth muscle cells, which play a significant role in graft rejection and immune regulation.

Table 2
Ligands Used for Receptor-Mediated Gene-Delivery Vectors

Ligand	Polycation	Receptor	Cell/tissue target	Reference
α1-Antitrypsin motif peptide	Polylysine, oligolysine	Serpin–enzyme complex receptor	Liver, brain	***105,106***
ASGP, asialoorosomucoid	Polylysine	ASGP receptor	Liver	***107,108***
EGF and anti-EGF	Polylysine, PEI	EGF receptor	Tumor cells	***79,89,109***
FGF	Polylysine	FGF receptor	Various	***110***
Folate	Polylysine, EPI	Folate receptor	Tumor cells	***42,111,113***
Galactosylated ligands (various, e.g., albumin)	Polylysine, oligolysine, histones	ASGP receptor	Liver	***114,118***
Insulin	Polylysine	Insulin receptor	Liver	***119,120***
Malarial circumsporozoite protein	Polylysine	Unknown	Erthyrocytes	***121***
RGD peptides	Oligolysine, PEI	Integrins	Multiple cell types	***77,97,122,125***
Synthetic ligands, galactosylated, lactosylated, or mannosylated ligands	Polylysine, PEI	Sugar-specific receptors (e.g., lectins, mannose receptor)	Liver, tumor, endothelium, monocytes, macrophages, lung, epithelium, etc.	***126,129***
Transferrin	Polylysine, protamine, PEI	Transferrin receptor	Rapidly dividing tissues, (e.g., tumors)	***74,78,130***

α-CD3 antibody	Polylysine, PEI	CD3	Peripheral blood mononuclear cells	***76***
Anti-CD5	Polylysine	CD5	Lymphocytes	***131***
Antibody ChCEy	Polylysine	ChCE7	Neuroblastoma	***132***
Anti-her2	Polylysine	Her2		***133***
Antisecretory component antibodies	Polylysine	Polymeric immunoglobulin receptor	Lund and live epithelium	***134***
Anti-thrombomodulin	Polylysine	Thrombomodulin	Neuroblastoma, endothelium, leukemic cells	***132, 135***
Anti-TGF	Polylysine	EGF receptor	Tumor cells	***136***
Anti-IgG	Polylysine	Surface immunoglobuin	lymphocytes	***137***
IgG	Polylysine	FcR	Macrophages	***138***

ASGP, asialoglycoprotein; EGF, epidermal growth factor; EPI, polyethyleneimine; FGF, fibroblast growth factor; RGD, arginine-glycine-aspartate; TGF, transforming growth factor; IgG, immuoglobulin G.

It must not be forgotten that in partner to the ligand, the receptor is an essential consideration in vector design. Ideally a receptor would be unique for a specific cell type or tissue to provide a highly specialized targeted delivery system. The binding affinity of the ligand to the receptor is important. If it is too high, it may prevent the ligand–DNA complexes from dissociating from the receptor following internalization, and they may be returned to the cell surface ***(62)***, but if it is too weak, it would reduce binding to the cell surface and corresponding internalization efficiency. Receptor targets for ligand-directed gene delivery are almost exclusively actively recycling receptor types that associate with coated pits.

The most attractive advantage of the receptor-mediated gene transfer system, however, is the targeting property of the ligand to the cell receptor that makes possible the development of a highly specific system. The cell also remains relatively unharmed because the process of cell entry exploits natural cellular uptake pathways. In particular, the design of peptides or structural motifs derived from larger molecules eliminates any unwanted side effects associated with the rest of the molecule, producing smaller vector complexes to aid in diffusion and reduce any potential immunogenicity.

Polylysine has been shown, in some circumstances, to induce an inflammatory response when injected into animals ***(63)***, but animals in which the DNA–ligand–polylysine complexes are introduced via receptor-mediated endocytosis have not shown any immunological response ***(64)***. This would make multiple administrations possible if necessary.

3.3. Organic Polymers

Polyethyleneimine (PEI), a polymer widely used in the manufacturing industry, has been more recently exploited in the gene-therapy field (reviewed in **ref. *65***). Available in both a linear and a branched form and in many different molecular weights (*see* **Fig. 1**), it has proved a valuable method of nonviral gene delivery.

PEI is a highly positively charged polymer, which allows rapid and effective DNA condensation into small, stable complexes protected from nuclease degradation under physiological conditions ***(66)***. The positive charge allows electrostatic binding to the cell surface followed by natural endocytic uptake processes. The high buffering capacity ("proton sponge") over a broad pH range, a result of the high number of protonable nitrogen groups, aids delivery of plasmid DNA to a variety of cell types in vitro and in vivo without the addition of any membrane-disruption agents ***(67,68)***.

Gene expression has been achieved in a number of in vivo models including rat kidneys ***(69)***, mouse brains ***(67, 70)***, mouse tumors ***(71,72)***, and rabbit lungs ***(73)***. Following systemic administration, transgene expression is found predominantly in the lungs, similar to cationic liposomes.

Toxicity has been associated with the use of PEI in vivo, thought to be caused by the excessive positive charges on the polymer ***(67)***. This can be significantly reduced by shielding PEI–DNA complexes with PEG ***(74)***, as has been shown with lipids. This shielding also diverts intravenous delivery of the complexes away from the lung and toward the liver ***(75)***, adding some degree of specificity to the PEI vector. The untargeted nature of PEI limits the suitability of the vector for clinical applications. Targeting has, however, been introduced by the addition of ligands, such as transferrin ***(76)***, RGD peptides ***(77)***, anti-CD3 ***(78)***, and epidermal growth factor ***(79)***, either with or without the added PEG shield.

Polyamidoamine cascade polymers, or Starburst dendrimers, were the first polycations to show high transfection potential without the need for additional endosomolytic agents. Dendrimers are spherical, highly branched polymers with varying degrees of branching forming different generations, many of which are commercially available (*see* **Fig. 1**). Like PEI, they are highly positively charged, with high densities of amines on the surface, which are able to electrostatically condense the DNA and internalize by endocytosis. The remaining inner amine residues are then available to neutralize the acid pH in the endosomal vesicles, allowing DNA to escape degradation ***(80)***.

Like liposomes and several polycation-delivery systems, dendrimers have been shown to transfect corneal endothelium and to deliver genes encoding soluble tumor necrosis factor receptor immunoglobulin (TNFR-Ig) to block TNF action and reduce corneal allograft rejection ***(81)***. Dendrimers have also been used in a murine cardiac transplantation model to deliver viral IL-10, resulting in prolongation of graft survival ***(82)***.

4. Barriers for Nonviral Gene Delivery

The administration of DNA complexes, and subsequent passage to the nucleus of a specific cell type for expression, is a path hampered by many obstacles (*see* **Fig. 3**). Barriers to successful transgene expression may be extracellular or intracellular.

4.1. Extracellular

The route of administration of the complexes is of particular importance. It is important to establish the intended tissue target and deliver accordingly. For example, aerosol delivery to the lung or direct intravascular delivery to the liver are far more direct, localized methods compared to intravenous delivery to target a distant tissue or organ. Further tissue specificity can be achieved by the inclusion of tissue-specific promoters and enhancers in the plasmid DNA to limit expression to the tissue of choice.

For transplantation purposes, ex vivo graft manipulation offers an attractive and highly targeted delivery method whether the vector is cell targeted or not.

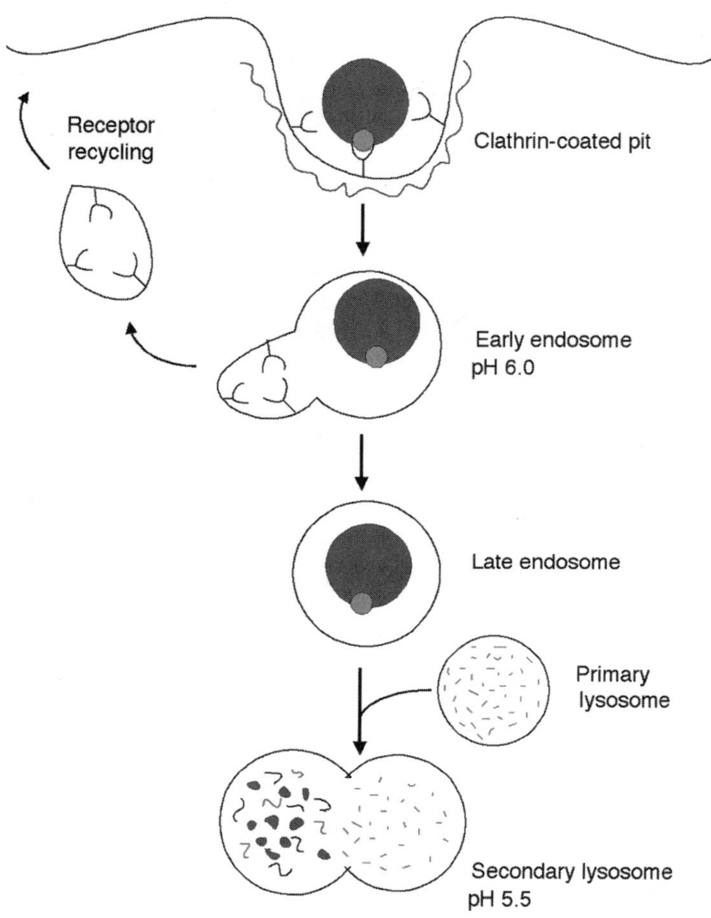

Fig. 3. Receptor-mediated endocytosis via clathrin-coated pits.

There is no possibility of unwanted gene delivery in distant organs or tissues, which often occurs following systemic delivery.

Almost all nonviral vectors are highly positively charged, which is beneficial for electrostatic attachment to cell-surface anionic molecules. When applied systemically, however, this leads to many nonspecific interactions with blood components and plasma proteins including albumin, fibronectin, and Ig *(83)*, leading to short circulation time and reduced cellular uptake. There is also the possibility of aggregation with erythrocytes, potentially resulting in vessel obstruction. It is thought that the high cationic charge, together with the size of some of the complexes, leads to complement activation in a number of situations, especially with large polylysine molecules and PEI *(84)*.

To address these potential hurdles, complexes have been sterically stabilized by the attachment of hydrophilic polymers, such as PEG *(40)* or human placental microsomal aromatase *(85)*, to shield the cationic charge in order to improve circulation stability, prevent aggregation, and reduce toxicity.

Diffusion through the tissues is strongly influenced by size, charge, and solubility of the DNA vector complexes. However, it is essential that complexes can be transported through capillaries, extravasate out of blood vessels, and be taken up by the cell. Extravasation through the endothelium is strictly limited by size, and it is only in some tissues such as liver, spleen, bone marrow, and some tumors that large fenestrations make it possible for particles of 100 nm or more to enter the parenchymal cells. In other tissues the natural defense system of the reticuloendothelium prevents access by any unwanted foreign particles.

4.2. Intracellular

4.2.1. Uptake by Target Cell

The membrane lipid bilayers selectively screen all foreign molecules entering the cell. Uptake through cellular membranes is dependent on the DNA complex surface charge and size. It is thought that the route of entry for cationic nonviral vectors is adsorptive or receptor-mediated endocytosis through clathrin-coated pits *(86)*. Although an innovative way to introduce gene-therapy vectors into the cell, it does have its disadvantages as it exposes the complexes to enzymatic degradation in the endosomal–lysosomal pathway (*see* **Fig. 3**).

The use of transduction domains from viral proteins such as HIV-TAT *(87)* or herpes simplex VP22 *(88)* is being investigated. Such proteins are capable of taking large molecules directly into the cytoplasm, circumventing the endocytic entry mechanisms.

4.2.2. Endosomal Release

Interruption of the endosomal–lysosomal pathway is thought to be the most rate-limiting step to successful nonviral gene delivery. Prevention of intraendosomal DNA degradation has been addressed in a number of ways, using both organic and natural agents.

PEI and dendrimers have been shown to have intrinsic endosomolytic properties resulting from their ability to become highly protonated in the acid lysosomal environment, leading to endosomal swelling and subsequent rupture —the "proton sponge" hypothesis *(67,80)*. They have thus effectively been used either alone or in combination with targeting ligands to achieve high transfection levels. Similarly, some cationic lipids have shown endosomolytic properties when used at very low levels, and these are able to enhance other nonviral vectors without any reported toxicity *(31)*.

Receptor-mediated polylysine-based delivery vehicles require assistance with endosomolysis, since they lack any buffering capacity during the pH drop. Original success was achieved by the simple addition of the organic lysosomotropic agent chloroquine. Chloroquine allows DNA to escape by preventing pH decrease and, hence, enzymatic degradation within the endosomes ***(89)***. The success of its use has been widely reported in vitro, but toxicity has limited its use in vivo and for any clinical applications.

One of the most sophisticated methods has been adapted from viruses. Destabilizing proteins are present in many viruses. The best studied is a 20-amino-acid peptide synthesized from the hemagglutinin protein of the influenza virus ***(90)***. Inside the lysosomal compartment, the peptide gains fusogenic activity following protonation in the acidic environment, resulting in a hydrophobic, helical structure that inserts and disrupts the vesicular membrane, releasing the contents. This is an elegant use of nature's evolutionary success in a nonviral system. Other synthetic peptides displaying similar properties have also been used, such as glutamic acid–alanine–leucine–alanine (GALA) ***(91)*** and lysine-alanine-leucine-alanine (KALA) ***(92)***. The immunogenic potential of these peptides is minimal because they are small.

Other membrane-disrupting methods employed include ultrasound ***(39)*** and a method called photochemical transfection, which uses photosensitizing compounds to accumulate in lysosomal membranes of a selected tissue, which disrupt the vesicle upon illumination ***(93)***.

4.2.3. Cytoplasm Stability

Transport across the cytoplasm is a relatively slow process, depending on the size of the complexes. A fine balance, however, is needed between the requirement for protection of the DNA from cytoplasmic nucleases and the ability of the complexes to disassemble, freeing the DNA for nuclear entry. Recently, intracellular release of DNA has been more specifically triggered by using polyplexes ***(85,94)*** or cationic lipids ***(95)*** containing disulfide bonds, which reduce and release the DNA in the cytoplasm. However, there is evidence of intact PEI–DNA complexes reaching the nucleus, so it may not be necessary to separate components prior to nuclear entry ***(86)***.

4.2.4. Transport to the Nucleus

DNA nuclear entry has been suggested to be dependent on cell division and nuclear envelope dissolution. However, this is not universal to all nonviral vectors, and certainly linear PEI ***(96)*** and RGD peptides ***(97,98)*** have been shown to successfully transfect postmitotic cells. It is thought that DNA is also able to enter through pores in the nuclear membrane.

It has been suggested that less than 1% of the plasmid DNA molecules in the cytoplasm actually reach the nucleus. These levels can be improved by incorporating a nuclear localizing signal (NLS) peptide to redirect DNA transport to the nucleus. Some vectors, including polylysine, the fusogenic peptide, and PEI, are thought to have intrinsic nuclear homing abilities. Some sequences within the plasmid DNA have been suggested to lead to nuclear import by binding to cellular proteins such as transcription factors ***(99)***.

Several NLSs have been isolated from proteins that are naturally synthesised in the cytoplasm but are required in the nucleus. Most are centered around a lysine or arginine motif. The most commonly used NLS is from the SV40 large T antigen ***(100)***.

5. Specificity and Longevity of Gene Expression

Gene delivery using nonviral vectors results in transient episomal expression of the plasmid. This has major advantages over integrating viral vectors, which have been shown to integrate into the host genome at sites of tumor suppression or oncogenic activation. However, expression with nonviral vectors is short lived, and, despite its low immunogenicity, which would enable multiple administration in vivo, for many clinical applications long-term expression would be favored. To address this issue, research has looked at a number of approaches. The inclusion of tissue-specific locus control regions ***(101,102)*** and similarly the addition of ubiquitous chromatin-opening elements in the DNA plasmids have been shown to improve longevity of expression by delaying gene silencing and holding the DNA in a more open, transcriptionally active conformation. The production of artificial chromosomes containing all of the features necessary to confer their own gene transcription and regulation independently of the cell's machinery (reviewed in **ref. *103***) is another avenue explored. More recently, a safer system for site-selective mammalian genome integration using transposons (e.g., Sleeping Beauty) has been developed ***(104)***.

6. Conclusion

Nonviral vectors have many distinct advantages over viruses, not least because they lack all potentially hazardous viral components. They can theoretically take a DNA piece of any size to a targeted type of cell or tissue for treatment of a specific disease. From a manufacturing point of view, they are readily standardized, easy to prepare, and relatively low in cost.

The major disadvantage of nonviral vectors is that, currently, the transfection efficiency is lower than that achieved with viruses and expression is only transient, although their relative nonimmunogenicity makes them ideally suited for repeat administration.

It is clear that there will never be a universal DNA vector applicable for all gene-therapy treatments. Delivery strategies need to be optimized on a disease-by-disease basis. While nonviral vectors have not yet reached clinical use, there are, to date, more than 80 clinical trials for a range of diseases including cystic fibrosis, arthritis, artery disease, and many cancers, all using nonviral vectors (http://www.wiley.co.uk/genetherapy). As a better understanding of extracellular and intracellular barriers to gene delivery is unleashed, we will in time develop a more refined nonviral design that will ultimately lead to successful gene-therapy treatment.

While still in its infancy, the application of gene therapy for transplantation holds great promise for modulating graft or host immune responses. It may eventually replace or at least substantially reduce the aggressive immunosuppressive regime that is currently essential to organ graft survival. Additionally, there is a possibility of furthering the genetic modification of organs to make them acceptable for xenotransplantation.

References

1. Marshall, E. (1999) Gene therapy death prompts review of adenovirus vector. *Science* **286**, 2244–2245.
2. Marshall, E. (2003) Gene therapy. Second child in French trial is found to have leukemia. *Science* **299**, 320.
3. Herweijer, H. and Wolff, J. A. (2003) Progress and prospects: naked DNA gene transfer and therapy. *Gene Ther.* **10**, 453–458.
4. Velaz-Faircloth, M., Cobb, A. J., Horstman, A. L., Henry, S. C., and Frothingham, R. (1999) Protection against *Mycobacterium avium* by DNA vaccines expressing mycobacterial antigens as fusion proteins with green fluorescent protein. *Infect. Immunol.* **67**, 4243–4250.
5. Geissler, E. K., Wang, J., Fechner, J. H. Jr., Burlingham, W. J., and Knechtle, S. J. (1994) Immunity to MHC class I antigen after direct DNA transfer into skeletal muscle. *J. Immunol.* **152**, 413–421.
6. Zhang, G., Vargo, D., Budker, V., Armstrong, N., Knechtle, S., and Wolff, J. A. (1997) Expression of naked plasmid DNA injected into the afferent and efferent vessels of rodent and dog livers. *Hum. Gene Ther.* **8**, 1763–1772.
7. Qin, L., Chavin, K. D., Ding, Y., et al. (1995) Multiple vectors effectively achieve gene transfer in a murine cardiac transplantation model. *Transplantation* **59**, 809–816.
8. Alexander, M. Y., Webster, K. A., McDonald, P. H., and Prentice, H. M. (1999) Gene transfer and models of gene therapy for the myocardium. *Clin. Exp. Pharmacol. Physiol* **26**, 661–668.
9. Yu, W. H., Kashani-Sabet, M., Liggitt, D., Moore, D., Heath, T. D., and Debs, R. J. (1999) Topical gene delivery to murine skin. *J. Invest. Dermatol.* **112**, 370–375.
10. Schwartz, B., Beonoist, C., Abdullah, B., et al. (1996) Gene transfer by naked DNA into adult mouse brain. *Gene Ther.* **3**, 405–411.
11. Meuli-Simmen, C., Liu, Y., Yeo, T. T., et al. (1999) Gene expression along the cerebral-spinal axis after regional gene delivery. *Hum. Gene Ther.* **10**, 2689–2700.

12. Yang, J.-P. and Huang, L. (1996) Direct gene transfer to mouse melanoma by intratumor injection of free DNA. *Gene Ther.* **3**, 542–548.
13. Zhang, G., Budker, V., Williams, P., Hanson, K., and Wolff, J. A. (2002) Surgical procedures for intravascular delivery of plasmid DNA to organs. *Methods Enzymol.* **346**, 125–133.
14. Kawabata, K., Takakura, Y., and Hashida, M. (1995) The fate of plasmid DNA after intravenous injection in mice: involvement of scavenger receptors in its hepatic uptake. *Pharm. Res.* **12**, 825–830.
15. Maruyama, H., Higuchi, N., Nishikawa, Y.,et al. (2002) High-level expression of naked DNA delivered to rat liver via tail vein injection. *J. Gene Med.* **4**, 333–341.
16. Maruyama, H., Higuchi, N., Nishikawa, Y., et al. (2002) Kidney-targeted naked DNA transfer by retrograde renal vein injection in rats. *Hum. Gene Ther.* **13**, 455–468.
17. Yang, N.-S., Burkholder, J., Roberts, B., Martinell, B., and McCabe, D. (1990) *In vivo* and *in vitro* gene transfer to mammalian somatic cells by particle bombardment. *Proc. Natl. Acad. Sci. USA* **87**, 9568–9572.
18. Sun, W. H., Burkholder, J. K., Sun, J., et al. (1995) *In vivo* cytokine gene transfer by gene gun reduces tumor growth in mice. *Proc. Natl. Acad. Sci. USA* **92**, 2889–2893.
19. Taniyama, Y., Tachibana, K., Hiraoka, K., et al. (2002) Development of safe and efficient novel nonviral gene transfer using ultrasound: enhancement of transfection efficiency of naked plasmid DNA in skeletal muscle. *Gene Ther.* **9**, 372–380.
20. Weaver, J. C. (1993) Electroporation: a general phenomenon for manipulating cells and tissues. *J. Cell. Biochem.* **51**, 426–435.
21. Somiari, S., Glasspool-Malone, J., Drabick, J. J., et al. (2000) Theory and in vivo application of electroporative gene delivery. *Mol. Ther.* **2**, 178–187.
22. Li, S. and Benninger, M. (2002) Applications of muscle electroporation gene therapy. *Curr. Gene Ther.* **2**, 101–105.
23. Mislick, K. A. and Baldeschwieler, J. D. (1996) Evidence for the role of proteoglycans in cation-mediated gene transfer. *Proc. Natl. Acad. Sci. USA* **93**, 12,349–12,354.
24. Felgner, P. L., Gadek, T. R., Holm, M., et al. (1987) Lipofection: a highly efficient, lipid-mediated DNA-transfection procedure. *Proc. Natl. Acad. Sci. USA* **84**, 7413–7417.
25. Zabner, J., Fasbender, A. J., Moninger, T., Poellinger, K. A., and Welsh, M. J. (1995) Cellular and molecular barriers to gene transfer by a cationic lipid. *J. Biol. Chem.* **270**, 18,997–19,007.
26. Felgner, P. L. and Ringold, G. M. (1989) Cationic liposome-mediated transfection. *Nature* **337**, 387–388.
27. Legendre, J.-Y. and Szoka, F. C. Jr. (1993) Cyclic amphipathic peptide-DNA complexes mediated high-efficiency transfection of adherent mammalian cells. *Proc. Natl. Acad. Sci. USA* **90**, 893–897.
28. Templeton, N. S. (2003) Cationic liposomes as in vivo delivery vehicles. *Curr. Med. Chem.* **10**, 1279–1287.

29. Niculescu-Duvaz, D., Heyes, J., and Springer, C. J. (2003) Structure-activity relationship in cationic lipid mediated gene transfection. *Curr. Med. Chem.* **10**, 1233–1261.
30. Farhood, H., Serbina, N., and Huang, L. (1995) The role of dioleoyl phosphatidylethanolamine in cationic liposome mediated gene transfer. *Biochim. Biophys. Acta* **1235**, 289–295.
31. Hafez, I. M., Maurer, N., and Cullis, P. R. (2001) On the mechanism whereby cationic lipids promote intracellular delivery of polynucleic acids. *Gene Ther.* **8**, 1188–1196.
32. Itano, H., Mora, B. N., Zhang, W., et al. (2001) Lipid-mediated ex vivo gene transfer of viral interleukin 10 in rat lung allotransplantation. *J. Thorac. Cardiovasc. Surg.* **122**, 29–38.
33. DeBruyne, L. A., Li, K., Chan, S. Y., Qin, L., Bishop, D. K., and Bromberg, J. S. (1998) Lipid-mediated gene transfer of viral IL-10 prolongs vascularised cardiac allograft survival by inhibiting donor-specific cellular and humoral immune responses. *Gene Ther.* **5**, 1079–1087.
34. Liu, Y., Liggitt, D., Zhong, W., Tu, G., Gaensler, K., and Debs, R. (1995) Cationic liposome-mediated intravenous gene delivery. *J. Biol. Chem.* **270**, 24,864–24,870.
35. Ishiwata, H., Suzuki, N., Ando, S., Kikuchi, H., and Kitagawa, T. (2000) Characteristics and biodistribution of cationic liposomes and their DNA complexes. *J. Control Release* **69**, 139–148.
36. Keogh, M.-C., Chen, D., Lupu, F., et al. (1997) High efficiency reported gene transfection of vascular tissue *in vitro* and *in vivo* using a cationic lipid-DNA complex. *Gene Ther.* **4**, 162–171.
37. Remy, J.-S., Kichler, A., Mordvinov, V., Schuber, F., and Behr, J.-P. (1995) Targeted gene transfer into hepatoma cells with lipopolyamine-condensed DNA particles presenting galactose ligands: A stage toward artificial viruses. *Proc. Natl. Acad. Sci. USA* **92**, 1744–1748.
38. Filion, M. C. and Phillips, N. C. (1997) Toxicity and immunomodulatory activity of liposomal vectors formulated with cationic lipids toward immune effector cells. *Biochim. Biophys. Acta* **1329**, 345–356.
39. Anwer, K., Kao, G., Proctor, B., Anscombe, I., Florack, V., Earls, R., Wilson, E., McCreery, T., Unger, E., Rolland, A., and Sullivan, S. M. (2000) Ultrasound enhancement of cationic lipid-mediated gene transfer to primary tumors following systemic administration. *Gene Ther.* **7**, 1833–1839.
40. Kim, J. K., Choi, S. H., Kim, C. O., Park, J. S., Ahn, W. S., and Kim, C. K. (2003) Enhancement of polyethylene glycol (PEG)-modified cationic liposome-mediated gene deliveries: effects on serum stability and transfection efficiency. *J. Pharm. Pharmacol.* **55**, 453–460.
41. Cheng, P. W. (1996) Receptor ligand facilitated gene transfer: enhancement of liposome-mediated gene transfer and expression by transferrin. *Hum. Gene Ther.* **7**, 285–282.
42. Hofland, H. E., Masson, C., Iginla, S., et al. (2002) Folate-targeted gene transfer in vivo. *Mol. Ther.* **5**, 739–744.

43. Hara, T., Aramaki, Y., Takada, S., Koike, K., and Tsuchiya, S. (1995) Receptor-mediated transfer of pSV2CAT DNA to mouse liver cells using asialofetuin-labeled liposomes. *Gene Ther.* **2**, 784–788.
44. Tan, P. H., Manunta, M., Ardjomand, N., et al. (2003) Antibody targeted gene transfer to endothelium. *J. Gene Med.* **5**, 311–323.
45. Gao, X. and Huang, L. (1996) Potentiation of cationic liposome-mediated gene delivery by polycations. *Biochem.* **35**, 1027–1036.
46. Vitiello, L., Chonn, A., Wasserman, J. D., Duff, C., and Worton, R. G. (1996) Condensation of plasmid DNA with polylysine improves liposome-mediated gene transfer into established and primary muscle cells. *Gene Ther.* **3**, 396–404.
47. Hart, S. L., Arancibia-Cárcamo, C. V., Wolfert, M. A., et al. (1998) Lipid-mediated enhancement of transfection by a nonviral integrin-targeting vector. *Hum. Gene Ther.* **9**, 575–585.
48. Li, J. M., Collins, L., Zhang, X., Gustafsson, K., and Fabre, J. W. (2000) Efficient gene delivery to vascular smooth muscle cells using a nontoxic, synthetic peptide vector system targeted to membrane integrins: a first step toward the gene therapy of chronic rejection. *Transplantation* **70**, 1616–1624.
49. Zhang, X., Collins, L., and Fabre, J. W. (2001) A powerful cooperative interaction between a fusogenic peptide and lipofectamine for the enhancement of receptor-targeted, non-viral gene delivery via integrin receptors. *J. Gene Med.* **3**, 560–568.
50. Dodds, E., Piper, T. A., Murphy, S. J., and Dickson, G. (1999) Cationic lipids and polymers are able to enhance adenoviral infection of cultured mouse myotubes. *J. Neurochem.* **72**, 2105–2112.
51. Kaneda, Y. (2001) Improvements in gene therapy technologies. *Mol. Urol.* **5**, 85–89.
52. Haensler, J. and Szoka, F. C. Jr. (1993) Synthesis and characterisation of a trigalactosylated bisacridine compound to target DNA to hepatocytes. *Bioconjug. Chem.* **4**, 85–93.
53. Soto, J., Bessodes, M., Pitard, B., Mailhe, P., Scherman, D., and Byk, G. (2000) Non-electrostatic complexes with DNA: towards novel synthetic gene delivery systems. *Bioorg. Med. Chem. Lett.* **10**, 911–914.
54. Fominaya, J. and Wels, W. (1996) Target cell specific DNA transfer mediated by a chimeric multidomain protein. *J. Biol. Chem.* **271**, 10,560–10,568.
55. Marquet, R., Wyart, A., and Houssier, C. (1987) Influence of DNA length on spermine-induced condensation. Importance of the bending and stiffening of DNA. *Biochim. Biophys. Acta.* **909**, 165–172.
56. Fritz, J. D., Herweijer, H., Zhang, G., and Wolff, J. A. (1996) Gene transfer into mammalian cells using histone-condensed plasmid DNA. *Hum. Gene Ther.* **7**, 1395–1404.
57. Sorgi, F. L., Bhattacharya, S., and Huang, L. (1997) Protamine sulfate enhances lipid-mediated gene transfer. *Gene Ther.* **4**, 961–968.
58. Wagner, E., Cotten, M., Foisner, R., and Birnstiel, M. L. (1991) Transferrin-polycation-DNA complexes: The effect of polycations on the structure of the complex and DNA delivery to cells. *Proc. Natl. Acad. Sci. USA* **88**, 4255–4259.

59. Wolfert, M. A. and Seymour, L. W. (1996) Atomic force microscopic analysis of the influence of the molecular weight of poly(L)lysine on the size of polyelectrolyte complexes formed with DNA. *Gene Ther.* **3**, 269–273.
60. Chiow, H. C., Tangco, M. V., Levine, S. M., et al. (1994) Enhanced resistance to nuclease degradation of nucleic acids complexes to asialoglycoprotein-polylysine carriers. *Nuc. Acid. Res.* **22**, 5439–5446.
61. Olins, D. E., Olins, A. L., and Von Hippel, P. H. (1986) Model nucleoprotein complexes: Studies on the interaction of cationic homopolypeptides with DNA. *J. Mol. Biol.* **24**, 157–176.
62. Lemoine, N. R. and Cooper, D. N. (1996) *Gene Therapy.* Bios Scientific Publishers, Oxford, UK.
63. Gill, T. J., Papermaster, D. S., Kunz, H. W., and Marfey, P. S. (1968) Studies on synthetic polypeptide antigens. *J. Biol. Chem.* **213**, 289–300.
64. Wilson, J. M., Grossman, M., Wu, C. H., Chowdhury, N. R., Wu, G. Y., and Chowdhury, J. R. (1992) Hepatocyte-directed gene transfer *in vivo* to transient improvement of Hypercholesterolemia in low density lipoprotein receptor-deficient rabbits. *J. Biol. Chem.* **267**, 963–967.
65. Kircheis, R., Wightman, L., and Wagner, E. (2001) Design and gene delivery activity of modified polyethylenimines. *Adv. Drug Deliv. Rev.* **53**, 341–358.
66. Goula, D., Remy, J.-S., Erbacher, P., et al. (1998) Size, diffusibilty and transfection performance of linear PEI/DNA complexed in the mouse central nervous system. *Gene Ther.* **5**, 712–717.
67. Boussif, O., Lezoualc'h, F., Zanta, M. A., et al. (1995) A versatile vector for gene and oligonucleotide transfer into cells in culture and *in vivo*: polyethylenimine. *Proc. Natl. Acad. Sci. USA* **92**, 7797–7301.
68. Kichler, A., Leborgne, C., Coeytaux, E., and Danos, O. (2001) Polyethylenimine-mediated gene delivery: a mechanistic study. *J. Gene Med.* **3**, 135–144.
69. Boletta, A., Benigni, A., Lutz, J., Remuzzi, G., Soria, M. R., and Monaco, L. (1997) Nonviral gene delivery to the rat kidney with polyethylenimine. *Hum. Gene Ther.* **8**, 1243–1251.
70. Lemkine, G. F., Goula, D., Becker, N., Paleari, L., Levi, G., and Demeneix, B. A. (1999) Optimisation of polyethylenimine-based gene delivery to mouse brain. *J. Drug Target* **7**, 305–312.
71. Coll, J. L., Chollet, P., Brambilla, E., Desplanques, D., Behr, J. P., and Favrot, M. (1999) In vivo delivery to tumors of DNA complexed with linear polyethylenimine. *Hum. Gene Ther.* **10**, 1659–1666.
72. Aoki, K., Furuhata, S., Hatanaka, K., et al. (2001) Polyethylenimine-mediated gene transfer into pancreatic tumor dissemination in the murine peritoneal cavity. *Gene Ther.* **8**, 508–514.
73. Ferrari, S., Pettenazzo, A., Garbati, N., Zacchello, F., Behr, J. P., and Scarpa, M. (1999) Polyethylenimine shows properties of interest for cystic fibrosis gene therapy. *Biochim. Biophys. Acta* **1447**, 219–225.
74. Ogris, M., Brunner, S., Schuller, S., Kircheis, R., and Wagner, E. (1999) PEGylated DNA/transferrin-PEI complexes: reduced interaction with blood com-

ponents, extended circulation in blood and potential for systemic gene delivery. *Gene Ther.* **6**, 595–605.
75. Nguyen, H. K., Lemieux, P., Vinogradov, S. V., et al. (2000) Evaluation of polyether-polyethyleneimine graft copolymers as gene transfer agents. *Gene Ther.* **7**, 126–138.
76. Kircheis, R., Kichler, A., Wallner, G., et al. (1997) Coupling of cell-binding ligands to polyethylenimine for targeted gene delivery. *Gene Ther.* **4**, 409–418.
77. Erbacher, P., Remy, J. S., and Behr, J. P. (1999) Gene transfer with synthetic virus-like particles via the integrin-mediated endocytosis pathway. *Gene Ther.* **6**, 138–145.
78. Kircheis, R., Kichler, A., Wallner, G., et al. (1997) Coupling of cell-binding ligands to polyethylenimine for targeted gene delivery. *Gene Ther.* **4**, 409–418.
79. Blessing, T., Kursa, M., Holzhauser, R., Kircheis, R., and Wagner, E. (2001) Different strategies for formation of pegylated EGF-conjugated PEI/DNA complexes for targeted gene delivery. *Bioconjug. Chem.* **12**, 529–537.
80. Tang, M. X., Redemann, C. T., and Szoka, F. C. Jr. (1996) In vitro gene delivery by degraded polyamidoamine dendrimers. *Bioconjug. Chem.* **7**, 703–714.
81. Hudde, T., Rayner, S. A., Comer, R. M., et al. (1999) Activated polyamidoamine dendrimers, a non-viral vector for gene transfer to the corneal endothelium. *Gene Ther.* **6**, 939–943.
82. Qin, L., Pahud, D. R., Ding, Y., et al. (1998) Efficient transfer of genes into murine cardiac grafts by Starburst polyamidoamine dendrimers. *Hum. Gene Ther.* **9**, 553–560.
83. Oupicky, D., Konak, C., Dash, P. R., Seymour, L. W., and Ulbrich, K. (1999) Effect of albumin and polyanion on the structure of DNA complexes with polycation containing hydrophilic nonionic block. *Bioconjug. Chem.* **10**, 764–772.
84. Plank, C., Mechtler, K., Szoka, F. C. Jr., and Wagner, E. (1996) Activation of the complement system by synthetic DNA complexes: a potential barrier for intravenous gene delivery. *Hum. Gene Ther.* **7**, 1437–1446.
85. Oupicky, D., Carlisle, R. C., and Seymour, L. W. (2001) Triggered intracellular activation of disulfide crosslinked polyelectrolyte gene delivery complexes with extended systemic circulation in vivo. *Gene Ther.* **8**, 713–724.
86. Godbey, W. T., Wu, K. K., and Mikos, A. G. (1999) Tracking the intracellular path of poly(ethylenimine)/DNA complexes for gene delivery. *Proc. Natl. Acad. Sci. USA* **96**, 5177–5181.
87. Ford, K. G., Souberbielle, B. E., Darling, D., and Farzaneh, F. (2001) Protein transduction: an alternative to genetic intervention? *Gene Ther.* **8**, 1–4.
88. Elliott, G. and O'Hare, P. (1997) Intercellular trafficking and protein delivery by a herpesvirus structural protein. *Cell* **88**, 223–233.
89. Tietz, P. S., Yamazaki, K., and LaRusso, N. F. (1990) Time-dependent effects of chloroquine on pH of hepatocyte lysosomes. *Biochem. Pharmacol.* **40**, 1419–1421.
90. Carr, C. M. and Kim, P. S. (1993) A spring loaded mechanism for the comformational change of influenza hemagglutinin. *Cell* **73**, 823–832.

91. Simoes, S., Slepushkin, V., Gaspar, R., de Lima, M. C., and Duzgunes, N. (1998) Gene delivery by negatively charged ternary complexes of DNA, cationic liposomes and transferrin or fusigenic peptides. *Gene Ther.* **5**, 955–964.
92. Lim, D. W., Yeom, Y. I., and Park, T. G. (2000) Poly(DMAEMA-NVP)-b-PEG-galactose as gene delivery vector for hepatocytes. *Bioconjug. Chem.* **11**, 688–695.
93. Hogset, A., Prasmickaite, L., Tjelle, T. E., and Berg, K. (2000) Photochemical transfection: a new technology for light-induced, site-directed gene delivery. *Hum. Gene Ther.* **11**, 869–880.
94. McKenzie, D. L., Kwok, K. Y., and Rice, K. G. (2000) A potent new class of reductively activated peptide gene delivery agents. *J. Biol. Chem.* **275**, 9970–9977.
95. Wetzer, B., Byk, G., Frederic, M., Airiau, M., Blanche, F., Pitard, B., and Scherman, D. (2001) Reducible cationic lipids for gene transfer. *Biochem. J.* **356**, 747–756.
96. Brunner, S., Furtbauer, E., Sauer, T., Kursa, M., and Wagner, E. (2002) Overcoming the nuclear barrier: cell cycle independent nonviral gene transfer with linear polyethylenimine or electroporation. *Mol. Ther.* **5**, 80–86.
97. Shewring, L. D., Collins, L., Lightman, S. L., Hart, S. L., Gustafsson, K., and Fabre, J. W. (1997) A nonviral vector system for efficient gene transfer to corneal endothelial cells via membrane integrins. *Transplantation* **64**, 763–769.
98. Collins, L., Asuni, A. A., Anderton, B. H., and Fabre, J. W. (2003) Efficient gene delivery to primary neuron cultures using a synthetic peptide vector system. *J. Neurosci. Methods* **125**, 113–120.
99. Vacik, J., Dean, B. S., Zimmer, W. E., and Dean, D. A. (1999) Cell-specific nuclear import of plasmid DNA. *Gene Ther.* **6**, 1006–1014.
100. Goldfarb, D. S., Gariépy, J., Schoolnik, G., and Kornberg, R. D. (1986) Synthetic peptides as nuclear localisation signals. *Nature* **322**, 641–644.
101. Miao, C. H., Thompson, A. R., Loeb, K., and Ye, X. (2001) Long-term and therapeutic-level hepatic gene expression of human factor IX after naked plasmid transfer in vivo. *Mol. Ther.* **3**, 947–957.
102. Miao, C. H., Ohashi, K., Patijn, G. A., et al. (2000) Inclusion of the hepatic locus control region, an intron, and untranslated region increases and stabilizes hepatic factor IX gene expression in vivo but not in vitro. *Mol. Ther.* **1**, 522–532.
103. Larin, Z. and Mejia, J. E. (2002) Advances in human artificial chromosome technology. *Trends Genet.* **18**, 313–319.
104. Kaminski, J. M., Huber, M. R., Summers, J. B., and Ward, M. B. (2002) Design of a nonviral vector for site-selective, efficient integration into the human genome. *FASEB J.* **16**, 1242–1247.
105. Ziady, A. G., Perales, J. C., Ferkol, T., Gerken, T., Beegen, H., Perlmutter, D. H., and Davis, P. B. (1997) Gene transfer into hepatoma cell lines via the serpin enzyme complex receptor. *Am. J. Physiol.* **273**, 545–552.
106. Patel, S., Zhang, X., Collins, L., and Fabre, J. W. (2001) A small, synthetic peptide for gene delivery via the serpin-enzyme complex receptor. *J. Gene Med.* **3**, 271–279.

107. Wu, G. Y. and Wu, C. H. (1987) Receptor-mediated in vitro gene transformation by a soluble DNA carrier system. *J. Biol. Chem.* **262**, 4429–4432.
108. Singh, M., Kisoon, N., and Ariatti, M. (2001) Receptor-mediated gene delivery to HepG2 cells by ternary assemblies containing cationic liposomes and cationized asialoorosomucoid. *Drug Deliv.* **8**, 29–34.
109. Chen, J., Gamou, S., Takayanagi, A., and Shimizu, N. (1994) A novel gene delivery system using EGF receptor-mediated endocytosis. *FEBS Lett.* **338**, 167–169.
110. Sosnowski, B. A., Gonzalez, A. M., Chandler, L. A., Buechler, Y. J., Pierce, G. F., and Baird, A. (1996) Targeting DNA to cells with basic fibroblast growth factor (FGF2) *J. Biol. Chem.* **271**, 33,647–33,653. ·
111. Leamon, C. P. and Low, P. S. (1991) Delivery of macromolecules into living cells: A method that exploits folate receptor endocytosis. *Proc. Natl. Acad. Sci. USA* **88**, 5572–5576.
112. Lee, R. J. and Low, P. S. (1994) Delivery of liposomes into cultured KB cells via folate receptor-mediated endocytosis. *J. Biol. Chem.* **269**, 3198–3204.
113. Guo, W. and Lee, R. L. (1999) Receptor-targeted gene delivery via folate-conjugated polyethylenimine. *AAPS. PharmSci.* **1**, E19.
114. Chen, J., Stickles, R. J., and Daichendt, K. A. (1994) Galactosylated histone-mediated gene transfer and expression. *Hum. Gene Ther.* **5**, 429–435.
115. Ferkol, T., Lindberg, G. L., Chen, J., Perales, J. C., Crawford, D. R., Ratnoff, O. D., and Hanson, R. W. (1993) Regulation of the phosphoenolpyruvate carboxykinase/human factor IX gene introduced into the livers of adult rats by receptor-mediated gene transfer. *FASEB J.* **7**, 1081–1091.
116. Plank, C., Zatloukal, K., Cotten, M., Mechtler, K., and Wagner, E. (1992) Gene transfer into hepatocytes using asialoglycoprotein receptor mediated endocytosis of DNA complexed with an artificial tetra-antennary galactose ligand. *Bioconjug. Chem.* **3**, 533–539.
117. Carlos Perales, J., Ferkol, T., Beegen, H., Ratnoff, O. D., and Hanson, R. W. (1994) Gene transfer *in vivo*: Sustained expression and regulation of genes introduced into the liver by receptor-targeted uptake. *Proc. Natl. Acad. Sci. USA* **91**, 4086–4090.
118. Nishikawa, M., Yamauchi, M., Morimoto, K., Ishida, E., Takakura, Y., and Hashida, M. (2000) Hepatocyte-targeted in vivo gene expression by intravenous injection of plasmid DNA complexed with synthetic multi-functional gene delivery system. *Gene Ther.* **7**, 548–555.
119. Huckett, B., Ariatti, M., and Hawtrey, A. O. (1990) Evidence for targeted gene transfer by receptor-mediated endocytosis. Stable expression following insulin-directed entry of NEO into HepG2 cells. *Biochem. Pharmacol.* **40**, 253–263.
120. Rosenkranz, A. A., Yachmenev, S. V., Jans, D. A., et al. (1992) Receptor-mediated endocytosis and nuclear transport of a transfecting DNA construct. *Exp. Cell. Res.* **199**, 323–329.
121. Ding, Z. M., Cristiano, R. J., Roth, J. A., Takacs, B., and Kuo, M. T. (1995) Malarial circumsporozoite protein is a novel gene delivery vehicle to primary hepatocyte cultures and cultured cells. *J. Biol. Chem.* **270**, 3667–3676.

122. Hart, S. L., Harbottle, R. P., Cooper, R. G., Miller, A. D., Williamson, R., and Coutelle, C. (1995) Gene delivery and expression mediated by an integrin-binding peptide. *Gene Ther.* **2**, 552–554.
123. Hart, S. L., Collins, L., Gustafsson, K., and Fabre, J. W. (1997) Integrin-mediated transfection with peptides containing arginine-glycine-aspartic acid domains. *Gene Ther.* **4**, 1225–1230.
124. Harbottle, R. P., Cooper, R. G., Hart, S. L., et al. (1998) An RGD-Oligolysine peptide: A prototype construct for integrin mediated gene delivery. *Hum. Gene Ther.* **9**, 1037–1047.
125. Collins, L., Sawyer, G. J., Zhang, X. H., Gustafsson, K., and Fabre, J. W. (2000) In vitro investigation of factors important for the delivery of an integrin-targeted nonviral DNA vector in organ transplantation. *Transplantation* **69**, 1168–1176.
126. Midoux, P., Mendes, C., Legrand, A., et al. (1993) Specific gene transfer mediated by lactosylated poly-l-lysine into hepatoma cells. *Nuc. Acid. Res.* **21**, 871–878.
127. Ferkol, T., Perales, J. C., Mularo, F., and Hanson, R. W. (1996) Receptor-mediated gene transfer into macrophages. *Proc. Natl. Acad. Sci. USA* **93**, 101–105.
128. Ferkol, T., Mularo, F., Hilliard, J., et al. (1998) Transfer of the human Alpha 1-antitrypsin gene into pulmonary macrophages in vivo. *Am. J. Respir. Cell Mol. Biol.* **18**, 591–601.
129. Diebold, S. S., Lehrmann, H., Kursa, M., Wagner, E., Cotten, M., and Zenke, M. (1999) Efficient gene delivery into human dendritic cells by adenovirus polyethylenimine and mannose polyethylenimine transfection. *Hum. Gene Ther.* **10**, 775–786.
130. Wagner, E., Zenke, M., Cotten, M., Beug, H., and Birnstiel, M. L. (1990) Transferrin- polycation conjugates as carriers for DNA uptake into cells. *Proc. Natl. Acad. Sci. USA* **87**, 3410–3414.
131. Merwin, J. R., Carmichael, E. P., Noell, G. S., et al. (1995) CD5-mediated specific delivery of DNA to T lymphocytes: compartmentalization augmented by adenovirus. *J. Immunol. Methods* **186**, 257–266.
132. Coll, J. L., Wagner, E., Combaret, V., et al. (1997) In vitro targeting and specific transfection of human neuroblastoma cells by chCE7 antibody-mediated gene transfer. *Gene Ther.* **4**, 156–161.
133. Foster, B. J. and Kern, J. A. (1997) HER2-targeted gene transfer. *Hum. Gene Ther.* **8**, 719–727.
134. Ferkol, T., Kaetzel, C. S., and Davis, P. B. (1993) Gene transfer into respiratory epithelial cells by targeting the polymeric immunoglobulin receptor. *J. Clin. Invest.* **92**, 2394–2400.
135. Thurnher, M., Wagner, E., Clausen, H., et al. (1994) Carbohydrate receptor-mediated gene transfer to human T leukaemic cells. *Glycobiology* **4**, 429–435.
136. Fominaya, J., Uherek, C., and Wels, W. (1998) A chimeric fusion protein containing transforming growth factor-α mediates gene transfer via binding to the ECF receptor. *Gene Ther.* **5**, 521–530.

137. Schachtschabel, U., Pavlinkova, G., Lou, D., and Kohler, H. (1996) Antibody-mediated gene delivery for B-cell lymphoma in vitro. *Cancer Gene Ther.* **3**, 365–372.
138. Rojanasakul, Y., Wang, L. Y., Malanga, C. J., Ma, J. K., and Liaw, J. (1994) Targeted gene delivery to alveolar macrophages via Fc receptor-mediated endocytosis. *Pharm. Res.* **11**, 1731–1736.

10

Detection and Clinical Relevance of Antibodies After Transplantation

John D. Smith and Marlene Rose

Summary

Until recently, the role of antibodies in graft failure has been hampered by poor methods of defining specificity. Development of solid phase assays using purified major histocompatibility complex (MHC) molecules has greatly advanced our ability to monitor anti-human leukocyte antigen (HLA) antibodies in patients and to distinguish between HLA and non-HLA antibodies. The purpose of this chapter is to describe the methods for detecting antibodies and what we have learned in recent years regarding the role of well-defined antibodies to HLA and non-HLA antigens. Use of the complement-dependent lymphocytotoxic test was instrumental in defining patients who are sensitized to donor HLA antigens, and it still plays a major role in avoiding transplantation of organs into sensitized patients. However, solid phase assays are more useful for following patients posttransplant. A major advance has been the demonstration that anti-MHC class II antibodies are made late after transplantation and contribute to late graft failure. This has been demonstrated for renal and lung transplantation, but has not yet been confirmed for other organs. Clearer definition of non-HLA antibodies has been achieved, such as the autoantigen vimentin and MHC I-related chain A. Experimental studies using minor mismatched strain combinations confirm that non-HLA antibodies bind to donor endothelial cells; these antibodies seem to cause apoptosis but not complement-mediated lysis.

Key Words: Antibodies; humoral rejection; non-HLA antigens; HLA; complement; antiendothelial antibodies.

1. Methodological Considerations

Human leukocyte antigen (HLA) antibodies can be detected by a number of different techniques that employ live cells or purified HLA molecules. Traditionally, cell-based techniques assessing cell viability were used, but newer methods utilizing purified HLA molecules bound to a solid surface giving

From: *Methods in Molecular Biology, vol. 333: Transplantation Immunology: Methods and Protocols*
Edited by: P. Hornick and M. Rose © Humana Press Inc., Totowa, NJ

greater sensitivity and specificity are now employed. Indeed, solid phase methods have revolutionized detection of antibodies and have led to greater recognition of their importance in posttransplant events.

1.1. Complement Dependent Cytotoxicity

The earliest method commonly used to detect HLA-specific antibodies was a microlymphocytotoxic assay known as the complement-dependent cytotoxicity (CDC) assay *(1)*. Briefly, viable lymphocytes are incubated with sera; during this stage, any antibodies present in the serum specific for the HLA molecules expressed on the surface of the target cells bind to the cell surface. Rabbit complement is added, and antibody bound to the cell surface activates the classical complement pathway, leading to production of the membrane attack complex of complement (C5-9), which ultimately causes lysis of the target cell. Staining of the cells is used to determine cell viability. The most commonly used stains are the cocktail of the fluorescent stains ethidium bromide and acridine orange.

In order to determine the frequency and specificity of HLA antibodies in antisera, a panel of HLA-typed lymphocytes are used as targets and the specificity determined by the patterns of reactivity. An adequate cell panel is necessary in order to be able to detect all HLA antibodies. The method of selection of a cell panel is an important consideration. Panels can be selected to cover the majority of known HLA specificities, which may not reflect the frequency of HLA antigens in the general population, or panels can be random, where sera are screened with a panel of cells that are representative of the population. For example, a serum containing antibodies directed against the HLA-A2 antigen may react with 40% of the cell panel if a random panel is used because the HLA-A2 antigen maybe present in approx 40% of the population one is using. However, if a selected cell panel is used, the reactivity may be much lower. The results from the CDC assay have therefore been reported as a percentage of the cell panel with which a serum has reacted, known as the percentage panel reactive antibody frequency (%PRA). Each laboratory will have produced its own panel, and because of the differences in panel composition, the PRA results from different laboratories cannot be compared. Therefore, the use of the term PRA is decreasing, with the majority of laboratories no longer using the phrase.

CDC assays are able to detect both immunoglobulin (Ig)G and IgM antibodies with the use of dithiothreitol (DTT) in the assay. Although relatively crude and insensitive, DTT breaks down disulfide bonds, and because IgM contains significantly more than IgG, the IgM reactivity is preferentially degraded.

Despite its widespread use in the past, the CDC assay has a number of limitations. First, an adequate cell panel is difficult to obtain and maintain. Second, cell viability and the source of complement can easily influence the specificity and sensitivity of the assay. In addition, only complement-dependent antibodies are detected, and not all antibody reactivity detected may be HLA specific.

Furthermore, false-positive results owing to the presence of IgM non-HLA autoreactive antibodies can also lead to misleading results. IgM non-HLA antibodies react with the majority of normal lymphocytes, but not with lymphocytes from chronic lymphocytic leukemia (CLL) patients. These antibodies have been shown to be irrelevant to transplant outcome in renal transplantation *(**2**)*, and therefore a patient should not be considered sensitized purely on the basis of percentage PRA. These antibodies are of the IgM class and will therefore be removed by treatment with DTT, and in order to determine the presence of HLA antibodies it is necessary to define an HLA specificity to the antibodies.

As HLA class II antigens are only found on B cells within the lymphocyte populations, the detection of HLA class II antibodies has always been problematic. Historically, this has been achieved by using lymphocytes isolated from the peripheral blood of patients with CLL, a B-cell lymphoma. However, the sensitivity and accuracy of the assay was limited, and identification of class II antibodies was almost certainly underestimated. For ethical reasons it is now difficult to obtain blood samples from CLL patients, and their use is thus limited.

Following transplantation, therapies used to combat rejection include the use of the monoclonal antibody (MAb) OKT3 and antithymocyte globulin, which are antibody preparations directed against T cells. Unfortunately, these antibodies are detectable in the serum of patients in the CDC assay demonstrated by an IgG response to all panel members' lymphocytes.

With the introduction of newer, more sensitive techniques, the use of CDC has declined, and it is now used as an additional test rather than a front-line method for the detection of HLA antibodies. Until the mid to late 1990s, the majority of all HLA antibody screening and published studies utilized CDC screening, and it was often difficult to determine the true nature and effect of HLA antibodies on the outcome of transplantation.

1.2. Flow Cytometry

Flow cytometry assays were originally developed to be more sensitive than the CDC assay. Rather than using panels comprised of individual cells, flow cytometry antibody screening used pools of cells designed to cover all of the major serological HLA specificities *(**3**)*. The cell types used included CLL cells, Epstein–Barr virus transformed lymphoblastoid cell lines, as well as peripheral blood lymphocytes (PBLs).

The assay involves an initial incubation of serum with target cells followed by a series of washes and incubation with a fluorescein isothiocyanate conjugated (FITC) MAb directed against human IgG. Following this, the cells are passed through the flow cytometer, and the number of positive cells and channel shift increase above negative controls is calculated. Screening sera with individual cell panels is cumbersome for initial antibody screening, but the use of pooled cells enables the initial detection of antibodies. Once it is established that a serum contains antibodies, screening against individual cells allows the identification of HLA specificities. As with CDC, there are problems associated with assigning a %PRA.

1.3. Solid Phase Assays

In recent years, advances have been made in the detection of HLA-specific antibodies with the introduction of assays utilizing purified HLA molecules. The HLA molecules are purified from either lymphoblastoid cell lines for class I and class II molecules or from platelets for class I *(4–6)*. Two distinct types of assay are available involving mixtures of HLA molecules from many (up to 100 individuals) cell lines to detect the presence or absence of HLA antibodies or HLA molecules purified from individual cell lines in order to determine the specificity of the antibodies. Three different types of solid phase assays are available.

1.3.1. Flow Cytometric Bead Assays

Flow cytometry microparticles coated with soluble HLA molecules are incubated with serum followed by a further incubation with an FITC MAb against human IgG. Beads coated with either mixtures of HLA molecules or individual molecules make possible detection of the presence of HLA antibodies or the identification of HLA specificities. Studies have shown these flow cytometry microparticles to be a more sensitive and specific test than CDC for the detection of HLA-specific antibodies *(7)*.

1.3.2. Enzyme-Linked Immunosorbent Assays

Enzyme-linked immunosorbent assays (ELISAs) also incorporate soluble HLA antigens coating the surface of plastic trays *(4,5)*. Two types of ELISA tests are available. The first uses mixtures of HLA molecules and allows the determination of the presence of HLA-specific antibody, whereas the second assay uses HLA molecules purified from individual cells coated into separate wells of the plastic tray, allowing the identification of specificity. These ELISA tests have the advantage that reactions are based on optical density readings and can be ranked in order of strength to allow determination of reactivity. It is generally considered that ELISA test kit sensitivity is greater than that of CDC, but less than that of flow cytometry.

1.3.3. Luminex Assays

The luminex bead system incorporates minute polystyrene beads that contain varying amounts of two different fluorochromes. The differing amounts of the two fluorochromes enable the separate identification of 100 different beads when passed through the flow cell of a specialized flow cytometer known as a luminex machine. Because the beads can be identified according to the amount of fluorochromes contained within the bead, many different bead types can be multiplexed in a single reaction. It is therefore possible to use panels of a large number of beads to identify antibody specificity. The advantage of the luminex assays is that they are extremely specific, highly sensitive (comparable to flow cytometry), and extremely rapid.

1.4. General Comments on Solid Phase Assays

Solid phase assays have several advantages over conventional CDC assays:

- There is no requirement for viable lymphocytes and complement.
- They detect only HLA-specific antibodies.
- They detect non-complement-fixing antibodies.
- They are objective and can be partially automated.
- They are commercially available.

Large studies of solid phase assays have found that they are extremely reliable in detecting IgG HLA antibodies, although the use of reagents to detect IgM antibodies appears to be less reliable. More recently, production of recombinant HLA molecules has enabled both flow cytometry and luminex beads to be coated with single HLA antigens, making the identification of HLA antibodies and, in the case of highly sensitized patients, the identification of HLA antigens to which the patient is not sensitized, simpler.

1.5. Crossmatching

Crossmatching for solid organ transplantation has traditionally been performed using the CDC test *(8)*. In 1969 Patel and Terasaki were able to demonstrate that 80% of patients with a positive crossmatch against donor lymphocytes experienced graft failure within 2 d of transplantation compared with just 4% of patients with a negative crossmatch *(9)*. It has been accepted since this time that renal transplantation should not proceed in the face of a positive crossmatch.

The CDC crossmatch involves incubation of donor lymphocytes (T cells, B cells, or a mixture of T and B cells) with recipient serum samples followed by the addition of rabbit complement. An increase in cell death over control wells indicates the presence of donor-specific antibodies and is considered a positive crossmatch. Many centers also perform the crossmatch in the presence of DTT, as it is now believed that IgG antibodies are those significantly associated with graft failure.

The recently developed flow cytometric crossmatch test is considered a highly sensitive method for detecting donor-specific HLA antibodies. Unfortunately, both the CDC and flow crossmatches detect not only HLA antibodies but non-HLA antibodies as well. The target cells for both techniques are donor lymphocytes commonly isolated from donor spleen, lymph node, or peripheral blood. More often, T cells are isolated for detection of class I antibodies and B cells for the detection of class I and class II antibodies by the CDC assay. The use of PBLs for crossmatching is less than ideal because PBLs contain relatively low numbers of B cells, which could affect the reliability of the test, particularly for detection of class II antibodies.

The crossmatch test, whether using CDC or flow cytometry, is always performed prior to renal transplantation, whereas in cardiothoracic transplantation, the limitations of time caused by the short ischemic time of the organs mean that crossmatching must be performed retrospectively (usually the following day) with recipient serum collected before transplantation. For sensitized patients undergoing cardiothoracic transplantation, a crossmatch against donor lymphocytes is usually performed prospectively with lymphocytes isolated from peripheral blood, with the transplant proceeding only if the result is negative.

A crossmatch result is either negative or positive. A positive result is usually due to the presence of donor-specific antibodies but, as with CDC screening, may also be the result of non-HLA antibodies. If the result is caused by IgM non-HLA antibodies, this is not generally considered a contraindication to transplantation.

As with CDC antibody screening, the CDC crossmatch suffers from a number of inherent problems. First, the test is relatively insensitive compared with flow cytometry and solid phase assays. Second, the requirement for viable cells of good quality is often a problem. Third, lymphocytes express many more molecules than HLA, and it is therefore possible that any reactivity detected may not necessarily be attributed to HLA antibodies.

1.6. Screening Strategies

It is essential that the histocompatibilty and immunogenetics (H&I) laboratory develop a comprehensive program for HLA antibody detection and identification when providing a service for solid organ transplant programs. It has been shown that fewer than half of the patients awaiting solid organ transplantation will have produced HLA antibodies ***(10)***. In the modern era it is necessary to have a test capable of rapidly detecting the presence of antibodies, followed by more extensive methods to define the specificity of the antibodies detected in the initial screen. The techniques outlined in the previous sections are all commercially available to the H&I laboratory and should not be considered alternative techniques. However, these techniques can all yield different information, and it is therefore advisable to devise screening strategies that utilize a combination of these techniques to maximize the information available to the clinician.

The crossmatch is the final test used before transplantation, and it is therefore essential that the screening techniques provide information predictive of the crossmatch test and have a comparable sensitivity and specificity.

1.7. Detection of Non-HLA Antibodies

Antibodies directed against a number of molecules and cell types have been detected and implicated in decreases in graft survival and function ***(11–17)***. Antibodies to cellular proteins are commonly described using ELISA techniques where the target protein is either bound directly to the ELISA plate or captured into the assay with MAbs specific for the protein bound to the surface of the plate. Patient serum would then be added, followed by detection with a MAb to human Igs conjugated to an enzymatic system such as horseradish peroxidase or alkaline phosphatase allowing a colorimetric detection.

Antibodies to particular cell types such as endothelial cells (ECs) or epithelial cells ***(14,18,19)*** are often detected using flow cytometric techniques. Either cell lines of the specific type or primary cultured cells are incubated with patient serum followed by a second incubation with an FITC antibody to human Igs (these can also be isotype-specific). The amount of fluoroscein binding is then measured in the flow cytometer.

2. Association Between Posttransplant Production of Antibodies and Rejection

It is universally accepted that transplantation of organs into patients with preformed antibodies to donor antigens can cause hyperacute rejection, and this situation is avoided whenever possible. However, more controversial is whether antibodies formed after transplantation have a pathogenic role. There are three major problems with ascribing a role for antibodies in graft deterioration: poor definition of antigen specificity, failure to localize antibodies in the graft, and lack of information regarding mechanisms of damage. Considerable progress has been made with regard to tissue-localization of antibodies, especially in the area of renal transplantation; e.g., deposition of C4d in the graft is one of the diagnostic citeria for humoral rejection following renal transplantation ***(20)***. More is now known about complement-independent pathways of antibody activation ***(21)***. This chapter focuses on the progress made in defining the specificity of antibodies made after transplantation and in particular the distinction between HLA and non-HLA antibodies.

Although antibodies can be damaging at any time after transplantation, the current interest in the long-term fate of grafts has helped to focus attention on antibodies. Many grafts fail or become dysfunctional because of a fibrogenic and obliterative disease affecting the main conduits, be they blood vessels or airways. Such complications are known as cardiac allograft vasculopathy (CAV), bronchiolitis obliterans syndrome (BOS), or chronic renal rejection following heart, lung, and renal transplantation, respectively.

Precise identification of antigen specificity is crucial to understanding the role of antibodies in graft failure, partly in order to obtain robust assays, the results of which can be compared between labs. Also, knowing the precise target of the antibody response could lead to therapeutic intervention.

2.1. Antibodies to Major Histocompatibility Complex Antigens

Until recently, live cells were used to measure antibody reactivity in patient sera, as described above. This was done using complement-dependent cytotoxicity or, alternatively, flow cytometry. However, using live cells underestimates antibodies to major histocompatibility complex (MHC) class II antigens, which are only expressed on monocytes and B cells in peripheral blood. Even specificities attributed to MHC class I antigens, which are abundantly expressed on the surface of leukocytes, were not always confirmed using blocking MAbs. Use of solid phase assays has been especially useful for defining reactivity to MHC class II antigens. It has been reported that a B-cell-positive crossmatch prior to transplantation is associated with more rejection episodes ***(22)*** or poor graft survival ***(23)***, but it is not known to what extent B-cell reactivity represented reactivity to MHC class II antigens. Human microvascular ECs constitutively express MHC class II antigens ***(24)***, and antibodies targeting ECs could be damaging. Palmer et al. have demonstrated a high association between *de novo* production of antibodies to donor-specific MHC antigens (using flow cytometric analysis of HLA-coated beads) and development of BOS after lung transplantation ***(25)***. They concluded that although *de novo* production of donor-specific anti-HLA antibodies is rare after lung transplantation (occurring in 10 of 90 patients), 8 of 10 patients developed BOS as opposed to only 38% of the flow-negative patients. Of considerable interest was the observation that in 90% of the flow-positive cases, antibody was to MHC class II antigens. Jaramillo et al. ***(26)*** also reported a strong association between antidonor antibodies and BOS after lung transplantation; these authors compared the ELISA method with complement-dependent cytotoxicity and found that only 2 of 15 BOS patients were antibody positive by complement-dependent cytotoxicity, but 10 of 15 were positive using the ELISA method. In contrast to Palmer et al. ***(25)***, none of the antibodies were against MHC class II antigens—they were all to class I antigens. The results of Palmer et al., along with recent studies from renal transplantation, suggest that anti-class II antigens are much more common than previously thought and are associated with late graft failure. Worthington et al. ***(27)*** studied 112 recipients of renal allografts that had failed within 5 yr. This group was compared with 123 recipients with functioning allografts who had been transplanted during the same time period. All recipients had been negative for donor HLA-specific antibodies before transplantation. After transplantation, 50.9% of the 112 patients in the failure group produced donor HLA-specific antibodies, compared with 1.6% of the 123 controls (p <0.0001). For 60% of the donor-specific antibody-positive patients, antibodies were detected before transplant failure. In 17 cases, these were MHC class I-specific, in 14 cases they were class II-specific, and in 3 cases they were specific for MHC class I and class II. Interestingly, a significant number of patients made antibody to DQ antigen in the absence of antibody to DR, demonstrating the importance of monitoring reactivity to DQ. In the studies of Palmer and Worthington, *de novo* production of antibodies and especially MHC class II antibodies sometimes became apparent many years after transplantation (1–8 yr) and still preceded organ failure or BOS. That antibodies to MHC class II tend to appear at later times than antibodies to MHC class I ***(27)*** may explain why such antibodies were not detected by Jaramillo et al., who only followed their patients for 2 yr. In the long-term study of renal transplant recipients by Pelletier et al. ***(28)***, it was shown that alloantibodies to MHC class II, but not class I antigens are an independent risk factor for chronic rejection. Our own studies have shown that 4 of 9 patients who required retransplantation had anti-class II donor-specific antibodies (Smith, J. D. and Rose, M. L., unpublished), suggesting that these antibodies also portend poor graft survival after heart transplantation. It is anticipated that widespread use of solid phase assays will more clearly define the role of MHC class II antibodies after transplantation.

Solid phase assays have been used to examine the specificity of the B-cell-positive crossmatch ***(29)***, which has commonly been thought to represent MHC class II reactivity. The authors examined 62 recipients of renal allografts transplanted across a B-cell-positive (T-cell-negative) crossmatch. Surprisingly, in only 23% of cases was this reactivity caused by anti-class II antigens, most of which were against donor DQ. In 16% activity was due to IgM autoantibodies, and in the remainder of cases (61%) the specificity of the response could not be determined. Whereas the clinical course of the autoantibody-positive patients did not differ from controls, patients with anti-class II antibodies prior to transplantation fared worse. Three of them with donor-specific anti-DQ antibodies lost their grafts within 3 mo because of vascular rejection. Overall, however, the 3-yr survival of the B cell$^+$ class II$^+$ patients was no worse than controls. In view of the detrimental effect of *de novo* production of MHC class II antibodies ***(25,27,28)***, it will be interesting to discover whether longer-term follow-up of these patients reveals an adverse effect of the class II-positive crossmatch.

2.2. Antibodies to Non-MHC Antigens

There is a long history of non-HLA antibodies being produced after renal or cardiac transplantation, in particular, anti-EC antibodies (AECAs). The initial interest in AECAs was stimulated by cases of hyperacute or accelerated rejection in patients who had been transplanted with a negative crossmatch to donor leukocytes. The early suggestion of a common polymorphic non-HLA antigen system between ECs and monocytes ***(12,30)*** has not been confirmed by biochemical identification of the relevant antigens. It also clear that renal graft failure can occur because of IgM or IgG antibodies against donor ECs that do not cross-react with donor monocytes, lymphocytes, or keratinocytes ***(31,32)***. Although cases of hyperacute rejection in the face of a negative leukocyte-specific crossmatch seem rarer these days, possibly owing to better crossmatch procedures, the story of non-HLA antibodies does not go away. Indeed, with more interest in the long-term fate of grafts and pathogenesis of chronic graft vasculopathy, there is increased interest in the role of non-HLA antibodies.

There is strong evidence that non-HLA antibodies, in particular AECAs, can be made at any time after transplantation and are associated with acute and chronic rejection. One of the earliest studies to show an association between AECAs and chronic cardiac allograft vasculopathy used Western blotting to measure AECAs ***(13)***. That AECAs correlate with chronic cardiac allograft vasculopathy has been confirmed using flow cytometry ***(18)*** and ELISA ***(33, 34)***. More recently, a syndrome of septal capillary injury, accompanied by endothelial localization of C1q, C3, C4d, and Ig deposition, has been associated with production of AECAs after lung transplantation ***(35)***. These patients were negative for PRAs at the time of diagnosis, but unfortunately this study did not investigate production of donor-specific antibodies. Bas-Bernardet et al., showed that 47% of renal transplant recipients who are presensitized to HLA antigens also have AECAs in their sera ***(36)***. Sera from these patients was absorbed against platelets (eliminating antibodies to MHC class I antigens) and tested against resting ABO- and HLA-matched aortic ECs. The AECAs of IgG isotype predominantly reacted with EC surface antigens upregulated by interferon (IFN)-γ and tumor necrosis factor-α; in contrast, AECAs of IgM isotype only reacted with untreated ECs. The EC antigens recognized by IgG were 35 and 50 kDa. Clinically, no significant effect of pretransplant AECAs on acute rejection or 5-yr graft survival was detected, but as the authors caution, only 52 patients were analyzed in this study.

Production of non-HLA antibodies is also associated with BOS after lung transplantation ***(14)***, in this case antibodies to epithelial cells. Thus, AECAs were found in 5 of 11 patients who developed BOS and 0 of 11 patients who remained free of BOS. In this study the serum had absorbed any anti-HLA antibodies, confirming that reactivity was not against HLA antigens. Interestingly, in this study, patients with BOS who were not producing non-HLA antibodies were making antibodies to HLA antigens ***(14)***.

As with the technical difficulties of monitoring antibodies to live cells described previously, the non-HLA story is complicated by the fact that groups use different methods of detecting AECAs, namely live, fixed, or processed ECs. Identification of antigen specificity not only gives one mechanistic insight, it usually leads to more reliable assays. Using two-dimensional gel electrophoretic separation of endothelial proteins, we were able to identify the most abundant immunoreactive endothelial antigen targeted by patient sera as the intermediate filament vimentin ***(37)***. Since then we have reported that use of a simple robust ELISA for anti-vimentin antibodies identifies patients at risk of developing CAV ***(15,38)***. Vimentin is the intermediate filament characteristic of ECs, fibroblasts, and leukocytes. Interestingly, although desmin is the main intermediate filament of quiescent smooth muscle cells, vimentin is co-expressed in smooth muscle cells, which are proliferating or migrating. Vimentin is therefore abundantly expressed in the intima of blood vessels with CAV. The question arises as to what the source of vimentin in the clinical setting is. We have shown that vimentin is not present on the surface of healthy ECs, but it is exposed at the surface of ECs that have been driven into apoptosis or necrosis (Holder and Rose, in preparation). It is also present on the cell surface of some cell lines. In view of the fact that apoptosis/necrosis occur at every stage after transplantation ***(39)***, the most likely explanation is that vimentin is exposed on apoptopic cells—these could be of donor (ECs) or recipient (infiltrating leukocytes) origin. As far as we know, vimentin is not a polymorphic antigen. The current view is that it is acting as an autoantigen. We would then suggest that apoptopic cells are recognized by recipient dendritic cells ***(40)*** and that antigens derived from the apoptopic cells are processed and presented to recipient T cells in an MHC self-restricted manner. Recently we have used vimentin peptides bound to A*0201 tetramers to demonstrate the presence of vimentin-specific self-restricted $CD8^+$ T cells in cardiac transplant patients ***(41)***, confirming that vimentin acts as an autoantigen after heart transplantation and that cross-priming, as described above, probably occurs.

Experimental studies have demonstrated that transplantation breaks tolerance to autoantigens ***(42)***. Clinically, there have been numerous descriptions of antibody responses to autoantigens after heart transplantation, including anticardiac myosin antibodies ***(43,44)***, antiphospholipid antibodies ***(45)***, and antibodies to oxidized low-density lipoprotein (LDL) ***(46)***. Such responses are associated with more rejection episodes. Collagen V has been identified as a major component in human bronchiolar lavage, and experimental studies have suggested that immune reactivity to collagen V may reduce survival of lung allografts ***(47,48)***. The majority of clinical studies have used antibody response as a readout of an autoimmune response.

Recent studies suggest that there may be a wide range of antigens that can act as autoantigens after transplantation; thus expression cloning using EC cDNA libraries from either human umbilical vein ECs or coronary artery ECs has identified a great diversity of putative autoantigens that are recognized by sera from patients with cardiac graft vasculopathy ***(49,50)***. These antigens include ribosomal proteins L7 and L9 ***(50)***, autoantigens that are also associated with autoimmune diseases such as systemic lupus erythematosus. Although most of the antigens identified were nuclear or cytoplasmic antigens, neuropilin-2 (np2), an antigen expressed on the surface of ECs, was also identified as a possible autoantigen after cardiac transplantation ***(49)***. This is interesting because np2 is a receptor for vascular endothelial growth factor (VEGF), suggesting that autoantibodies to np2 might be able to activate VEGF, thus causing EC growth, which might contribute to the diffuse and concentric narrowing of coronary arteries characteristic of cardiac graft vasculopathy. Further studies are in progress to test this hypothesis. A working hypothesis for involvement of autoimmune responses after cardiac transplantation would be that organs are damaged at every stage after transplantation (including prior to implantation), leading to release or exposure of putative autoantigens.

There is interest in the role of apoptopic cells as reservoirs of autoantigens ***(51)***. Cytosolic and nuclear antigens are disorganized during apoptosis, resulting in exposure of cryptic epitopes ***(52)***; for example, ribosomal proteins are expressed as blebs at the surface of apoptopic keratinocytes, suggesting a possible stimulating source for the antiribosomal protein antibodies we have found in some of the cardiac transplant patients ***(50)***. Similarly, expression of phosphatidyl serine could lead to production of antiphospholipid antibodies, which occurs after clinical heart transplantation ***(45)***. Indeed, immunization of mice with apoptopic cells results in autoantibody production ***(53)***. The fact that the indirect pathway of antigen presentation comes to dominate immune responsiveness in long-term transplant patients ***(54)*** also gives support to this hypothesis. Whereas the majority of studies have used peptides derived from HLA antigens to detect the indirect pathway, there is no reason why peptides derived from autoantigens cannot be processed and presented by recipient antigen-presenting cells to potentially autoreactive T and B cells.

Another advance in the area of non-HLA antibodies has been use of B-lymphoblastoid cell lines transfected with MHC class I-related A (MICA) or MHC class I-related B (MICB) antigens ***(17)*** to screen for antibodies. MICA and MICB genes are located in close proximity to the HLA-B-locus on chromosome 6 and encode 62-kDa cell surface glycoproteins, which share limited sequence homologies with HLA class I ***(55)***. ECs and monocytes may express MICA ***(56)***, whereas lymphocytes do not. A recent study of 748 sera from 139 renal transplant patients showed that the presence of anti-MICA antibodies (before or after transplantation) correlated with rejection episode and early graft loss ***(17)***. Importantly, the antibodies causing graft loss were formed in the absence of donor-specific antibodies. This interesting study raises the possibility that reactivity to MICA antigen, expressed on ECs, may explain some of the earlier reports of graft loss in patients with a negative crossmatch to donor leukocytes ***(11,31,32)*** as well as positive binding of sera to the cell surface of live ECs ***(18,34)***. It must be said that Sumitran-Karuppan et al. ***(32)*** reported their endothelial antigen to be 97–110 kDa, which suggests it is not MICA or MICB. The study of Jaramillo et al. ***(26)*** reported that antibodies to epithelial cells did not react with ECs, excluding MICA as an antigen. However, these authors did report their epithelial antigen to be a 60-kDa cytosolic molecule that was present on the surface of some but not all cell lines. This raises the possibility that it could be vimentin, which we have found to be expressed on the surface of some EC lines (A. Holder, M. Rose, unpublished data).

2.3. Mechanism of Damage of HLA and Non-HLA Antibodies

Traditionally, complement-mediated lysis has been considered to be the major mechanism whereby IgG antibodies binding MHC class I antigens cause damage. It is now clear that complement-independent mechanisms are also involved. There is little published about how antibodies to MHC class II antigens are damaging. Although we know that anti-MHC class II antibodies cause activation of leukocytes, far less is known about their effects on parenchymal cells such as endothelial or epithelial cells. Recently, it has been shown that ligation of IFN-γ-treated human fibroblasts with MAb to HLA-DR causes secretion of Rantes, interleukin (IL)-8, monocyte chemoattractant protein-1, and IL-6 ***(57)***. In the context of transplantation, it will be important to know whether alloantibodies to MHC class II antigens cause activation (pro-inflammatory or apoptopic?) or lysis of parenchymal cells. This is likely to be an area of rapid advancement it the next few years.

As far as non-HLA antibodies are concerned, there is not going to be a single or common mechanism of damage. The wide diversity of specificities of non-HLA antibodies means that mechanisms of damage are likely to vary accordingly. It is more straightforward to understand the mechanism of damage if the antigens are expressed on the cell surface, such as MICA and neuropilin (discussed earlier). Antibodies to MICA cause complement-dependent lysis of donor kidney microvascular ECs and MICA-transfected cells ***(17)***. In the absence of complement, they induce tissue factor and plasminogen activator inhibitor of microvascular ECs. Similarly, antibodies that bind to a 60-kDa antigen expressed on epithelial cell lines cause signal transduction, resulting in epithelial cell proliferation and upregulation of transforming growth factor-β ***(14)***. These antibodies were derived from lung transplant recipients with BOS. The target of anti-vimentin antibodies is currently not known, but the recent report that activated platelets express cell surface vimentin ***(58)*** suggests that anti-vimentin antibodies may cause platelet aggregation and initiate thrombosis. Although titers of antibodies to oxidized low-density lipoprotein (LDL) correlate with impaired coronary artery endothelial vasodilation in heart transplant recipients ***(46)***, the reason for this correlation may not be directly linked to antibodies. It may be that levels of antibodies in this case reflect the load of oxidized LDL in the arteries. $F(ab)_2$ fragments of AECAs from a patient with Kawasaki disease have been shown to activate human ECs to secrete IL-6 and show enhanced expression of adhesion molecules ***(59)***, but the precise cell surface antigen target was not elucidated. Indeed, it was suggested that AECAs may contain multiple target antigens, a situation that would apply equally to transplantation. It is difficult to attribute a damaging role to antibodies when the target antigen is cytosolic, but it is likely that some autoantibodies cross-react with cell surface antigens. Experimental studies that transplant across minor-mismatch MHC combinations ***(60–62)*** are valuable because they provide unambiguous evidence that non-HLA antibodies bind to donor ECs. Antigalactose antibodies, raised in $Gal^{-/-}$ mice, bind to $Gal^{+/+}$ ECs and cause rejection of xenografted rat hearts transplanted into mice. Interestingly, the ability to cause rapid rejection was not restricted to complement-fixing antigalactose antibodies; IgG1 antibodies, which poorly fix complement, also cause rapid rejection ***(62)***. Wu et al. concluded that, although non-HLA antibodies bind to donor ECs, they are not efficient at fixing complement; nevertheless non-HLA AECAs transfer chronic graft vasculopathy in vivo and cause apoptosis of donor ECs in vitro ***(61)***. Interestingly, Bas-Bernardet et al. ***(36)*** confirm using human sera that IgG AECAs from renal transplant recipients induce apoptosis of human ECs but do not cause complement-mediated lysis. The biological effects of these in vitro assays still need to be ascertained by in vivo experiments. Why AECAs are so inefficient at lysing ECs by complement fixation is not known; it could be a function of the relative resistance of ECs to complement-mediated lysis or the isotype of the binding antibody. This issue is yet to be resolved.

3. Conclusion

There is good evidence that *de novo* production of antibodies to MHC and non-MHC antigens contribute to graft deterioration at all times after transplantation. Recent studies suggest an important role for anti-MHC class II antibodies in late graft failure. There are multiple mechanisms of antibody-mediated injury depending on the nature of the antigen and the tissues that express the antigens. Some of the non-HLA antigens may be part of a polymorphic system (such as MICA), while others may represent minor antigen mismatches and others appear to be autoantigens. Although complement-mediated lysis is the conventional way to measure antibody-mediated damage, it is likely that non-HLA antibodies cause chronic damage to target parenchymal cells by multiple mechanisms including pro-inflammatory cell activation, induction of growth factors, fibrogenesis, thrombotic events, and apoptosis. Regular monitoring of posttransplant antibody production using solid phase antigen-binding assays will continue to clarify the role of antibodies in graft deterioration.

References

1. Terasaki, P. I. and McClelland, J. D. (1964) Microdroplet assay of human serum cytotoxins. *Nature* **204**, 998–1000.
2. Ting, A. (1983) The lymphocytotoxic crossmatch test in clinical renal transplantation. *Transplantation* **35**, 403–407.
3. Harmer, A. W., Sutton, M., Bayne A., Vaughan, R. W., and Welsh. K. I. (1993) A highly sensitive, rapid screening method for the detection of antibodies directed against HLA class I and II antigens. *Transplant. Int.* **6**, 277–280.
4. Baier, K. A., Meyer J. A., O'Brien, B. J., et al. (1994) Solubilized HLA class I antigen enzyme-linked immunoassay to identify HLA-typing reagents. *Hum. Immunol.* **40**, 187–190.
5. Kao, K. J., Scornik J. C., and Small, S. J. (1993) Enzyme-linked immunoassay for anti-HLA antibodies—an alternative to panel studies by lymphocytotoxicity. *Transplantation* **55**, 192–196.
6. Pei, R., Lee, J. H., Shih, N. J., Chen, M., and Terasaki, P. I. (2003) Single human leukocyte antigen flow cytometry beads for accurate identification of human leukocyte antigen antibody specificities. *Transplantation* **75**, 43–49.
7. Pei, R., Lee, J., Chen, T., Rojo S., and Terasaki, P. I. (1999) Flow cytometric detection of HLA antibodies using a spectrum of microbeads. *Hum. Immunol.* **60**, 1293–1302.
8. Brand, D. L., Ray, J. G., Hare, D. B., Kayhoe D. E., and McClelland, J. D. (1970) Preliminary trials towards standardisation of leukocyte typing, in *Histocompatibilty Testing* (P. I. Terasaki, ed), Munskaard, Copenhagen, pp. 357–367.
9. Patel, R. and Terasaki, P. I. (1969) Significance of the positive crossmatch test in kidney transplantation. *N .Engl. J. Med.* **280**, 735–739.
10. Lucas, D. P., Paparounis, M. L., Myers, L., Hart, J. M. and Zachary, A. A. (1997) Detection of HLA class I-specific antibodies by the QuikScreen enzyme-linked immunosorbent assay. *Clin. Diagn. Lab. Immunol.* **4**, 252–257.
11. Brasile, L., Zerbe, T., Rabin, B., Clarke, J., Abrams, A., and Cerilli, J. (1985) Identification of the antibody to vascular endothelial cells in patients undergoing cardiac transplantation. *Transplantation* **40**, 672–675.
12. Cerilli, J., Bay, W., and Brasile, L. (1983) The significance of the monocyte crossmatch in recipients of living-related HLA identical kidney grafts. *Hum. Immunol.* **7**, 45–50.
13. Dunn, M. J., Crisp, S. J.,, Rose, M. L., Taylor, P. M., and Yacoub, M. H. (1992) Anti-endothelial antibodies and coronary artery disease after cardiac transplantation. *Lancet* **339**, 1566–1570.

14. Jaramillo, A., Naziruddin, B., Zhang, L., et al. (2001) Activation of human airway epithelial cells by non-HLA antibodies developed after lung transplantation: a potential etiological factor for bronchiolitis obliterans syndrome. *Transplantation* **71**, 966–976.
15. Jurcevic, S., Ainsworth, M. E., Pomerance A., , et al. (2001) Anti-vimentin antibodies are an independent predictor of transplant-associated coronary artery disease after cardiac transplantation. *Transplantation* **71**, 886–892.
16. Latif, N., Rose, M. L., Yacoub, M. H., and Dunn, M. J. (1995) Association of pretransplantation antiheart antibodies with clinical course after heart transplantation. *J. Heart Lung Transplant.* **14**, 119–126.
17. Sumitran-Holgersson, S., Wilczek, H. E., Holgersson J., and Soderstrom, K. (2002) Identification of the nonclassical HLA molecules, mica, as targets for humoral immunity associated with irreversible rejection of kidney allografts. *Transplantation* **74**, 268–277.
18. Ferry, B. L., Welsh, K. I., Dunn, M. J., et al. (1997) Anti-cell surface endothelial antibodies in sera from cardiac and kidney transplant recipients: association with chronic rejection. *Transplant. Immunol.* **5**, 17–24.
19. Shenton, B. K., Bal, W., Bell, A. E., et al. (1995) The value of flow cytometric crossmatching in lung transplantation: relevance of pretransplant antibodies to lung epithelial cells. *Transplant. Proc.* **27**,1295–1297.
20. Watschinger, B. (2002) Capillary C4d deposition as a marker of humoral immunity in renal allograft rejection. *J. Am. Soc. Nephrol.* **13**, 2420-2423.
21. Lepin, E. J., Jin, Y. P., Barwe, S. P., Rozengurt, E., and Reed, E. F. (2004) HLA class I signal transduction is dependent on Rho GTPase and ROK12. *Biochem. Biophys. Res. Commun.* **323**, 213–217.
22. Itescu, S., Tung, T. C., Burke, E. M., et al. (1998) Preformed IgG antibodies against major histocompatibility complex class II antigens are major risk factors for high-grade cellular rejection in recipients of heart transplantation. *Circulation* **98**, 786–793.
23. Smith, J. D., Danskine, A. J., Laylor, R. M., Rose, M. L., and Yacoub, M. H. (1993) The effect of panel reactive antibodies and the donor specific crossmatch on graft survival after heart and heart-lung transplantation. *Transplant. Immunol.* **1**, 60–65.
24. Page, C., Rose, M., Yacoub, M., and Pigott, R. (1992) Antigenic heterogeneity of vascular endothelium. *Am. J. Pathol.* **141**, 673–683.
25. Palmer, S. M., Davis, R. D., Hadjiliadis, D., et al. (2002) Development of an antibody specific to major histocompatibility antigens detectable by flow cytometry after lung transplant is associated with bronchiolitis obliterans syndrome. *Transplantation* **74**, 799–804.
26. Jaramillo, A., Smith, M. A., Phelan, D., et al. (1999) Development of ELISA-detected anti-HLA antibodies precedes the development of bronchiolitis obliterans syndrome and correlates with progressive decline in pulmonary function after lung transplantation. *Transplantation* **67**, 1155–1161.
27. Worthington, J. E., Martin, S., Al Husseini, D. M., Dyer, P. A., and Johnson, R. W. (2003) Posttransplantation production of donor HLA-specific antibodies as a predictor of renal transplant outcome. *Transplantation* **75**, 1034–1040.

28. Pelletier, R. P., Hennessy, P. K., Adams, P. W., VanBuskirk, A. M., Ferguson, R. M., and Orosz, C. G. (2002) Clinical significance of MHC-reactive alloantibodies that develop after kidney or kidney-pancreas transplantation. *Am. J. Transplant.* **2**, 134–141.
29. Bas-Bernardet, S., Hourmant, M., Valentin, N., et al. (2003) Identification of the antibodies involved in B-cell crossmatch positivity in renal transplantation. *Transplantation* **75**, 477–482.
30. Moraes, J. R. and Stastny, P. (1977) Human endothelial cell antigens: molecular independence from HLA and expression in blood monocytes. *Transplant. Proc.* **9**, 605–607.
31. Perrey, C., Brenchley, P. E., Johnson, R. W., and Martin, S. (1998) An association between antibodies specific for endothelial cells and renal transplant failure. *Transplant. Immunol.* **6**, 101–106.
32. Sumitran-Karuppan, S., Tyden, G., Reinholt, F., Berg, U., and Moller, E. (1997) Hyperacute rejections of two consecutive renal allografts and early loss of the third transplant caused by non-HLA antibodies specific for endothelial cells. *Transplant. Immunol.* **5**, 321–327.
33. Faulk, W. P., Rose, M., Meroni, P. L., et al. (1999) Antibodies to endothelial cells identify myocardial damage and predict development of coronary artery disease in patients with transplanted hearts. *Hum. Immunol.* **60**, 826–832.
34. Fredrich, R., Toyoda, M., Czer, L. S., et al. (1999) The clinical significance of antibodies to human vascular endothelial cells after cardiac transplantation. *Transplantation* **67**, 385–391.
35. Magro, C. M., Deng, A., Pope-Harman, A., et al. (2002) Humorally mediated posttransplantation septal capillary injury syndrome as a common form of pulmonary allograft rejection: a hypothesis. *Transplantation* **74**, 1273–1280.
36. Bas-Bernardet, S., Hourmant, M., Coupel, S., et al. (2003) Non-HLA-type endothelial cell reactive alloantibodies in pre-transplant sera of kidney recipients trigger apoptosis. *Am. J. Transplant* **3**, 167–177.
37. Wheeler, C. H., Collins, A., Dunn, M. J., Crisp, S. J., Yacoub, M. H., and Rose, M. L. (1995) Characterization of endothelial antigens associated with transplant-associated coronary artery disease. *J. Heart Lung Transplant.* **14**, S188–S197.
38. Danskine, A. J., Smith, J. D., Stanford, R. E., Newell, H., and Rose, M. L. (2002) Correlation of anti-vimentin antibodies with acute and chronic rejection following cardiac transplantation. *Hum. Immunol.* **63**, S30–S31.
39. Miller, L. W., Granville, D. J., Narula, J., and McManus, B. M. (2001) Apoptosis in cardiac transplant rejection. *Cardiol. Clin.* **19**, 141–154.
40. Propato, A., Cutrona, G., Francavilla, V., et al. (2001) Apoptotic cells overexpress vinculin and induce vinculin-specific cytotoxic T-cell cross-priming. *Nat. Med.* **7**, 807–813.
41. Barber, L. D., Whitelegg, A.. Madrigal, J. A.. Banner, N. R., and Rose, M. L. (2004) Detection of vimentin-specific autoreactive CD8+ T cells in cardiac transplant patients. *Transplantation* **77**, 1604–1609.

42. Fedoseyeva, E. V., Tam, R. C., Popov, I. A, Orr, P. L., Garovoy, M. R., and Benichou, G. (1996) Induction of T cell responses to a self-antigen following allotransplantation. *Transplantation* **61**, 679–683.
43. Dunn, M. J., Rose, M. L., Latif, N., et al. (1991) Demonstration by western blotting of antiheart antibodies before and after cardiac transplantation. *Transplantation* **51**, 806–812.
44. Warraich, R. S., Pomerance, A., Stanley, A., Banner, N. R., Dunn, M. J., and Yacoub, M. H. (2000) Cardiac myosin autoantibodies and acute rejection after heart transplantation in patients with dilated cardiomyopathy. *Transplantation* **69**, 1609–1617.
45. Laguens, R. P., Argel, M. I., Chambo, J. G., et al. (1996) Anti-skeletal muscle glycolipid antibodies in human heart transplantation as markers of acute rejection. Correlation with endomyocardial biopsy. *Transplantation* **62**, 211–216.
46. Fang, J. C., Kinlay, S., Behrendt, D., et al. (2002) Circulating autoantibodies to oxidized LDL correlate with impaired coronary endothelial function after cardiac transplantation. *Arterioscler.Thromb. Vasc. Biol.* **22**, 2044–2048.
47. Haque, M. A., Mizobuchi, T., Yasufuku, K., et al. (2002) Evidence for immune responses to a self-antigen in lung transplantation: role of type V collagen-specific T cells in the pathogenesis of lung allograft rejection. *J. Immunol.* **169**, 1542–1549.
48. Yasufuku, K., Heidler, K. M., Woods, K. A., et al. (2002) Prevention of bronchiolitis obliterans in rat lung allografts by type V collagen-induced oral tolerance. *Transplantation* **73**, 500–505.
49. Bates, R. L., Frampton, G., Rose, M. L., and Murphy, J. J. (2003) High diversity of non-human leukocyte antigens in transplant-associated coronary artery disease. *Transplantation* **75**, 1347–1350.
50. Linke, A. T., Marchant, B., Marsh, P., Frampton, G., Murphy, J., and Rose, M. L. (2001) Screening of a HUVEC cDNA library with transplant-associated coronary artery disease sera identifies RPL7 as a candidate autoantigen associated with this disease. *Clin. Exp. Immunol.* **126**, 173–179.
51. Rosen, A. and Casciola-Rosen, L. A. (1999) Autoantigen as substrates for apoptopic proteases: implications for the pathogenesis of systemic autoimmune diseases. *Cell Death Diff.* **6**, 6–12.
52. Casciola-Rosen, L. A., Anhalt, G., and Rosen, A. (1994) Autoantigens targeted in systemic lupus erythematosus are clustered in two populations of surface structures on apoptotic keratinocytes. *J. Exp. Med.* **179**, 1317–1330.
53. Mevorach, D., Zhou, J. L., Song, X., and Elkon, K. B. (1998) Systemic exposure to irradiated apoptotic cells induces autoantibody production. *J. Exp. Med* **188**, 387–392.
54. Baker, R. J., Hernandez-Fuentes, M. P., Brookes, P. A., Chaudhry, A. N., Cook, H. T., and Lechler, R. I. (2001) Loss of direct and maintenance of indirect alloresponses in renal allograft recipients: implications for the pathogenesis of chronic allograft nephropathy. *J. Immunol.* **167**, 7199–7206.
55. Bahram, S. (2000) MIC genes: from genetics to biology. *Adv. Immunol.* **76**, 1–60.

56. Zwirner, N. W., Fernandez-Vina, M. A., and Stastny, P. (1998) MICA, a new polymorphic HLA-related antigen, is expressed mainly by keratinocytes, endothelial cells, and monocytes. *Immunogenetics* **47**, 139–148.
57. Meguro, M., Nishimura, F., Ohyama, H., Takashiba, S., Murayama, Y., and Matsushita, S. (2003) Ligation of IFN-[gamma]-induced HLA-DR molecules on fibroblasts induces RANTES expression via c-Jun N-terminal kinase (JNK) pathway. *Cytokine* **22**, 107–115.
58. Podor, T. J., Singh, D., Chindemi, P., et al. (2002) Vimentin exposed on activated platelets and platelet microparticles localizes vitronectin and plasminogen activator inhibitor complexes on their surface. *J. Biol. Chem.* **277**, 7529–7539.
59. Grunebaum, E., Blank, M., Cohen, S., et al. (2002) The role of anti-endothelial cell antibodies in Kawasaki disease—in vitro and in vivo studies. *Clin. Exp. Immunol.* **130**, 233–240.
60. Diujvestijn, A. M., Derhaag, J. G., and Breda Vriesman, P. J. (2000) Complement activation by anti-endothelial cell antibodies in MHC-mismatched and MHC-matched heart allograft rejection: anti-MHC-, but not anti non-MHC alloantibodies are effective in complement activation. *Transplant. Int.* **13**, 363–371.
61. Wu, G. D., Jin, Y. S., Salazar, R., et al. (2002) Vascular endothelial cell apoptosis induced by anti-donor non-MHC antibodies: a possible injury pathway contributing to chronic allograft rejection. *J. Heart Lung Transplant.* **21**, 1174–1187.
62. Xu, H., Yin, D., Naziruddin, B., et al. (2003) The in vitro and in vivo effects of anti-galactose antibodies on endothelial cell activation and xenograft rejection. *J. Immunol.* **170**, 1531–1539.

11

Reprogramming the Immune System Using Antibodies

Luis Graca and Herman Waldmann

Summary

Tolerance induction induced by monoclonal antibodies or co-receptor blockade is robust enough to resist breakdown by adoptive transfer of lymphocytes. Such resistance, the hallmark of dominant tolerance, is mediated by CD4$^+$ regulatory T cells. CD4$^+$CD25$^+$ T cells inhibit lymphopenia-mediated accumulation of T cells in vivo, but caution should be exerted when investigating antigen-specific regulation in replete mice. A number of different deletional and tolerogenic processes following antibody-induced tolerance are discussed in this chapter, including activation-induced cell death, immunosuppressive cytokines, and immunopriveleged sites. The possibility of spreading tolerance to other cells, including parenchymal cells, is also discussed. This chapter emphasizes recent evidence that shows that self-tolerance does not rely on several mechanisms running independently, but rather a continuum of synergistic and overlapping mechanisms.

Key Words: Transplantation; tolerance; regulatory T cells; antibodies; immuno-regulation; CD4; CD25.

1. Introduction

The immune system has evolved as a mechanism to protect the body against foreign pathogens while being harmless to self-constituents of the body. As a consequence, the exquisite ability the immune system has developed to react against foreign antigens has become the major hurdle for clinical transplantation. In current clinical practice, alloresponses are prevented by use of immunosuppressive drugs that penalize the whole of the immune system. There is a need for strategies that, by reprogramming the immune system, can lead to long-term tolerance or, at least, to the minimization of immunosuppression. The use of monoclonal antibodies (MAbs) has proved promising in reprogramming the immune system toward transplantation tolerance in experimental animals.

From: *Methods in Molecular Biology, vol. 333: Transplantation Immunology: Methods and Protocols*
Edited by: P. Hornick and M. Rose © Humana Press Inc., Totowa, NJ

2. The Use of Monoclonal Antibodies in Transplantation

The emergence of clinically useful MAbs has been slower than many have anticipated. During the more than 25 yr since their discovery, only a small number of MAbs have been licensed for clinical use as immunosuppressive agents. One important reason has been the realization that the inherent immunogenicity of MAbs can limit their efficacy. As a consequence, the use of MAbs as agents to reprogram the immune system in the context of transplantation cannot be uncoupled from the problem of eliminating their own immunogenicity.

The first MAbs routinely used in clinical transplantation have been administered with the aim, at least in part, of eliminating T-cell populations. The idea of eliminating lymphocytes in transplant patients is not new, as demonstrated by old experimental methods such as the placement of a catheter collecting lymph from the thoracic duct or the use of polyclonal antilymphocyte sera *(1,2)*. The specificity of MAbs has allowed better control of the targeted cell populations. Such is the case for CD3, CD25, or CAMPATH-1H MAbs. The anti-CD3 MAb OKT3, also known as muromab, was the first MAb licensed to be used to prevent rejection episodes *(3)*. However, its own immunogenicity and the triggering of a cytokine release syndrome have limited its use. A MAb targeting CD25, the α-chain of the interleukin (IL)-2 receptor (IL-2R), offered the perspective of specific elimination of only the activated T cells *(4)*. However, recent evidence suggests that such MAbs may be also targeting a population of T cells with known regulatory function *(5,6)*. More recently, there is evidence that by targeting the most abundant surface antigen on the T-cell surface, namely the CD52 antigen with the humanized MAb CAMPATH-1H, one can prevent graft rejection with minimal maintenance immunosuppressive drugs *(7,8)*.

In addition to the usefulness of MAbs in eliminating cell populations in vivo, there is compelling evidence that some MAbs can reprogram the immune system towards tolerance. Such MAbs, when given short term following transplantation in experimental animals, frequently allow indefinite survival of the transplanted tissues *(9,10)*. Among these are MAbs that target co-receptor molecules, such as CD4, CD3 or CD45; co-stimulatory molecules, such as CD40-ligand (CD40L or CD154) or CD28; or adhesion molecules, such as leukocyte function antigen (LFA)-1 or intercellular adhesion molecule (ICAM)-1 (**Table 1**).

3. Antibody-Induced Transplantation Tolerance

The initial demonstrations that peripheral tolerance can be induced following short-term treatment with MAbs were published in the mid-1980s *(11,12)*. It was demonstrated that immune responses toward foreign immunoglobulins could be prevented by a short course of anti-CD4 MAbs. Shortly thereafter, it was proven that depletion of $CD4^+$ cells was not required, because similar results could be

Table 1
Monoclonal Antibodies Effective in Prolonging Allograft Survival or Inducing Transplantation Tolerance

Antibody	Comments
CD4 + CD8 + CD154	Tolerance to MHC-mismatched skin
CD4 + CD8 (nondepleting)	Tolerance to MHC-mismatched heart
CD154 + hCTLA-4-Ig	Long-term survival of MHC-mismatched skin
CD154 + CD8 depletion	Dominant tolerance to minor antigen-mismatched skin
CD3 (nonmitogenic)	Tolerance to minor antigen-mismatched skin
CD4	Tolerance to MHC-mismatched heart
hCTLA-4-Ig	Tolerance to MHC-mismatched heart
CD45	Tolerance to MHC-mismatched islets
LFA1 + ICAM1	Tolerance to MHC-mismatched hearts

CTLA, cytotoxic T-lymphocyte-associated antigen; LFA, leukocyte function antigen; ICAM, intercellular adhesion molecule; MHC, major histocompatability complex. (Adapted from **ref. *10***.)

observed using F(ab')2 fragments ***(13–15)***, nondepleting isotypes ***(16)***, or nondepleting doses of synergistic pairs of anti-CD4 MAbs ***(17)***.

A short treatment with nondepleting anti-CD4 MAbs was also shown to generate long-term acceptance of skin grafts differing in multiple minor transplantation antigens ***(16)***, even in presensitized recipients ***(18)***. The same outcome was seen for heart grafts across major histocompatibility complex barriers ***(19,20)*** or concordant xenografts ***(19)***. The treated animals accepted the transplanted tissues indefinitely without the need for prolonged immunosuppression and remained fully competent to reject unrelated (third-party) grafts. Clearly, antibody treatment had rendered them tolerant of antigens of the transplanted tissue (**Fig. 1**).

Following these observations, it became clear that MAbs other than anti-CD4 could be used to impose peripheral transplantation tolerance. Transplantation tolerance or long-term graft survival were reported following treatment with anti-LFA1 MAbs alone ***(13)*** or in combination with anti-ICAM1 ***(21)***; with anti-CD2 and anti-CD3 MAbs ***(22)***; with anti-CD45RB ***(23)***; or with co-stimulation blockade of CD28 ***(24)***, CD40L ***(25,26)***, or both in combination ***(27)***. These findings have recently been extended to nonhuman primates ***(28,29)***.

Transplantation tolerance induced with co-receptor blockade (nondepleting anti-CD4 and anti-CD8 MAbs) or co-stimulation blockade (nondepleting anti-CD154 MAbs) can be robust enough to resist breakdown by the adoptive transfer of lymphocytes from a nontolerant donor ***(16,30,31)***. Such "resistance" that is, the capacity to prevent transfused cells to mediate graft rejection, is the hallmark of dominant tolerance and is mediated by $CD4^+$ regulatory T cells ***(31–***

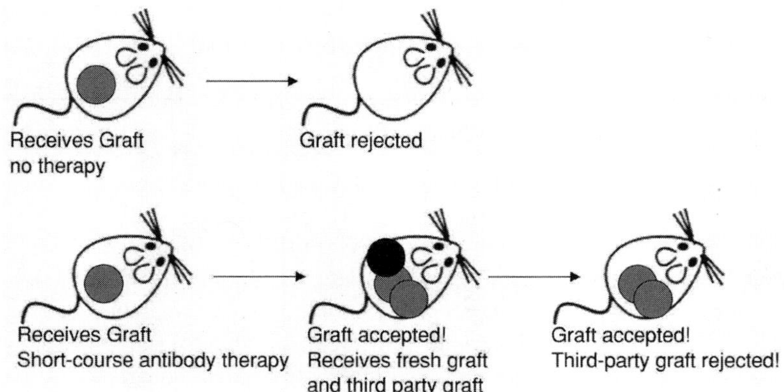

Fig. 1. Induction of transplantation tolerance with antibody treatment. Mice accept a second challenge with a graft of the same type, but readily reject third-party grafts. Although some alloreactive cells are likely to undergo apoptosis, some cells reactive to transplantation antigens, as demonstrated by proliferation assays, are present at any time point.

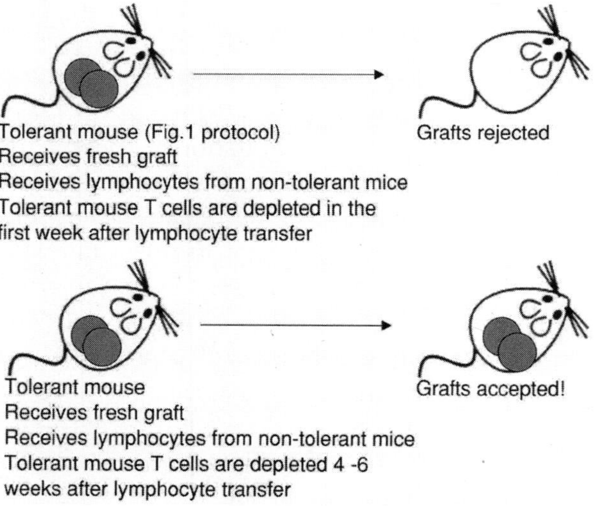

Fig. 2. Infectious transplantation tolerance. When nontolerant lymphocytes are allowed to coexist with the regulatory cells in a tolerant host, with time, regulatory properties emerge in the initially nontolerant population.

33). When nontolerant (naive) T cells are allowed to coexist with regulatory CD4+ T cells, the naive cells can themselves acquire regulatory properties, a process that we have named "infectious tolerance" ***(31–33)*** **(Fig. 2)**.

4. Dominant Transplantation Tolerance

Almost two decades have passed since the initial demonstrations that long-term tolerance can be induced following a brief treatment with MAbs (for a historical perspective, *see* **ref. *34***). However, the mechanisms by which tolerance is induced and maintained are not yet fully understood. The development of human therapies based on antibody-induced tolerance will be greatly facilitated by a better characterization of the mechanisms involved and may lead to the development of much-needed diagnostic tests for tolerance.

4.1. Regulatory T Cells

Since the early 1990s, it has been known that $CD4^+$ regulatory T cells are necessary to achieve dominant transplantation tolerance. However, studies of specific subpopulations have been delayed by the lack of adequate reagents and in vitro assays. Recently, the field of T-cell regulation has acquired respectability following the identification of cell-surface markers that allow the isolation of $CD4^+$ T-cell populations enriched in regulatory T cells. Initially, an isoform of CD45 (CD45RClow in rats or CD45RBlow in mice) ***(35)*** and, more recently, CD25 have been used to purify regulatory T cells ***(36)***. Not only can cells with this phenotype prevent in vitro T-cell proliferation, but they are also capable of preventing autoimmunity, inflammatory pathology, and transplant rejection when co-injected into lymphopenic hosts together with nonregulatory T cells ***(37–39)***. These same cells have also been shown to have a deleterious effect on the development of protective immunity in the context of infectious disease (*Leishmania* and *Pneumocystis*) and tumor immunity ***(40,41)***.

The α chain of the IL-2R—the CD25 molecule—is not an exclusive marker for regulatory T cells. It has been known to be present on the surface of activated lymphocytes and is targeted by therapeutic MAbs aiming for the depletion of activated cells, as discussed earlier. An attempt has been made by several groups to define more useful markers that uniquely identify the regulatory cells from within the $CD4^+CD25^+$ lymphocytes ***(42–46)***. Several have been found to be associated with, but not exclusive to, regulatory cells. These include cytotoxic T-lymphocyte-associated antigen 4 (CTLA-4) ***(47,48)***, glucocorticoid-induced tumor necrosis factor receptor (GITR) ***(43,44,49)***, L-selectin (CD62L) ***(50–52)***, and αEβ7 integrin (CD103) ***(43,45,53,54)***. Recently, much interest has been generated by the identification of the gene *Foxp3*, which encodes a forkhead-winged-helix transcription factor, which seems to be present exclusively on regulatory T cells ***(55–57)***. Viral transfection of nonregulatory T cells with *Foxp3* renders them functionally and phenotypically identical to $CD4^+CD25^+$ regulatory T cells ***(55)***. In humans a *Foxp3* mutation is associated with immune dysregulation, polyendocrinopathy, enteropathy, X-linked syndrome or X-linked autoimmunity-allergic dysregulation syndrome ***(55)***.

Despite this knowledge, we still lack incontrovertible proof that dominant transplantation tolerance is the responsibility of CD4$^+$CD25$^+$ regulatory T cells alone. In fact, there is evidence suggesting this is not the case. When the regulatory potency of the CD4$^+$CD25$^+$ and CD4$^+$CD25$^-$ T-cell populations was investigated, it became apparent that both populations have a similar regulatory potency in relation to their physiological proportions (i.e., the average regulatory potency of one CD4$^+$CD25$^+$ T cell is similar to that of 10 CD4$^+$CD25$^-$ cells) ***(58)***.

It is clear that CD4$^+$CD25$^+$ regulatory T cells can suppress transplant rejection when co-transferred with effector cells into lymphopenic mice (reviewed in **ref. *6***). What is not so clear is whether strategies to induce dominant tolerance (mediated by regulatory T cells) lead to the expansion of CD4$^+$CD25$^+$ regulatory cells specific for the alloantigen or rather to the expansion of other types of donor antigen-specific regulatory cells, probably similar to the Tr1 cells ***(59)***, or indeed both.

4.2. Antigen Specificity of Regulatory T Cells

Recent reports have claimed that CD4$^+$CD25$^+$ T cells from mice tolerized to transplants acquire the ability to mediate antigen-specific regulation ***(60–62)***. This issue has to remain open because none of these studies was conducted with a criss-cross analysis. Furthermore, where titration of (regulatory to naive) cell ratios was performed, "specific" suppression was seen only at a single ratio of effectors to regulators ***(62)***. In the absence of criss-cross studies, apparent specificity may be a consequence of the higher "rejectability" of the third-party tissues when compared with the tolerated ones. Small titration effects may simply reflect a reduction of aggressive cells by activation-induced cell death (AICD) from within the CD25$^+$ population.

Our own results suggest that, at least under lymphopenic conditions, CD4$^+$CD25$^+$ regulatory T cells from tolerized mice do not behave differently from cells with the same phenotype obtained from naive mice or mice whose tolerance was induced through mixed hematopoietic chimerism, where dominant regulation cannot be demonstrated ***(63)***. The apparent alloantigen nonspecificity of CD4$^+$CD25$^+$ T cells may be a consequence of their thymic lineage and commitment to prevention of self-reactivity. Any expansion of donor-alloantigen-specific CD4$^+$CD25$^+$ T cells may be masked by the large proportion of the cells preoccupied with self-antigens shared by the allograft. Alternatively, one can envisage that natural regulatory T cells can collaborate with induced regulators, possibly with both a CD25$^+$ and a CD25$^-$ phenotype, leading to the antigen-specific dominant regulation that is characteristic of lymphocyte-replete mice tolerized with MAbs (**Fig. 3**). We have recently published our findings that, in addition to the thymic lineage of CD4$^+$CD25$^+$

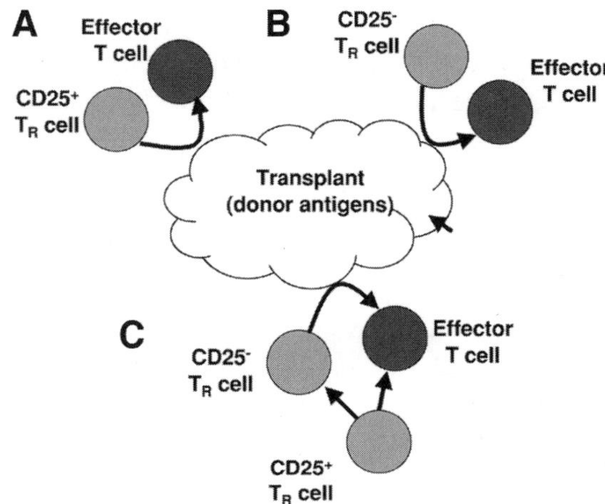

Fig. 3. The antigen-specificity problem. The current mainstream view postulates that CD4+CD25+ regulatory T cells directly mediate antigen-specific suppression (**A**). However, alternative hypotheses cannot at the present be excluded. First, it is possible that antigen-specific suppression is an exclusive property of CD25- regulatory T cells, whereas CD4+CD25+ regulatory T cells are involved in nonspecific suppression that may be irrelevant in transplantation tolerance in nonlymphopenic conditions (**B**). Second, CD4+CD25+ regulatory T cells may modulate, in an antigen-nonspecific manner, both effector T cells and CD25- regulatory T cells. In this case, although specificity would come from the CD25- cells, both populations acting in concert would be required for the overall specificity (**C**).

regulatory T cells, regulatory T cells with the same phenotype can be induced in the periphery following CD4 MAb tolerization *(64)*.

An alternative hypothesis has been suggested by Stockinger and colleagues *(65)* based on their observation that T-cell competition under lymphopenic conditions may appear as T-cell regulation *(66)*. In their experiments nonregulatory T cells, which under lymphopenic conditions are pathogenic, become harmless when co-injected with regulatory T cells, with T-cell clones having a proliferative advantage, or when injected in larger numbers. Given the striking capacity of CD4+CD25+ T cells to inhibit lymphopenia-driven accumulation of T cells in vivo *(67, 69)* and the propensity of lymphopenic environments to promote rejection *(69)*, one should be careful in comparing antigen-specific regulation in a T-cell-replete animal with homeostatic effects under lymphopenic conditions.

Other CD4+ T-cell populations, distinct from the CD4+CD25+ regulatory T cells, have also been shown to have suppressive properties in vitro and in vivo. Such is the case for IL-10-secreting Tr1 cells *(70)* and the Th3 cells that secrete transforming growth factor (TGF)-β in addition to IL-10 and IL-4 *(71)*. Whereas Th1 and Th2 T-cell clones can mediate transplant rejection when transfused into lymphopenic hosts *(72)*, rejection can be prevented by prior transfer of Tr1 cell clones with the same antigen specificity *(43)*. The antigen specificity of these cell populations is also poorly characterized in the context of transplantation, although a recent report has suggested that cells with a Tr1 phenotype may be antigen-specific regulators in the context of human diabetes *(73)*.

CD4$^-$ regulatory T cells have also been described *(74–76)*. However, although such cells may be important for the regulation of certain immune responses, it is unlikely that they will have a major role in antibody-induced transplantation tolerance, in which tolerance can be broken by removal of CD4$^+$ T cells.

5. Control of Alloreactive Clones in Antibody-Induced Tolerance

There is now strong evidence suggesting that alloreactive T-cell clones are controlled in three different ways in the course of antibody-induced tolerance: they can be deleted, or survive and become anergic, or become subject to regulation. Deletion of alloreactive clones may occur in the initial days following the tolerogenic treatment and results from AICD and in some instances the direct effect of the MAb, as appears to be the case with anti-CD40L *(77,78)*. Tolerance induction can be abrogated in mice where AICD is prevented *(79,80)*. It is important to note that AICD of alloreactive clones requires IL-2 signaling, being abrogated when cyclosporine is administered *(80)*. This observation raises the concern that when anti-CD25 MAbs are given peri-transplantation to investigate the role of CD4$^+$CD25$^+$ regulatory T cells in tolerance induction, the anti-CD25 MAbs may contribute to rejection by interfering with IL-2-dependent AICD of alloreactive clones.

However, even when tolerance is successfully induced, it has been shown that some alloreactive cells escape AICD and are prevented from rejecting grafts through dominant regulation mediated by regulatory T cells, as evidenced by restoration of rejection after deletion of CD4$^+$ T cells (containing the regulatory cells) *(31)*. Such regulatory cells are likely to have a reduced susceptibility to AICD, perhaps through expression of antiapoptotic genes such as Bag-1 *(81)*.

Other alloreactive cells may escape deletion and become anergic cells refractory to further antigenic stimulation in transplanted mice treated with anti-CD4 MAbs *(82,83)*. It is possible that such anergic cells may functionally behave as active regulators simply by co-localizing with other alloreactive cells and competing for elements in the microenvironment (e.g., cytokines or adhesion molecules). As a consequence, by preventing adequate "help" from being generated, the anergic cells could suppress the proliferation and effector function of naive T cells, a model known as the "civil service model" *(84)*.

Much has recently been published on the difficulty of inducing transplantation tolerance in situations where memory cells are present ***(85)*** or where host T cells experience lymphopenic-driven proliferation ***(69)***. Although it is clear that the presence of donor-antigen-reactive memory cells increases the stringency of the system, it is still possible, using co-receptor blockade with nondepleting CD4 and CD8 MAbs, to tolerize mice previously primed to alloantigens ***(18)***. Furthermore, although lymphopenia creates a hurdle to tolerance induction with MAbs that target co-stimulatory molecules, it has already been shown that T-cell-depleting MAbs can facilitate tolerance induction to fully mismatched skin allografts ***(86)***.

6. Suppressive Mechanisms

The manner in which regulatory T cells keep effector cells under control is also an issue awaiting clarification. There is evidence that inhibition of proliferation, one of the favorite in vitro readouts for regulatory function, may not be the key mechanism of regulation. Allospecific $CD8^+$ T cells, once adoptively transferred, can proliferate and accumulate in tolerant mice to the same extent as in naïve controls ***(87)***. Yet, in tolerant mice they do not lead to graft rejection. This effect seems to be owing to "disarming" of the effector cells: they do not produce interferon (IFN)-γ or generate cytotoxic T lymphocytes (CTLs). Another example of differences between in vitro and in vivo conditions is the observation that inhibition of $CD4^+$ proliferation and IFN-γ secretion can be observed following co-culture with alloantigen-specific T helper (Th)1, Th2, or Tr1 clones ***(88)***. Although suppression mediated by Th1 clones could be abrogated by addition of nitric oxide synthase (NOS), in vitro suppression mediated by Th2 and Tr1 clones was NOS independent. Interestingly, when the suppressive capacity of the same clones was assessed by in vivo capacity to prevent transplant rejection, only the Tr1 clone was found to have regulatory properties ***(43)***.

Many different cytokines have been implicated as having a key role in dominant tolerance. Yet consensus has not been achieved. The contribution of IL-4 and IL-10 has been extensively studied, and, although in some circumstances neutralization of such molecules can abrogate tolerance, albeit partially in some cases ***(89–91)***, other studies have described no effect ***(58,92)***, even when IL-4 and IL-10 are simultaneously neutralized ***(58)***. TGF-β has been considered to be a suppressive mediator essential for in vivo prevention of inflammatory bowel disease ***(47,93)***, but other assays have shown regulation to be independent of TGF-β ***(94)***. Recently, TGF-β-dependent mechanisms were shown to be important for the restoration of self-tolerance in autoimmune diabetic mice treated with anti-CD3 MAbs ***(95,96)***. We have also found that blockade of TGF-β with MAbs prevents the induction of transplantation tolerance with anti-CD4 MAbs in T-cell receptor (TCR) transgenic mice ***(63)***.

The role of surface molecules such as CTLA-4 or GITR in antibody-induced tolerance still requires confirmation. Following reports that CTLA-4 blockade could inhibit regulation mediated by $CD4^+CD25^+$ T cells ***(47,48)***, two studies have shown that CTLA-4 blockade with MAbs could prevent transplantation tolerance ***(60,97)***. However, our own results have failed to confirm a role for CTLA-4 blockade in preventing dominant transplantation tolerance ***(58)***. Similarly, antibodies to GITR blocked the suppressive function of $CD4^+CD25^+$ T cells both in vitro and in vivo in autoimmunity models ***(44,49)***. However, the role of GITR in dominant transplantation tolerance remains to be clarified.

Two reports suggested that T-cell regulation may involve contact-dependent mechanisms, as well as contact-independent ones ***(98,99)***. In these reports, $CD4^+CD25^+$ T cells can render co-cultured $CD4^+CD25^-$ cells anergic through a contact-dependent, yet-unidentified mechanism. The anergized $CD4^+CD25^-$ T cells acquire suppressive function, working in a contact-independent way through the production of cytokines. The two reports disagree, however, on the nature of the cytokine that mediates the secondary suppression: one claims it is IL-10 and not TGF-β ***(98)***, whereas the other claims the opposite ***(99)***. It is important to note that the experimental systems do not depend on antigen-presenting cells (APCs) and use polyclonal T-cell populations. Yet tolerance in vivo is clearly antigen-specific and dependent on how antigen is presented. Until we fully understand the microenvironment basis of dominant tolerance, we cannot assume that any current in vitro model will provide meaningful data on the behavior of regulatory T cells.

7. Induction of Immunoprivilege in Tolerated Tissues

The observation that a regulatory T-cell population can suppress T cells in vivo can be explained without the need to propose direct T-cell–T-cell interaction. One can imagine that the regulatory effect may be mediated, at least in part, by third-party cells that need not even be hematopoietic. The demonstration that tolerated allografts harbor T cells with regulatory properties and that express *Foxp3* is compatible with this view ***(63,100)***. It is possible that such regulatory T cells empower the local microenvironment with a time-limited capacity to prevent T-cell aggression. It is conceivable that the spreading of tolerance to other T cells through linked suppression or infectious tolerance can operate through this indirect route (**Fig. 4**).

Perhaps it is time to stop considering the transplanted tissue as a passive participant in rejection and tolerance and to acknowledge that it may have an active role in these processes ***(101,102)***.

There are now many examples of how local tissue (i.e., not lymphocytes) contributes to its own defense. For example, endothelial expression of heme oxygenase-1 is induced in accommodated rat heart grafts, leading to local pro-

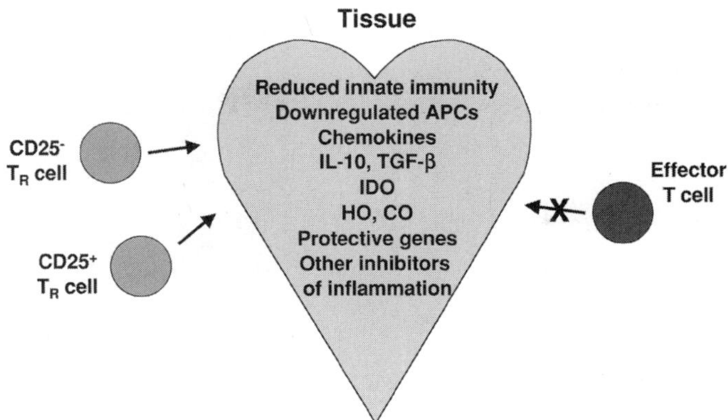

Fig. 4. Regulatory T cells conferring immunoprivilege. Regulatory T cells may exert their suppressive activity indirectly by inducing the deployment of protective mechanisms by peripheral tissues. APC, antigen-presenting cell; IL, interleukin; TGF, transforming growth factor; IDO, indoleamine 2,3-dioxygenase.

duction of carbon monoxide, which protects the transplant from being rejected ***(103)***. Moreover, tolerance induced with nondepleting anti-CD4 MAbs in rats is associated with changes in the matrix components that may contribute to a rejection-resistant environment ***(104)***. Other studies have suggested that expression of suppressor of cytokine-signaling 1 or indoleamine 2,3-dioxygenase by APCs may promote a tolerogenic environment ***(105–108)***.

It has been reported that a close relationship between immunoprivilege and dominant regulation can occur in the context of the anterior chamber-associated immune deviation ***(109)***. Antigens placed in the anterior chamber of the eye are transported by APCs into the marginal zone of the spleen, where they drive the emergence of antigen-specific $CD4^+$ and $CD8^+$ regulatory T cells. The $CD4^+$ regulatory cells can then exert their suppressive effect in secondary lymphoid organs, whereas the $CD8^+$ regulatory cells act in the periphery ***(110,111)***. It is also important to consider the impact of regulatory cells within the graft on the components of the innate immune system that might contribute to or dampen an immune response. Recent reports suggest that interactions between regulatory T cells and the innate immune system do occur ***(112–114)***. It is particularly relevant to note that by secreting IL-5, T cells may recruit eosinophils to the graft, with these cells themselves contributing to graft rejection ***(115,116)***. It is not inconceivable that other cell types may be recruited or even excluded by regulatory lymphocytes as part of a self-defense mechanism. Consistent with this is the intriguing association of mast cells with regulatory T cells mediating skin graft tolerance ***(88)***. In this respect, gene expression studies of transplanted tissue may prove informative ***(117,118)***.

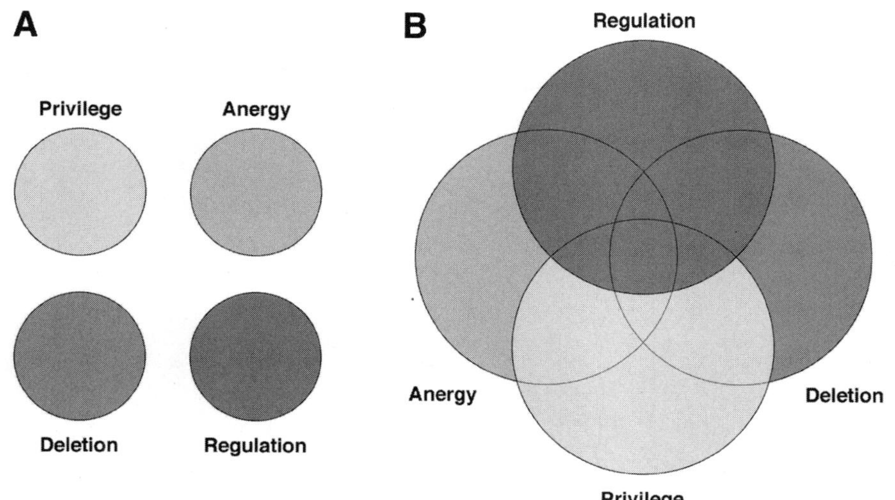

Fig. 5. A revised view of tolerance mechanisms. Classically different tolerance mechanisms have been studied as distinct phenomena (**A**). It is becoming clear that these mechanisms are a continuum of interrelated processes (**B**).

The interactions established between T cells and APCs, dendritic cells (DCs) in particular, may be important not only for a better understanding of how tolerance operates, but also for therapeutic modulation of the immune response ***(119,120)***. Host DCs, through indirect presentation, are critical both for rejection and for dominant regulation ***(121)***. This phenomenon may provide an explanation for infectious tolerance in that continuous presentation of donor antigens by host DCs in a tolerogenic environment may drive the recruitment of additional regulatory T cells. As a consequence, it may become possible to explore the tolerogenic properties of DCs, for example, with genetically modified DCs derived from embryonic stem cells ***(122,123)***.

8. A Revised View of Tolerance Mechanisms

Over the years, immunologists have neatly created discrete categories of mechanisms that mediate self-tolerance: deletion, anergy, dominant regulation, immune privilege, and ignorance (**Fig. 5**). As discussed in a recent review ***(124)***, it is becoming evident that self-tolerance does not rely on several mechanisms running independently, but rather on a continuum of synergistic and overlapping mechanisms, e.g., cells that regulate may be capable of creating immunoprivileged sites ***(109)***, an immunoprivileged environment may promote the development of regulatory or anergic cells or even cell deletion ***(125)***, anergic cells may be able to regulate ***(126,127)***, and so on.

We all need to be increasingly aware that tolerance is maintained by several mechanisms operating in concert. Reductionist approaches may be useful in identifying components but will necessarily miss the overall picture.

9. Conclusions

Current immunosuppressive agents, although the best option available, are far from ideal drugs. However, their known efficacy in preventing acute allograft rejection makes it ethically difficult to displace them in clinical trials of potential tolerogenic drugs. Safe clinical trials of experimental tolerogenic regimens will be greatly facilitated when tolerance can be monitored in vitro, allowing the use of conventional immunosuppressive drugs as soon as there is evidence of tolerance failure and before irreversible damage occurs. We therefore anticipate that some of the most important advances in the field of antibody-induced transplantation tolerance will be in the identification of diagnostic tests for the tolerant state. In this respect, the study of cellular and molecular characteristics of therapeutic-induced tolerance may identify cell populations, molecules, or gene transcripts whose presence or absence correlates with the maintenance of tolerance.

Furthermore, it may be in the patient's best interest not to aim for full tolerance but rather near tolerance *(7,8)*. If a low-impact reprogramming with tolerizing MAbs allows long-term graft survival with low doses of immunosuppressive drugs, it may prove to be an effective way to prevent transplant rejection with few side effects and good clinician and patient compliance. A recent uncontrolled study has shown that cadaveric kidney recipients treated with two doses of 20 mg of CAMPATH-1H could be maintained on a low dose of cyclosporine in the absence of other immunosuppressive agents such as steroids *(7)*. These patients have maintained good renal function with a low incidence of rejection episodes.

It is likely that the use of tolerogenic MAbs, such as those targeting CD4, will prove useful in extending graft survival in the absence of side effects, even if small doses of immunosuppressive drugs are also administered in a near-tolerance protocol.

References

1. Woodruff, M. F. and Anderson, N. A. (1963) Effect of lymphocyte depletion by thoracic duct fistula and administration of antilymphocytic serum on the survival of skin homografts in rats. *Nature* **200**,702.
2. Franksson, C., Lundgren, G., Magnusson, G., and Ringden, O. (1976) Drainage of thoracic duct lymph in renal transplant patients. *Transplantation* **21**, 133–140.
3. Cosimi, A. B., Colvin, R. B., Burton, R. C., et al. (1981) Use of monoclonal antibodies to T-cell subsets for immunologic monitoring and treatment in recipients of renal allografts. *N. Engl. J. Med.* **305**, 308–314.

4. Kahan, B. D., Rajagopalan, P. R., and Hall, M. (1999) Reduction of the occurrence of acute cellular rejection among renal allograft recipients treated with basiliximab, a chimeric anti-interleukin-2-receptor monoclonal antibody. United States Simulect Renal Study Group. *Transplantation* **67**, 276–284.
5. Graca, L., Le Moine, A., Cobbold, S. P., and Waldmann, H. (2003) Antibody-induced transplantation tolerance: the role of dominant regulation. *Immunol. Res.* **28**, 181–191.
6. Wood, K. J., Ushigome, H., Karim, M., Bushell, A., Hori, S., and Sakaguchi, S. (2003) Regulatory cells in transplantation. *Novartis Found. Symp.* **252**, 177–188.
7. Calne, R., Moffatt, S. D., Friend, P. J., et al. (1999) Campath IH allows low-dose cyclosporine monotherapy in 31 cadaveric renal allograft recipients. *Transplantation* **68**, 1613–1616.
8. Waldmann, H., Cobbold, S. P., Fairchild, P., and Adams, E. (2001) Therapeutic aspects of tolerance. *Curr. Opin. Pharmacol.* **1**, 392–397.
9. Waldmann, H. and Cobbold, S. (1998) How do monoclonal antibodies induce tolerance? A role for infectious tolerance? *Annu. Rev. Immunol.* **16**, 619–644.
10. Waldmann, H. and Cobbold, S. (2001) Regulating the immune response to transplants: a role for CD4+ regulatory cells? *Immunity* **14**, 399–406.
11. Benjamin, R. J. and Waldmann, H. (1986) Induction of tolerance by monoclonal antibody therapy. *Nature* **320**, 449–451.
12. Gutstein, N. L., Seaman, W. E., Scott, J. H., and Wofsy, D. (1986) Induction of immune tolerance by administration of monoclonal antibody to L3T4. *J. Immunol.* **137**, 1127–1132.
13. Benjamin, R. J., Qin, S. X., Wise, M. P., Cobbold, S. P,. and Waldmann, H. (1988) Mechanisms of monoclonal antibody-facilitated tolerance induction: a possible role for the CD4 (L3T4) and CD11a (LFA-1) molecules in self-non-self discrimination. *Eur. J. Immunol.* **18**, 1079–1088.
14. Carteron, N. L., Wofsy, D., and Seaman, W. E. (1988) Induction of immune tolerance during administration of monoclonal antibody to L3T4 does not depend on depletion of L3T4+ cells. *J. Immunol.* **140**, 713–716.
15. Carteron, N. L., Schimenti, C. L., and Wofsy, D. (1989) Treatment of murine lupus with F(ab')2 fragments of monoclonal antibody to L3T4. Suppression of autoimmunity does not depend on T helper cell depletion. *J. Immunol.* **142**, 1470–1475.
16. Qin, S. X., Wise, M., Cobbold, S. P., et al. (1990) Induction of tolerance in peripheral T cells with monoclonal antibodies. *Eur. J. Immunol.* **20**, 2737–2745.
17. Qin, S., Cobbold, S., Tighe, H., Benjamin, R., and Waldmann, H. (1987) CD4 monoclonal antibody pairs for immunosuppression and tolerance induction. *Eur. J. Immunol.* **17**, 1159–1165.
18. Marshall, S. E., Cobbold, S. P., Davies, J. D., Martin, G. M., Phillips, J. M., and Waldmann, H. (1996) Tolerance and suppression in a primed immune system. *Transplantation* **62**, 1614–1621.
19. Chen, Z., Cobbold, S., Metcalfe, S., and Waldmann, H. (1992) Tolerance in the mouse to major histocompatibility complex-mismatched heart allografts, and to

rat heart xenografts, using monoclonal antibodies to CD4 and CD8. *Eur. J. Immunol.* **22**, 805–810.
20. Onodera, K., Lehmann, M., Akalin, E., Volk, H. D., Sayegh, M. H., and Kupiec-Weglinski, J. W. (1996) Induction of infectious tolerance to MHC-incompatible cardiac allografts in CD4 monoclonal antibody-treated sensitized rat recipients. *J. Immunol.* **157**, 1944–1950.
21. Isobe, M., Yagita, H., Okumura, K., and Ihara, A. (1992) Specific acceptance of cardiac allograft after treatment with antibodies to ICAM-1 and LFA-1. *Science* **255**, 1125–1127.
22. Chavin, K. D., Qin, L., Lin, J., Yagita, H., and Bromberg, J. S. (1993) Combined anti-CD2 and anti-CD3 receptor monoclonal antibodies induce donor-specific tolerance in a cardiac transplant model. *J. Immunol.* **151**, 7249–7259.
23. Basadonna, G. P., Auersvald, L., Khuong, C. Q., et al. (1998) Antibody-mediated targeting of CD45 isoforms: a novel immunotherapeutic strategy. *Proc. Natl. Acad. Sci. USA* **95**, 3821–3826.
24. Lenschow, D. J., Zeng, Y., Thistlethwaite, J. R., et al. (1992) Long-term survival of xenogeneic pancreatic islet grafts induced by CTLA4lg. *Science* **257**, 789–792.
25. Parker, D. C., Greiner, D. L., Phillips, N. E., et al. (1995) Survival of mouse pancreatic islet allografts in recipients treated with allogeneic small lymphocytes and antibody to CD40 ligand. *Proc. Natl. Acad. Sci. USA* **92**, 9560–9564.
26. Honey, K., Cobbold, S. P., and Waldmann, H. (1999) CD40 ligand blockade induces CD4+ T cell tolerance and linked suppression. *J. Immunol.* **163**, 4805–4810.
27. Larsen, C. P., Elwood, E. T., Alexander, D. Z., et al. (1996) Long-term acceptance of skin and cardiac allografts after blocking CD40 and CD28 pathways. *Nature* **381**, 434–438.
28. Kirk, A. D., Burkly, L. C., Batty, D. S., et al. (1999) Treatment with humanized monoclonal antibody against CD154 prevents acute renal allograft rejection in nonhuman primates. *Nat. Med.* **5**, 686–693.
29. Kenyon, N. S., Chatzipetrou, M., Masetti, M., et al. (1999) Long-term survival and function of intrahepatic islet allografts in rhesus monkeys treated with humanized anti-CD154. *Proc. Natl. Acad. Sci. USA* **96**, 8132–8137.
30. Scully, R., Qin, S., Cobbold, S., and Waldmann, H. (1994) Mechanisms in CD4 antibody-mediated transplantation tolerance: kinetics of induction, antigen dependency and role of regulatory T cells. *Eur. J. Immunol.* **24**, 2383–2392.
31. Graca, L., Honey, K., Adams, E., Cobbold, S. P., and Waldmann, H. (2000) Cutting edge: anti-CD154 therapeutic antibodies induce infectious transplantation tolerance. *J. Immunol.* **165**, 4783–4786.
32. Chen, Z. K., Cobbold, S. P., Waldmann, H., and Metcalfe, S. (1996) Amplification of natural regulatory immune mechanisms for transplantation tolerance. *Transplantation* **62**, 1200–1206.
33. Qin, S., Cobbold, S. P., Pope, H., et al. (1993) Infectious transplantation tolerance. *Science* **259**, 974–977.
34. Waldmann, H. (2002) Reprogramming the immune system. *Immunol. Rev.* **185**, 227–235.

35. Powrie, F. and Mason, D. (1990) OX-22high CD4+ T cells induce wasting disease with multiple organ pathology: prevention by the OX-22low subset. *J. Exp. Med.* **172**, 1701–1708.
36. Sakaguchi, S., Sakaguchi, N., Asano, M., Itoh, M., and Toda, M. (1995) Immunologic self-tolerance maintained by activated T cells expressing IL-2 receptor alpha-chains (CD25). Breakdown of a single mechanism of self-tolerance causes various autoimmune diseases. *J. Immunol.* **155**, 1151–1164.
37. Sakaguchi, S. (2000) Regulatory T cells: key controllers of immunologic self-tolerance. *Cell* **101**, 455–458.
38. Shevach, E. M. (2002) CD4+ CD25+ suppressor T cells: more questions than answers. *Nat. Rev. Immunol.* **2**, 389–400.
39. Cobbold, S. P., Graca, L., Lin, C. Y., Adams, E., and Waldmann, H. (2003) Regulatory T cells in the induction and maintenance of peripheral transplantation tolerance. *Transplant. Int.* **16**, 66–75.
40. Gallimore, A. and Sakaguchi, S. (2002) Regulation of tumour immunity by CD25+ T cells. *Immunology* **107**, 5–9.
41. Mittrucker, H. W. and Kaufmann, S. H. (2004) Mini-review: regulatory T cells and infection: suppression revisited. *Eur. J. Immunol.* **34**, 306–312.
42. Lechner, O., Lauber, J., Franzke, A., Sarukhan, A., von Boehmer, H., and Buer, J. (2001) Fingerprints of anergic T cells. *Curr. Biol.* **11**, 587–595.
43. Zelenika, D., Adams, E., Humm, S., et al. (2002) Regulatory T cells over-express a subset of Th2 gene transcripts. *J. Immunol.* **168**, 1069–1079.
44. McHugh, R. S., Whitters, M. J., Piccirillo, C. A., et al. (2002) CD4(+)CD25(+) Immunoregulatory T cells. Gene expression analysis reveals a functional role for the glucocorticoid-induced TNF receptor. *Immunity* **16**, 311–323.
45. Gavin, M. A., Clarke, S. R., Negrou, E., Gallegos, A., and Rudensky, A. (2002) Homeostasis and anergy of CD4(+)CD25(+) suppressor T cells in vivo. *Nat. Immunol.* **3**, 33–41.
46. Cobbold, S. P., Adams, E., Graca, L. M., and Waldmann, H. (2003) Serial analysis of gene expression provides new insights into regulatory T cells. *Semin. Immunol.* **15**, 209–214.
47. Read, S., Malmstrom, V., and Powrie, F. (2000) Cytotoxic T lymphocyte-associated antigen 4 plays an essential role in the function of CD25(+)CD4(+) regulatory cells that control intestinal inflammation. *J. Exp. Med.* **192**, 295–302.
48. Takahashi, T., Tagami, T., Yamazaki, S., et al. (2000) Immunologic self-tolerance maintained by CD25(+)CD4(+) regulatory T cells constitutively expressing cytotoxic T lymphocyte-associated antigen 4. *J. Exp. Med.* **192**, 303–310.
49. Shimizu, J., Yamazaki, S., Takahashi, T., Ishida, Y., and Sakaguchi, S. (2002) Stimulation of CD25+CD4+ regulatory T cells through GITR breaks immunological self-tolerance. *Nat. Immunol.* **3**, 135–142.
50. Chatenoud, L., Salomon, B., and Bluestone, J. A. (2001) Suppressor T cells—they're back and critical for regulation of autoimmunity! *Immunol. Rev.* **182**, 149–163.

51. Szanya, V., Ermann, J., Taylor, C., Holness, C., and Fathman, C. G. (2002) The subpopulation of CD4+CD25+ splenocytes that delays adoptive transfer of diabetes expresses L-selectin and high levels of CCR7. *J. Immunol.* **169**, 2461–2465.
52. Fu, S., Yopp, A. C., Mao, X., et al. (2004) CD4+ CD25+ CD62+ T-regulatory cell subset has optimal suppressive and proliferative potential. *Am. J. Transplant.* **4**, 65–78.
53. McHugh, R. S. and Shevach, E. M. (2002) Cutting edge: depletion of CD4+CD25+ regulatory T cells is necessary, but not sufficient, for induction of organ-specific autoimmune disease. *J. Immunol.* **168**, 5979–5983.
54. Banz, A., Peixoto, A., Pontoux, C., Cordier, C., Rocha, B., and Papiernik, M. (2003) A unique subpopulation of CD4+ regulatory T cells controls wasting disease, IL-10 secretion and T cell homeostasis. *Eur. J. Immunol.* **33**, 2419–2428.
55. Hori, S., Nomura, T., and Sakaguchi, S. (2003) Control of regulatory T cell development by the transcription factor FOXP3. *Science* **299**, 1057–1061.
56. Fontenot, J. D., Gavin, M. A., and Rudensky, A. Y. (2003) Foxp3 programs the development and function of CD4(+)CD25(+) regulatory T cells. *Nat. Immunol.* **4**, 330–336.
57. Khattri, R., Cox, T., Yasayko, S. A., and Ramsdell, F. (2003) An essential role for Scurfin in CD4(+)CD25(+) T regulatory cells. *Nat. Immunol.* **4**, 337–342.
58. Graca, L., Thompson, S., Lin, C.-Y., Adams, E., Cobbold, S. P., and Waldmann, H. (2002) Both CD4+CD25+ and CD4+CD25- regulatory cells mediate dominant transplantation tolerance. *J. Immunol.* **168**, 5558–5567.
59. Roncarolo, M. G., Bacchetta, R., Bordignon, C., Narula, S., and Levings, M. K. (2001) Type 1 T regulatory cells. *Immunol. Rev.* **182**, 68–79.
60. Kingsley, C. I., Karim, M., Bushell, A. R., and Wood, K. J. (2002) CD25+CD4+ regulatory T cells prevent graft rejection: CTLA-4- and IL-10- dependent immunoregulation of alloresponses. *J. Immunol.* **168**, 1080–1086.
61. van Maurik, A., Herber, M., Wood, K. J., and Jones, N. D. (2002) Cutting edge: CD4(+)CD25(+) alloantigen-specific immunoregulatory cells that can prevent CD8(+) T cell-mediated graft rejection: implications for anti-CD154 immunotherapy. *J. Immunol.* **169**, 5401–5404.
62. Sanchez-Fueyo, A., Tian, J., Picarella, D., et al. (2003) Tim-3 inhibits T helper type 1-mediated auto- and alloimmune responses and promotes immunological tolerance. *Nat. Immunol.* **4**, 1093–1101.
63. Graca, L., Le Moine, A., Lin, C. Y., Fairchild, P. J., Cobbold, S. P., and Waldmann, H. (2004) Donor-specific transplantation tolerance: the paradoxical behavior of CD4+CD25+ T cells. *Pro.c Natl. Acad. Sci. USA* **101**, 10,122–10,126.
64. Cobbold, S. P., Castejon, R., Adams, E., et al. (2004) Induction of foxP3+ regulatory T cells in the periphery of T cell receptor transgenic mice tolerized to transplants. *J. Immunol.* **172**, 6003–6010.
65. Stockinger, B., Barthlott, T., and Kassiotis, G. (2001) T cell regulation: a special job or everyone's responsibility? *Nat. Immunol.* **2**, 757–758.
66. Barthlott, T., Kassiotis, G., and Stockinger, B. (2003) T cell regulation as a side effect of homeostasis and competition. *J. Exp. Med.* **197**, 451–460.

67. Annacker, O., Pimenta-Araujo, R., Burlen-Defranoux, O., Barbosa, T. C., Cumano, A., and Bandeira, A. (2001) CD25+ CD4+ T cells regulate the expansion of peripheral CD4 T cells through the production of IL-10. *J. Immunol.* **166**, 3008–3018.
68. Almeida, A. R., Legrand, N., Papiernik, M., and Freitas, A. A. (2002) Homeostasis of peripheral CD4+ T cells: IL-2R alpha and IL-2 shape a population of regulatory cells that controls CD4+ T cell numbers. *J. Immunol.* **169**, 4850–4860.
69. Wu, Z., Bensinger, S. J., Zhang, J., et al. (2004) Homeostatic proliferation is a barrier to transplantation tolerance. *Nat. Med.* **10**, 87–92.
70. Groux, H., Bigler, M., de Vries, J. E., and Roncarolo, M. G. (1996) Interleukin-10 induces a long-term antigen-specific anergic state in human CD4+ T cells. *J. Exp. Med.* **184**, 19–29.
71. Chen, Y., Kuchroo, V. K., Inobe, J., Hafler, D. A., and Weiner, H. L. (1994) Regulatory T cell clones induced by oral tolerance: suppression of autoimmune encephalomyelitis. *Science* **265**, 1237–1240.
72. Zelenika, D., Adams, E., Mellor, A., et al. (1998) Rejection of H-Y disparate skin grafts by monospecific CD4+ Th1 and Th2 cells: no requirement for CD8+ T cells or B cells. *J. Immunol.* **161**, 1868–1874.
73. Arif, S., Tree, T. I., Astill, T. P., et al. (2004) Autoreactive T cell responses show proinflammatory polarization in diabetes but a regulatory phenotype in health. *J. Clin. Invest.* **113**, 451–463.
74. Ciubotariu, R., Colovai, A. I., Pennesi, G., et al. (1998) Specific suppression of human CD4+ Th cell responses to pig MHC antigens by CD8+CD28- regulatory T cells. *J. Immunol.* **161**, 5193–5202.
75. Gilliet, M. and Liu, Y. J. (2002) Generation of human CD8 T regulatory cells by CD40 ligand-activated plasmacytoid dendritic cells. *J. Exp. Med.* **195**, 695–704.
76. Zhang, Z. X., Yang, L., Young, K. J., DuTemple, B., and Zhang, L. (2000) Identification of a previously unknown antigen-specific regulatory T cell and its mechanism of suppression. *Nat. Med.* **6**, 782–789.
77. Sanchez-Fueyo, A., Domenig, C., Strom, T. B., and Zheng, X. X. (2002) The complement dependent cytotoxicity (CDC) immune effector mechanism contributes to anti-CD154 induced immunosuppression. *Transplantation* **74**, 898–900.
78. Monk, N. J., Hargreaves, R. E., Marsh, J. E., et al. (2003) Fc-dependent depletion of activated T cells occurs through CD40L-specific antibody rather than costimulation blockade. *Nat. Med.* **9**, 1275–1280.
79. Wells, A. D., Li, X. C., Li, Y., et al. (1999) Requirement for T-cell apoptosis in the induction of peripheral transplantation tolerance. *Nat. Med.* **5**, 1303–1307.
80. Li, Y., Li, X. C., Zheng, X. X., Wells, A. D., Turka, L. A., and Strom, T. B. (1999) Blocking both signal 1 and signal 2 of T-cell activation prevents apoptosis of alloreactive T cells and induction of peripheral allograft tolerance. *Nat. Med.* **5**, 1298–1302.
81. Sawitzki, B., Lehmann, M., Vogt, K., et al. (2002) Bag-1 up-regulation in anti-CD4 mAb treated allo-activated T cells confers resistance to apoptosis. *Eur. J. Immunol.* **32**, 800–809.

82. Qin, S. X., Cobbold, S., Benjamin, R., and Waldmann, H. (1989) Induction of classical transplantation tolerance in the adult. *J. Exp. Med.* **169**, 779–794.
83. Alters, S. E., Shizuru, J. A., Ackerman, J., Grossman, D., Seydel, K. B. and Fathman, C. G. (1991) Anti-CD4 mediates clonal anergy during transplantation tolerance induction. *J. Exp. Med.* **173**, 491–494.
84. Waldmann, H., Qin, S., and Cobbold, S. (1992) Monoclonal antibodies as agents to reinduce tolerance in autoimmunity. *J. Autoimmun.* **5(Suppl. A)**, 93–102.
85. Adams, A. B., Williams, M. A., Jones, T. R., et al. (2003) Heterologous immunity provides a potent barrier to transplantation tolerance. *J. Clin. Invest.* **111**, 1887–1895.
86. Cobbold, S. P., Martin, G., and Waldmann, H. (1990) The induction of skin graft tolerance in major histocompatibility complex-mismatched or primed recipients: primed T cells can be tolerized in the periphery with anti-CD4 and anti-CD8 antibodies. *Eur. J. Immunol.* **20**, 2747–2755.
87. Lin, C. Y., Graca, L., Cobbold, S. P., and Waldmann, H. (2002) Dominant transplantation tolerance impairs CD8(+) T cell function but not expansion. *Nat. Immunol.* **3**, 1208–1213.
88. Zelenika, D., Adams, E., Humm, S., Lin, C.-Y., Waldmann, H., and Cobbold, S. P. (2001) The role of CD4+ T cell subsets in determining transplantation rejection and tolerance. *Immunol. Rev.* **182**, 164–179.
89. Davies, J. D., Martin, G., Phillips, J., Marshall, S. E., Cobbold, S. P., and Waldmann, H. (1996) T cell regulation in adult transplantation tolerance. *J. Immunol.* **157**, 529–533.
90. Onodera, K., Hancock, W. W., Graser, E., et al. (1997) Type 2 helper T cell-type cytokines and the development of "infectious" tolerance in rat cardiac allograft recipients. *J. Immunol.* **158**, 1572–1581.
91. Hara, M., Kingsley, C. I., Niimi, M., et al. (2001) IL-10 is required for regulatory T cells to mediate tolerance to alloantigens in vivo. *J. Immunol.* **166**, 3789–3796.
92. Hall, B. M., Fava, L., Chen, J., et al. (1998) Anti-CD4 monoclonal antibody-induced tolerance to MHC-incompatible cardiac allografts maintained by CD4+ suppressor T cells that are not dependent upon IL-4. *J. Immunol.* **161**, 5147–5156.
93. Powrie, F., Carlino, J., Leach, M. W., Mauze, S., and Coffman, R. L. (1996) A critical role for transforming growth factor-beta but not interleukin 4 in the suppression of T helper type 1-mediated colitis by CD45RB(low) CD4+ T cells. *J. Exp. Med.* **183**, 2669–2674.
94. Piccirillo, C. A., Letterio, J. J., Thornton, A. M., et al. (2002) CD4(+)CD25(+) regulatory T cells can mediate suppressor function in the absence of transforming growth factor beta1 production and responsiveness. *J. Exp. Med.* **196**, 237–246.
95. Belghith, M., Bluestone, J. A., Barriot, S., Megret, J., Bach, J. F., and Chatenoud, L. (2003) TGF-beta-dependent mechanisms mediate restoration of self-tolerance induced by antibodies to CD3 in overt autoimmune diabetes. *Nat. Med.* **9**, 1202–1208.

96. Bommireddy, R. and Doetschman, T. (2004) TGF-beta, T-cell tolerance and anti-CD3 therapy. *Trends Mol. Med.* **10**, 3–9.
97. Sanchez-Fueyo, A., Weber, M., Domenig, C., Strom, T. B., and Zheng, X. X. (2002) Tracking the immunoregulatory mechanisms active during allograft tolerance. *J. Immunol.* **168**, 2274–2281.
98. Dieckmann, D., Bruett, C. H., Ploettner, H., Lutz, M. B., and Schuler, G. (2002) Human CD4(+)CD25(+) regulatory, contact-dependent T cells induce interleukin 10-producing, contact-independent type 1-like regulatory T cells. *J. Exp. Med.* **196**, 247–253.
99. Jonuleit, H., Schmitt, E., Kakirman, H., Stassen, M., Knop, J., and Enk, A. H. (2002) Infectious tolerance: human CD25(+) regulatory T cells convey suppressor activity to conventional CD4(+) T helper cells. *J. Exp. Med.* **196**, 255–260.
100. Graca, L., Cobbold, S. P., and Waldmann, H. (2002) Identification of regulatory T cells in tolerated allografts. *J. Exp. Med.* **195**, 1641–1646.
101. Pratt, J. R., Basheer, S. A., and Sacks, S. H. (2002) Local synthesis of complement component C3 regulates acute renal transplant rejection. *Nat. Med.* **8**, 582–587.
102. Hancock, W. W., Wang, L., Ye, Q., Han, R., and Lee, I. (2003) Chemokines and their receptors as markers of allograft rejection and targets for immunosuppression. *Curr. Opin. Immunol.* **15**, 479–486.
103. Soares, M. P., Brouard, S., Smith, R. N., and Bach, F. H. (2001) Heme oxygenase-1, a protective gene that prevents the rejection of transplanted organs. *Immunol. Rev.* **184**, 275–285.
104. Coito, A. J. and Kupiec-Weglinski, J. W. (2000) Extracellular matrix proteins in organ transplantation. *Transplantation* **69**, 2465–2473.
105. Nakagawa, R., Naka, T., Tsutsui, H., et al. (2002) SOCS-1 participates in negative regulation of LPS responses. *Immunity* **17**, 677–687.
106. Munn, D. H., Sharma, M. D., Lee, J. R., et al. (2002) Potential regulatory function of human dendritic cells expressing indoleamine 2,3-dioxygenase. *Science* **297**, 1867–1870.
107. Mellor, A. L., Keskin, D. B., Johnson, T., Chandler, P., and Munn, D. H. (2002) Cells expressing indoleamine 2,3-dioxygenase inhibit T cell responses. *J. Immunol.* **168**, 3771–3776.
108. Kinjyo, I., Hanada, T., Inagaki-Ohara, K., et al. (2002) SOCS1/JAB is a negative regulator of LPS-induced macrophage activation. *Immunity* **17**, 583–591.
109. Streilein, J. W. (2003) Ocular immune privilege: therapeutic opportunities from an experiment of nature. *Nat. Rev. Immunol.* **3**, 879–889.
110. Stein-Streilein, J. and Streilein, J. W. (2002) Anterior chamber associated immune deviation (ACAID): regulation, biological relevance, and implications for therapy. *Int. Rev. Immunol.* **21**, 123–152.
111. Streilein, J. W., Masli, S., Takeuchi, M., and Kezuka, T. (2002) The eye's view of antigen presentation. *Hum. Immunol.* **63**, 435–443.
112. Maloy, K. J., Salaun, L., Cahill, R., Dougan, G., Saunders, N. J., and Powrie, F. (2003) CD4+CD25+ T(R) cells suppress innate immune pathology through cytokine-dependent mechanisms. *J. Exp. Med.* **197**, 111–119.

113. Pasare, C. and Medzhitov, R. (2003) Toll pathway-dependent blockade of CD4+CD25+ T cell-mediated suppression by dendritic cells. *Science* **299**, 1033–1036.
114. Caramalho, I., Lopes-Carvalho, T., Ostler, D., Zelenay, S., Haury, M., and Demengeot, J. (2003) Regulatory T cells selectively express toll-like receptors and are activated by lipopolysaccharide. *J. Exp. Med.* **197**, 403–411.
115. Le Moine, A., Surquin, M., Demoor, F. X., et al. (1999) IL-5 mediates eosinophilic rejection of MHC class II-disparate skin allografts in mice. *J. Immunol.* **163**, 3778–3784.
116. Le Moine, A., Flamand, V., Demoor, F. X., et al. (1999) Critical roles for IL-4, IL-5, and eosinophils in chronic skin allograft rejection. *J. Clin. Invest.* **103**, 1659–1667.
117. Saiura, A., Mataki, C., Murakami, T., et al. (2001) A comparison of gene expression in murine cardiac allografts and isografts by means DNA microarray analysis. *Transplantation* **72**, 320–329.
118. Christopher, K., Mueller, T. F., Ma, C., Liang, Y., and Perkins, D. L. (2002) Analysis of the innate and adaptive phases of allograft rejection by cluster analysis of transcriptional profiles. *J. Immunol.* **169**, 522–530.
119. Fairchild, P. J. and Waldmann, H. (2000) Dendritic cells and prospects for transplantation tolerance. *Curr. Opin. Immunol.* **12**, 528–535.
120. Jonuleit, H., Schmitt, E., Steinbrink, K., and Enk, A. H. (2001) Dendritic cells as a tool to induce anergic and regulatory T cells. *Trends Immunol.* **22**, 394–400.
121. Wise, M. P., Bemelman, F., Cobbold, S. P., and Waldmann, H. (1998) Linked suppression of skin graft rejection can operate through indirect recognition. *J. Immunol.* **161**, 5813–5816.
122. Fairchild, P. J., Brook, F. A., Gardner, R. L., et al. (2000) Directed differentiation of dendritic cells from mouse embryonic stem cells. *Curr. Biol.* **10**, 1515–1518.
123. Fairchild, P. J., Nolan, K. F., Cartland, S., Graca, L., and Waldmann, H. (2003) Stable lines of genetically modified dendritic cells from mouse embryonic stem cells. *Transplantation* **76**, 606–608.
124. Waldmann, H., Graca, L., Cobbold, S., Adams, E., Tone, M., and Tone, Y. (2004) Regulatory T cells and organ transplantation. *Semin. Immunol.* **16**, 119–126.
125. Arnold, B. (2003) Parenchymal cells in immune and tolerance induction. *Immunol. Lett.* **89**, 225–228.
126. Lombardi, G., Sidhu, S., Batchelor, R., and Lechler, R. (1994) Anergic T cells as suppressor cells in vitro. *Science* **264**, 1587–1589.
127. Chai, J. G., Bartok, I., Chandler, P., et al. (1999) Anergic T cells act as suppressor cells in vitro and in vivo. *Eur. J. Immunol.* **29**, 686–692.

12

In Vitro Assays for Immune Monitoring in Transplantation

Maria P. Hernandez-Fuentes and Alan Salama

Summary

Because immune responses to transplant allografts are the main drivers of rejection, the ability to accurately quantitate antidonor immunity is an important goal in clinical transplantation. These allow for the prediction of presensitization to the transplanted tissue and the identification of rejection without needing more invasive tests.

In this chapter, we will review three methods currently used in transplantation research. Limiting dilution assays are a traditional tool. The evolution of these assays has brought about the ELISpot. Developments in flow cytometry are also contributing to the understanding of the composition of the cells involved in these immune responses.

We can therefore obtain a deeper understanding of the process of rejection and tolerance and their evolution with time. This chapter reviews in vitro assays in the context of transplantation, but the scientific applications of sensitive, accurate, and specific immune-monitoring reach well beyond this field of research.

Key Words: Immune monitoring; mixed lymphocyte reaction; limiting dilution assays (LDAs); ELISpot; carboxyfluorescein succinimidyl ester (CFSE); lymphocyte division; cytokine secretion assay; regulatory T cells; immunological tolerance; T-cell responses; allogeneic responses; transplant monitoring; alloreactivity; direct and indirect pathways of allorecognition.

1. Introduction

The development of assays that would allow monitoring of the current state of an alloimmune response is of interest for several reasons. They would have the potential to identify rejection without resorting to invasive tests. More importantly, a reliable index of the immune status could allow immunosuppressive drug prescribing to be individualized. In some cases the identification of immu-

From: *Methods in Molecular Biology, vol. 333: Transplantation Immunology: Methods and Protocols*
Edited by: P. Hornick and M. Rose © Humana Press Inc., Totowa, NJ

nological tolerance could allow the partial or complete cessation of immunosuppressants, a highly desirable goal given the morbidity and mortality associated with long-term administration of such therapy. It is also clear that such assays will bring with them a more complete understanding of the mechanisms underlying the generation of tolerance and rejection, which will open the door to new and better targeted therapeutic interventions.

1.1. Managing the Transplant Recipient

Monitoring the allogeneic effector response may help us understand the mechanisms that result in graft rejection. Assays that are able to identify key steps in the process might ultimately be used as predictors of potentially detrimental events, prior to their clinical manifestation. This would allow intervention at a much earlier stage in the rejection process. Increased antidonor responses have been measured in association with rejection in solid organ transplantation ***(1–3)***, but these results have not been consistent ***(4,5)***. No large prospective studies have been conducted that evaluate clinically useful antidonor responses, probably the result of the lack of definition of an assay that can be easily conducted in a large number of patients, requires acceptably small volumes of blood, and can be repeated on several occasions.

The efficacy of immunosuppression over the past two decades have led to a considerable improvement in the short-term survival of organ transplants. Notwithstanding this, almost all transplanted patients have to endure immunosuppression for the rest of their lives. Long-term immunosuppressive drug treatment is associated with significant morbidity and mortality, mainly due to cardiovascular disease, opportunistic infections, and an increased incidence of malignancy. The ultimate goal in the management of transplanted patients is the induction of donor-specific tolerance—antigen-specific immunological unresponsiveness that is sustained in the absence of chronic immunosuppression. Immunological monitoring could contribute by quantitating pro-inflammatory and anti-inflammatory components of the antidonor response. If reliable assays were available, it would be possible to monitor the evolution of antidonor responses in individual patients and to determine the effectiveness of potentially tolerogenic therapeutic strategies. As new drugs and biological agents are introduced, such assays are vitally important in determining whether they are tolerance promoting or whether they impede the development of immune tolerance. In patients who have already received a transplant, the assays would be used to identify those in whom tolerance had developed and, therefore, whose immunosuppression could be weaned, avoiding much of its detrimental effects.

We can define immunological monitoring as the *ex vivo* measurement of pro-inflammatory and anti-inflammatory responses with clinical utility. Examples of such assays that conform to this definition will be the subject of this review.

Although monitoring immune responses in transplant recipients could be through analysis of genes or proteins in the urine, blood, or within the graft, traditional methods were limited to the study of lymphocytes. It can be argued that the responses of cells from the peripheral blood do not necessarily mirror what happens in the tissue, as this is regulated by infiltrating lymphocytes. To address this question, Orosz et al. used an elegant model of an allograft made of polyurethane sponges bearing allogeneic splenocytes *(6)*. Donor-reactive cytotoxic T cells represented up to 0.2% of the cells recovered from these allografts, which are similar to the frequencies found in limiting dilution assays (LDAs) on peripheral blood using completely mismatched human samples *(7)*. While acknowledging that peripheral blood is not the ideal source of information reflecting the situation in the graft, these data argue that there are reasons to believe it is good enough. Most of the assays described relate to studying T-lymphocyte responses, as these are the orchestrators of the allogeneic immune response. It is important to note that, almost certainly, no single assay will provide all the answers; rather, each will analyze the immune response in a subtly different fashion. Combining the results of several assays should allow the determination of the fingerprint of the immune response at any given time in a given individual.

1.2. Animal Transplantation

Although individual kinetic assessment of alloreactivity by different methods is feasible in human peripheral blood, in murine systems peripheral blood is a poor source of cells, and, thus, individual kinetic assessment of alloreactivity in the same individual can be challenging. The advantage is that transplantation groups can be bigger and the variation from one individual to the next in littermates is so small that the kinetic studies can be performed on different individuals. Moreover, graft-infiltrating lymphocytes are available for study, arguably providing the most interesting source of information. Most of the assays described here can be applied in rodents using the appropriate reagents. However, many reports using animal models of transplantation assess alloreactivity simply by graft survival, and accurate quantitation of responses to donor antigens is surprisingly scarce in the literature. Where in vitro assays have been informative in rodent systems, we have added them in their section.

2. Biological Basis for Immune Assays to Monitor Responses to Grafts

To understand the basis of assays to monitor antidonor T-cell immunity, several concepts have to be considered. First, the molecules responsible for the immune response to allogeneic tissues are encoded by genes found in the major histocompatibility complex (MHC) locus on the short arm of chromosome 6 in humans (chromosome 17 in mice). The protein products of MHC genes have

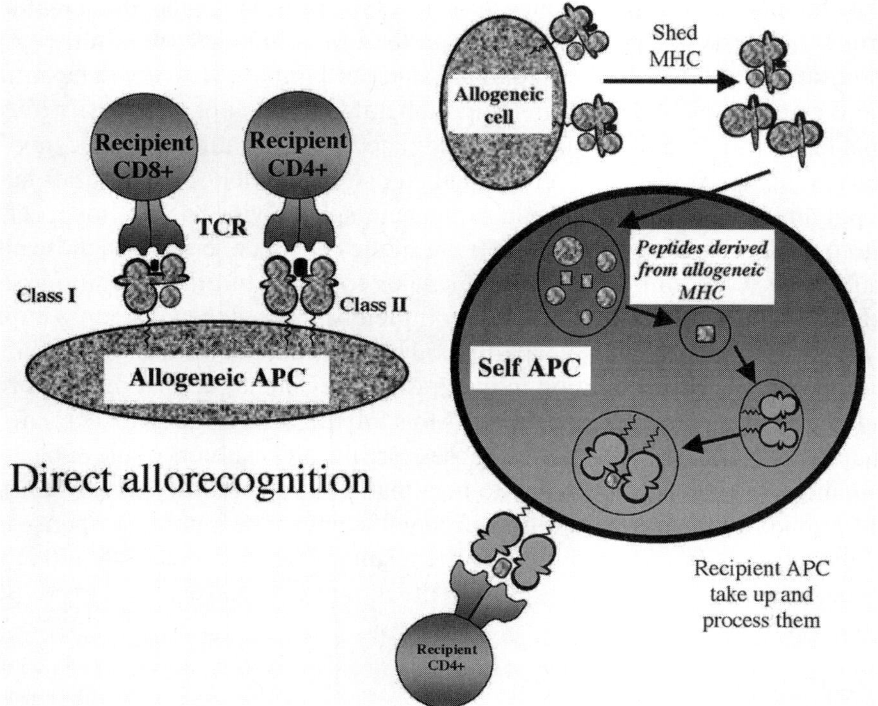

Fig. 1. Direct and indirect pathways of allorecognition. In direct allorecognition, T cells recognize and are activated by intact allogeneic MHC molecules on the donor cells. $CD8^+$ T cells are activated by recognition of class I molecules of the MHC complex, whereas $CD4^+$ cells are activated by the recognition of class II molecules. In the indirect pathway allogeneic MHC molecules are shed from the graft, taken up, processed by the recipient APCs, and presented as allo-peptides on the surface of recipient's MHC molecules. MHC, major histocompatibility complex; APC, antigen-presenting cell.

been divided into two major groups: class I and class II molecules. The class I molecules are human leukocyte antigens (HLAs)-A, -B, and -C in humans and H2-K, -D, and -L in mice, and they are expressed by all nucleated cells in an organism. The class II molecules are HLA-DR, -DP, and -DQ in humans and H2-A and -E in mice. These are constitutively expressed only by bone-marrow-derived antigen-presenting, such as macrophages, dendritic cells, and B lymphocytes, and by thymic epithelial cells *(8)*.

Second, there are two pathways of T-cell alloreactivity (**Fig. 1**). The direct pathway requires the recognition of intact donor MHC alloantigens on the surface of donor cells by recipient T cells. The cells stimulating the direct pathway most efficiently are passenger dendritic cells from the donor that migrate to draining lymphoid tissues shortly after transplantation. Thereafter, the direct pathway is stimulated mainly by allogeneic MHC molecules on the graft cells themselves. The second pathway of MHC allorecognition, the indirect pathway, involves the internalization, processing, and presentation of alloantigens as peptides bound to recipient MHC molecules. There is sufficient evidence now to support that indirect allorecognition is an important driver of transplant rejection ***(7,9–12)*** and that the induction of tolerance in this pathway is a requirement for long-term transplant survival ***(13,14)***.

Third, regulatory T cells may be vital in holding the antidonor immune response in check. The evidence for such cells is long-standing and comes from adoptive transfer studies in which tolerance can be transferred to a naïve recipient by $CD4^+$ T cells. Although the mechanisms of this regulation remain incompletely understood, some progress has been made in defining the phenotype of this regulatory population. A group of these cells have the same phenotype, $CD4^+CD25^+$, as the spontaneously arising population that plays a vital role in the prevention of autoimmune disease. Depletion of these $CD4^+CD25^+$ prevents the transfer of tolerance by $CD4^+$ T cells from a transplant-bearing animal ***(15)***. Over the past decade, an ever-increasing body of data in both human and animal models has established the role of these and other naturally occurring regulatory cells (e.g., natural killer cells) in transplantation. Several authors have recently reviewed this phenomenon ***(16–18)***. The picture of the mechanisms underlying the regulatory function of these cells is far from completely defined, but it does appear that this population of T cells plays an important role in the maintenance of experimental ***(17)*** and possibly clinical ***(19)*** transplantation tolerance.

The assays here described attempt to quantify the frequencies of lymphocytes recognizing donor antigen. Frequently, only the direct pathway has been considered when measuring these responses. The primary in vitro response to the direct recognition of allogeneic molecules occurs in the mixed lymphocyte reaction (MLR) where mixtures of allogeneic lymphocytes are placed in culture. This reaction was first described in the 1960s and has been extensively used to study antidonor responses. However, in its conventional form, proliferative MLR bulk cultures have very little predictive value in the context of transplantation ***(20)***. For this reason, alternative assays have been developed to obtain information regarding immunological responses that are of greater clinical utility.

To measure indirect pathway responses, some modifications in the culture conditions have to be set in place for almost all the assays. This requires the presentation of alloantigen as protein preparations rather than whole cells. Several preparations have been used, namely freeze–thawed donor cells ***(21)***, membrane protein preparations of donor cells *(7)*, or peptides derived from the hypervariable regions of MHC molecules *(22)*. The special challenge that measuring indirect pathway responses poses is caused by the low frequency of T cells with this specificity. In many instances these responses are near the limit of detection of the assays described. Therefore, it is essential that steps are taken to increase the sensitivity of the assays, as this will help in the ability to accurately measure such responses and any subtle variations that may occur. It is important to note that in allogeneic mixed lymphocyte reactions, where the donor and the recipient share HLA molecules (e.g., siblings), the assumption is that both direct and indirect responses are being detected simultaneously in these cultures. To be able to measure one or the other, purified populations are required in the culture.

3. Limiting Dilution Assays

LDAs allow the estimation of frequencies of antigen-specific cells participating in an immune response *(23,24)*. They have become a standard experimental tool for estimating frequencies of cells with defined function within a population of cells (**Fig. 2**).

Traditionally, measuring frequencies of proliferating or cytokine-secreting cells has been considered to measure helper T-lymphocyte precursor frequencies (HTLps), whereas when measuring cytotoxicity we describe them as cytotoxic T lymphocyte precursor frequencies (CTLps). LDA assays have been shown to be specific and reproducible as a measurement of alloreactivity *(25)*. A number of refinements have been described to increase the specificity and sensitivity in the measurement of interleukin (IL)-2-secreting HTLps *(26–28)*, as well as for CTLp frequencies *(29)*. Different cytokines derived from both Th1 and Th2 polarized cells can be detected in these cultures; the most frequently found are interferon (IFN)-γ, IL-5, IL-4, or even IL-10 *(30–32)*. The clinical utility of antidonor frequency measurement has been extensively demonstrated for IL-2 *(33,34)* and CTLp in bone marrow transplant recipients *(35–39)*. However, in solid organ transplants the picture is less clear, and conflicting data have been reported regarding the ability of CTLp measurements to predict rejection *(40–42)*. Further development in the detection of cytokines may help in dissecting mechanisms of tolerance and rejection.

Recent data have emphasized the critical role of regulatory cells and the complex interactions between them and effector cells in the generation of an immune response. It has therefore become very important to include the study of such regulatory cells. The absence of a clear phenotypic marker for these cells further complicates the issue. LDAs have a unique advantage in that they allow the study of complex responses at a population level. When the responder population contains cells (such as regulatory cells) that affect the response of other cells, LDAs can reveal their presence. These complex responses usually

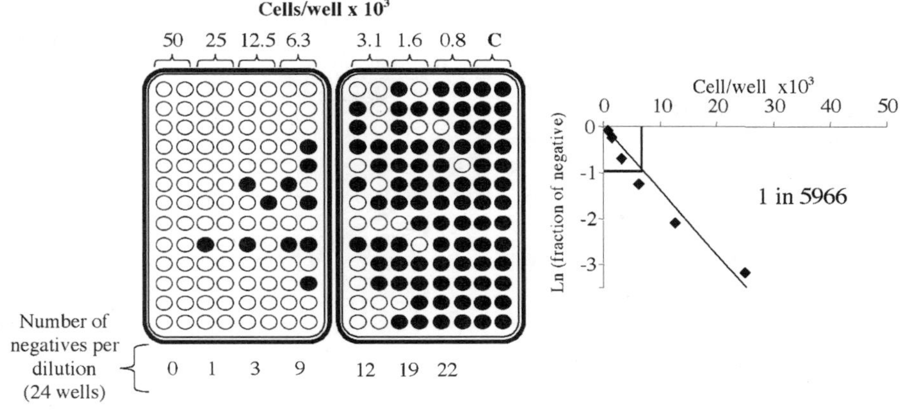

Fig. 2. Limiting dilution analysis: general protocol for use in allotransplantation assays. At least 24 replicates of responder cells (peripheral blood mononuclear cells, CD4+, CD8+, etc.) at no fewer than seven doubling dilutions are aliquoted in U-bottom sterile plates. Culture medium alone is added to the 24 control wells (C). Stimulation can be in the form of allogeneic cells (direct pathway) or antigen-presenting cells (APCs) pulsed with different preparations of allogeneic antigen (peptides, cell lysates, sonicated cells, etc.—this is the indirect pathway). Stimulator cells are irradiated (30 Gy) prior to addition to all the wells. After optimal culture conditions, supernatants can be collected for the detection of cytokines (determined by ELISA or a bioassay), proliferation, and measured by adding thymidine-H^3 12–18 h before the end of culture. A special situation arises if cytotoxic precursors are to be measured. Stimulator and responders are cultured for 9 d, and wells are supplemented with interleukin-2 after 3 and 6 d. On day 9 ^{51}chromium-labeled stimulator cells are added to each well followed by 4-h incubation; γ-radiation is then measured in the supernatant. For all of the measurable outcomes, wells are scored positive when the measure of choice is higher than the mean + 3 standard deviations of the control wells, in which only stimulators are added. As the concentration of the responder cells increases, the proportion of negative wells will tend to be less; the relation between the number of negative wells and the mean number of precursors can be plotted and a frequency obtained *(24, 78)*. The ability of an limiting dilution assay assay to predict the frequency of precursors depends on the number of replicates and the number of responder cells added per dilution *(79)*. An important issue concerns the statistical method used to estimate the unknown frequency. A number of methods are available to estimate the effector frequency from the experimental data: least-squares, weighted means, minimum c-square, and maximum likelihood. Extensive evaluation of the methods using artificial data concluded that the last three were useful *(80)*. We have favored a maximum likelihood-based method that introduces bias reduction *(81)*.

manifest themselves as deviations from the single-hit kinetics and graphically give rise to the zigzag curves when cell dose is plotted against fraction of negative cultures *(43)* (*see* **Fig. 3** for further explanation of this concept).

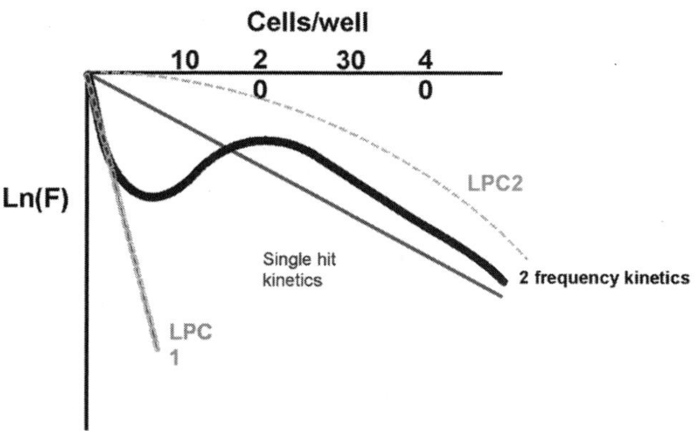

Fig. 3. Single-hit and multiple kinetics in limiting dilution assays (LDAs). Single- and multiple-hit LDA curves are represented. An experiment with only one population of cells responding results in a straight line when cell number and the fraction of negative wells are plotted (single-hit kinetics, dark grey thin line). In contrast, an experiment in which the population of responding cells is mixed results in a classic "humped" curve (thick black line) (adapted from **ref.** ***43***). In this model, several assumptions are made when deriving a curve. The most important is that one of the populations acts only as responders, while another can act as a regulatory population at low cell number and as an effector at high cell numbers. This model has been found to best fit the experimental data ***(45)***.

In isolation the responder population would be represented by LPC1 (light grey dotted line), which follows single-hit kinetics. At low cell numbers there is a sharp decrease in the number of responding wells. In contrast, the regulatory population is represented by LPC2 (light grey broken line), where at low cell numbers, cells remain unresponsive but as the number increases those cells begin to proliferate, thus producing a curve. If the populations are mixed (thick black line), at a low frequency the responders predominate, but as the number of cells per well increases, the regulatory cells can exert their suppressive effect and inhibit the responders proliferating, resulting in more wells scoring negative, hence the "hump." The wells will not score positive again until there are both enough regulators to start proliferating and an excess of responders to prevent suppression. Once this happens, the "hump" is overcome and the line tends towards a straight line. The actual frequency of the two populations can be derived from the gradients of LPC1 and LPC2.

Indeed, in LDA experiments, if one of these regulatory populations, namely $CD4^+CD25^+$ cells, is added back to a culture with the effector $CD4^+CD25^-$ fraction, there is a dose-dependent effect between the percentage of $CD4^+CD25^+$ cells and the deviation of the data from single-hit kinetics ***(44)***. Dozmorov et al. have developed mathematical models for the accurate estimation of the frequencies of two separate interacting cells types in such mixed populations ***(45)***.

More recently, a French group has proposed a novel theoretical approach for quantifying the frequency of suppressor cells in a responding population. This method allows the simultaneous estimation of the frequencies of both proliferating and suppressor cells and is based on LDA data modeling ***(46)***.

Several aspects support LDA as a valuable tool to monitor donor-specific responses, particularly if aided by computerized calculations. No other assay to date has surpassed their specificity and relationship to clinical outcome. It is the only assay so far that allows measurement of regulatory cell frequencies. Furthermore, the range of readouts that can be measured will ensure its ongoing usefulness in the near future. Notwithstanding, they are labor-intensive and require complex data analysis.

4. ELISpot

The ELISpot assay allows the detection of soluble products from single cells after stimulation with mitogens or antigens ***(47,48)***. The secreted product is detected by specific monoclonal antibodies, and the cells producing it are revealed by the generation of discrete spots. The number of spots reflects the number of product-secreting cells ***(49)*** (**Fig. 4**). Automated video image analysis has helped develop the potential use of this assay ***(50)*** by reducing its labor-intensiveness. The main use of this assay at the moment is to study the production of signature Th1 and Th2 cytokines (IFN-γ and IL-4) after stimulation in samples from targeted patients. Presently it is widely used in monitoring antigen-specific responses in the context of vaccine development for infectious diseases ***(51)***, cancer ***(52)***, and autoimmunity ***(53,54)***. In the context of transplantation, it has been used to identify the presence of donor-specific T cells in patients prior to surgery ***(55)*** and to assess the indirect pathway in patients with evidence of chronic rejection ***(22)***.

ELISpot frequencies have been found to correlate with LDA precursor frequencies of varied effector functions ***(56,57)***. ELISpot has also been used to assess direct and indirect allogeneic responses in murine models ***(10)*** and in renal transplant recipients ***(19)***. Recently a modification of the ELISpot, namely the Lysispot, has been published to assess antigen-specific perforin-dependent cytotoxicity ***(58)***. ELISpot results, unlike those of LDA, are not dependent on clonal expansion. The assay is less labor-intensive, and results can be analyzed after 48 h (vs 7 d for LDA) in conjunction with an image analyzer. This assay has great potential for clinical application. However, disadvantages include the need to invest in an image analyzer and the chance of error due to subjectivity in the interpretation of results, because a threshold for the size, intensity, and gradient of the spots is user-defined. The near future may bring about a comparison of results using different ELISpot readers. Standardization across laboratories and readers of parameters that define a positive

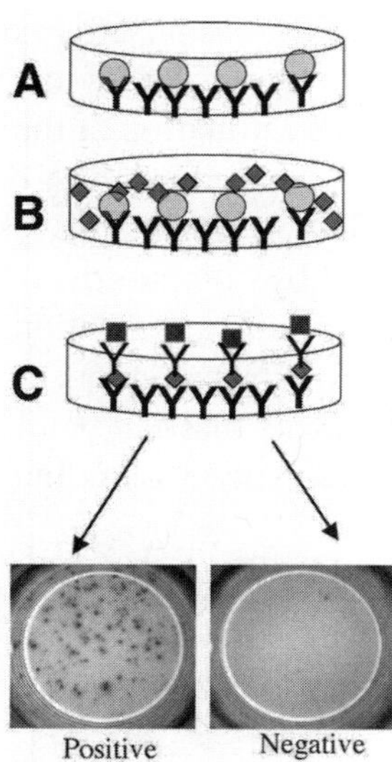

Fig. 4. ELISpot general protocol. Special plates should be used with high-protein-binding membranes, such as Immobilon P (Millipore, Bedford, MA). Paired antibodies developed for ELISpot or ELISA can be used. **(A)** Capture antibody (4–15 mg/mL) diluted in sterile buffer (phosphate-buffered saline [PBS] or $NaHCO_3$, pH = 8.0–9.6) is added to the wells. To allow binding, incubate antibody for 4–6 h at room temperature or overnight at 4°C. Under sterile conditions wash the plate with PBS, then add cells and stimuli (*see* below for culture conditions). **(B)** Cultures are incubated for 24–48 h while the cytokine is produced by the cells. Cells are then removed from the plate and washed extensively with PBS. The cytokine will remain bound to the antibody. **(C)** A detection biotinylated antibody is then added (1 mg/mL) diluted in PBS containing 0.5–1% protein (albumin or bovine serum). Another extensive washing step is followed by the addition of a conjugate of an enzyme (horseradish peroxidase or alkaline phosphatase) and streptavidin. In the final step, the substrate is added (BCIP/NBT or AEC), which precipitates where the secondary antibody was bound, forming spots that correspond to cells producing the cytokine. Spots can be counted manually with magnifying microscope or using an automatic counter in conjuctions with video image analysis. Culture conditions: the concept of measurement is different from standard tissue culture plates as the outcome is the number of cytokine-producing cells or frequency of responders. The researcher must ensure that the number and/or concentration of stimulators is well in excess for the number of cells added in each well. Different dilutions of responder cells should be used to accurately confirm the frequency of spot-forming cells.

spot will be required for reproducibility as well. The increasing use of this assay to monitor immune responses in different clinical situations is generating a wealth of literature, and it will be interesting to find out if this assay meets the expectations it is generating.

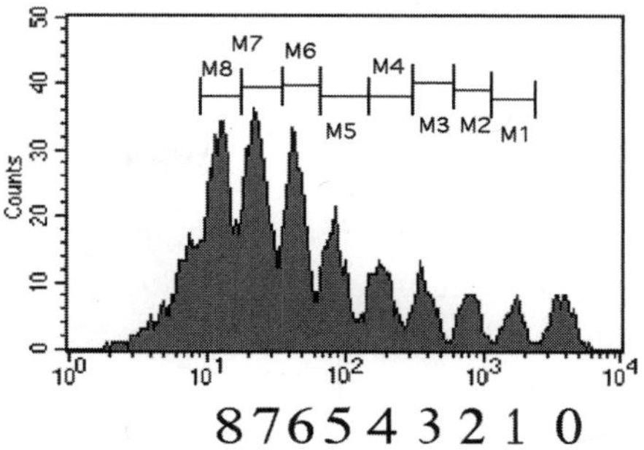

Number of cell divisions

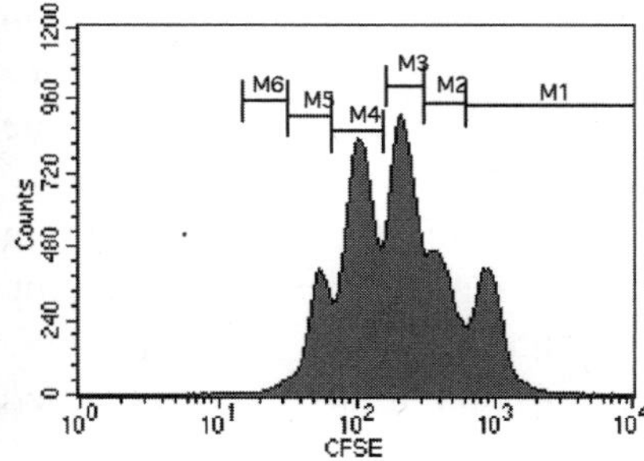

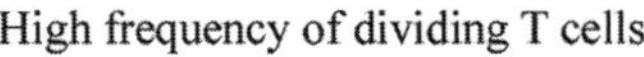

High frequency of dividing T cells

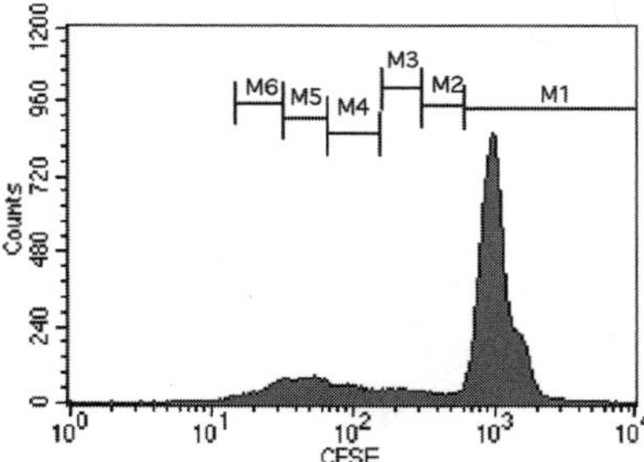

Low frequency of dividing T cells

Fig. 5. Flow cytometry analysis of cell division: carboxyfluorescein succinimidyl sster (CFSE) labeling. Lymphocytes are labeled with a 1- to 5-m*M* solution of CFSE (green fluorochrome) in PBS and then washed prior to setting up the culture. Following lymphocyte activation and proliferation, each cell division results in a halving of the fluorescence intensity. Green fluorescence intensity of the population can be measured using a flow cytometer. A histogram plot produces the classical image of groups of cells that have divided a certain number of times. In T lymphocytes, up to eight cell divisions can accurately be distinguished. Accurate quantitation of dividing cells can be achieved by the use of internal standards such as microspheres that allow enumeration of absolute cell numbers as opposed to percentages ***(82)***. This way we can calculate the number of precursors that have undergone division. By relating precursors to the number of cells seeded, a frequency of proliferating precursors can be obtained.

5. Flow Cytometry and Immunological Monitoring

A recent development for studying cell division following antigen encounter involves the use of fluorescent dyes, which also allows tracking of cellular migration. The most widely used dye, carboxyfluorescein succinimidyl ester (CFSE), is an intracellular fluorescent label that divides equally between daughter cells following cellular division ***(59,60)*** **(Fig. 5)**. Recently, a method was developed using this dye to quantify alloreactive T-cell responses *(61)*. A combination of LDA and CFSE labeling has also been described to measure alloactivation in CD8+ cells *(62)*. Using this enumeration method, antigen-specific frequencies have been measured with high sensitivity and reproducibility (Hernandez-Fuentes, manuscript in preparation). The advantage of this method, as with other flow-cytometric methods, is that different phenotypically defined subsets of cells can be studied simultaneously *(63)*. In combination with intracellular staining, the quantity of secreted cytokine or other cytoplasmic proteins can be measured. It also allows for the study of individual cell populations within mixed cultures, such as dendritic cells and T lymphocytes or regulatory and effector cells.

The use of CFSE labeling to assess allogeneic responses in vivo has been widely used in murine systems, chiefly bcause the CFSE-labeled cells remain identifiable for a prolonged period of time. The limit of detection of the dividing cells is the number of divisions they have undergone, which dilutes out the fluorescent dye. Through the adoptive transfer of CFSE-labeled cells, the number of responding cells can be calculated *(61)* and the mechanisms of rejection and tolerance in vivo studied *(64)*. It has proven invaluable in understanding issues related to cell migration, such as localization of sites of lymphocyte activation and antigen presentation. Moreover, this technique can also be used to determine the kinetics of immune responses, track proliferation in minor subsets of cells and follow the acquisition of differentiation markers or internal proteins linked to cell division *(65)*.

We have compared different methods of calculating CD4+ antigen-specific T-cell frequencies in healthy human controls and have found them to be reproducible over time. In addition, using a mouse model specifically designed to compare the accuracy of these alternative approaches, ELISpot was found to be marginally superior to LDA or CFSE labeling and flow cytometry in accurately calculating alloreactive T-cell frequencies (Hernandez-Fuentes, manuscript in preparation). Given the speed and relative ease of performing ELISpot assays, this clearly makes it an attractive option for translation into the clinic.

5.1. Flow-Cytometric Detection of Cytokines

Two flow cytometry methods for detection and measurement of lymphocyte cytokine production have been used in relation to immunological monitoring. The first is the cytokine secretion assay, in which an artificial affinity matrix on the cell surface specific for the secreted product of interest is created **(Fig. 6)**. This method has been shown to correlate with the number of tetramer-binding CD8+ T cells, reacting to a melanoma-associated peptide, Melan-A *(66)*. However, measuring responses to influenza peptides in healthy volunteers, this method did not correlate with results obtained with either ELISpot or intracellular cytokine staining *(67)*. This method was initially designed to isolate func-

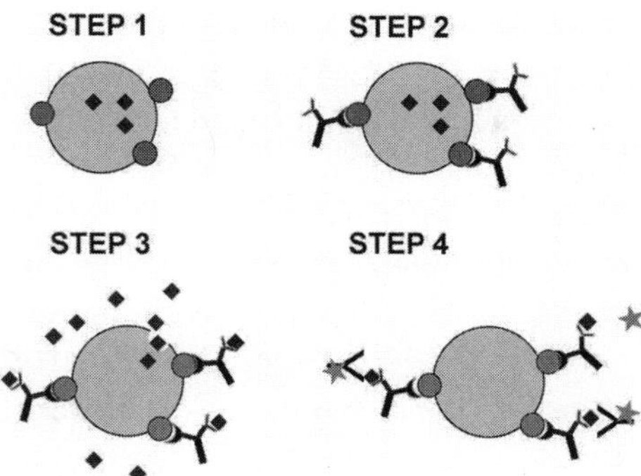

Fig. 6. Cytokine secretion assay (Miltenyi®). Step 1: T cells are stimulated for 16–20 h in normal culture conditions with the antigen of choice. Step 2: A cell affinity matrix is generated by attaching a bispecific antibody to the cell surface. This means that an antibody that binds CD45 on lymphocytes will cover the surface of the cell and the second specificity will detect a cytokine, such as IFN-γ or IL-4. By binding CD45 on the surface, the second specificity of the antibody localizes secreted IFN-γ to the surface of secreting cells. Step 3: Once the matrix is added, the cells are allowed to secrete the cytokine for a defined time period, and the secreted product is then "captured" in the matrix. The incubation time is short, usually 45 min, with cell mixing required. This ensures that cells are not aggregating and cytokines secreted originate only from the stimulated cell. Step 4: The cells are subsequently labeled with specific fluorescent antibody. This allows them to be identified using a flow cytometer. Cells can also be isolated using magnetic bead separation and a magnetic column ***(68)***.

tional cytokine-producing T cells specific for a target antigen, and in this respect it has been successful, even when the frequency of antigen-specific cells was low ***(68)***. For measuring frequencies of antigen-specific T cells, our experience and that of Asemissen et al. ***(67)*** is that this assay shows some nonspecific binding of the secondary anti-IFN-γ antibody, hence, background staining is often a problem and the noise-to-signal ratio leads to a lack of sensitivity.

An alternative flow-cytometry-based cytokine-detection method involves intracellular cytokine staining ***(69)***. Specific activation procedures are required to allow the detection of cytokines, notably with phorbol esters (such as phorbol myristate acetate) and ionomycin; moreover, it generally involves the addition of inhibitors of intracellular transport (such as brefeldin or monensin) ***(70)***. This method allows the characterization of large numbers of cells. With multiparameter staining it can demonstrate exclusive or mutual co-expression of different cytokines within individual cells. It therefore allows for the categorization of T-cell subsets, such as Th1 or Th2, rather than relying only on cell-surface markers, which can also be achieved with ELISpot. Frequencies calculated by this method have been shown to correlate with the number of tetramer-binding cells in patients infected with the HIV *(57)*, although in patients with metastatic melanoma, such a correlation was not found *(71)*. Moreover, it appears to correlate with ELISpot frequencies when using influenza-specific T cells *(67)* and to exceed the frequency obtained by LDA using cytotoxicity as a readout for Epstein-Barr virus and allogeneic responses *(72)*.

6. Past Experience and the Future of Immune Monitoring

Traditionally, donor-specific immunity or tolerance has been monitored in vitro using LDAs with different readouts (proliferation, cytokine production, or cytotoxicity). The largest clinically useful experience in immune monitoring has been carried out in the context of hematopoietic cell transplantation from unrelated donors with a view to predicting graft-vs-host disease as well as for donor selection. There is vast experience in the usefulness of CTLp calculated by LDA for these purposes *(25,35–37,39)*. Furthermore, IL-2 HTLp frequencies have been shown to correlate with graft outcome in bone marrow transplant recipients *(33,36,39,73,74)*. Functional assays will have a lasting role in bone marrow transplantation even in the era of high-resolution typing in that these assays can define permissible mismatches and identify less immunogenic donors in the absence of a perfectly matched donor (a comparison can be found in Table 1).

The experience in solid organ transplantation is less extensive, although a renewed effort is underway to dissect mechanisms of tolerance and rejection (reviewed in **ref.** *75*). Generally, monitoring has demonstrated that the hyporesponsiveness of direct-pathway donor-specific responses ensues shortly after transplantation *(5,41,76)*, whereas raised indirect-pathway antidonor reactivity appears to correlate with the presence of chronic transplant rejection. The implications are that abolition of only the direct pathway will not achieve allograft tolerance, while strategies that promote tolerance in the indirect pathway should improve allograft survival, as has been demonstrated in animal models *(77)*.

As we develop a deeper understanding of how our immune system works and how to specifically stimulate effector functions within subsets of cells, immunological monitoring is gaining increasing importance. Innovative immunotherapies are being tested in targeted groups of patients, in particular, in the study of immune responses to new vaccines or T-cell therapies in infectious diseases and the boosting of immune responses in response to malignant tumors (e.g., melanoma).

The goal yet to be achieved is the identification and perhaps even quantification of tolerance. The crucial point here will be to differentiate in vitro tolerance from a lack of response or assay insensitivity. So far a single or a small

Table 1
Current and Potential Future Assays for Clinical Alloimmune Monitoring

Measured in blood/serum	Using
Direct and indirect T-cell alloreactivity	• Proliferation (LDA)* • Cytokine analysis (LDA, ELISPOT, CSA)* • Cell division (CFSE)* • Trans-vivo delayed type hypersensitivity
Expression profiling using lymphocyte activation markers	• Real-time PCR* • Microarrays
Humoral immune responses	• Cytotoxic or flow cytometric antibody detection *
Soluble lymphocyte activation markers	• ELISA for soluble factors (e.g., sCD30)*

Measured in transplant	Using
Graft damage, inflammation *(biopsy required)*	• Histology * • Immunohistochemistry (e.g., C4d staining)*
Expression profiling (in graft or draining from graft; e.g., urine) *(biopsy may be required)*	• PCR • Microarrays • Proteomics } defining immune gene polymorphisms, "tolerance genes or proteins"

Note: Assays marked with an * indicate the currently most practical for clinical use.

group of assays of definitive clinical usefulness has not been identified or standardized. Collaborative research initiatives are being set up in Europe and the United States in order to find the "fingerprint" of tolerance. Their results will provide very useful information both for the design of tolerance-promoting protocols and for guiding decisions about immunosuppression withdrawal. There is now reason to be optimistic about the possibility of quantitating the effectiveness of immune interventions of clinical utility.

References

1. Reader, J. A., Burke, M. M., Counihan, P., et al. (1990) Noninvasive monitoring of human cardiac allograft rejection. *Transplantation* **50**, 29–33.
2. Fisher, P. E., Suciu-Foca, N., Ho, E., Michler, R. E., Rose, E. A., and Mancini, D. (1995) Additive value of immunologic monitoring to histologic grading of heart allograft biopsy specimens: implications for therapy. *J. Heart Lung Transplant.* **14**, 1156–1161.
3. Beik, A. I., Higgins, R. M., Lam, F. T., and Morris, A. G. (1997) Clinical significance of selective decline of donor-reactive IL-2-producing T lymphocytes after renal transplantation. *Transplant. Immunol.* **5**, 89–96.
4. Weston, L. E., Sullivan, J. S., Keogh, A. M., and Geczy, A. F. (2000) Interleukin-2-producing helper T lymphocyte precursor frequency and rejection: a longitudinal cellular study after cardiac transplantation. *Immunol. Cell Biol.* **78**, 272–279.
5. de Haan, A., van der Gun, I., Hepkema, B. G., et al. (2000) Decreased donor-specific cytotoxic T cell precursor frequencies one year after clinical lung transplantation do not reflect transplantation tolerance: a comparison of lung transplant recipients with or without bronchiolitis obliterans syndrome. *Transplantation* **69**, 1434–1439.
6. Orosz, C. G., Zinn, N. E., Sirinek, L. P., and Ferguson, R. M. (1986) In vivo mechanisms of alloreactivity. II. Allospecificity of cytotoxic T lymphocytes in sponge matrix allografts as determined by limiting dilution analysis. *Transplantation* **41**, 84–92.
7. Baker, R. J., Hernandez-Fuentes, M. P., Brookes, P. A., Chaudhry, A. N., Cook, H. T., and Lechler, R. I. (2001) Loss of direct and maintenance of indirect alloresponses in renal allograft recipients: implications for the pathogenesis of chronic allograft nephropathy. *J. Immunol.* **167**, 7199–7206.
8. Abbas, A., Lichtman, A., and Pober, J. (1995) *The Major Histocompatibility Complex. Cellular and Molecular Immunology*, Vol. 3, McGraw-Hill, New York, pp. 96–114.
9. Vella, J. P., Spadafora-Ferreira, M., Murphy, B., et al. (1997) Indirect allorecognition of major histocompatibility complex allopeptides in human renal transplant recipients with chronic graft dysfunction. *Transplantation* **64**, 795–800.
10. Benichou, G., Valujskikh, A., and Heeger, P. S. (1999) Contributions of direct and indirect T cell alloreactivity during allograft rejection in mice. *J. Immunol.* **162**, 352–358.

11. SivaSai, K. S., Smith, M. A., Poindexter, N. J., et al. (1999) Indirect recognition of donor HLA class I peptides in lung transplant recipients with bronchiolitis obliterans syndrome. *Transplantation* **67**, 1094–1098.
12. Hornick, P. I., Mason, P. D., Baker, R. J., et al. (2000) Significant frequencies of T cells with indirect anti-donor specificity in heart graft recipients with chronic rejection. *Circulation* **101**, 2405–2410.
13. Azuma, H., Chandraker, A., Nadeau, K., et al. (1996) Blockade of T-cell costimulation prevents development of experimental chronic renal allograft rejection. *Proc. Natl. Acad. Sci. USA* **93**, 12,439–12,444.
14. Yamada, A., Chandraker, A., Laufer, T. M., Gerth, A. J., Sayegh, M. H., and Auchincloss, H., Jr. (2001) Recipient MHC class II expression is required to achieve long-term survival of murine cardiac allografts after costimulatory blockade. *J. Immunol.* **167**, 5522–5526.
15. Hall, B. M., Pearce, N. W., Gurley, K. E., and Dorsch, S. E. (1990) Specific unresponsiveness in rats with prolonged cardiac allograft survival after treatment with cyclosporine. III. Further characterization of the CD4+ suppressor cell and its mechanisms of action. *J. Exp. Med.* **171**, 141–157.
16. Lechler, R. I., Garden, O. A., and Turka, L. A. (2003) The complementary roles of deletion and regulation in transplantation tolerance. *Nat. Rev. Immunol.* **3**, 147–158.
17. Wood, K. J. and Sakaguchi, S. (2003) Regulatory T cells in transplantation tolerance. *Nat. Rev. Immunol.* **3**, 199–210.
18. Garin, M. I. and Lechler, R. I. (2003) Regulatory T cells. *Curr. Opin. Organ Transplant.* **8**, 7–12.
19. Salama, A. D., Najafian, N., Clarkson, M. R., Harmon, W. E., and Sayegh, M. H. (2003) Regulatory CD25(+) T cells in human kidney transplant recipients. *J. Am. Soc. Nephrol.* **14**, 1643–1651.
20. Segall, M., Noreen, H., Edwins, L., Haake, R., Shu, X. O., and Kersey, J. (1996) Lack of correlation of MLC reactivity with acute graft-versus-host disease and mortality in unrelated donor bone marrow transplantation. *Hum. Immunol.* **49**, 49–55.
21. Yamada, K., Sachs, D. H., and DerSimonian, H. (1995) Human anti-porcine xenogeneic T cell response. Evidence for allelic specificity of mixed leukocyte reaction and for both direct and indirect pathways of recognition. *J. Immunol.* **155**, 5249–5256.
22. Najafian, N., Salama, A. D., Fedoseyeva, E. V., Benichou, G., and Sayegh, M. H. (2002) Enzyme-linked immunosorbent spot assay analysis of peripheral blood lymphocyte reactivity to donor HLA-DR peptides: potential novel assay for prediction of outcomes for renal transplant recipients. *J. Am. Soc. Nephrol.* **13**, 252–259.
23. Lefkovits, I. (1972) Induction of antibody-forming cell clones in microcultures. *Eur J. Immunol.* **2**, 360–366.
24. Lefkovits, I., and Waldmann, H. (1984) Limiting dilution analysis of the cells of immune system I. The clonal basis of the immune response. *Immunol. Today* **5**, 265–268

25. Sharrock, C. E., Kaminski, E., and Man, S. (1990) Limiting dilution analysis of human T cells: a useful clinical tool. *Immunol. Today* **11**, 281–286.
26. Orosz, C. G., Adams, P. W., and Ferguson, R. M. (1987) Frequency of human alloantigen-reactive T lymphocytes. II. Method for limiting dilution analysis of alloantigen-reactive helper T cells in human peripheral blood. *Transplantation* **43**, 718–724.
27. Moretti, L., Giuliodori, L., Stramigioli, S., Luchetti, F., Baldi, A., and Sparaventi, G. (1992) Limiting dilution analysis of IL-2 producing cells: I. Studies of normal human peripheral blood. *Haematologica* **77**, 463–469.
28. Hornick, P. I., Brookes, P. A., Mason, P. D., et al. (1997) Optimizing a limiting dilution culture system for quantifying the frequency of interleukin-2-producing alloreactive T helper lymphocytes. *Transplantation* **64**, 472–479.
29. Kaminski, E., Hows, J., Goldman, J., and Batchelor, R. (1991) Optimising a limiting dilution culture system for quantitating frequencies of alloreactive cytotoxic T lymphocyte precursors. *Cell Immunol* **137**, 88–95.
30. Kelso, A. and Macdonald, H. R. (1982) Precursor frequency analysis of lymphokine-secreting alloreactive T lymphocytes. Dissociation of subsets producing interleukin 2, macrophage-activating factor, and granulocyte-macrophage colony-stimulating factor on the basis of Lyt-2 phenotype. *J. Exp. Med.* **156**, 1366–1379.
31. Kelso, A. (1990) Frequency analysis of lymphokine-secreting CD4+ and CD8+ T cells activated in a graft-versus-host reaction. *J. Immunol.* **145**, 2167–2176.
32. Jordan, W. J. and Ritter, M. A. (2002) Optimal analysis of composite cytokine responses during alloreactivity. *J. Immunol. Methods* **260**, 1–14.
33. Schwarer, A. P., Jiang, Y. Z., Brookes, P. A., Bet al. (1993) Frequency of anti-recipient alloreactive helper T-cell precursors in donor blood and graft-versus-host disease after HLA-identical sibling bone-marrow transplantation. *Lancet* **341**, 203–205.
34. Theobald, M., Hoffmann, T., Bunjes, D., and Heit, W. (1990) Frequency, specificity, and phenotype of clonally growing human alloreactive interleukin-2-secreting helper T lymphocyte precursors. *Transplantation* **50**, 850–856.
35. Kaminski, E., Hows, J., Man, S., et al. (1989) Prediction of graft versus host disease by frequency analysis of cytotoxic T cells after unrelated donor bone marrow transplantation. *Transplantation* **48**, 608–613.
36. Schwarer, A. P., Jiang, Y. Z., Deacock, S., et al. (1994) Comparison of helper and cytotoxic antirecipient T cell frequencies in unrelated bone marrow transplantation. *Transplantation* **58**, 1198–1203.
37. Spencer, A., Brookes, P. A., Kaminski, E., et al. (1995) Cytotoxic T lymphocyte precursor frequency analyses in bone marrow transplantation with volunteer unrelated donors. Value in donor selection. *Transplantation* **59**, 1302–1308.
38. Speiser, D. E., Loliger, C. C., Siren, M. K., and Jeannet, M. (1996) Pretransplant cytotoxic donor T-cell activity specific to patient HLA class I antigens correlating with mortality after unrelated BMT. *Br. J. Haematol.* **93**, 935–939.
39. Keever-Taylor, C. A., Passweg, J., Kawanishi, Y., Casper, J., Flomenberg, N., and Baxter-Lowe, L. A. (1997) Association of donor-derived host-reactive cytolytic

and helper T cells with outcome following alternative donor T cell-depleted bone marrow transplantation. *Bone Marrow Transplant.* **19**, 1001–1009.
40. Hu, H., Robertus, M., de Jonge, N., et al. (1994) Reduction of donor-specific cytotoxic T lymphocyte precursors in peripheral blood of allografted heart recipients. *Transplantation* **58**, 1263–1268.
41. Mestre, M., Massip, E., Bas, J., et al. (1996) Longitudinal study of the frequency of cytotoxic T cell precursors in kidney allograft recipients. *Clin. Exp. Immunol.* **104**, 108–114.
42. Steinmann, J., Kaden, J., May, G., Schroder, K., Herwartz, C., and Muller-Ruchholtz, W. (1994) Failure of in vitro T-cell assays to predict clinical outcome after human kidney transplantation. *J. Clin. Lab. Anal.* **8**, 157–162.
43. Dozmorov, I., Eisenbraun, M. D., and Lefkovits, I. (2000) Limiting dilution analysis: from frequencies to cellular interactions. *Immunol. Today* **21**, 15–18.
44. Game, D. S., Hernandez-Fuentes, M. P., Chaudhry, A. N., and Lechler, R. I. (2003) CD4(+)CD25(+) Regulatory T cells do not significantly contribute to direct pathway hyporesponsiveness in stable renal transplant patients. *J. Am. Soc. Nephrol.* **14**, 1652–1661.
45. Dozmorov, I. M., Lutsenko, G. V., Sidorov, L. A., and Miller, R. A. (1996) Analysis of cellular interactions in limiting dilution cultures. *J. Immunol. Methods* **189**, 183–196.
46. Bonnefoix, T., Bonnefoix, P., Mi, J. Q., Lawrence, J. J., Sotto, J. J., and Leroux, D. (2003) Detection of suppressor T lymphocytes and estimation of their frequency in limiting dilution assays by generalized linear regression modeling. *J. Immunol.* **170**, 2884–2894.
47. Taguchi, T., McGhee, J. R., Coffman, R. L., et al. (1990) Detection of individual mouse splenic T cells producing IFN-gamma and IL-5 using the enzyme-linked immunospot (ELISPOT) assay. *J. Immunol. Methods* **128**, 65–73.
48. Miyahira, Y., Murata, K., Rodriguez, D., et al. (1995) Quantification of antigen specific CD8+ T cells using an ELISpot assay. *J. Immunol. Methods* **181**, 45–54.
49. Czerkinsky, C., Andersson, G., Ekre, H. P., Nilsson, L. A., Klareskog, L., and Ouchterlony, O. (1988) Reverse ELISpot assay for clonal analysis of cytokine production. I. Enumeration of gamma-interferon-secreting cells. *J. Immunol. Methods* **110**, 29–36.
50. Herr, W., Linn, B., Leister, N., Wandel, E., Meyer zum Buschenfelde, K. H., and Wolfel, T. (1997) The use of computer-assisted video image analysis for the quantification of CD8+ T lymphocytes producing tumor necrosis factor alpha spots in response to peptide antigens. *J. Immunol. Methods* **203**, 141–152.
51. Smith, J. G., Levin, M., Vessey, R., et al. (2003) Measurement of cell-mediated immunity with a Varicella-Zoster Virus- specific interferon-gamma ELISPOT assay: responses in an elderly population receiving a booster immunization. *J. Med. Virol.* **70**, S38–41.
52. Asai, T., Storkus, W. J., Mueller-Berghaus, J., et al. (2002) In vitro generated cytolytic T lymphocytes reactive against head and neck cancer recognize multiple

epitopes presented by HLA-A2, including peptides derived from the p53 and MDM-2 proteins. *Cancer Immun.* **2**, 3.

53. Pelfrey, C. M., Rudick, R. A., Cotleur, A. C., Lee, J. C., Tary-Lehmann, M., and Lehmann, P. V. (2000) Quantification of self-recognition in multiple sclerosis by single-cell analysis of cytokine production. *J. Immunol.* **165**, 1641–1651.
54. Salama, A. D., Chaudhry, A. N., Holthaus, K. A., et al. (2003) Regulation by $CD25^+$ lymphocytes of autoantigen-specific T-cell responses in Goodpasture's (anti-GBM) disease. *Kidney Int.* **64**, 1685–1694.
55. Heeger, P. S., Greenspan, N. S., Kuhlenschmidt, S., et al. (1999) Pretransplant frequency of donor-specific, IFN-gamma-producing lymphocytes is a manifestation of immunologic memory and correlates with the risk of posttransplant rejection episodes. *J. Immunol.* **163**, 2267–2275.
56. Scheibenbogen, C., Romero, P., Rivoltini, L., et al. (2000) Quantitation of antigen-reactive T cells in peripheral blood by IFNgamma-ELISPOT assay and chromium-release assay: a four-centre comparative trial. *J. Immunol. Methods* **244**, 81–89.
57. Goulder, P. J., Tang, Y., Brander, C., et al. (2000) Functionally inert HIV-specific cytotoxic T lymphocytes do not play a major role in chronically infected adults and children. *J. Exp.Med.* **192**, 1819–1832.
58. Snyder, J. E., Bowers, W. J., Livingstone, A. M., Lee, F. E., Federoff, H. J., and Mosmann, T. R. (2003) Measuring the frequency of mouse and human cytotoxic T cells by the Lysispot assay: independent regulation of cytokine secretion and short-term killing. *Nat. Med.* **9**, 231–235.
59. Lyons, A. B., and Parish, C. R. (1994) Determination of lymphocyte division by flow cytometry. *J. Immunol. Methods* **171**, 131–137.
60. Wells, A. D., Gudmundsdottir, H., and Turka, L. A. (1997) Following the fate of individual T cells throughout activation and clonal expansion. Signals from T cell receptor and CD28 differentially regulate the induction and duration of a proliferative response. *J. Clin. Invest.* **100**, 3173–3183.
61. Suchin, E. J., Langmuir, P. B., Palmer, E., Sayegh, M. H., Wells, A. D., and Turka, L. A. (2001) Quantifying the frequency of alloreactive T cells in vivo: new answers to an old question. *J. Immunol.* **166**, 973–981.
62. Dengler, T. J., Johnson, D. R., and Pober, J. S. (2001) Human vascular endothelial cells stimulate a lower frequency of alloreactive CD8+ pre-CTL and induce less clonal expansion than matching B lymphoblastoid cells: development of a novel limiting dilution analysis method based on CFSE labeling of lymphocytes. *J. Immunol.* **166**, 3846–3854.
63. Allez, M., Brimnes, J., Dotan, I., and Mayer, L. (2002) Expansion of CD8+ T cells with regulatory function after interaction with intestinal epithelial cells. *Gastroenterology* **123**, 1516–1526.
64. Sanchez-Fueyo, A., Weber, M., Domenig, C., Strom, T. B., and Zheng, X. X. (2002) Tracking the immunoregulatory mechanisms active during allograft tolerance. *J. Immunol.* **168**, 2274–2281.
65. Lyons, A. B. (2000) Analysing cell division in vivo and in vitro using flow cytometric measurement of CFSE dye dilution. *J. Immunol. Methods* **243**, 147–154.

66. Oelke, M., Kurokawa, T., Hentrich, I., et al. (2000) Functional characterization of CD8(+) antigen-specific cytotoxic T lymphocytes after enrichment based on cytokine secretion: comparison with the MHC-tetramer technology. *Scand J. Immunol.* **52**, 544–549.
67. Asemissen, A. M., Nagorsen, D., Keilholz, U., et al. (2001) Flow cytometric determination of intracellular or secreted IFNgamma for the quantification of antigen reactive T cells. *J. Immunol. Methods* **251**, 101–108.
68. Manz, R., Assenmacher, M., Pfluger, E., Miltenyi, S., and Radbruch, A. (1995) Analysis and sorting of live cells according to secreted molecules, relocated to a cell-surface affinity matrix. *Proc. Natl. Acad. Sci. USA* **92**, 1921–1925.
69. Pala, P., Hussell, T., and Openshaw, P. J. (2000) Flow cytometric measurement of intracellular cytokines. *J. Immunol. Methods* **243**, 107–124.
70. Dinter, A. and Berger, E. G. (1998) Golgi-disturbing agents. *Histochem. Cell Biol.* **109**, 571–590.
71. Whiteside, T. L., Zhao, Y., Tsukishiro, T., Elder, E. M., Gooding, W., and Baar, J. (2003) Enzyme-linked immunospot, cytokine flow cytometry, and tetramers in the detection of T-cell responses to a dendritic cell-based multipeptide vaccine in patients with melanoma. *Clin. Cancer Res.* **9**, 641–649.
72. Koehne, G., Smith, K. M., Ferguson, T. L., et al. (2002) Quantitation, selection, and functional characterization of Epstein- Barr virus-specific and alloreactive T cells detected by intracellular interferon-gamma production and growth of cytotoxic precursors. *Blood* **99**, 1730–1740.
73. Theobald, M., Nierle, T., Bunjes, D., Arnold, R., and Heimpel, H. (1992) Host-specific interleukin-2-secreting donor T-cell precursors as predictors of acute graft-versus-host disease in bone marrow transplantation between HLA-identical siblings. *N. Engl. J. Med.* **327**, 1613–1617.
74. Winandy, M., Lewalle, P., Deneys, V., Ferrant, A., and De Bruyere, M. (1999) Pretransplant helper T-lymphocyte determination in bone marrow donors: acute graft-versus-host disease prediction and relation with long-term survival. *B.r J. Haematol.* **105**, 288–294.
75. Hernandez-Fuentes, M. P., Warrens, A. N., and Lechler, R. I. (2003) Immunologic monitoring. *Immunol. Rev.* **196**, 247–264.
76. Hornick, P. I., Mason, P. D., Yacoub, M. H., Rose, M. L., Batchelor, R., and Lechler, R. I. (1998) Assessment of the contribution that direct allorecognition makes to the progression of chronic cardiac transplant rejection in humans. *Circulation* **97**, 1257–1263.
77. Sayegh, M. H., Perico, N., Gallon, L., et al. (1994) Mechanisms of acquired thymic unresponsiveness to renal allografts. Thymic recognition of immunodominant allo-MHC peptides induces peripheral T cell anergy. *Transplantation* **58**, 125–132.
78. Taswell, C. (1981) Limiting dilution assays for the determination of immunocompetent cell frequencies. I. Data analysis. *J. Immunol.* **126**, 1614–1619.
79. Strijbosch, L. W., Buurman, W. A., Does, R. J., Zinken, P. H., and Groenewegen, G. (1987) Limiting dilution assays. Experimental design and statistical analysis. *J. Immunol. Methods* **97**, 133–140.

80. Strijbosch, L. W., Does, R. J., and Buurman, W. A. (1988) Computer aided design and evaluation of limiting and serial dilution experiments. *Int. J. Biomed. Comput.* **23**, 279–290.
81. Mehrabi, Y. and Matthews, J. N. S. (1995) Likelihood-based methods for bias reduction in limiting dilution assays. *Biometrics* **51**, 1543–1549
82. Prieto, A., Reyes, E., Diaz, D., et al. (2000) A new method for the simultaneous analysis of growth and death of immunophenotypically defined cells in culture. *Cytometry* **39**, 56–66.

13

Proteomics and Laser Microdissection

Emma McGregor and Ayesha De Souza

Summary

Two-dimensional gel electrophoresis (2-DE) combined with protein identification by mass spectrometry (MS) is currently the method of choice in the majority of proteomic projects. Novel gel-free technologies have been developed but 2-DE remains the technique of choice for quantitative expression profiling of large sets of complex protein mixtures such as whole cell/tissue lysates.

Solubilized proteins are separated in the first dimension according to their charge properties (isoelectric point, p*I*) by isoelectric focusing (IEF) under denaturing conditions, followed by their separation in the second dimension by sodium dodecyl sulfate-polyacrylamide gel electrophoresis (SDS-PAGE), according to their relative molecular mass (M_r). 2-DE can resolve more than 5000 proteins simultaneously (~2000 proteins routinely) and can detect less than 1 ng of protein per spot. Furthermore, it delivers a map of intact proteins, which reflects changes in protein expression level, isoforms or posttranslational modifications.

In this chapter we describe the various steps in the 2-DE proteomics workflow, namely sample preparation, solubilization, 2-D gel electrophoresis, protein detection and visualization, and protein identification by mass spectrometry. The use of 2-DE in conjunction with laser microdissection microscopy is presented and discussed.

Key Words: Laser microdissection; two-dimensional gel electrophoresis (2-DE); isoelectric focusing; cardiovascular research; blood vessels; cardiac myocytes; left ventricle.

1. Introduction

In 2001, a major milestone was reached with the publication of the draft sequence of the human genome ***(1,2)***. The human genome contains fewer open reading frames (~30,000 open reading frames) encoding functional proteins than was generally predicted and, like all other completed genomes, contains many

From: *Methods in Molecular Biology, vol. 333: Transplantation Immunology: Methods and Protocols*
Edited by: P. Hornick and M. Rose © Humana Press Inc., Totowa, NJ

novel genes with no ascribed functions. It is now widely known and accepted that one gene does not encode a single protein, as a result of alternative mRNA splicing, RNA editing and posttranslational protein modification (e.g., phosphorylation, sulfation, glycosylation, hydroxylation, *N*-methylation, carboxymethylation, acetylation, prenylation and *N*-myristolation). As a result of these processes, the functional complexity of an organism far exceeds that indicated by its genome sequence alone. The global study of the products of gene expression, including transcriptomics, proteomics and metabolomics, plays a major role in elucidating the functional role of the many novel genes and their products and in understanding their involvement in biologically relevant phenotypes in health and disease. Despite this, tissue heterogeneity and the need for specific cell enrichment prior to sample analysis represents a major barrier in the study of normal vs diseased tissue.

In this chapter, we describe how we have used laser microdissection in conjunction with proteomics to investigate cardiac proteins.

2. Proteomics

The concept of mapping the human complement of protein expression was first proposed more than 25 yr ago ***(3,4)*** with the development of a technique in which large numbers of proteins could be separated simultaneously by two-dimensional polyacrylamide gel electrophoresis (2-DE) ***(5,6)***. However, it was not until 1995, that the term *proteome*, defined as the protein complement of a genome, was first coined by Wilkins working as part of a collaborative team at Macquarie (Australia) and Sydney Universities (Australia) ***(7,8)***. Since then, the term *proteomics* has evolved to include alternative gel-free techniques based on mass spectrometry (MS) or protein arrays for high-throughput proteomics.

2.1. Sample Preparation

The most important step in a proteomics experiment is sample preparation. Any artifacts introduced during sample preparation can often be magnified with the potential to impair the validity of the results. No single method for sample preparation can be applied universally owing to the diverse nature of samples that are analyzed by 2-DE ***(9)***, but some general considerations can be mentioned. Detection of subtle posttranslational modifications such as phosphorylation is possible because of the high resolution capacity of 2-DE. 2-DE will also readily reveal artefactual modifications such as protein carbamylation that can be induced by heating of samples in the presence of urea. Additionally, proteases present within samples can readily result in artifactual spots, so that samples should be subjected to minimal handling and kept cold at all times. It is possible to add cocktails of protease inhibitors during sample preparation.

2.2. Protein Solubilization

Ideally, solubilization of proteins prior to 2-DE would result in the disruption of all non-covalently bound protein complexes and aggregates into a solution of individual polypeptides *(9)*. If this is not successfully achieved, persistent protein complexes in the sample are likely to result in new spots in the 2-D profile, with a concomitant reduction in the intensity of those spots representing the single polypeptides. In addition, the solubilization method must permit the removal of substances such as salts, lipids, polysaccharides and nucleic acids that can interfere with the 2-DE separation. Finally, the sample proteins must remain soluble during the 2-DE process. For the foregoing reasons sample solubility is one of the most critical factors for successful protein separation by 2-DE.

The original and still the most popular method for protein solubilization prior to 2-DE remains that described by O'Farrell *(6)* using a mixture of 9.5 *M* urea, 4% w/v of the nonionic detergent NP-40 or the zwitterionic detergent 3-[(3-cholamidopropyl)-dimethylammonio]-1-propane sulfonate (CHAPS), 1% w/v of the reducing agent dithiothreitol (DTT) and 2% w/v of synthetic carrier ampholyte in the appropriate pH range ("lysis buffer"). This method can be applied to many sample types, but it is not universally applicable, with membrane proteins representing a particular challenge *(10)*. Protein solubilization can be improved by varying solubilization buffer constituents. Newly developed detergents such as sulfobetaines *(11)*, additional denaturing agents such as thiourea *(12)*, and alternative reducing agents such as trubutyl phosphine *(13)*, can help to improve protein solubilization and hence the concentration of extracted protein for certain sample types. It is of paramount importance that the choice of solubilization buffer be optimized for each sample type to be analyzed by 2-DE (*see* **ref. *14*** for an example of optimizing the solubilization of human myocardium).

2.3. Two-Dimensional Gel Electrophoresis

2-DE involves the separation of solubilized proteins by isoelectric focusing (IEF) according to their charge properties (isoelectric point, p*I*), under denaturing conditions, in the first dimension, followed by separation in the second dimension according to relative molecular mass (M_r) by sodium dodecyl sulphate (SDS)-PAGE. Charge and mass properties of proteins are effectively independent parameters, thus, an orthogonal combination of charge (p*I*) and size (M_r) separations results in the sample proteins being distributed across the two-dimensional gel profile (**Fig. 1**).

The recent introduction of immobilized pH gradients (IPGs) (Amersham Biosciences), used in the first dimension, has served to increase the resolution of 2-DE and improve the reproducibility of protein separations *(15,16)*. IPGs are

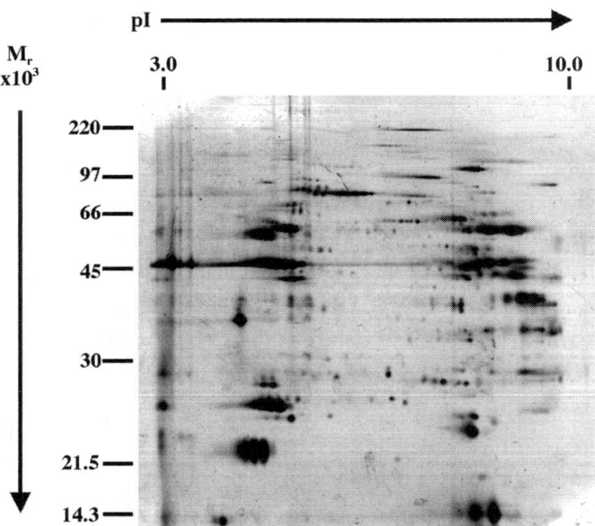

Fig. 1. A two-dimensional electrophoretic separation of heart (ventricle) proteins. The first dimension comprised an 18-cm nonlinear pH 3.0–10.0 immobilized pH gradient (IPG) subjected to isoelectric focusing. The second dimension was a 21-cm 12% sodium dodecylsulphate polyacrylamide gel electrophoresis (SDS-PAGE) gel. Proteins were detected by silver staining. The non-linear pH range of the first-dimension IPG strip is indicated along the top of the gel, acidic pH to the left. The M_r (relative molecular mass) scale can be used to estimate the molecular weights of the separated proteins.

generated using immobiline reagents ***(17)*** to replace the synthetic carrier ampholytes (SCAs) previously used to generate the pH gradients required for IEF. As a result IPGs are immune to the effects of electroendosmosis which results in cathodic drift with the consequent loss of basic proteins from 2-D gel profiles generated using SCA IEF. IPGs are commercially available as a range of different pH gradients. Standard gradients include pH 3.0–10.0, 4.0–7.0 and 6.0–9.0, but if increasing proteomic coverage of a sample is required (i.e., "pulling apart" protein profiles), protein samples can be separated using narrow-range IPGs (e.g., pH 4.0–5.0, 4.5–5.5, 5.0–6.0, 5.5–6.7), thus increasing resolution.

First-dimension IEF of protein samples is carried out on individual gel strips (IPGs), 3–5mm wide, cast on a plastic support. This can be done using either the IPGphor (Amersham Biosciences) or Multiphor (Amersham Biosciences). For the purpose of the experiments described in this chapter, first-dimension IEF was performed on a Multiphor (Amersham Biosciences) using 180-mm, pH 3.0–10.0 nonlinear (NL) IPGs.

Following steady-state IEF, strips are equilibrated and then applied to the surface of either vertical or horizontal slab SDS-PAGE gels ***(18)***. It is possible to routinely separate up to 2000 proteins from whole-cell and tissue extracts using 18-cm IPG strips with standard format SDS gels (20 × 20 cm). Resolution can be significantly enhanced (separation of 5000–10,000 proteins) using large-format (40 × 30 cm) 2D gels ***(19)***. However, gels of this size are very rarely used due to the handling problems associated with such large gels. The longest commercial IPG IEF gels have a length of 24 cm ***(20)***. Mini-gels (7 × 7 cm) can be run using 7-cm IPG strips. These gels will only separate a few hundred proteins but can be very useful for rapid screening purposes. Second-dimension SDS-PAGE is usually carried out using apparatus capable of running simultaneously multiple large-format 2-D gels (e.g., Ettan DALT 2, 12 gels, Amersham Biosciences; Protean Plus Dodeca Cell, 12 gels, Bio-Rad). Large numbers of 2-D protein separations can be performed using this type of apparatus, but the procedure is very time-consuming and labor-intensive.

2.4. Protein Detection and Visualization

Proteins must be visualized at high sensitivity following separation by electrophoresis. Ideally detection methods should combine properties of a high dynamic range (i.e., the ability to detect proteins present in the gel at a wide range of relative abundance), linearity of staining response (to facilitate rigorous quantitative analysis), and if possible compatibility with subsequent protein identification by MS. Coomassie brilliant blue (CBB) has for many years been a standard staining method for protein detection following gel electrophoresis. However its limited sensitivity (~100 ng protein) motivated the development of a more sensitive (~10 ng protein) method utilizing CBB in a colloidal form ***(21)***. Since its first description in 1979 ***(22)***, silver staining has often been the method of choice for protein detection on 2-D gels because of its high sensitivity (~0.1 ng protein). However, silver staining suffers from significant inherent disadvantages; it has a limited dynamic range, it is susceptible to saturation and negative staining effects that compromise quantitation, and most protocols are not compatible with subsequent protein identification by MS. This is because glutaraldehyde, included in many protocols as a sensitizing reagent, causes extensive cross-linking through reaction with both ε- and α-amino groups. To achieve compatibility with MS, glutaraldehyde must be omitted ***(23,24)***, but at the expense of increased background and reduced sensitivity. In the study presented here we have utilized the silver-staining method of Yan ***(24)***.

Detection methods based on the postelectrophoretic staining of proteins with fluorescent compounds have the potential of increased sensitivity combined with an extended dynamic range for improved quantitation. The most commonly used reagents are the SYPRO series of dyes from Molecular Probes ***(25)***. In addition to these the development of 2-D difference gel electrophoresis by Unlu ***(26)*** using fluorescent Cy dyes (Cy3, Cy5, and Cy2) has made it possible to detect and quantitate differences between experimentally paired protein samples resolved on the same 2-D gel. Fluorescent staining methods do not interfere with subsequent protein identification by MS *(25,27)*.

2.5. Protein Identification

MS is currently the technique of choice for protein identification as the methods involved are very sensitive, require small amounts of sample (femtomole to attomole concentrations) and have the capacity for high sample throughput *(28–30)*. Peptide mass fingerprinting (PMF) is typically the primary tool for protein identification. It is based on the finding that a set of peptide masses obtained by MS analysis of a protein digest (usually trypsin) provides a characteristic mass fingerprint of that protein. The protein is then identified by comparison of the experimental mass fingerprint with theoretical peptide masses generated in silico using protein and nucleotide sequence databases. PMF can be very effective when trying to identify proteins from species whose genomes are completely sequenced, but is not so reliable for organisms whose genomes have not been completed. This difficulty can be overcome effectively by improving PMF by adopting an orthogonal approach combined with amino acid compositional analysis *(31)*.

If identification of a protein becomes impossible based on PMF alone, amino acid sequence information is then key to obtaining identification. Conventional automated chemical Edman microsequencing is capable of generating this information but this is most readily accomplished using tandem MS (MS/MS). MS/MS takes advantage of two-stage MS instruments, either MALDI-MS with postsource decay (PSD), MALDI-TOF-TOF-MS/MS or ESI-MS/MS triple-quadropole, ion-trap, or Q-TOF machines, to induce fragmentation of peptide bonds. One approach is to generate a short partial sequence or tag which is used in combination with the mass of the intact parent peptide ion to provide significant additional information for the homology search *(32)*. A second approach uses the database-searching algorithm SEQUEST *(33)* to match uninterpreted experimental MS/MS spectra with predicted fragment patterns generated in silico from sequences in protein and nucleotide databases.

3. Laser Microdissection

Laser microdissection represents a breakthrough technology that allows rapid one-step procurement of selected homogeneous populations of intact cells from a section of complex, heterogeneous tissue, thus focusing on individual genes or proteins from a particular subset. In 1996 Emmert-Buck first described laser capture microdissection (LCM) *(34)*, and this technique has since become widely used in the world of both genomics *(35–38)* and proteomics *(39–43)*. Laser microdissection is an easy, extremely fast and versatile method for the isolation of morphologically or immunohistochemically defined cell populations. This combined with the ability to readily confirm the nature of the captured material is a great advantage of this technique.

There are three commercially available microscopes on the market for laser microdissection. The first LCM setup was developed at the National Cancer Institute of the National Institutes of Health and is commercially available from Arcturus Engineering (Mountain View, CA). To date, this is the most widely used system. The Arcturus system uses a laser beam and a special thermoplastic transfer film which is bound to the underside of a transfer cap. The cap is placed on the surface of the tissue and a laser pulse is sent through the transparent cap, which expands the thermoplastic film. The adherence of the tissue to the activated film exceeds the adhesion to the glass slide and thus allows the removal of the specified cells. The selected material is then collected by lifting the cap, which is then transferred to a tube containing the solubilization/lysis buffer required for the isolation of the desired proteins.

The second is the PALM laser-microbeam system (P.A.L.M, Wolfratshausen, Germany). Using the PALM, selected cells can be isolated from the surrounding tissue using a focused nitrogen laser. To collect the selected cells of interest, the energy of the laser is increased and the microdissected area is catapulted by a single laser shot. The detached material is then collected in a microcentrifuge cap containing lysis buffer, which is mounted above the slide. The efficiency of this procedure is verified by visualizing the collected samples under a second microscope.

We are currently using the Leica AS LMD (Leica Microsystems, UK). The Leica uses a maintenance-free, pulsed, nitrogen laser at a wavelength of 337 nm. In order to excise the structure of interest, the pulsed laser follows a predrawn line, ablating the material only in the region of the defined line. This method of dissection ensures that the specimen is not heated and endures no mechanical contact; therefore the risk of contamination is eliminated. After dissection, the sample falls by gravity into a precisely positioned polymerase chain reaction tube cap. Following capture, the cap can be automatically examined to visualize the excised material. **Figure 2** shows an example of the microdissection of a blood vessel and a group of cardiac myocytes from an 8-μm section of left ventricular tissue using the Leica AS LMD.

The precision of microdissection depends on the ability to distinguish specific cell types. Unfortunately, one of the major disadvantages of laser microdissection is that it is necessary to use dehydrated sections in the absence of a coverslip. This leads to a significant decrease in the optical resolution, which may alter the ease of this technique and may require various staining techniques to be employed. Another disadvantage is the initial cost of the microscope and accompanying computer hardware and software (~£75,000–100,000), with the

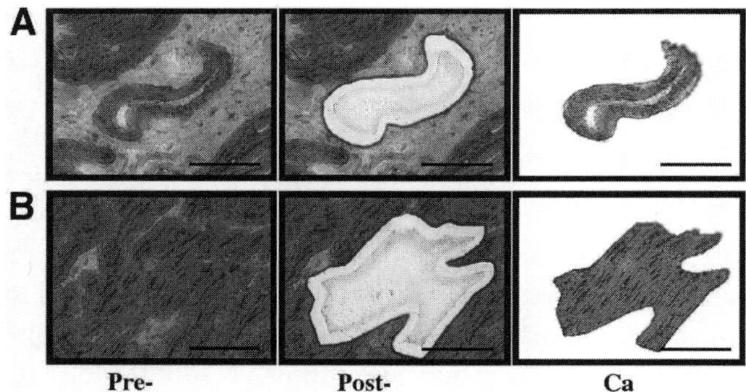

Fig. 2. Laser microdissection of left ventricular section. The appearance of a hematoxylin-and-eosin stained left ventricular section (×400 magnification) is illustrated prior to dissection and following dissection, and the dissected material is present in the cap. (**A**) Microdissection of a blood vessel; (**B**) dissection of a group of cardiac myocytes. The horizontal bar represents 100 μm.

additional cost of specially designed consumables, (e.g., slides, caps) depending on the microdissection system used. Finally, although LCM is extremely fast at excising the cell or group of cells of interest, depending on the downstream processing of the captured material, this technique can be considerably time-consuming. The amount of material needed for protein analysis is much greater than that for RNA analysis, because protein, unlike RNA, cannot be amplified. For this reason, days to weeks may be spent at the microscope in order to excise enough material for the extraction of a sufficient amount of protein. Even though this is the case, there are several important reasons for focusing on the analysis of proteins. mRNA expression may not correlate with the amount of active protein in a cell, the gene sequence does not describe posttranslational modifications that may be essential for protein function and activity, and the study of the genome does not provide information on dynamic cellular processes. The application of proteomics can be expected to provide an integrated view of an individual disease process at the protein level. Proteomics can be expected to show changes in the protein-expression profile occurring during both the development and the progression of disease, thus leading to the identification of new protein markers of disease and potential therapeutic targets.

3.1. Proteomics and Laser Microdissection

We are using laser microdissection to isolate myocytes and blood vessels from human cardiac tissue for proteomic analysis. We have performed a feasibility study to investigate the effects of fixation and staining on cardiac proteins separated by 2-DE. In brief, 20 8-μm sections of control ventricles were used in six groups ($n = 4$).

- Group 1: sections cut and placed into lysis buffer (7 *M* urea, 2 *M* thiourea, 2% (w/v) CHAPS, 1% (w/v) DTT, 0.8 % (v/v) Pharmalyte pH 3.0–10.0, 1 complete protease inhibitor cocktail tablet per 10 mL).
- Groups 2–6: sections cut onto glass slides and scraped into lysis buffer following fixation and staining. Group 2—unfixed and unstained. Groups 3 and 4—ethanol fixed followed by hematoxylin and eosin (H&E) staining with and without xylene respectively. Groups 5 and 6—ethanol and acetone fixed, respectively, followed by antibody staining for smooth muscle α-actin. Proteins (50 μg) were separated by two-dimensional gel electrophoresis using (18-cm) IPG pH 3–10 NL strips in the first dimension, followed by 12% SDS-PAGE in the second dimension. Protein spots were visualized by silver staining and the number of detected spots evaluated using Progenesis, a specialized 2-DE image analysis software package (Nonlinear Dynamics).

Analysis by 2-DE showed that contractile proteins were preserved in all groups. All methods resulted in some loss of soluble proteins, although no significant differences were found. However, there were differences in the visual quality of the gel patterns. These findings are similar to those found by Craven ***(41)***, who found that all staining protocols investigated were compatible with protein analysis although there was variation in the quality of the protein profiles obtained. In contrast to these studies, Mouledous ***(44)*** found that H&E staining greatly reduced protein recovery when compared with unstained material and this was seriously detrimental to the protein profile. Although our group and Craven et al. ***(41)*** found no changes in protein profiles under varying staining protocols, it is important to investigate each tissue type individually, because a staining protocol that works with one tissue, may not necessarily be compatible with another.

H&E staining without xylene provided the best morphology for our tissue and thus this staining method was used for further investigations. This staining method was performed using a modified rapid protocol for LCM ***(40)***. In brief, sections were fixed (70% ethanol for 1 min), H&E stained (Mayer's hematoxylin for 30 s, MQ water for 20 s, eosin for 20 s, [MQ] water for 20 s), and dehydrated (70% ethanol for 30 s, 100% ethanol for 1 min). H&E solutions contained complete protease inhibitor cocktail tablets. We have shown that the electrophoretic profiles of proteins from human cardiac tissue showed little change following the laser microdissection procedure. **Figure 3** shows 2-D gels for two left ventricle sections stained with H&E in the absence of xylene, then either scrapped or excised using laser microdissection and protein-extracted in lysis buffer ***(45)***. Using Progenesis, 346 protein spots were detected in the scrapped group compared with 361 in the laser-microdissected group. Using this staining protocol in conjunction with laser microdissection, we have successfully isolated enough blood vessels and cardiac myocytes to run large-format (18 × 24 cm) 2-D gels ***(45)***. **Figure 4** shows the protein profiles for proteins

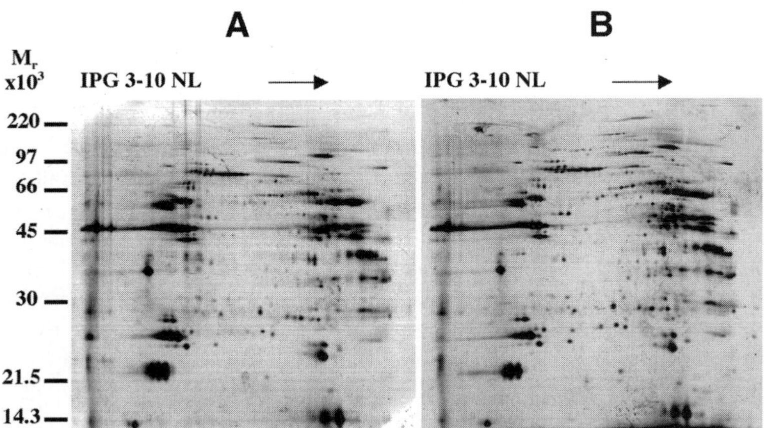

Fig. 3. Two-dimensional electrophoretic separation of control sections taken from human left ventricle. Proteins were separated by isoelectric focusing in the first dimension using a pH 3.0–10.0 NL, 18-cm, IPG DryStrip (Amersham Biosciences). The pH gradient of the strip is illustrated across the top of the two-dimensional gel with the most acidic pH to the left and the most basic pH to the right of the gel image. Proteins were then separated in the second dimension by SDS-PAGE through a 12% acrylamide gel (large format, 18 × 24 cm). Standard molecular weight markers (Amersham Biosciences), ranging from 14.3 to 97.4 kDa were run on the same gel and are annotated in the figure. Visualization of proteins was achieved using silver staining. Two-dimensional gel separations from hematoxylin and eosin-stained sections either scrapped (**A**) or laser microdissected (**B**).

extracted from cardiac myocytes and blood vessels. Collection of this material took 70 h, and represented approx 2800 blood vessels and 17,000 cardiac myocytes. In order to prevent protein degradation it is important when extracting protein that either the slides with the sections are kept on dry ice and thawed prior to fixing or that sections are cut onto slides as they are needed. Using Progenesis, 481 spots were found in the myocyte group and 206 in the blood vessel group. By comparing protein profiles between the two groups, it is clear that there was no contamination when microdissection was carried out. This is confirmed by the absence of the proteins cardiac tropomyosin and the cardiac light chains I and II from the blood vessel profile, which are clearly visible in the protein profile from cardiac myocytes (labeled 1, 2, and 3, respectively).

In conclusion, laser microdissection is a practical method for the rapid and efficient isolation of specific populations of cells. This technique however, may be extremely time-consuming depending on the desired downstream sample processing. The combination of laser microdissection and proteomics provides a powerful tool in studying the underlying changes in normal and

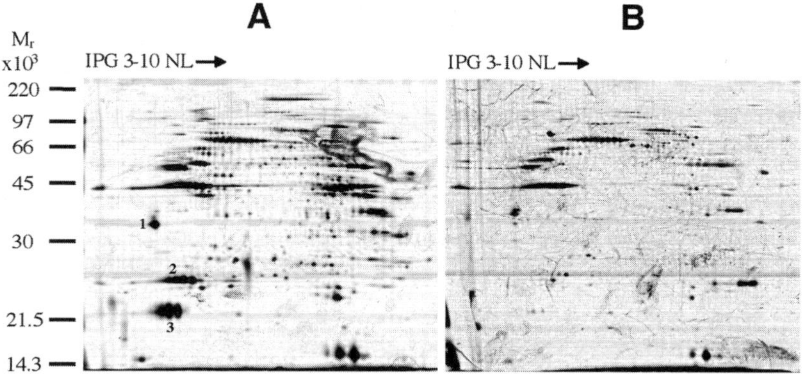

Fig. 4. Two-dimensional electrophoretic separation of isolated cells and blood vessels. Proteins were separated by isoelectric focusing in the first dimension using a pH 3.0–10.0 NL, 18-cm, IPG DryStrip (Amersham Biosciences). The pH gradient of the strip is illustrated across the top of the two-dimensional gel with the most acidic pH to the left and the most basic pH to the right of the gel image. Proteins were then separated in the second dimension by SDS-PAGE through a 12% acrylamide gel (large format, 18 × 24 cm). Standard molecular weight markers (Amersham Biosciences) ranging from 14.3 to 97.4 kDa were run on the same gel and are annotated on the far left of the figure. Visualization of proteins was achieved using silver staining. (**A**) Cardiac myocytes: (**B**) blood vessels isolated from human ventricular tissue by laser microdissection. 1, Cardiac tropomyosin; 2, cardiac light chain I; 3, cardiac light chain II.

diseased states. It has the potential to isolate and identify new protein markers and potential therapeutic targets of disease.

References

1. Lander, E. S. (2001) Initial sequencing and analysis of the human genome. *Nature* **409**, 860–921.
2. Venter, J. C. (2001) The sequence of the human genome. *Science* **291**, 1304–1351.
3. Anderson, N. G., Matheson, A., and Anderson N. L. (2001) Back to the future: the human protein index (HPI) and the agenda for post-proteomic biology. *Proteomics* **1**, 3–12.
4. Anderson, N. G. and Anderson, L. (1982) The human protein index. *Clin. Chem.* **28**, 739–748.
5. Klose, J. (1975) Protein mapping by combined isoelectric focusing and electrophoresis of mouse tissues. A novel approach to testing for induced point mutations in mammals. *Humangenetik* **26**, 231–243.
6. O'Farrell, P. H. (1975) High resolution two-dimensional electrophoresis of proteins. *J. Biol. Chem.* **250**, 4007–4021.

7. Wasinger, V. C., Cordwell, S. J., Cerpa-Poljak, A., et al. (1995) Progress with gene-product mapping of the Mollicutes: Mycoplasma genitalium. *Electrophoresis* **16**, 1090–1094.
8. Wilkins, M. R., Sanchez, J. C., Gooley, A. A., R. et al. (1996) Progress with proteome projects: why all proteins expressed by a genome should be identified and how to do it. *Biotechnol. Genet. Eng. Rev.* **13**, 19–50.
9. Dunn, M. J., and Gorg, A. (2001) Two-dimensional polyacrylamide gel electrophoresis for proteome analysis, in *Proteomics, From Protein Sequence to Function* (Pennington, S. R., and Dunn, M. J., eds.), BIOS Scientific Publishers Ltd, pp. 43–63.
10. Santoni, V., Kieffer, S., Desclaux, D., Masson, F., and Rabilloud, T. (2000) Membrane proteomics: use of additive main effects with multiplicative interaction model to classify plasma membrane proteins according to their solubility and electrophoretic properties. *Electrophoresis* **21**, 3329–3344.
11. Luche, S., Santoni, V., and Rabilloud, T. (2003) Evaluation of nonionic and zwitterionic detergents as membrane protein solubilizers in two-dimensional electrophoresis. *Proteomics* **3**, 249–253.
12. Rabilloud, T. (1998) Use of thiourea to increase the solubility of membrane proteins in two-dimensional electrophoresis. *Electrophoresis* **19**, 758–760.
13. Herbert, B. R., Molloy, M. P., Gooley, A. A., Walsh, B. J., Bryson, W. G., and Williams, K. L. (1998) Improved protein solubility in two-dimensional electrophoresis using tributyl phosphine as reducing agent. *Electrophoresis* **19**, 845–851.
14. Stanley, B. A., Neverova, I., Brown, H. A., and Van Eyk, J. E. (2003) Optimizing protein solubility for two-dimensional gel electrophoresis analysis of human myocardium. *Proteomics* **3**, 815–820.
15. Blomberg, A., Blomberg, L., Norbeck, J., et al. (1995) Interlaboratory reproducibility of yeast protein patterns analyzed by immobilized pH gradient two-dimensional gel electrophoresis. *Electrophoresis* **16**, 1935–1945.
16. Corbett, J. M., Dunn, M. J., Posch, A., and Gorg, A. (1994) Positional reproducibility of protein spots in two-dimensional polyacrylamide gel electrophoresis using immobilised pH gradient isoelectric focusing in the first dimension: an interlaboratory comparison. *Electrophoresis* **15**, 1205–1211.
17. Bjellqvist, B., Ek, K., Righetti, P. G., et al. (1982) Isoelectric focusing in immobilized pH gradients: principle, methodology and some applications. *J. Biochem. Biophys. Methods* **6**, 317–339.
18. Gorg, A., Obermaier, C., Boguth, G., et al. (2000) The current state of two-dimensional electrophoresis with immobilized pH gradients. *Electrophoresis* **21**, 1037–1053.
19. Klose, J. and Kobalz, U. (1995) Two-dimensional electrophoresis of proteins: an updated protocol and implications for a functional analysis of the genome. *Electrophoresis* **16**, 1034–1059.
20. Gorg, A., Obermaier, C., Boguth, G., and Weiss, W. (1999) Recent developments in two-dimensional gel electrophoresis with immobilized pH gradients: wide pH

gradients up to pH 12, longer separation distances and simplified procedures. *Electrophoresis* **20**, 712–717.

21. Neuhoff, V., Arold, N., Taube, D., and Ehrhardt, W. (1988) Improved staining of proteins in polyacrylamide gels including isoelectric focusing gels with clear background at nanogram sensitivity using Coomassie brilliant blue G-250 and R-250. *Electrophoresis* **9**, 255–262.
22. Switzer, R. C., III, Merril, C. R., and Shifrin, S. (1979) A highly sensitive silver stain for detecting proteins and peptides in polyacrylamide gels. *Anal. Biochem.* **98**, 231–237.
23. Shevchenko, A., Wilm, M., Vorm, O., and Mann, M. (1996) Mass spectrometric sequencing of proteins silver-stained polyacrylamide gels. *Anal. Chem.* **68**, 850–858.
24. Yan, J. X., Wait, R., Berkelman, T., et al. (2002) A modified silver staining protocol for visualization of proteins compatible with matrix-assisted laser desorption/ionization and electrospray ionization-mass spectrometry. *Electrophoresis* **21**, 3666–3672.
25. Patton, W. F. (2000) A thousand points of light: the application of fluorescence detection technologies to two-dimensional gel electrophoresis and proteomics. *Electrophoresis* **21**, 1123–1144.
26. Unlu, M., Morgan, M. E., and Minden, J. S. (1997) Difference gel electrophoresis: a single gel method for detecting changes in protein extracts. *Electrophoresis* **18**, 2071–2077.
27. Lauber, W. M., Carroll, J. A., Dufield, D. R., Kiesel, J. R., Radabaugh, M. R., and Malone, J. P. (2001) Mass spectrometry compatibility of two-dimensional gel protein stains. *Electrophoresis* **22**, 906–918.
28. Patterson, S. D. and Aebersold, R. (1995) Mass spectrometric approaches for the identification of gel-separated proteins. *Electrophoresis* **16**, 1791–1814.
29. Yates, J. R., III (1998) Mass spectrometry and the age of the proteome. *J. Mass Spectrom.* **33**, 1–19.
30. Byers,H. L. and Ward, M. A. (2003) Mass spectrometry—a powerful analytical tool, in *Proteomic and Genomic Analysis of Cardiovascular Disease* (Van Eyk, J. E. and Dunn, M. J. eds.), Wiley-VCH GmbH & Co., KGaA, pp. 195–211.
31. Wheeler, C. H., Berry, S. L., Wilkins, M. R., et al. (1996) Characterisation of proteins from two-dimensional electrophoresis gels by matrix-assisted laser desorption mass spectrometry and amino acid compositional analysis. *Electrophoresis* **17**, 580–587.
32. Mann, M. and Wilm, M. (1994) Error-tolerant identification of peptides in sequence databases by peptide sequence tags. *Anal. Chem.* **66**, 4390–4399.
33. Eng, J. K. (1994) An approach to correlate tandem mass spectral data of peptides with amino acid sequences in a protein database. *J. Am. Soc. Mass Spec.* **5**, 976–989.
34. Emmert-Buck, M. R., Bonner, R. F., Smith, P. D., et al. (1996) Laser capture microdissection. *Science* **274**, 998–1001.
35. Fend, F., Emmert-Buck, M. R., Chuaqui, R. F., Cole, K., Lee, J., Liotta, L. A., and Raffeld, M. (1999) Immuno-LCM: laser capture microdissection of immunostained frozen sections for mRNA analysis. *Am. J. Pathol.* **154**, 61–66.

36. Goldsworthy, S. M., Stockton, P. S., Trempus, C. S., Foley, J. F., and Maronpot, R. R. (1999) Effects of fixation on RNA extraction and amplification from laser capture microdissected tissue. *Mol. Carcinog.* **25**, 86–91.
37. Stagliano, N. E., Carpino, A. J., Ross, J. S., and Donovan, M. (2001) Vascular gene discovery using laser capture microdissection of human blood vessels and quantitative PCR. *Ann. NY Acad. Sci.* **947**, 334–349.
38. Parlato, R., Rosica, A., Cuccurullo, V., et al. (2002) A preservation method that allows recovery of intact RNA from tissues dissected by laser capture microdissection. *Anal. Biochem.* **300**, 139–145.
39. Craven, R. A. and Banks, R. E. (2001) Laser capture microdissection and proteomics: Possibilities and limitation. *Proteomics* **1**, 1200–1204.
40. Banks, R. E., Dunn, M. J., Forbes, M. A., et al. (1999) The potential use of laser capture microdissection to selectively obtain distinct populations of cells for proteomic analysis–preliminary findings. *Electrophoresis* **20**, 689–700.
41. Craven, R. A., Totty, N., Harden, P., Selby, P. J., and Banks, R. E. (2002) Laser capture microdissection and two-dimensional polyacrylamide gel electrophoresis. *Am. J. Pathol.* **160**, 815–822.
42. Brown Jones, M., Krutzsch, H., Shu, H., et al. (2002) Proteomic analysis and identification of new biomarkers and therapeutic targets for invasive ovarian cancer. *Proteomics* **2**, 76–84.
43. Lawrie, L. C., Curran, S., McLeod, H. L., Fothergill, J. E., and Murray, G. I. (2001) Application of laser capture microdissection and proteomics in colon cancer. *J. Clin. Pathol. Mol. Pathol.* **54**, 253–258.
44. Mouledous, L., Hunt, S., Harcourt, R., Harry, J. L., Williams, K. L., and Gutstein, H. B. (2002) Lack of compatibility of histological staining methods with proteomic analysis of laser-captured microdissected brain samples. *J. Biomol. Tech.* **13**, 288–264.
45. De Souza, A. I., McGregor, E., Dunn, M. J., and Rose, M. L. (2004) Preparation of human heart for laser microdissection and proteomics. *Proteomics* **4**, 578–586.

14

Real-Time Quantitative Polymerase Chain Reaction in Cardiac Transplant Research

Leanne E. Felkin, Anne B. Taegtmeyer, and Paul J. R. Barton

Summary

The real-time quantitative polymerase chain reaction (PCR), an increasingly popular technique for the detection of DNA, combines a high degree of accuracy with extreme sensitivity. In this chapter we describe the use of real-time quantitative PCR in transplantation research in two areas in which this method is commonly applied: the accurate quantification of mRNA in tissue samples and genotyping of DNA. These are described in the context of cardiac transplantation, but they are of equal relevance to other areas of transplant biology.

Key Words: Real-time PCR; quantitative PCR; mRNA quantification; TaqMan; RiboGreen; RNA degradation; genotyping; single-nucleotide polymorphism (SNP); polymorphism; myocardial biopsy.

1. Introduction

Since the first description of the principles of the 5'-nuclease assay *(1)* and the consequent development of the method to include increasingly sophisticated chemistries and detection systems *(2–4)*, real-time polymerase chain reaction (PCR) has offered exceptionally high accuracy and sensitivity. The general principles of real-time PCR have been described in a number of excellent reviews *(5–7)* and an especially useful source of information is www.gene-quantification.com). A number of platforms and chemistries for real-time PCR are available. We describe here the use of TaqMan real-time PCR for measuring mRNA abundance in human myocardial samples and for single-nucleotide polymorphism (SNP) genotyping of cardiac transplant patients and their donors.

From: *Methods in Molecular Biology, vol. 333: Transplantation Immunology: Methods and Protocols*
Edited by: P. Hornick and M. Rose © Humana Press Inc., Totowa, NJ

2. Real-Time PCR and mRNA Quantification

2.1. Overview

The accurate measurement of mRNA abundance remains an important prerequisite for analyzing gene expression *(8)*. Traditional methods such as Northern blotting and ribonuclease protection assay offer reasonable accuracy and specificity but consume significant quantities of RNA. Methods based on PCR offer the distinct advantage of requiring only small amounts of starting material. While this may be less important when considering research on organs removed at the time of transplantation where tissue is readily available, it offers a significant advantage when considering analysis where tissue is limited, as is the case with surgical samples *(9)*, endomyocardial biopsies *(10)*, fetal heart samples *(11)*, or material derived by laser microdissection. Initial PCR-based methods were "final-product" methods derived from the ability to establish retrospectively the point at which amplification was exponential. However, these were complicated by the need for complex and often time-consuming validation in order to achieve conditions of accurate quantification. Typically, this would involve serial dilution experiments to determine a linear working range, the use of a titrated exogenous RNA standard, or construction of artificial DNA constructs to act as internal competition reference targets. More recently, the approach of analyzing PCR products cycle-by-cycle in real time has led to the development of a variety of instruments with a range of analysis speeds, sample throughput, and cost (**Table 1**). Useful sources of information comparing currently available instruments can be found at www.biocom pare.com and www.gene-quantification.com.

2.2. Principles of Real-Time PCR

As with the detection instruments, a number of chemistries are available for real-time PCR, each of which offers distinct advantages and disadvantages (for a review *see* www.gene-quantification.com). Two of the more commonly used chemistries are Applied Biosystems' TaqMan assay *(2,3)*, described in more detail below, and SYBR Green detection, which uses a double-stranded DNA-binding dye *(12,13)*. Whatever the system used, the general principles are largely the same. During real-time PCR, a fluorescent signal is generated that is directly proportional to the amount of accumulating PCR product. This signal is detected, calibrated, and used to provide a measure of initial target abundance. In the case of the ABI Prism 7700, fluorescent signal is collected from each reaction every 7 s. Thus, over the course of a 40-cycle PCR lasting 1 h and 56 min, a total of 994 measurements will be made for every reaction. When the data are plotted against time, a picture of how the fluorescence accumulates in real time during the PCR emerges (**Fig. 1**). Displaying the kinetics of the real-

Table 1
Real-Time PCR Instrumentation

Supplier	Number of available instruments	Features
Applied Biosystems www.appliedbiosystems.com	5	96- and 384-well formats available, single or multicolor detection, SNP autocalling, facility automation possible
Roche Diagnostics www.roche-applied-science.com	3	32-, 96-, and 384-well formats, multicolor detection, SNP autocalling facility, high-speed cycling
Corbett Research www.corbettresearch.com	1	36- and 72-well formats available, multicolor detection, SNP autocalling facility, high-speed cycling
Cepheid www.cepheid.com	2	96 independently programmable wells, multicolor detection
Biorad www.bio-rad.com	3	96- and 384-well formats available, single or multicolor detection, SNP autocalling facility
Stratagene www.stratagene.com	3	96- well and 384-formats, multicolor detection, SNP autocalling facility
MJ Research www.mjr.com	4	96-well format, single or multicolor detection, SNP autocalling facility

time PCR reaction in this way clearly identifies the exponential, linear, and plateau phases of the reaction.

2.2.1. PCR Kinetics

PCR amplification is only truly exponential in the early phases of the reaction. As the reaction progresses, reagents are depleted and become limiting. By the time the product becomes readily detectable by gel electrophoresis, its abundance is often affected not only by the amount of initial starting template, but also by the increasingly impaired PCR efficiency. The principal advantage of real-time PCR analysis over all other PCR-based quantification techniques is the ability to reveal all phases of PCR for every sample, making possible quantification of the product early during the exponential phase.

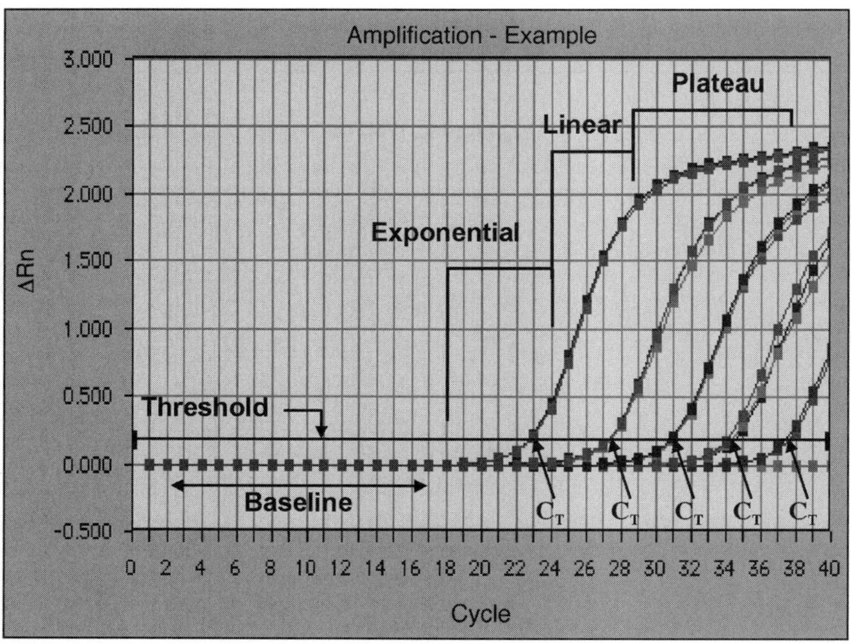

Fig. 1. Detection of amplification product by real-time PCR. The graph shows the fluorescence signal (ΔRn) detected during the course of a series of PCR reactions loaded with increasing quantities of target sequence. At the start of PCR, signal is below detectable level (baseline). Initial detection above threshold shows doubling of product with each cycle (exponential phase). As PCR progresses, reagents become limiting (linear phase), resulting eventually in depletion (plateau phase). Note that each reaction will go to completion and the amount of product near the plateau phase is not proportional to input starting template. In real-time PCR, data is collected throughout the entire reaction, allowing the operator to select data from the exponential phase of each reaction. The C_T value is the cycle at which signal first becomes detected over background.

2.2.2. The Cycle Threshold

The basic measurement in real-time PCR is the cycle threshold (C_T), also known as the crossing point in some systems. The C_T is the cycle at which fluorescence generated by the accumulating PCR product exceeds a fixed threshold **(Fig. 1)**. The threshold is placed in the exponential phase of the amplification curve and may be set automatically or by the user. In this way the C_T value indicates the number of cycles required to detect appearance of product above background. The greater the abundance of target mRNA in the starting material, the sooner the threshold fluorescence level is reached; in other words,

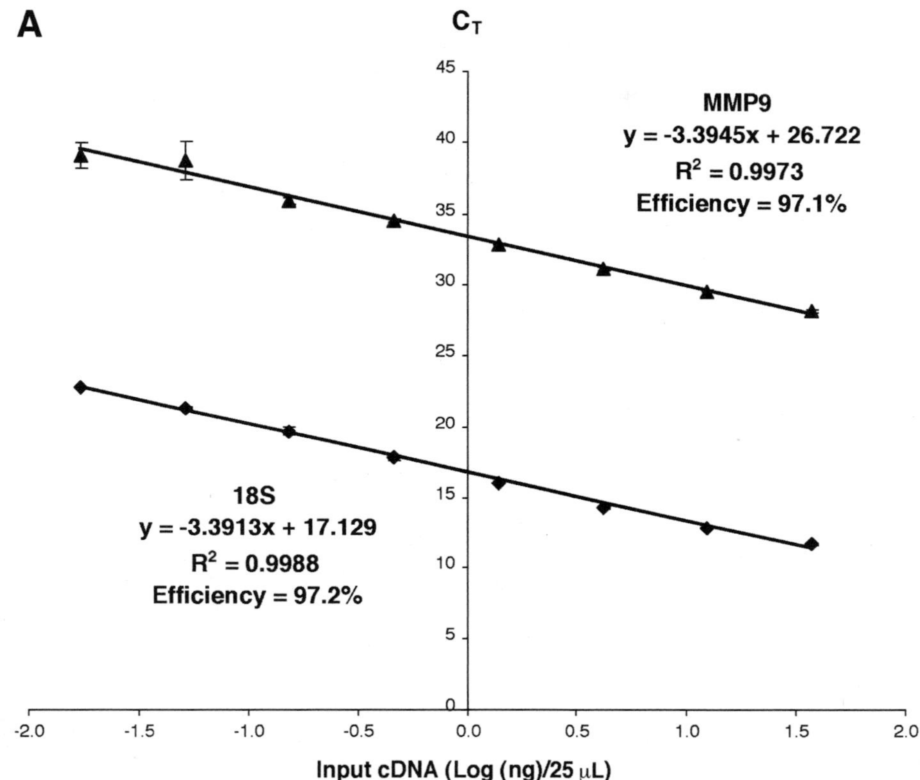

Fig. 2. Determination of real-time PCR efficiency. **(A)** Efficiency analysis. A threefold dilution series of cDNA prepared from human bone marrow RNA was analyzed by real-time PCR using TaqMan probes and primer sets for matrix metalloproteinase 9 (MMP9) and 18S rRNA. Mean C_T values are plotted against log input amount of cDNA. The slope of the graph is determined by linear regression and can be used to calculate the efficiency of the amplification: PCR efficiency = $100 \times (10^{(-1/\text{slope})} - 1)$. Note the similarity in the slope of the lines for MMP9 and 18S, which indicates similar PCR efficiencies. Error bars represent standard deviation; $n = 3$ PCR replicates. *(Continued on next page)*

the higher the target abundance, the lower the C_T. Because PCR amplification is exponential, the C_T value is proportional to the log concentration of the target DNA or, in the case of reverse transcriptase (RT)-PCR, of the target RNA **(Fig. 2A)**. It is therefore necessary to calibrate and log transform the C_T to get the final result. It is also important to note that the C_T is not an absolute measure of target abundance, as its value will vary depending on where the threshold is set.

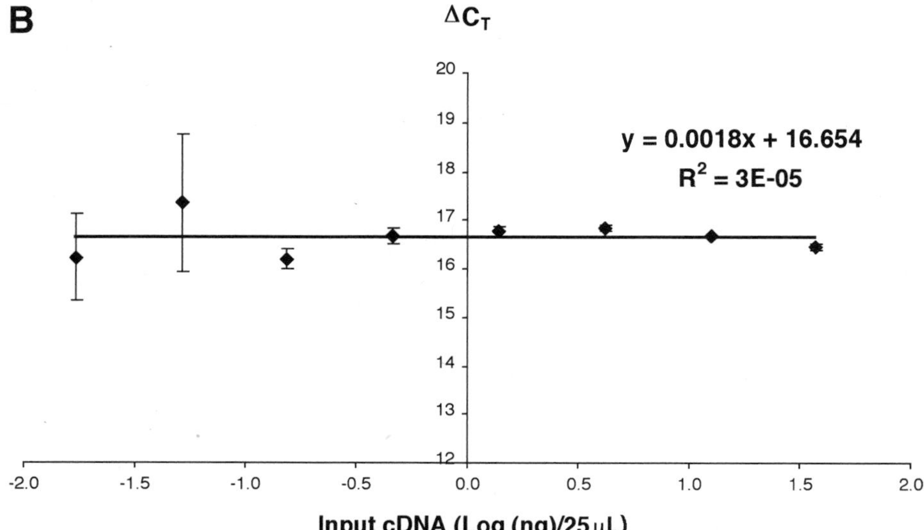

Fig. 2. *(continued)* **(B)** Validation plot for the $\Delta\Delta C_T$ method. ΔC_T values ($\Delta C_T = C_T$ MMP9 - C_T 18S) were calculated for each dilution point shown in **A** and plotted against log input amount of cDNA. The absolute value of the slope was calculated by linear regression and shown to be less than 0.1, thereby confirming that PCR assays for MMP9 and 18S have equal efficiencies and validating the use of the $\Delta\Delta C_T$ method of analysis (*see* text). Error bars represent standard deviation; $n = 3$ PCR replicates.

2.3. Experimental Considerations

2.3.1. Assay Design

When beginning a real-time PCR experiment, a significant part of user input is directed towards assay design. In addition to the usual pair of PCR primers, TaqMan assays require a sequence-specific fluorescently labeled probe, which is flanked by the primers. The primers and probe should be contained within a target amplicon of 150 bp, preferably straddling an exon–exon junction. The melting temperatures (*Tm*) of the two primers should be within 1°C of each other and between 58 and 60°C. The *Tm* of the TaqMan probe should be 10°C greater than that of the primers. Primer and probe selection requires detailed sequence analysis using specialist software such as Applied Biosystems' proprietary design package, Primer Express ***(14)***, or MIT's free design program, Primer3 (www.genome.wi.mit.edu/cgi-bin/primer/primer3_www.cgi). Following design and synthesis, primer and probe concentrations are optimized and amplification efficiencies determined (see below) prior to use. As alternatives to in-house primer and probe design, sequences designed and published by others or the increasingly commercially available preoptimized assays can be used, such as Applied Biosystems' off-the-shelf TaqMan Gene Expression Assays ***(15)*** or their personalized Custom TaqMan Gene Expression Assays ***(16)***. A catalog of available TaqMan Gene Expression Assays can be found at www.allgenes.com. It is important to note that whatever the source of the assay to be used, it is imperative to consider in detail the mRNA being targeted. Many genes are subject to complex alternative splicing, and the specificity of real-time PCR is such that only the specified target sequence will be detected. For example, if the assay is designed over an alternative splice junction, only this splice variant will be detected.

2.3.2. Tissue Collection and Storage for mRNA Quantification

Procedures for tissue collection and storage can easily be overlooked when beginning a real-time PCR project. At the time of collection, priority is not necessarily given to immediate tissue storage. However, if samples are destined for mRNA analysis, measures to protect the sample need to be considered, as RNA is both thermolabile and susceptible to rapid degradation by endoribonucleases (RNases). In vivo, RNA degradation can also be influenced by its sequence, especially in the 3'-untranslated region, and many transcripts, particularly cytokines and other signaling molecules, contain sequences specifically designed to enhance degradation ***(17)***. As illustrated in **Fig. 3**, mRNAs degrade rapidly in excised tissue held at room temperature due primarily to the breakdown of intracellular compartmentalization and the release of ribonucleases. Moreover, different transcripts degrade at differing rates, making their relative quantification inaccurate. It is therefore essential to establish the degradation rate of the target genes if analysis is to be attempted on partially degraded material ***(18)***. Wherever possible, protection and correct storage of tissue should occur immediately after collection. This can best be achieved by snap freezing the sample in liquid nitrogen. Where this is not possible, tissue can be placed in a suitable protective solution such as RNAlater (Ambion, Crawley, UK). Note, however, that for this method to be successful, the sample size must be small enough to enable adequate diffusion of the protective solution through the sample.

2.3.4. RNA Preparation

RNA isolation using off-the-shelf extraction kits, such as the RNeasy kit (Qiagen, Crawley, UK) and the RNAqueous kit (Ambion, Huntingdon, UK) is convenient, rapid, and obviates the need for phenol. Samples are disrupted and homogenized in a buffer containing guanidinium salts, which simultaneously lyses cells and inactivates endogenous RNases. Ethanol is added to the lysate and the solution passed through a silica-based filter to which RNA binds while other cellular components pass through. Finally, the filter is washed to remove contaminants, and the RNA is eluted.

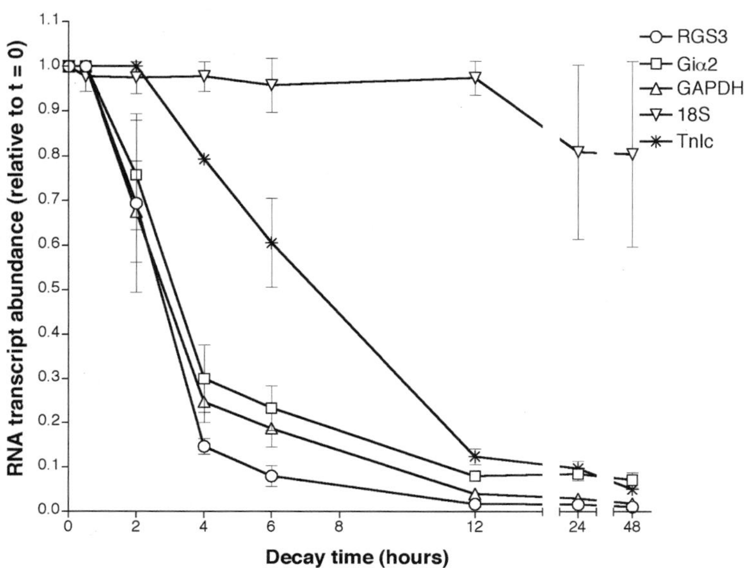

Fig. 3. Effect of time at room temperature on RNA degradation in cardiac tissue. Samples of left ventricular myocardium were left at room temperature for the times shown prior to RNA extraction. 300 ng of RNA was used in a 30-µL reverse transcription (RT) reaction, and the cDNA equivalent of 4 ng of RNA was analyzed by real-time PCR for RGS3, Giα2 *(49)*, TnIc (*see* **Table 4**), GAPDH and 18S rRNA (cat. nos. 402869 and 4310893E, respectively, Applied Biosystems, Warrington, UK). Note the stability of the 18S rRNA target in intact tissue. Error bars = standard deviation.

RNA recovery using filter-based protocols is determined by the RNA-binding capacity of the filter and is thus influenced by the amount of starting material. When working with endomyocardial biopsies (typically ranging in size from 0.3 to 20 mg), it is unlikely that the capacity of the filter will be exceeded. However, using standard manufacturers' protocols we found varying levels of protein contamination, DNA co-purification, and RNA yield. The choice of disruption and homogenization technique is an important factor (**Tables 2** and **3**). In our hands the most efficient disruption and homogenization protocol for endomyocardial biopsies is sample disruption in lysis buffer in a 1.5-mL microtube using a disposable fitted pestle (cat. no. 749520-0090; Anachem, Luton, UK), followed by homogenization in a 2.0-mL microtube using a hand-held Ultra Turrax T8 homogenizer with a 5-mm probe (cat. nos. 406/0319/00 and 406/0319/10, respectively; VWR International, Lutterworth, UK) and further homogenization using Qiagen's QiaShredder (cat. no. 79654; Qiagen, Crawley, UK). Contaminating protein and DNA can be removed by including proteinase K and DNase I (e.g., Qiagen's RNase-free DNase set, cat. no. 79254; Qiagen, Crawley, UK) treat-

Table 2
Comparison of RNA Yield From Biopsy-Sized Myocardium Samples Using Different Extraction Techniques

Homogenization technique	Average RNA yield (ng) per 1.0 mg tissue ± SD	*n*
Electric homogenizer + QiaShredder	327.1 ± 194.8	8
Electric homogenizer only	173.6 ± 40.3	4
QiaShredder only	229.9 ± 81.6	3

Table 3
Comparison of RNA Quality From Myocardium and Myocyte Cell Culture Samples Using Different Extraction Techniques

Tissue source	Homogenization technique	Proteinase K treatment	Mean sample purity (A_{260}/A_{280}) ± SD	*n*
Rat myocardium (biopsy-sized sample)	Electric homogenizer + QiaShredder	Yes	1.95 ± 0.05	4
	Electric homogenizer only	Yes	1.93 ± 0.08	4
	QiaShredder only	Yes	1.87 ± 0.05	4
Cultured neonatal rat cardiomyocytes	QiaShredder only	No	1.37 ± 0.06	12

ment steps. The beneficial effect of proteinase K incubation on resulting RNA purity is shown in **Table 3**. DNase I treatment is included because reliable RNA quantification is essential, in samples prepared using commercial filter columns, DNA can account for up to 50% of the purified nucleic acid ***(6)***.

2.3.5. RNA Quantification

Reliable RNA quantification is important for real-time PCR because it enables equal and appropriate loading of both RT and PCR reactions, thereby generating predictable and reproducible measurements of internal control levels. The most common method of measuring RNA concentration is ultraviolet (UV) absorption spectroscopy. While this method is quick and simple to perform, it is comparatively insensitive, with minimum nucleic acid concentrations of 1 μg/mL typically required to obtain reliable measurements. Ethidium-bromide-based protocols are more sensitive than UV absorption spectroscopy and are also routinely used to measure RNA concentration, but a superior alternative is to use RiboGreen RNA quantification reagent (cat. no. R11490; Molecular Probes Europe BV, Leiden, The Netherlands). RiboGreen is a RNA-binding dye that exceeds the sensitivity of ethidium-bromide-based assays and UV absorbance spectrophotometry by 200- and 1000-fold, respectively *(19)*. The excitation and emission maxima for RiboGreen reagent bound to RNA are approx 500 and 525 nm, respectively. Conventionally, RiboGreen reagent is used with a fluorescence microplate reader, standard spectrofluorometer, or filter fluorometer. However, the reagent may also be used on any real-time PCR instrument by selecting the SYBR dye layer (SYBR Green I: excitation maximum = 497 nm, emission maximum = 521 nm), an important caveat being that other dye options (e.g., TAMRA and ROX) have been deselected. While the RiboGreen commercial protocol advocates the use of a high-range (20 ng/mL to 1 µg/mL) and a low-range (1–50 ng/mL) assay for sample quantification, we find the assay to be linear between 10 and 500 ng/mL when performed on an ABI Prism 7700 in a 200-µL reaction volume with RiboGreen reagent at a final dilution of 1 in 400 (**Fig. 4**).

High-quality RNA extraction and strict quantification give consistently reproducible real-time data. Moreover, using accurately quantified input RNA, predictable internal control measurements can be seen, thereby allowing problematic RNAs to be readily identified. For example, **Fig. 5** shows the 18S rRNA levels measured using real-time PCR in cDNA samples prepared from 86 human left ventricular myocardial samples ranging in size from less than 1 mg to more than 90 mg. C_T values for 18S rRNA are tightly clustered, and a single sample is visible as an outlier indicating a degraded or otherwise unreliable sample.

2.3.6. Reverse Transcriptase Reaction

Reverse transcription (RT) of RNA is necessary because RNA cannot act as a template for PCR. The RT reaction may be carried out immediately before the PCR in the same tube (using either one or two enzymes) or as a separate reaction. Single-tube RT-PCR is reportedly less sensitive than two-tube RT-PCR *(6)* and also requires that samples be stored as RNA. In contrast, two-tube RT-PCR generates a stock of stable cDNA that is more suitable for long-term storage.

When performing two-tube RT-PCR, deciding which type of primer to use for initiating reverse transcription is important. Random hexamers, gene-specific, and oligo dT primers are all suitable options, but as yet there is no broad agreement as to which is the most efficient or sensitive *(7,20,21)*. Indeed, first-strand cDNA can be synthesized in the absence of exogenous primers, most likely owing to self-priming events. In a two-tube RT-PCR reaction, gene-specific primers confine analysis to the single gene specified by the initial RT primer. In contrast, using random hexamers, oligo dT, or a combination of the two, as primers will allow amplification of the whole mRNA population. Note, however, that ribosomal RNA transcripts (e.g., 18S), often used as normalizing internal standards, will not be represented in oligo-dT-primed cDNA since they lack a poly-A tail. In this case the use of random hexamers is recommended.

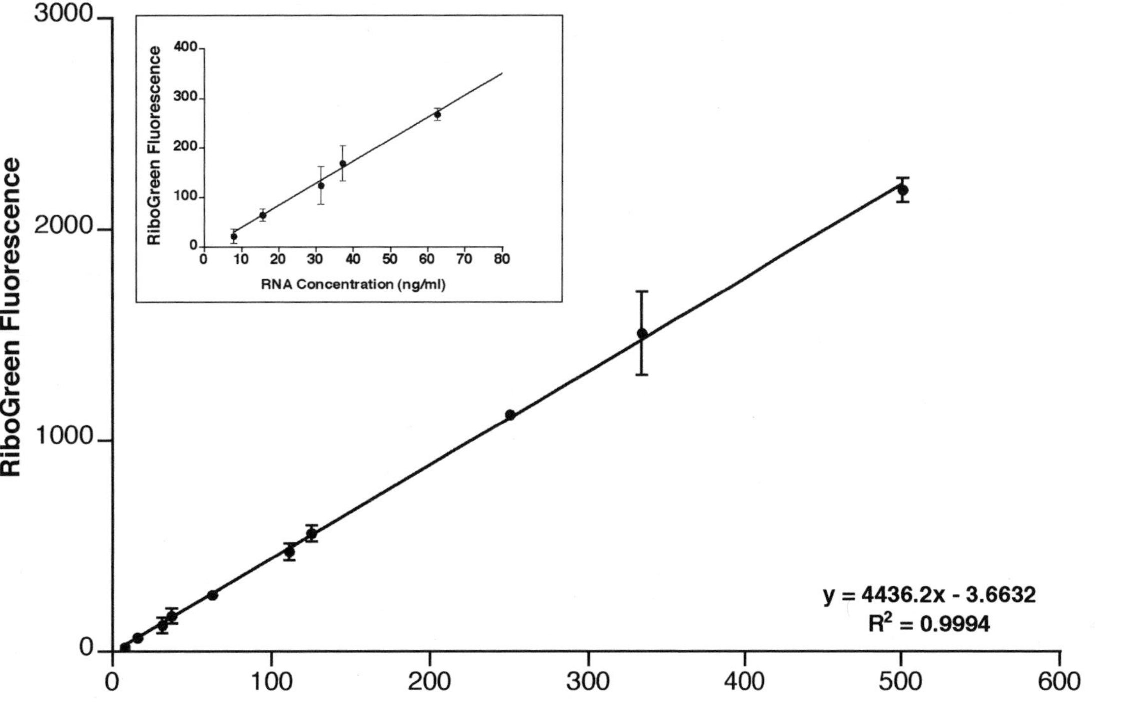

Fig. 4. Quantification of RNA using RiboGreen. Two independent dilution series (three- and twofold) were prepared from total RNA with RNA-grade TE buffer (pH 7.5) and combined to form a single set of quantity standards. The manufacturer's RiboGreen high-range assay protocol (Molecular Probes Europe BV, Leiden, The Netherlands) was followed and fluorescence measured on the ABI Prism 7700. Plotting the mean fluorescence against RNA standard concentration shows the RiboGreen assay to be linear between 10 and 500 ng/mL. An expansion of the lower portion of the graph is inset. Error bars = standard deviation; $n = 3$.

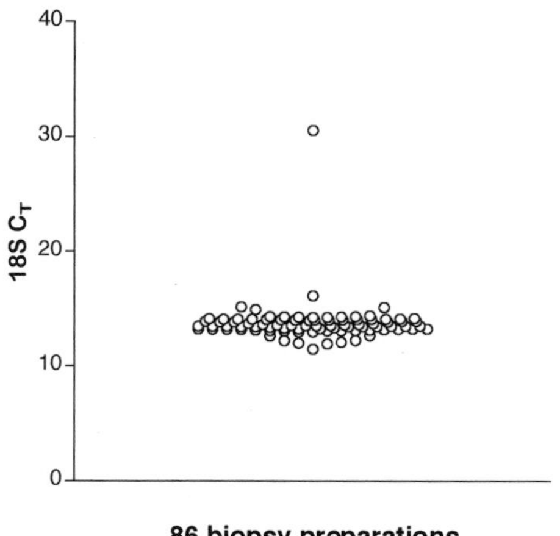

Fig. 5. Determination of 18S rRNA abundance by real-time PCR. Total RNA was extracted from human ventricular myocardial samples and quantified using the protocols described (*see* text). Myocardial sample sizes were 25.44 mg ± 20.37 mg, range 1–90 mg. RNA yield was 538 ± 362 ng/mg tissue. RT reactions were accurately loaded with either 60 or 300 ng RNA, depending on sample yields. Resulting cDNAs were diluted to the equivalent of 2 ng of RNA per μL and a total of 5 ng used in a 25-μL PCR with primers and TaqMan probe for 18S rRNA. Mean 18S C_T was 13.78 ± 1.96. Note the outlying data point is readily identified.

2.3.7. Choice of Quantification Strategy

There are two basic approaches to the quantification of mRNA transcript levels using real-time PCR: absolute quantification, in which the precise number of mRNAs per cell, unit of RNA, or unit of tissue is determined, and relative quantification, where mRNA abundance is calculated relative to a calibrator sample or control group.

2.3.7.1. Absolute Quantification

Absolute quantification requires the preparation of a set of quantity standards for which the number of copies of target sequence per unit of sample is accurately known for each dilution point. To compensate for variation introduced during the RT step, the standard curve may be prepared from RNA copies of the target amplicon sequence. These may be generated by in vitro transcription of the amplicon ***(2,5,22,23)*** or by purchasing custom synthesized RNA oligonucleotides ***(24)***. In practice, many authors use standard curves derived from dilution of a DNA copy of the target amplicon and have shown them to be an acceptable alternative ***(5,22)***. However, although this may be a quick and convenient way of deriving an accurate correlation between C_T and DNA abundance, it may not correlate directly with mRNA abundance, as the efficiency of mRNA to cDNA conversion during the RT reaction will be unknown.

2.3.7.2. Relative Quantification

In many cases absolute quantification is not required and relative quantification of mRNA can be used. There are several methods of relative quantification, including the use of standard curves, but one of the most frequently used is the comparative C_T method. Here, expression of the abundance of a target mRNA in a test sample is normalized to an internal standard (often 18S rRNA) and related to the expression level in a control sample (e.g., normal donor myocardium). The difference between the C_T value of the target mRNA and that of the internal standard is represented as C_T (target mRNA) – C_T (internal standard) = ΔC_T. The expression of the target gene in the test sample relative to the control sample is therefore given as ΔC_T (test) – ΔC_T(control) = $\Delta\Delta C_T$.* Where the efficiency of PCR is close to 100% (i.e., close to a doubling of product per cycle), the relative abundance of the target RNA between the two samples becomes $2^{-\Delta CT}$. The advantage of the comparative C_T method is that standard curves do not need to be constructed, allowing more samples to be analyzed per plate, saving time and money. However, it should be noted that for this form of comparative analysis, the PCR amplification efficiencies for both the target gene and the internal standard need to be equal. The PCR efficiency must be demonstrated for each assay and is assessed by observing how C_T varies with template dilution (**Fig. 2A**). When efficiencies for each PCR are equal, the ΔC_T value will be the same no matter the dilution (*see* **Fig. 2B**). Specifically, Applied Biosystems stipulate that the comparative C_T method can only be reliably used when the gradient of the ΔC_T plot is less than 0.1 *(25)*. In the event that equal PCR efficiencies cannot be demonstrated, new primers may need to be designed to improve efficiency, quantification performed using the relative standard curve method, or a refined comparative C_T calculation used. In recognition of the difficulties encountered with unequal efficiencies, new strategies have been developed where the actual efficiencies of PCR amplifications are included in the quantification calculation *(26–31)*. In addition to minimizing assay optimization and validation, the advantage of such strategies is that they do not assume 100% PCR efficiency. Furthermore, some strategies estimate PCR efficiency for each reaction from the actual data used to create the amplification plot rather than an external standard curve *(26–*

---

*The amount of target mRNA recorded at any time during a PCR is influenced by the amount of target mRNA at the start of PCR, the efficiency of PCR, and by the number of PCR cycles performed. This is described by the equation: $X_n = X_0 \times (1 + E_X)^n$, where X_n is the amount of target mRNA at cycle n, X_0 is the initial amount of target mRNA, E_X is the efficiency of target amplification, and n is the number of cycles performed. The comparative C_T method expands this equation to give the formula: $2^{-\Delta C_t}$ (*see* Applied Biosystem's User Bulletin no. 2 *[25]*).

28). Such strategies do not assume that the PCR efficiencies of the standard curve and of the cDNA samples are identical. Neither do they assume that individual cDNA samples will have similar PCR efficiencies and can therefore be represented with a single efficiency value. Instead, analysis is based entirely upon the kinetics of the experimental samples.

2.3.8. Choice of Internal Control for Normalization

The importance of choosing a suitable internal control for normalization of the target mRNA cannot be overstated, and some researchers advocate the use of a minimum of three and up to five independent internal controls ***(32,33)***. Most importantly, expression of the internal control must be unaffected by the variable being investigated. This cannot be assumed and should always be established empirically ***(5,32–34)***. A list of useful standard internal control RNAs is given in **Table 4**. For analysis using tissue extracts, it is also important to consider potential bias resulting from differences in the cellular origins of target and internal control transcripts. For example, in the case of 18S rRNA, all cells present in the sample under investigation will contribute to the resulting signal, whereas a cell-type specific transcript will not. When cardiac myocyte gene expression is being analyzed in endomyocardial biopsies where the proportion of different cell types may vary between samples, it may be more appropriate to use a cell-specific internal standard such as myocyte-specific cardiac troponin I ***(35)***.

It is possible to measure both the target gene of interest and the internal control simultaneously in the same reaction by color coding the independent reactions using TaqMan probes labeled with different fluorescent dyes ***(36)***. Multiplexing reactions in this way not only prevents errors introduced by repeated pipetting, but also minimizes the amount of samples, time, and reagents needed to complete the study. The disadvantage of multiplexing assays is an increase in the initial time required to optimize both PCRs together and ensure that neither reaction predominates.

3. Real-Time PCR and Allelic Discrimination

3.1. Overview

Since the completion of the Human Genome Project, much attention has been focused on genetic variation. The simplest type of genetic variant is the SNP, where one nucleotide is substituted for another. Approximately 3 million SNPs have already been cataloged in the National Institutes of Health SNP database (http://www.ncbi.nlm.nih.gov/SNP). SNPs causing changes in promoter regions or in amino acid coding sequences have been identified in many genes and are a logical starting point when considering the impact of genetic variation between individuals, as they may affect gene regulation, protein structure, and/or function.

Table 4
Common Internal Controls Used in Real-Time PCR

Name	Symbol	Function	Abundance across a general tissue panel	Comment
18S ribosomal RNA	18S	Facilitates ribosome assembly	Very high	Reported pseudogenes
β-Actin	ACTB	Cytoskeletal protein	High/moderate[a]	Reported pseudogenes
Glyceraldehyde-3-phosphate dehydrogenase	GAPDH	Carbohydrate metabolism	High[a]	Reported pseudogenes
β_2-Microglobulin	B2M	β-Chain of major histo-compatibility complex class I molecules	High/moderate[a]	
Hypoxanthine phosphoribosyl-transferase-1	HRPT	Purine metabolism	Low/undetectable[a]	Reported pseudogenes
Acidic ribosomal phosphoprotein	PO	Component of 60S subunit of the ribosome	High[b]	Reported pseudogenes and splice variants
Cardiac troponin I	TnIc	Regulatory subunit of the cardiac contractile apparatus	Cardiac myocyte specific	Forward: 5' tcctccaactaccgcgctta Reverse: 5' ctcgctccagctcttgcttt Probe: 5' agcagagtcttcagctgcaattttctcgag

[a] From **ref. *50***.
[b] From GeneCards at http://bioinformatics.weizmann.ac.il/cards/.

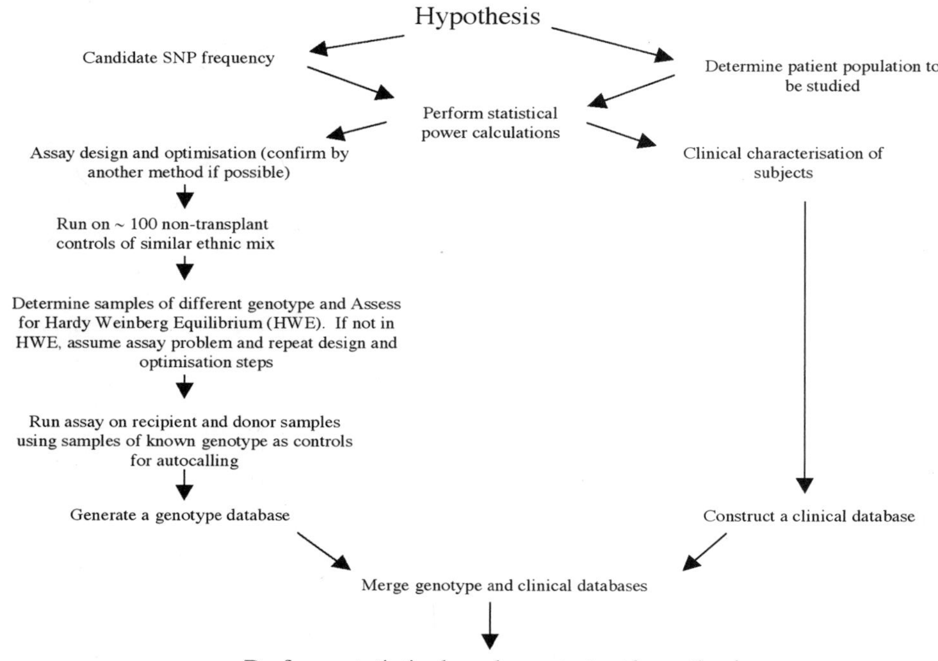

Fig. 6. Steps involved in carrying out a single-nucleotide polymorphism association study in cardiac transplantation.

In transplantation, several pathways exist where recipient or donor organ SNPs (or genotype) might affect the clinical outcome. SNP association may therefore provide valuable information on the prediction of complications after transplantation. Several studies to date have examined associations between SNPs in genes encoding immunological proteins as potential determinants of acute and chronic rejection. Other pathways relevant to cardiac transplantation include those involved in immunosuppressant and lipid metabolism and susceptibility to infection. A number of recent studies are summarized in **Table 5**.

The attraction of SNP association studies in transplantation compared to non-transplant chronic diseases includes shorter time to the occurrence of clinical events, regular clinical assessments, and the study of both recipient and donor genotypes. In studying recipient genotypes, the systemic effect of a particular SNP is being examined, whereas when studying their donor's genotype, the local effect is being examined. A significant limitation of SNP association studies in cardiac transplantation, however, is the small group size at a single center, which, in addition to reduction of statistical power, makes the study of rare SNPs impossible (*see* **Table 5** for typical sample sizes). **Figure 6** outlines the steps involved in conducting an SNP association study in cardiac transplantation.

Table 5
Examples of Single-Nucleotide Polymorphism Association Studies in Cardiac Transplantation

Topic	SNPs examined	Pathway	Total number	Association	Reference
Acute rejection	IL-10 G-1082A G-819T C-592A	IL-10 is an immunomodulator	70 recipients 61 donors	No association	***51***
	TNF-α TGF-β IL-10 IL-6 IFN-γ		90 recipients	TGF-β coding SNPs associated with time to first rejection	***52***
Transplant coronary artery disease	IL-10 IL-1082 IL -819 IL-592	IL-10: anti-inflammatory cytokine	148 recipients, 135 donors	No association	***53***
	IL-1B, IL-1R1, IL-1RN, I-L6, IL-10, TNF-α, TGF-β1, and FCGRIIA		179 recipients	IL-1R1 SNP associated with long-term graft survival	***54***

(Continued on next page)

Table 5 *(Continued)*
Examples of Single-Nucleotide Polymorphism Association Studies in Cardiac Transplantation

Topic	SNPs examined	Pathway	Total number	Association	Reference
Transplant coronary artery disease *(continued)*	β-Fibrinogen Factor V Prothrombin Factor XIII PAI-1 GPIIIa GPI a GPIbα	Pathways involved in hemostatis	53 recipients, 53 donors	Donor PAI-1 and factor XIII SNPs associated with development of transplant coronary artery disease	***55***
Pharmacokinetics	MDR1 C3435T and G2677T CYP 3A5	Calcineurin inhibitor uptake and metabolism	63 pediatric recipients	MDR1 C3435T TT and G2677T TT associated with lower tacrolimus dose requirements to achieve desired concentrations	***56***
Hyperlipidemia	Apo-A-I promoter polymorphism	Apolipoprotein is a component of high-density lipoprotein	103 recipients	Subjects possessing the A allele have higher triglyceride and LDL cholesterol levels	***57***

3.2. Real-Time PCR and Genotyping

Real-time PCR can be used to study SNPs by providing a useful method of genotyping. The method is based on the same overall principles described above but makes use of the ability to discriminate between the two alleles by use of two differently labeled probes. Primers flanking the polymorphic site and probes complementary to each of the two alleles, each with a unique reporter dye of different fluorescent wavelength, are designed. Typically, the reporter dyes FAM (518 nm) and VIC (525 nm) are used. In the PCR reaction, the probes hybridize preferentially to their complementary alleles so that fluorescence is only generated where perfect nucleotide matching has occurred. Wild-type homozygous DNA therefore produces one fluorescent wavelength, whereas mutant homozygous produces the other. DNA containing both alleles (heterozygous) produces emission of both fluorescent wavelengths. Fluorescence at the two wavelengths is detected by the integral fluorometer, in this case, the Sequence Detection System (SDS) of the ABI Prism 7700, which also dampens background signals and inequalities due to variations in initial DNA concentrations. Most systems can also be set up to perform autocalling of genotype by comparison with the spectral fluorescent emissions of control standards of known genotype (*see* **Fig. 7**). Genotypes may also be ascribed by hand by examining the raw spectral data. Using the ABI Prism 7700, it is possible to genotype between 84 and 96 individuals (using autocalling and manual methods, respectively) for one SNP in 2.5 h, making this a medium throughput genotyping method. The ABI Prism 7900HT has a 384-well block, so throughput can be four times higher.

3.3. Experimental Considerations

3.3.1. Assay Design

The usefulness of real-time PCR and TaqMan chemistry in genotyping is largely dictated by the sequence of the gene concerned. Unlike mRNA quantification, in which the position of TaqMan probe and flanking primers is largely at the discretion of the operator, for genotyping the position of the TaqMan probe is fixed by the SNP under study. In some cases it can prove difficult to design suitable probes. For optimal assay performance, primers and probes must be designed according to strict criteria. In particular, Applied Biosystems stipulate that the probe should contain the SNP in its middle third, be less than 20 nucleotides long, and have a salt-adjusted melting temperature (*Tm*) of 65–67°C. Where this proves difficult, for example, if the SNP of interest lies in an AT-rich region, TaqMan minor groove binder (MGB) probes may be used (cat. no. 4316034, Applied Biosystems, Warrington, UK). Conjugation of an MGB complex to an oligonucleotide dramatically increases its *Tm* by stabilizing the nucleic acid duplex *(37–39)*. Attaching an MGB to a TaqMan probe therefore

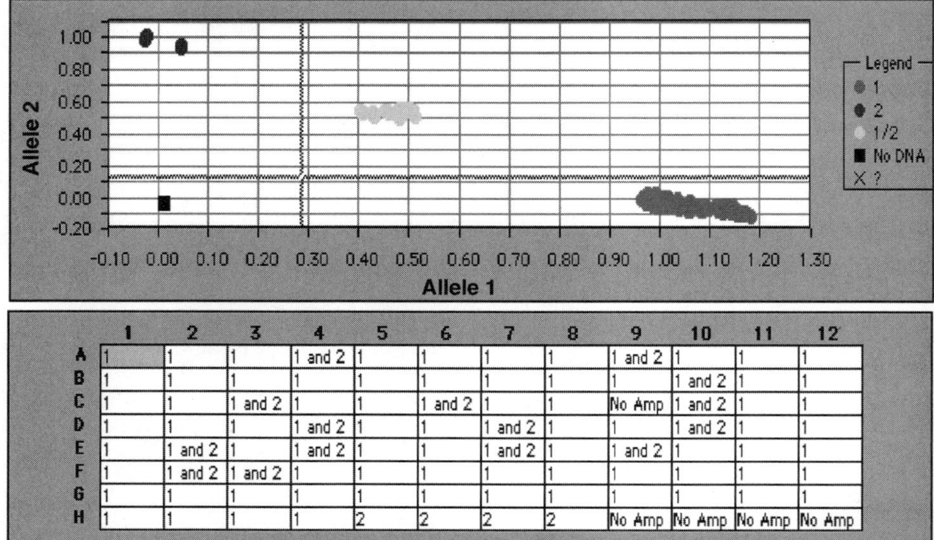

	1	2	3	4	5	6	7	8	9	10	11	12
A	1	1	1	1 and 2	1	1	1	1	1 and 2	1	1	1
B	1	1	1	1	1	1	1	1	1	1 and 2	1	1
C	1	1	1 and 2	1	1	1 and 2	1	1	No Amp	1 and 2	1	1
D	1	1	1	1 and 2	1	1	1 and 2	1	1	1 and 2	1	1
E	1	1 and 2	1	1 and 2	1	1	1 and 2	1	1 and 2	1	1	1
F	1	1 and 2	1 and 2	1	1	1	1	1	1	1	1	1
G	1	1	1	1	1	1	1	1	1	1	1	1
H	1	1	1	1	2	2	2	2	No Amp	No Amp	No Amp	No Amp

Fig. 7. Autocalling of AMPD-1 C34T genotypes. In the upper panel, individuals are sorted according to fluorescence characterisation as 1, 2, and 1/2. Each dot represents a single result. The lower panel gives details of each individual sample. In this example, allele 1 refers to the AMPD-1 C34T C allele and allele 2 to the T allele. Control DNA was placed in row H of the plate (No Amp refers to no-template controls) and DNA of unknown genotype in rows A–G. 1, CC homozygotes; 1/2, CT heterozygotes; 2, TT homozygotes.

means that shorter sequences (13- to 20-mers) can be used to obtain probes with an optimal *Tm*. Because single-nucleotide mismatches become more disruptive as probe length decreases, the opportunity to minimize probe length is particularly valuable in SNP analysis. Primers flanking the polymorphic site that create an amplicon ideally between 80 and 200 bp long are designed according to the criteria outlined by Applied Biosystems ***(40)***. Assay optimization is then performed in order to determine the primer and probe concentrations at which allelic discrimination is clearest.

As with mRNA detection assays, designing and optimizing probe and primer sets is often the most time-consuming part of any real-time PCR genotyping project. Off-the-shelf assays, such as Applied Biosystems' TaqMan SNP genotyping assays ***(41)*** or personalized products like Custom TaqMan SNP Genotyping Assays ***(42)***, can remove or substantially reduce the time spent on design. To search available TaqMan SNP genotyping assays visit www.allsnps.com.

3.3.2. Sources of DNA and Optimization

DNA for use in genotyping can be isolated from a variety of sources, including whole blood or spleen (often the case for donor DNA) using standard extraction methods and stored until use at –20°C in deionized, sterile water. In the setting of transplantation, DNA may be available for analysis as a byproduct of DNA-based routine tissue typing. DNA may also be isolated from stored myocardial samples *(43)*. Each genotyping reaction requires in the region of 0.01–0.1 µg of DNA.

The first step of a genotyping project is to identify DNA samples representing each of the genotypes being analyzed (i.e., AA, AB, and BB genotype). These will serve both as control templates for PCR optimization and as reference standards during subsequent analysis. Identifying DNA samples representing the three genotypes may have to be done by screening a large range of DNA samples essentially at random. Where the polymorphism is relatively frequent, as in the case of adenosine monophosphate deaminase (AMPD)-1 (described later), an initial screen of 1–200 DNA samples should reveal all genotypes. Alternatively, artificial target sequences can be synthesized and diluted appropriately for use. Once samples of all three genotypes have been detected, these can be included as controls against which the SDS software compares emissions from wells of unknown sample type and so ascribes the correct genotype. This feature is known as autocalling, and because 12 wells are required for samples of known genotype (3 for each of both homozygous genotypes, 3 for heterozygous genotypes, and 3 no-template controls), the genotypes of only 84 samples can be determined per 96-well plate.

3.4. AMPD-1 Genotyping Using Real-Time PCR

Because of its likely role in cardioprotection *(44,45)*, we have examined the C34T SNP (Gln12STOP) of (AMPD-1) in 392 cardiac transplant recipients, 377 of their donors, and 294 unrelated Caucasian controls using a real-time PCR-based allelic discrimination assay *(46)*. The method used for this and other similar projects, outlined in **Fig. 6,** included confirmation of genotype by single-stranded conformational polymorphism (SSCP) analysis in 10% of samples. All results were concordant between the two methods. Previous studies showed that approx 21% of Caucasians carry the C34T T allele, and heart failure patients possessing this allele have been shown to survive longer without need for transplantation (mean 7.6 vs 3.2 yr; $p < 0.001$) *(44)*. Carriers of the C34T T allele have substantially reduced cardiac AMPD activity *(47)*, which through increasing adenosine may contribute to cardioprotection. We found an association between possession of the C34T T allele in cardiac donors with reduced pre-donation inotrope requirements *(48)* suggesting a cardioprotective effect in the setting of donor organ function.

4. Conclusion

Since the launch of the original chemistry and instrumentation, quantitative real-time RT-PCR has become commonplace in laboratories worldwide, and its popularity has ensured the development of a large variety of chemistries and instruments to suit every budget and throughput requirement. The exceptional accuracy and sensitivity easily achievable with real-time PCR make it the method of choice for mRNA quantification, especially from limited tissue samples. When beginning a real-time RT-PCR project, it is important to remember that the technique is based entirely on the assumption that the amount of cDNA amplified and detected is an accurate reflection of the corresponding mRNA levels in the starting material and thus to consider how each aspect of the protocol may bias this assumption and consequently the conclusions. Genotyping using real-time PCR technology is also an accurate and useful method for single nucleotide polymorphism association studies in cardiac transplantation.

Acknowledgments

We thank Antony Mullen for his initial assistance in setting up real-time PCR and the Magdi Yacoub Institute, British Heart Foundation, and the Royal Brompton and Harefield NHS Trust for financial support.

References

1. Holland, P. M., Abramson, R. D., Watson, R., and Gelfand, D. H. (1991) Detection of specific polymerase chain reaction product by utilizing the 5'-3' nuclease actively of Thermus aquaticus DNA polymerase. *Proc. Natl. Acad. Sci. USA* **88**, 7276–7280.
2. Gibson, U. E. M., Heid, C. A., and Williams, P. M. (1996) A novel method for real time quantitative RT-PCR. *Genome Res.* **6**, 995–1001.
3. Heid, C. A., Stevens, J., Livak, K. J., and Williams, P. M. (1996) Real time quantitative PCR. *Genome Res.* **6**, 986–994.
4. Livak, K. J., Flood, S. J., Marmaro, J., Giusti, W., and Deetz, K. (1995) Oligonucleotides with fluorescent dyes at opposite ends provide a quenched probe system useful for detecting PCR product and nucleic acid hybridization. *PCR Methods Appl.* **4**, 357–362.
5. Bustin, S. A. (2000) Absolute quantification of mRNA using real-time reverse transcription polymerase chain reaction assays. *J. Mol. Endocrinol.* **25**, 169–193.
6. Bustin, S. A. (2002) Quantification of mRNA using real-time reverse transcription PCR (RT-PCR): trends and problems. *J. Mol. Endocrinol.* **29**, 23–39.
7. Ginzinger, D. G. (2002) Gene quantification using real-time quantitative PCR: an emerging technology hits the mainstream. *Exp. Hematol.* **30**, 503–512.
8. Brand, N. J. and Barton, P. J. R. (2002) Myocardial molecular biology: an introduction. *Heart* **87**, 284–293.

9. Barton, P. J. R., Birks, E. J., Felkin, L. E., Cullen, M. E., Koban, M. U., and Yacoub, M. H. (2003) Increased expression of extracellular matrix regulators TIMP1 and MMP1 in deteriorating heart failure. *J. Heart Lung Transplant.* **22**, 738–744.
10. De Souza, A. I., Felkin, L. E., Barton, P. J. R., Banner, N. R., and Rose, M. L. (2003) Sequential expression of three known protective genes in cardiac biopsies after transplantation.J. Heart Lung Transplant. **22(1)**, S163.
11. Barton, P. J. R., Felkin, L. E., Koban, M. U., Cullen, M. E., Brand, N. J., and Dhoot, G. K. (2004) The slow skeletal muscle troponin T gene is expressed in developing and diseased human heart. *Mol. Cell. Biochem.* **263**, 81–90.
12. SYBR Green PCR Master Mix and RT-PCR. (2004) Applied Biosystems Protocol: Rev C Part 4310251C.
13. Morrison, T. B., Weis, J. J., and Wittwer, C. T. (1998) Quantification of low-copy transcripts by continuous SYBR Green I monitoring during amplification. *BioTechniques* **24**, 954–958, 960, 962.
14. Primer Express Software v1.5 Applications-based primer design software. (2004) Applied Biosystems User's Manual: Rev D Part 4303014D.
15. TaqMan Gene Expression Assays. (2004) Applied Biosystems Protocol Rev B 4333458B.
16. Assays-by-Design service for gene expression assays. (2004) Applied Biosystems Protocol Part 4334429C.
17. van Hoof, A. and Parker, R. (2003) Messenger RNA degradation: beginning at the end. *Curr. Biol.* **12**, R285–R287.
18. Tong, D., Schneeberger, C., Leodolter, S., and Zeillinger, R. (1997) Quantitative determination of gene expression by competitive reverse transcription-polymerase chain reaction in degraded RNA samples. *Anal. Biochem.* **251**, 173–177.
19. Jones, L. J., Yue, S. T., Cheung, C. Y., and Singer, V. L. (1998) RNA quantitation by fluorescence-based solution assay: RiboGreen reagent characterization. *Anal. Biochem.* **265**, 368–374.
20. Stahlberg, A., Hakansson, J., Xian, X., Semb, H., and Kubista, M. (2004) Properties of the reverse transcription reaction in mRNA quantification. *Clin. Chem.* **50(3)**, 509–515.
21. Deprez, R. H. L., Fijnvandraat, A. C., Ruijter, J. M., and Moorman, A. F. M. (2002) Sensitivity and accuracy of quantitative real-time polymerase chain reaction using SYBR green I depends on cDNA synthesis conditions. *Anal. Biochem.* **307**, 63–69.
22. Pfaffl, M. W. and Hageleit, M. (2001) Validities of mRNA quantification using recombinant RNA and recombinant DNA external calibration curves in real-time RT-PCR. *Biotechnol. Lett.* **23**, 275–282.
23. Depre, C., Shipley, G. L., Chen, W., et al. (1998) Unloaded heart *in vivo* replicates fetal gene expression of cardiac hypertrophy. *Nat. Med.* **4**, 1269–1275.
24. Uray, I. P., Connelly, J. H., Thomazy, V., et al. (2002) Left ventricular unloading alters receptor tyrosine kinase expression in the failing human heart. *J. Heart Lung Transplant.* **21**, 771–782.

25. Relative quantitation of gene expression: ABI PRISM 7700 Sequence detection system. (1997) Applied Biosystems User Bulletin #2: Rev B Part 4304859B, pp. 1–36.
26. Peirson, S. N., Butler, J. N., and Foster, R. G. (2003) Experimental validation of novel and conventional approaches to quantitative real-time PCR data analysis. *Nucleic Acids Res.* **31**, e73.
27. Ramakers, C., Ruijter, J. M., Deprez, R. H. L., and Moorman, A. F. M. (2003) Assumption-free analysis of quantitative real-time polymerase chain reaction (PCR) data. *Neurosci. Lett.* **339**, 62–66.
28. Liu, W. and Saint, D. A. (2002) A new quantitative method of real time reverse transcription polymerase chain reaction assay based on simulation of polymerase chain reaction kinetics. *Anal. Biochem.* **302**, 52–59.
29. Liu, W. and Saint, D. A. (2002) Validation of a quantitative method for real time PCR kinetics. *Biochem. Biophys. Res. Commun.* **294**, 347–353.
30. Pfaffl, M. W., Horgan, G. W., and Dempfle, L. (2002) Relative expression software tool (REST) for group-wise comparison and statistical analysis of relative expression results in real-time PCR. *Nucleic Acids Res.* **30**, e36.
31. Pfaffl, M. W. (2001) A new mathematical model for relative quantification in real-time RT-PCR. *Nucleic Acids Res.* **29**, e45.
32. Vandesompele, J., De Preter, K., Pattyn, F., et al. (2002) Accurate normalization of real-time quantitative RT-PCR data by geometric averaging of multiple internal control genes. *Genome Biol.* **3**, 1–2.
33. Pfaffl, M. W., Tichopad, A., Prgomet, C., and Neuvians, T. P. (2004) Determination of stable housekeeping genes, differentially regulated target genes and sample integrity: BestKeeper—Excel-based tool using pair-wise correlations. *Biotechnol. Lett.* **26**, 509–515.
34. Livak, K. J. and Schmittgen, T. D. (2001) Analysis of relative gene expression data using real-time quantitative PCR and the 2(-delta delta C(T)) method. *Methods* **25**, 402–408.
35. Razeghi, P., Young, M. E., Cockrill, T. C., Frazier, O. H., and Taegtmeyer, H. (2002) Downregulation of myocardial myocyte enhancer factor 2C and myocyte enhancer factor 2C-regulated gene expression in diabetic patients with nonischemic heart failure. *Circulation* **106**, 407–411.
36. Multiple PCR with TaqMan VIC probes: ABI PRISM 7700 sequence detection system. Applied Biosystems User Bulletin 5: Rev B Part 4306236B, 2004.
37. Afonina, I. A., Reed, M. W., Lusby, E., Shishkina, I. G., and Belousov, Y. S. (2002) Minor groove binder-conjugated DNA probes for quantitative DNA detection by hybridization-triggered fluorescence. *BioTechniques* **32**, 940–949.
38. Afonina, I., Zivarts, M., Kutyavin, I., Lukhtanov, E., Gamper, H., and Meyer, R. B. (1997) Efficient priming of PCR with short oligonucleotides conjugated to a minor groove binder. *Nucleic Acids Res.* **25**, 2657–2660.
39. Kutyavin, I. V., Lukhtanov, E. A., Gamper, H. B., and Meyer, R. B. (1997) Oligonucleotides with conjugated dihydropyrroloindole tripeptides: base composition and backbone effects on hybridization. *Nucleic Acids Res.* **25**, 3718-3723.

40. Primer express v 1.5 and TaqMan MGB probes for allelic discrimination: All PCR instruments. (2000) Applied Biosystems User Bulletin Part 4317594A, pp. 1–28.
41. Assays-on-Demand SNP genotyping products. (2004) Applied Biosystems Protocol Rev A Part 4332856A.
42. Assays-by-Design Service for SNP Assays. (2004) Applied Biosystems Protocol Rev C Part 4334431C.
43. Cunningham, D. A., Crisp, S. J., Barbir, M., Lazem, F., Dunn, M. J., and Yacoub, M. H. (1998) Donor ACE gene polymorphism: A genetic risk factor for accelerated coronary sclerosis following cardiac transplantation. *Eur. Heart J.* **19**, 319–325.
44. Loh, E., Rebbeck, T. R., Mahoney, P. D., Denofrio, D., Swain, J. L., and Holmes, E. W. (1999) Common variant in AMPD1 gene predicts improved clinical outcome in patients with heart failure. *Circulation* **99**, 1422–1425.
45. Anderson, J. L., Habashi, J., Carlquist, J. F., et al. (2000) A common variant of the AMPD1 gene predicts improved cardiovascular survival in patients with coronary artery disease. *J. Am. Coll. Cardiol.* **36**, 1248–1252.
46. Taegtmeyer, A. B., Breen, J. B., Smith, J. D., et al. (2004) Increased incidence of acute rejection among cardiac transplant recipients possessing the Gln12STOP variant of AMPD-1. *Am. J. Transplant.* **4(8)**, 311.
47. Kalsi, K. K., Yuen, A. H., Rybakowska, I. M., et al. (2003) Decreased cardiac activity of AMP deaminase in subjects with the AMPD1 mutation-A potential mechanism of protection in heart failure. *Cardiovasc. Res.* **59**, 678–684.
48. Taegtmeyer, A. B., Breen, J., Smith, J. D., Banner, N. R., Yacoub, M. H., and Barton, P. J. (2004) Increased frequency of adenosine monophosphate deaminase 1 C34TT allele in cardiac donors is associated with reduced pre-donation inotrope. *J. Heart Lung Transplant.* **23(2)**, S89.
49. Owen, V. J., Burton, P. B. J., Mullen, A. J., Birks, E. J., Barton, P. J. R., and Yacoub, M. H. (2001) Expression of RGS3, RGS4 and Gi alpha 2 in acutely failing donor hearts and end-stage heart failure. *Eur. Heart J.* **22**, 1015–1020.
50. Radonic, A., Thulke, S., Mackay, I. M., Landt, O., Siegert, W., and Nitsche, A. (2004) Guideline to reference gene selection for quantitative real-time PCR. *Biochem. Biophys. Res. Commun.* **313**, 856–862.
51. Bijlsma, F. J., Bruggink, A. H., Hartman, M., et al. (2001) No association between IL-10 promoter gene polymorphism and heart failure or rejection following cardiac transplantation. *Tissue Antigens* **57**, 151–153.
52. Gourley, I. S., Denofrio, D., Rand, W., Desai, S., Loh, E., and Kamoun, M. (2004) The effect of recipient cytokine gene polymorphism on cardiac transplant outcome. *Hum. Immunol.* **65**, 248–254.
53. Densem, C. G., Hutchinson, I. V., Yonan, N., and Brooks, N. H. (2003) Influence of interleukin-10 polymorphism on the development of coronary vasculopathy following cardiac transplantation. *Transplant. Immunol.* **11**, 223–228.
54. Vamvakopoulos, J. E., Taylor, C. J., Green, C., et al. (2002) Interleukin 1 and chronic rejection: possible genetic links in human heart allografts. *Am. J. Transplant.* **2**, 76–83.

55. He, J. Q., Gaur, L. K., Stempien-Otero, A., et al. (2002) Genetic variants of the hemostatic system and development of transplant coronary artery disease. *J. Heart Lung Transplant.* **21**, 629–636.
56. Zheng, H., Webber, S., Zeevi, A., et al. (2003) Tacrolimus dosing in pediatric heart transplant patients is related to CYP3A5 and MDR1 gene polymorphisms. *Am. J. Transplant.* **3**, 477–483.
57. Gonzalez-Amieva, A., Lopez-Miranda, J., Marin, C., et al. (2003) The apo A-I gene promoter region polymorphism determines the severity of hyperlipidemia after heart transplantation. *Clin. Transplant.* **17**, 56–62.

15

Organ Preservation

Mark Hicks, Alfred Hing, Ling Gao, Jonathon Ryan, and Peter S. MacDonald

Summary

The success of organ transplantation is critically dependent on the quality of the donor organ. Donor organ quality, in turn, is determined by a variety of factors including donor age and preexisting disease, the mechanism of brain death, donor management prior to organ procurement, the duration of hypothermic storage, and the circumstances of reperfusion. It has been recognized for some time that both the short- and long-term outcomes after cadaveric organ transplantation are significantly inferior to those obtained when the transplanted organ is obtained from a living donor, regardless of whether the donor is related or unrelated to the recipient. Brain death results in a series of hemodynamic, neurohormonal, and pro-inflammatory perturbations, all of which are thought to contribute to donor organ dysfunction. The process of transplantation exposes the donor organ to an obligatory period of ischemia and reperfusion. Traditionally, hypothermic storage of the donor organ has been used to protect it from ischemic injury, but donor organs differ markedly in their capacity to withstand hypothermic ischemia. Data from the Registry of the International Society for Heart and Lung Transplantation indicate that the risk of primary graft failure and death rises dramatically for both the heart and lung as ischemic time increases. Based on these data, maximum recommended ischemic times for the donor heart and lung are 6 and 8 h, respectively. In this chapter, strategies aimed at minimizing the adverse consequences of brain death and ischemia/reperfusion injury to the donor heart and lung are discussed. These strategies are likely to become increasingly important as the reliance on marginal donors increases to meet the growing demand for organ transplantation.

Key Words: Brain death; neurohormonal changes; intensive care; catecholamines; hormonal therapy; reperfusion therapy.

1. Introduction

The success of organ transplantation is critically dependent on the quality of the donor organ. Donor organ quality, in turn, is determined by a variety of

From: *Methods in Molecular Biology, vol. 333: Transplantation Immunology: Methods and Protocols*
Edited by: P. Hornick and M. Rose © Humana Press Inc., Totowa, NJ

factors including donor age and preexisting disease, the mechanism of brain death, donor management prior to organ procurement, the duration of hypothermic storage, and the circumstances of reperfusion. As demand for solid organ transplantation has increased, so has the use of marginal donors (e.g., those obtained from older donors or from donors with evidence of chronic organ disease or dysfunction prior to brain death) *(1)*. Thus, many cadaveric organs offered for transplantation have preexisting disease or dysfunction prior to the onset of brain death, and although results obtained with marginal doors are generally regarded as acceptable (at least in relation to the waiting list mortality), it is clear that both short- and long-term posttransplant outcomes are not as good when compared with organs obtained from conventional donors *(2,3)*. Furthermore, although the use of marginal donors has led to an increase in the potential donor pool, it has also led to an increased discard rate of cadaveric organs offered for transplantation. For example, as reported by Rosendale et al. *(1)*, "the discard rate of kidneys procured from the cadaver donor in USA has been increasing to an alarming level of more than 15% of those kidneys recovered for transplantation." The discard rate for other organs is even higher. Approximately 25% of livers and 60% of hearts and lungs from cadaveric donors are not transplanted due to poor donor organ quality *(4,5)*.

Another factor that adversely affects donor organ quality is brain death. It has been recognized for some time that both the short- and long-term outcomes after cadaveric organ transplantation are significantly inferior to those obtained when the transplanted organ is obtained from a living donor whether the donor is related or unrelated to the recipient *(6)*. Brain death results in a series of hemodynamic, neurohormonal, and pro-inflammatory perturbations, all of which are thought to contribute to donor organ dysfunction.

Finally, the process of transplantation exposes the donor organ to an obligatory period of ischemia and reperfusion. Traditionally, hypothermic storage of the donor organ has been used to protect it from ischemic injury, but donor organs differ markedly in their capacity to withstand hypothermic ischemia. Data from the Registry of the International Society for Heart and Lung Transplantation indicate that the risk of primary graft failure and death rises dramatically for both the heart and lung as ischemic time increases *(2,3)*. Based on these data, the maximum recommended ischemic times for the donor heart and lung are 6 and 8 h, respectively.

In this chapter, strategies aimed at minimizing the adverse consequences of brain death and ischemia/reperfusion (I/R) injury to the donor heart and lung are discussed. These strategies are likely to become increasingly important as the reliance on marginal donors increases to meet the growing demand for organ transplantation.

2. Management of the Brain-Dead Donor

2.1. The Hemodynamic, Neurohumoral, and Immunological Consequences of Brain Death

2.1.1. Hemodynamic Changes

Brain death is accompanied by a series of complex hemodynamic, neurohormonal, and immunological changes. The time course and severity of these changes may vary according to the tempo and nature of the neurological insult leading to brain death. The most severe changes are usually seen in the setting of acute onset of brain death (such as occurs with severe intracranial hemorrhage), which is associated typically with an acute and intense autonomic discharge, characterized by initial bradycardia (parasympathetic discharge) followed by extreme tachycardia and hypertension (sympathetic discharge). Potential donor organs suffer an ischemic insult during this phase—the heart as a result of a massive increase in workload *(7)* and the peripheral organs caused by intense peripheral vasoconstriction *(8)*. This autonomic storm has its onset within the first few minutes and usually passes within 15 min. The autonomic storm is also characterized by a sudden increase in cytosolic calcium, which in turn activates enzymes such as lipase, protease, endonuclease, nitric oxide (NO) synthase, and xanthine oxidase *(8)*. These enzymatic changes disrupt normal adenosyl triphosphate (ATP) utilization and generate oxygen-free radicals, which contribute to organ failure. Thereafter, there is a loss of sympathetic tone associated with persistent tachycardia and hypotension. The loss of autonomic tone also results in impaired vascular autoregulation with diminished blood supply and oxygen delivery to organs and tissues. Both initial and late circulatory changes can lead to severe ischemic damage in donor organs before their removal, causing deterioration of the quality of the transplanted graft.

2.1.2. Neurohormonal Changes

Although most investigators accept a link between brain death and disruption of the hypothalamic–pituitary axis, there are conflicting data regarding the hormonal changes that occur during and after central nervous system injury and their influence on hemodynamic parameters and organ quality ***(9–11)***. In animal models the hormonal changes fall into two categories: those associated with the autonomic storm represent a transient and massive increase in circulating catecholamines, and those associated with hypothalamic–pituitary failure lead to neurogenic diabetes insipidus and a marked decrease in levels of thyroid hormones and cortisol, at least in animal models ***(12,13)***. Metabolic abnormalities associated with these hormonal perturbations include impaired aerobic metabolism despite normal O_2 delivery. This has been demonstrated both globally ***(14)*** and in specific organs including the heart ***(12)*** and kidney ***(15)***. The consequent reliance on anaerobic metabolism results in lactic acidosis ***(12,14,15)*** and rapid depletion of high-energy substrates such as ATP ***(12)***. Progressive depletion of high-energy stores has been reversed successfully by a combination of T3, cortisol, and insulin administration, suggesting that hormonal changes are the major cause of mitochondrial dysfunction with impaired energy production at the cellular level ***(16)***.

Some investigators, however, have demonstrated only minor hormonal changes in humans after the onset of brain death ***(17,18)***. An extensive survey of studies on brain-dead human donors indicates that a reduction in the level of free triiodothyronine (T3) has almost always been documented, but changes in other hormone levels (such as thyroid-stimulating hormone, thyroxine [T4], and cortisol) are variable ***(17–21)***. Levels of reverse T3 have been found to be normal or increased after brain death, consistent with a "sick euthyroid" state. Differences between experimental and some clinical findings may be explained by the fact that the former are determined with a uniform mechanism of brain death in highly controlled systems in contrast to the latter group, in which patients suffer brain death by a variety of mechanisms.

2.1.3. Immunological/Inflammatory Changes

Studies investigating the relation between brain death and immunological activation of peripheral organs have demonstrated that the explosive increase in intracranial pressure followed by systemic hypotension upregulates various lymphocyte- and macrophage-derived cytokines on solid organs in rats ***(22)***. The hypothesis that brain death increases the immunogenicity of solid organs is further supported by findings that kidneys and hearts transplanted from brain-dead donor animals experience accelerated acute rejection compared to those from living donors ***(23)***. Early adhesion molecules (selectins) not present on the vascular cell surface under resting conditions but upregulated rapidly after injury seem to trigger subsequent events. Adherent leukocyte populations express other classes of adhesion molecules (intercellular adhesion molecule; vascular cell adhesion molecule; lymphocyte-function associated antigen-1) and release proinflammatory lymphokines (tumor necrosis factor-α, interferon [IFN]-γ). Expression of major histocompatibility complex (MHC) class I and II molecules is increased. The upregulation of MHC on graft cells is mediated primarily by IFN-γ, itself increased by the brain-death–I/R insult. The mediators of immunological activation of donor organs after brain death have not been determined. The deleterious changes in endothelial surfaces and the increasing immunogenicity of solid organs begin promptly after massive central injury, and it has been suggested that these changes can be partly explained by excessive catecholamine release ***(8)***. This hypothesis is further supported by the experimental observation that even short-term administration of catecholamines in brain-dead donors is followed by reduced survival and poor initial function after renal allotransplantation in pigs *(24)*.

2.2. Intensive Care Unit Management of the Brain-Dead Organ Donor

Donor management has been described as "the most neglected area of transplant medicine" *(25)*. In one study it was estimated that failure to provide adequate physiological support to potential donors accounted for at least 25% of lost donor organs *(26)*. Data from the Australia & New Zealand Organ Donation registry *(27)* reveals that more than 90% of brain-dead individuals develop hypotension and receive some form of inotropic/pressor support, most commonly noradrenaline. Other inotropic/pressor agents used include adrenaline, dopamine, dobutamine, and metaraminol. The choice of agent is likely to reflect local preferences, but currently there is little evidence to support the use of any single catecholamine over others. The duration of pressor support varies considerably, but 90% of brain-dead donors receive support for between 6 and 24 h, prior to donor organ removal.

The impact of the administration of catecholamines to the brain-dead donor on subsequent graft outcome remains unclear. Experimental studies in solid organ transplantation and clinical studies in heart transplantation have generally demonstrated worse outcomes when the donor has received catecholamines *(24,28–32)*. On the other hand, several clinical studies, including a recent meta-analysis, found that that graft outcomes after kidney transplantation were better when donor kidneys were obtained from donors who had received catecholamines *(32)*. In this same meta-analysis, heart transplant outcomes were worse and liver transplant outcomes were unaffected by donor catecholamine treatment. At present, it is unknown whether these differences in transplanted organ outcomes reflect differences in the type of donors that receive catecholamines, the direct effects of catecholamines on different donor organs, or indirect effects (such as better maintenance of blood flow to the kidney in donors receiving catecholamine infusions). Regardless of the explanation, this observation creates an immediate dilemma for the intensive care physician caring for the brain-dead donor. Does he or she administer a drug that appears to benefit one potential donor organ but harms another?

A series of observations reported by Rosendale et al. *(1)* suggest that it may not be necessary to optimize preservation of one organ at the expense of another. In a large retrospective review of the Organ Procurement and Transplantation Network database, they noted that 15% more kidneys were transplanted from donors whose heart was transplanted: 91 vs 76% ($p < 0.001$). Furthermore, kidneys from heart donors had a lower incidence of delayed graft function: 18 vs 25% ($p < 0.001$) and better 1-yr survival: 91 vs 87% ($p < 0.001$). These data suggest that donor treatments that optimize the function of the donor heart (and cardiac output) are likely to benefit donor kidney function as well (and presumably the function of other donor organs).

2.3. Hormonal Resuscitation of the Brain-Dead Donor

Generally accepted principles of donor management include correction of any fluid imbalance by intravenous fluid replacement, treatment of diabetes insipidus, maintenance of blood pressure using vasoconstrictors (usually) or vasodilators, with maintenance of adequate ventilation and electrolyte homeostasis ***(33–35)***. However, there is no consensus regarding correction of hormonal abnormalities in the brain-dead donor other than treatment of diabetes insipidus. The use of vasopressin or its synthetic analog desmopressin is contentious because both have been reported to impair perfusion of the donor pancreas ***(36)***. On the other hand, there is a paucity of data on the effects of other vasopressor agents on perfusion of the donor pancreas or other intra-abdominal organs.

Almost 50 yr ago, Wagner and Braunwald demonstrated that patients with autonomic failure were exquisitely sensitive to the vasoconstrictor effects of vasopressin, whereas minimal vasopressor effects were demonstrable in normal subjects ***(37)***. In 1986, Yoshioka and colleagues demonstrated that brain-dead subjects could be maintained in a stable hemodynamic state for an average of 23 d using a combination of low-dose vasopressin and adrenaline ***(38)***. In the same study, brain-dead subjects treated with adrenaline alone all progressed to cardiac arrest at an average of 24 h after brain death. More recently, several investigators have demonstrated that low-dose vasopressin is effective in restoring blood pressure and systemic vascular resistance in hemodynamically unstable brain-dead donors ***(39,40)***. Low-dose vasopressin has been shown to be effective in maintaining hepatic energy metabolism after brain death in experimental dogs ***(41)***. Furthermore, human studies have shown that renal and hepatic function are well preserved in brain-dead patients supported with low-dose vasopressin infusions ***(38,42,43)***.

Clinical trials of thyroid hormone administration to the brain-dead donor have shown variable efficacy ***(44–47)***. There are several possible explanations for the discordant results observed in clinical trials to date. In general, studies in which the brain-dead donor has been treated with thyroid hormone alone (either T3 or T4) have generally failed to demonstrate any hemodynamic benefit associated with this treatment ***(45,46,48)***. In contrast, studies of hormonal replacement in which thyroid hormone has been administered in combination with cortisol ***(44,49)*** or as part of a multihormone "cocktail" have demonstrated favorable effects on donor hemodynamic status ***(16,50)***. The extent of hormonal disturbance and the impact this has on donor organ quality may vary among donors, depending on the clinical circumstances leading to brain death. Retrospective analysis of these studies suggests that combined hormonal therapy is most useful in hemodynamically unstable donors, those with impaired left ventricular function on echocardiography, or those requiring prolonged vasopressor support.

Perhaps the most supportive clinical study for combined hormonal therapy was that performed by Wheeldon and colleagues ***(50)***. Based on the experimental work of Novitzky and colleagues ***(12,16,51,52)***, they developed a combined infusion of T3, methylprednisolone, vasopressin, and insulin, which has subsequently become known as the Papworth cocktail. They reported that in 150 consecutive multiorgan donors, 52 hearts were unacceptable for transplantation based on conventional selection criteria. Forty-four of these (92%) became acceptable after institution of Swan–Ganz monitoring, hemodynamic "optimization," and administration of combined hormonal therapy. Importantly, similar posttransplant outcomes were observed after transplantation of these resuscitated hearts compared with organs that initially met "acceptable" criteria. Largely based on the results of this study, a recent consensus meeting of various stakeholders in the United States developed a uniform cadaveric donor management protocol **(Fig. 1)** that incorporates invasive hemodynamic monitoring and hormonal resuscitation (HR) for donors who are hemodynamically unstable ***(4)***.

Recently, Rosendale et al. ***(53)*** published the findings of a large retrospective analysis of all brain-dead donors recovered in the United States from January 1, 2000, to September 30, 2001. Of 10,292 consecutive brain-dead donors analyzed, 701 (7%) received three-drug HR (T3 or L-thyroxine, methylprednisolone, and vasopressin). Univariate analysis showed that the mean number of organs from HR donors (3.8) was 22.5% greater than that from non-HR resuscitation donors (3.1) ($p < 0.001$). Multivariate analyses showed that HR was associated with the following statistically significant increased probabilities of an organ being transplanted from a donor: kidney 7.3%, heart 4.7%, liver 4.9%, lung 2.8%, and pancreas 6.0%. Extrapolation of these probabilities to the 5921 brain-dead donors recovered in 2001 was calculated to yield a total increase of 2053 organs.

2.4. Anti-Inflammatory Treatment of the Brain-Dead Donor

Another potential approach to improving the quality of cadaveric donor organs involves the use of specific or nonspecific anti-inflammatory treatments aimed at blunting or reversing the upregulation of pro-inflammatory cytokines, adhesion molecules, and donor specific antigens. The administration of high-dose steroids to brain-dead donors has been shown experimentally to improve the survival of renal and cardiac allografts ***(54,55)*** and clinically to improve donor

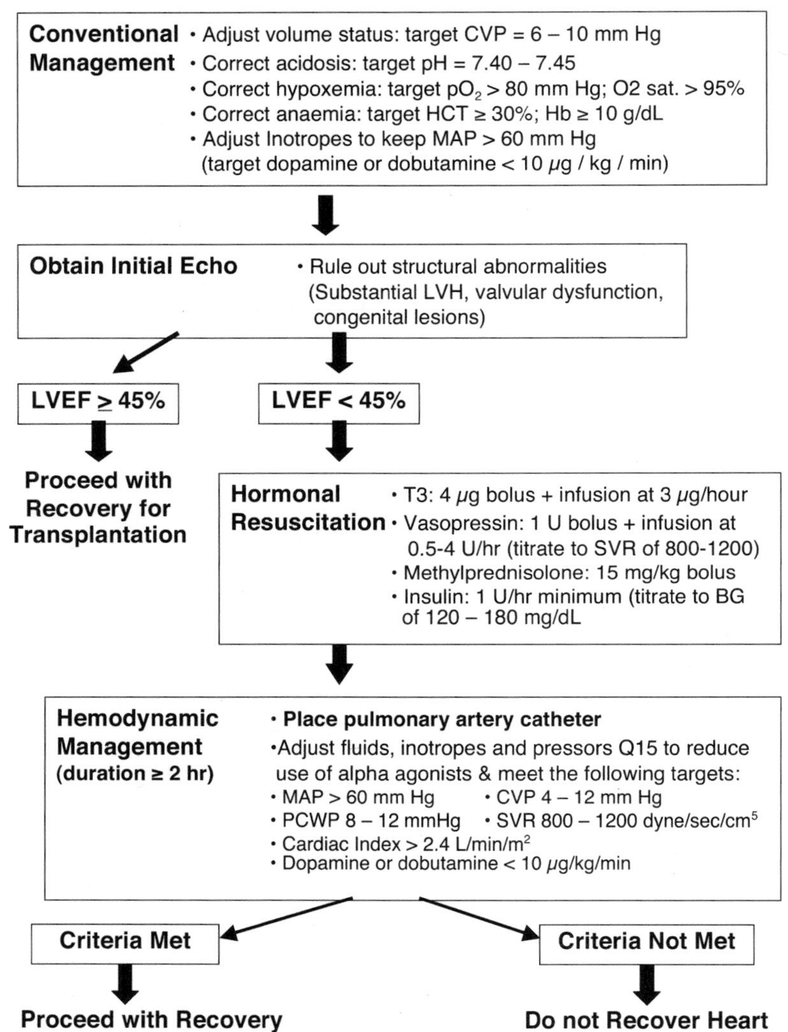

Fig. 1. Crystal City recommendations for cardiac donor management, which have been adopted into the United Network for Organ Sharing Critical Pathway. (From **ref. *5***.)

lung function, resulting in an increased number of transplanted lung allografts ***(56)***. It is noteworthy that the steroid doses of the combined hormone resuscitation protocols used in the above-mentioned studies were very high, indicating that the hormone cocktail is likely to be playing an anti-inflammatory as well as a hormone-replacement role ***(44,50,53)***.

Based on available experimental and clinical trial data reviewed above, the United Network for Organ Sharing and other stakeholders in the United States

Table 1
Lung Donor Management Recommendations

The airway
Bronchoscopy
Frequent suctioning and aspiration precautions
Albuterol therapy for wheezing (may improve lung fluid clearance)
Mechanical ventilation
Adequate oxygenation
PO_2 > 100 mmHg, FIO_2 = 0.40 or O_2 saaturation > 95%
Adequate ventilation
Maintain pH 7.35–7.45 and PCO_2 30-35 mmHg
PEEP+ 5 cm H2O
Tidal volume 10-12 mL/kg
Peak airway pressures < 30 mmHg
Fluid Management and Monitoring
CVP at a minimum; PA catheter desirable
Arterial line and pulse oximetry
Judicious fluid resuscitation to ensure end-organ perfusion
CVP 6–8 mmHg, Pcwp 8–12 mmHg
Urine output 1 mL/kg/h
Colloid as the fluid of choice for volume resuscitation
Albumin (normal serum) with normal PT, PTT; FFP with coagulopathy
Hemoglobin > 100 g/L

PO_2, partial pressure of oxygen; PIO_2, fractional concentration of O_2 in inspired gas; PCO_2, partial pressure of carbon dioxide; PEEP, positive end-expiratory pressure; CVP, central venous pressure; Pcwp, pulmonary capillary wedge pressure; PI, intrathorcic pressure; PTT, partial thromboplastin time; FFP, fresh frozen plasma.

From **ref. *4***.

have now endorsed the use of hemodynamic monitoring and combined HR in all brain-dead donors who are hemodynamically unstable, require high doses of inotropic/pressor agents, or show evidence of impaired cardiac function on echocardiography ***(4,5)***. Brain-dead donors who demonstrate one or more of these features probably account for between one-quarter and one-third of multi-organ donors. Routine administration of combined HR to these donors is likely to increase the yield of all donor organs ***(53,57)***. An algorithm for the management of the brain-dead donor developed by the Heart Working Group of the Consensus Meeting is shown in **Fig. 1**.

Additional recommendations were made by the Lung Working Group of the Consensus Meeting in relation to optimizing lung function and the suitability of the lungs for transplantation ***(4)***. These recommendations are summarized in **Table 1**. Of particular importance are management of the airway and ventilation.

Regular airway suctioning should be performed to clear bronchial secretions, and any donor with clinical or radiological signs of retained sputum or impaired alveolar ventilation should undergo bronchoscopy with bronchial toilet to clear the airways and collect specimens for microscopy and culture. Ventilator settings should be adjusted to maintain adequate oxygenation (arterial $pO_2 > 100$ mmHg or O_2 saturation > 95%) and ventilation (pH 7.35–7.45 with arterial pCO_2 30–35 mmHg) Target ventilator settings are $FiO_2 < 0.40$, PEEP $^+5$ cmH_2O, tidal volume 10–12 mL/kg, and peak airway pressure less than 30 mmHg. Major deviations from these ventilator settings should prompt the performance of a chest x-ray and bronchoscopy with corrective measures determined by the findings *(35)*.

3. Preservation of the Heart

3.1. Excision of the Donor Heart and Storage Conditions

More than 80% of cadaveric donors are multiorgan donors. Under these circumstances, the donor heart is procured during a procedure in which the lungs, liver, kidneys, and/or pancreas are also excised. After venting the venous circulation, the ascending aorta is cross-clamped and cold preservation solution is rapidly infused into the aortic root to produce rapid cooling and electromechanical arrest of the heart. Usually the donor heart is then excised and placed in a plastic bag containing approx 1 L of preservation solution. The plastic bag is then sealed and placed in an insulated container packed with ice (between 0 and 4°C), in which it is stored until implantation.

An alternative to static hypothermic ischemic storage is continuous ex vivo perfusion of the donor heart, a process that involves the continuous infusion of an oxygenated cold preservation fluid through the coronary circulation ***(58)***. Continuous ex vivo perfusion has been used to preserve donor kidneys since the 1960s. Experimental studies of continuous perfusion of the explanted heart have found that high flow rates can cause myocardial edema and early graft dysfunction ***(59–61)***. This tendency may be reduced by the addition of high-molecular-weight vascular impermeants (colloids) such as hydroxyethyl starch, polyethylene glycol, or dextran 40 to the perfusion fluid to prevent the accumulation of fluid in the interstitial space by exerting colloidal oncotic pressure in the intravascular space ***(60)***.

Alternatively, continuous low-flow or micro-perfusion has been shown experimentally to provide superior results to static hypothermic storage during extended preservation times. Indeed, excellent preservation of the donor rabbit heart for storage times up to 24 hr has been demonstrated with this technique ***(60)***. Despite the strong experimental data in support of its superior efficacy, the clinical uptake of continuous ex vivo perfusion of the donor heart has been very limited. There are several likely reasons for this. First, acceptable transplant outcomes have been obtained with static hypothermic storage of the donor heart for periods of up to 6 hr. Second, continuous perfusion systems are perceived as being costly and cumbersome. Third, the perfusion system requires close monitoring to ensure that the perfusate is bubble-free and is being delivered into the coronary circulation at the appropriate flow rate.

3.2. Cardiac Injury During Storage and Transplantation

3.2.1. Hypothermic Ischemia: The Good and the Bad

A common feature of all methods of donor heart preservation described to date has been the use of hypothermia, which markedly reduces myocardial energy consumption and slows the loss of high-energy substrates. According to the van't Hoff equation, the activity of enzymatic reactions is reduced by approx 50% for every 10°C reduction in temperature ***(62)***. For static ischemic storage, profound hypothermia (1–4°C in a standard ice chest) has been found to produce satisfactory myocardial protection for up to 6 h in clinical heart transplantation ***(63)***. Equivalent levels of myocardial preservation have been reported after 4 h of storage of the canine heart at 4 and 12°C ***(64)***. With continuous ex vivo perfusion, excellent myocardial protection may be achieved with lesser degrees of hypothermia ***(65)***.

The benefits of hypothermia, however, come at a cost. A major hazard of hypothermia is cell swelling. Normally, the cationic composition of intracellular (high K^+, low Na^+) and extracellular fluid (high Na^+, low K^+) is maintained by the membrane Na,K-ATPase pump, which uses energy (ATP) derived from oxidative phosphorylation in mitochondria. The total intracellular colloid osmotic pressure derived from the intracellular proteins and impermeable anions is approx 110–140 mOsm/kg ***(62)***. Anaerobic–hypothermic preservation suppresses the Na,K-ATPase pump. Sodium and chloride diffuse into the cell down their ionic concentration gradients, and the water that follows leads to cell swelling. Hence, in order to prevent cell swelling, impermeable substances must be added to the preservation solution to generate the same amount of osmotic pressure present in the intracellular compartment. Examples include the intravascular impermeants mentioned above. Other impermeants that can be used for this purpose are saccharides such as lactobionate, raffinose, glucose, and mannitol or anions such as citrate, phosphate, sulfate, and gluconate.

Another consequence of hypothermic ischemic storage is intracellular Ca^{2+} accumulation. Under normothermic conditions, myocyte handling of Ca^{2+} is an energy-dependent process, in which Ca^{2+} is removed from the cytoplasm (directly and indirectly) by the action of ATPases. Inactivation of these ATPases together with activation of the Na^+-H^+ exchanger (*see* below) during hypothermic storage allows Ca^{2+} to accumulate within the cytoplasm, resulting in Ca^{2+} overload during storage.

Hypothermia markedly slows myocardial energy consumption but does not arrest it completely. Under hypothermic ischemic storage conditions, the energy-dependent processes required to maintain cell viability can only be sustained through anaerobic glycolysis. This results in rapid depletion of high-energy substrates, lactic acid production, and intracellular acidosis. High levels of intracellular lactic acid not only injure cellular organelles, but also can activate macrophages. This, in turn, can lead to cytokine production and the initiation of an inflammatory response ***(62)***.

The accumulation of intracellular H^+ ion during hypothermic ischemic storage activates a membrane-bound Na-H ion exchanger or antiporter ***(66)*** **(Fig. 2)**. This ion exchanger, while quiescent under normal conditions, is activated by a decrease in intracellular pH and is driven by the transmembrane ionic gradients for Na^+ and H^+ in an energy-independent process. The Na-H antiporter exchanges intracellular H^+ for extracellular Na^+. With inactivation of the Na,K-ATPase pump by hypothermia, the resultant accumulation of intracellular Na^+ reverses the direction of a second membrane ion exchanger (the Na-Ca antiporter), which exchanges intracellular Na^+ for extracellular Ca^{2+}. Hence, the net effect of intracellular acidosis during ischemia is an accumulation of intracellular Ca^{2+} ***(66)***. One method to prevent acidosis during hypothermia is the addition of hydrogen ion buffers to the preservation solution. Hydrogen ion buffers used for cardiac preservation include potassium phosphate, sodium bicarbonate, magnesium sulfate, and histidine. One of the distinguishing characteristics of Bretschneider (HTK) solution, for example, is its extremely high concentration of histidine in comparison with other organ-preservation solutions **(Table 2)**. An alternative (and possibly more effective) approach to preventing the harmful effects of acidosis is via pharmacological inhibition of the Na-H exchanger ***(67)***.

3.2.2. Reperfusion Injury

Although restoration of oxygenated blood flow is essential to the survival of ischemic tissue, the process of reperfusion can paradoxically lead to further tissue injury ***(68)***. The severity of this reperfusion injury is directly related to the severity and duration of the ischemic insult that preceded it. Reperfusion injury results in myocyte damage through myocardial stunning, microvascular and endothelial injury, and irreversible cell damage or necrosis (lethal reperfusion injury). The major chemical mediators are thought to be oxygen-derived free radicals and Ca^{2+} ***(68)***. In addition, there is evidence that white blood cells directly contribute to reperfusion injury after periods of prolonged ischemia ***(69)***.

3.2.2.1. Oxygen-Derived Free Radicals

Restoration of oxygen to tissues that have accumulated anaerobic metabolites leads to a burst in the production of oxygen-derived free radicals and oxi-

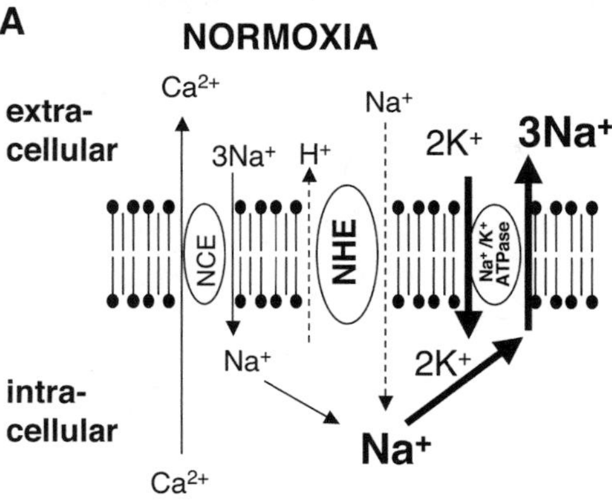

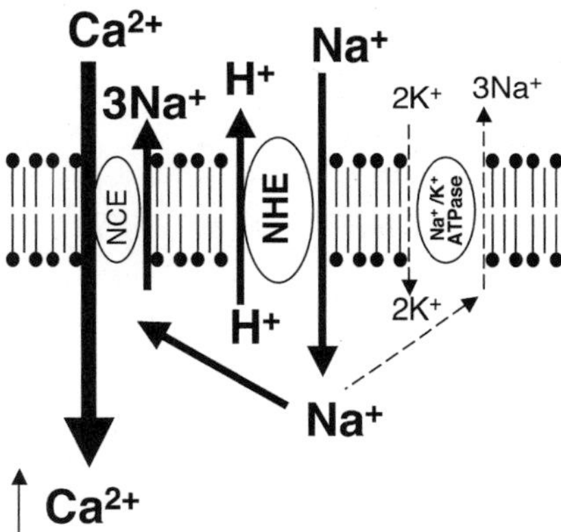

Fig. 2. Activity of the sodium hydrogen exchanger under normal conditions and during ischaemia reperfusion. Under normoxic conditions (Panel A), ATP supply is nonlimiting. Internal sodium is extruded via Na^+/K^+ ATPase, calcium is extruded via the sodium/calcium exchanger and the sodium/hydrogen exchanger is quiescent. As a consequence of ischaemia (Panel B), ATP is depleted and the Na^+/K^+ ATPase becomes inactive. Accumulation of H^+ as a result of glycolysis, activates the sodium hydrogen exchanger, resulting a large influx of sodium. This sodium is now cleared by the sodium/calcium exchanger resulting in a dangerous intracellular accumulation of calcium which may cause electrical instability, contractile dysfunctions and myocyte death.

dants. These include superoxide anion, hydrogen peroxide, hypochlorous acid, hydroxyl radical, and peroxynitrite. Small amounts of oxygen-derived free radicals are produced as a normal byproduct of a number of essential cellular processes (e.g., mitochondrial energy production and cell-to-cell signaling) but are prevented from causing cell injury by a variety of cellular antioxidant mecha-

Table 2
Composition and Clinical Usage of Some Commercial Preservation Solutions

Component	UW	m-EC	HTK	Stanford	STHS2	Celsior	Perfadex
Ionic Compositin							
Na^+ (mmol/L)	30	10	10	25	120	100	138
K^+ (mmol/L)	120	115	10	30	16	15	6
Cl (mmol/L)	0	15	50	30	203	41.5	142
Mg^{2+} (mmol/L)	5	0	4	0	16	13	0.8
Ca^{2+} (mmol/L)	0	0	0.015	0	1.2	0.25	0.3
Acid-Base Buffers							
Bicarbonate (mmol/L)	0	10	0	25	10	0	0
Phospage (mmol/L)	25	57.5	0	0	0	0	0.8
Sulphate (mmol/L)	4	0	0	0	0	0	00.8
Histidine	0	0	180	0	0	30	0
Impermeants							
Lactobionate (mmol/L)	100	0	0	0	0	80	0
Raffinose (mmol/L)	30	0	0	0	0	0	0
Hydroxyethyl starch (g/L)	50	0	0	0	0	0	0
Dextran 40 (g/L)	0	0	0	0	0	0	50
Mannitol (mmol/L)	0	0	30	12.5	0	60	0
Glucose (mmol/L)	0	214	0	50	0	0	5
Metabolic Agents							
Adenosine (mmol/L)	5	0	0	0	0	0	0
Glutamate (mmol/L)	0	0	0	0	0	20	0
Ketoglutarate (mmol/L)	0	0	1	0	0	0	0
Tryptophan (mmol/L)	0	0	2	0	0	0	0
Anti-Oxidants							
Glutathione (mmol/L)	2	0	0	0	0	3	0
Allopurinol (mmol/L)	1	0	0	0	0	0	0
pH 7.4	7.4	7.2	8.1–8.4	7.8	7.3	7.4	
Osmolality (mOsm/L)	320	375	310	440	324	360	302

Clinical usage	UW	m-EC	HTK	Stanford	STHS2	Celsior	Perfadex
Organ							
Kidney	+++	+/–	++	–	–	+	–
Liver	+++	+/–	++	–	–	+	–
Heart	+	–	++	+	+	++	–
Lung	+	+	++	+/–	–	++	+++
Pancreas	+++	+/–	++	–	–	+	–

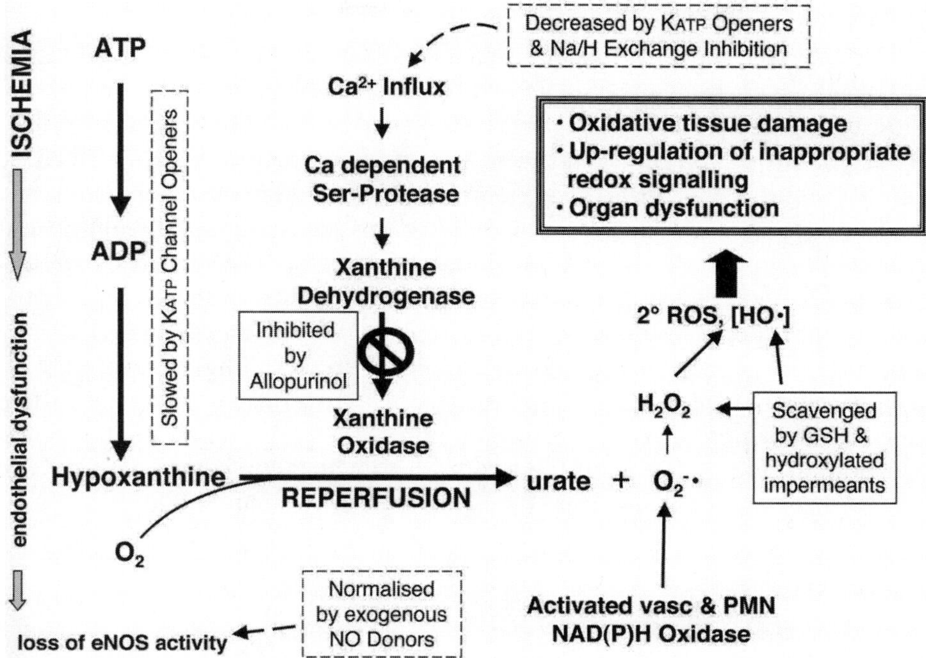

Fig. 3. Outline of some of the potential free radical consequences of ischaemia reperfusion during organ harvest, storage, re-implantation and reperfusion. Some experimental approaches to minimize various elements of the process are shown in red dashed boxes. Approaches incorporated into commercially available storage solutions are shown in solid boxes.

nisms. The abrupt increase in cellular levels of oxygen-derived free radicals that occurs during reperfusion after prolonged ischemia is due in part to excess production of free radicals via reaction of xanthine and hypoxanthine with xanthine oxidase. In addition, prolonged ischemia depletes the cell of its antioxidant reserves so that it is less capable of scavenging any excess free radicals generated during reperfusion. Oxygen-derived free radicals contribute to cell injury through a wide variety of chemical reactions including lipid peroxidation, abnormal crosslinking, and cleavage of proteins and DNA disruption. Potential approaches to the prevention of the burst in oxygen-derived free radical accumulation during organ storage and reperfusion (**Fig. 3**) include the addition to the preservation solution of a pharmacological inhibitor of xanthine oxidase, such as allopurinol, and the addition of antioxidant free radical scavengers. Examples include reduced glutathione, mannitol, superoxide dismutase, desferrioxamine, and 21-aminosteroids.

3.2.2.2. Ca^{2+} Overload During Reperfusion

As described previously, there is an accumulation of intracellular Ca^{2+} during hypothermic ischemic storage due to coupled activation of the Na-H and Na-Ca exchangers. Reperfusion with oxygenated blood initially leads to further activation of the Na-H exchanger resulting in further Ca^{2+} influx ***(67)***. In addition to increased Ca^{2+} influx, Ca^{2+} reuptake into the sarcoplasmic reticulum is reduced as a result of depressed activity of the sarcoplasmic reticulum Ca^{2+} pump (following depletion of intracellular ATP levels). The sustained increase in diastolic Ca^{2+} has two potentially lethal consequences for the myocyte: sustained contraction (contracture) of actin–myosin proteins and sustained activation of Ca^{2+}-dependent enzymes within mitochondria resulting in mitochondrial failure. Potential approaches to prevention of Ca^{2+} overload during reperfusion include a reduction in the Ca^{2+} concentration of the preservation fluid, supplementation of the preservation fluid with Mg^{2+}, which competes with Ca^{2+} for Ca^{2+} exchangers and pumps, and the addition of drugs that inhibit Ca^{2+} influx. These include Ca^{2+} channel blockers and Na-H exchange inhibitors.

3.2.2.3. White Blood Cells

White blood cells are another potential source of oxygen-derived free radicals. Ischemic injury to the vascular endothelium leads to upregulation of various adhesion molecules, which initiate sticking and activation of circulating white cells and platelets to the vessel lumen ***(69)***. In addition to release of free radicals, white cells may physically plug the lumens of microscopic vessels within the reperfused organ, leading to the no-reflow phenomenon ***(70)***. The use of white blood cell filters at the time of reperfusion has been shown experimentally and clinically to reduce evidence of reperfusion injury and graft dysfunction ***(71,72)***.

3.2.2.4. Endothelial Injury During Ischemia and Reperfusion

Under normal physiological conditions, the vascular endothelium synthesizes compounds that induce vascular relaxation and inhibit white cell and platelet adherence to the vessel wall. These compounds include NO, endothelium-dependent hyperpolarization factor, and prostacyclin. Ischemic injury to endothelial cells inhibits production of these compounds upregulating of prothrombotic and pro-inflammatory adhesion molecules as a consequence. Oxygen-derived free radicals generated on reperfusion may further damage the vascular endothelium. For example, superoxide reacts directly with NO, leading to loss of the physiological activity of NO and formation of peroxynitrite, a potent cytotoxic-free radical. Nitric oxide and prostacyclin are potent vasodilators and possess cytoprotective properties that may be beneficial for preservation of allograft function during and after cold ischemic storage. Prostacyclin and related prostanoids have been used to produce maximal vasodilatation within the vascular bed of the donor organ either via prior intravenous administration ***(73–76)*** or by addition to the preservation solution ***(73,77,78)***. Similarly, NO donors (e.g., glyceryl trinitrate and diazenium diolates—NONOates) have been added to preservation solutions to offset the loss of endogenous NO that occurs during hypothermic storage and reperfusion ***(79–81)***.

Endothelial injury caused by I/R injury has been implicated as a factor in the development of both acute allograft dysfunction and chronic allograft vasculopathy. Another potential source of endothelial injury is the high K^+ concentration of some intracellular preservation solutions such as University of Wisconsin (UW) solution, although this remains controversial. Several clinical studies suggest that the development of coronary allograft vasculopathy may differ according to the type of preservation solution used at the time of transplantation, with two studies reporting higher rates when the heart was stored in UW solution ***(82,83)***.

3.3. Formulation of Preservation Solutions

Such is the complexity of the molecular and cellular mechanisms that mediate I/R injury that it is unlikely that any single approach or treatment will provide maximal protection to the donor organ during ischemic storage and reperfusion. Rather a combination of therapeutic approaches is likely to be required. In the context of myocardial preservation, three general principles have guided the formulation of cardioplegic and preservation solutions: (1) rapid reduction of tissue metabolic rate by profound hypothermia and electromechanical arrest of the heart, (2) provision of a biochemical medium that maintains tissue viability and structural integrity, and (3) prevention of reperfusion injury.

Many different myocardial preservation solutions have been developed and are in use for clinical heart transplantation. In one survey it was reported that at least 167 different types of preservation fluids were used for heart transplantation in the United States ***(84)***. This in itself is a reflection of the current uncertainties regarding the optimal strategy for myocardial preservation. Some (e.g., Bretschneider [HTK, Custodial], Celsior, St Thomas solution [STS, Plegisol], and UW solution [UW, Viaspan]) are commercially available solutions, but many are locally produced noncommercial solutions ***(84,85)***. In some centers, the same solution is used for both flush (cardioplegia) and storage, whereas other centers have elected to use separate solutions for initial cardioplegia and subsequent cold storage and transport of the cardiac allograft. With currently available preservation solutions, the maximum recommended storage time for cardiac allografts is approx 6 h. **Table 2** lists the electrolyte composition, chemical additives, and common clinical uses of a number of commercially available organ-preservation solutions.

3.3.1. Electrolyte Composition of Preservation Solutions

Preservation solutions differ in terms of both their electrolyte composition and additives. Most solutions can be divided into two broad categories—extracellular and intracellular—based on their Na^+ and K^+ concentrations. Preservation solutions that mimic extracellular fluid contain a high Na^+ concentration (≥70 mmol/L) and a K^+ concentration in the range of 5–30 mmol/L. Preservation solutions that mimic intracellular fluid contain a low Na^+ concentration (≤70 mmol/L) and K^+ concentration in the range of 30–125 mmol/L. Examples of intracellular and extracellular preservation solutions are shown in **Table 1**. Celsior (Na^+ 100, K^+ 15 mmol/L) and UW solutions (Na^+ 30, K^+ 125 mmol/L) are examples of extracellular and intracellular preservation solutions that have been used for clinical heart transplantation ***(82,86–88)***.

The primary rationale for intracellular preservation solutions is that the presence of similar concentrations of Na^+ and Cl^- in the intracellular and extracellular compartments minimizes the passive fluxes of these ions into the cell (and hence cell swelling) during hypothermia. Another potential advantage of intracellular solutions is that the high K^+ concentration in the preservation solution facilitates cardiac arrest while the low Na^+ concentration reduces the drive for the Na-H exchanger. On the other hand, a significant concern with intracellular preservation solutions, particularly with regard to myocardial preservation, is the potential for high K^+ concentrations to cause coronary endothelial cell injury. This is a controversial issue as there is contradictory experimental evidence ***(89–92)***. The damaging effects of hyperkalemia on the endothelial cell may be temperature dependent. Several investigators have noted that UW solution provided excellent endothelial cell preservation at 4°C but caused endothelial injury at higher temperatures ***(93,94)***. This observation suggests that if UW solution is used to preserve the donor heart, the preservation solution should be completely rinsed from the heart before any cardiac rewarming occurs at the time of implantation.

A further limitation of hyperkalemic preservation solutions, whether intracellular or extracellular, relates to their depolarizing action, which results in continuing transmembrane fluxes and the consequent maintenance of high-energy phosphate metabolism, even during hypothermic ischemia ***(89)***. A potentially beneficial alternative to hyperkalemic cardioplegia is to arrest the heart in a "hyperpolarized" or "polarized" state, which maintains the membrane potential of the arrested myocardium at or near to the resting membrane potential. At these potentials, transmembrane fluxes will be minimized and there should be little metabolic demand, resulting in improved myocardial protection. Recent studies have explored these alternative concepts for myocardial protection ***(89,95)***. The use of compounds such as adenosine or ATP-sensitive potassium channel openers, which are thought to induce hyperpolarized arrest, has demonstrated improved protection after normothermic, or short periods of hypothermic, ischemia when compared to hyperkalemic (depolarized) arrest. Similarly, the sodium channel blockers tetrodotoxin and lignocaine were used to induce polarized arrest (demonstrated by direct measurement of membrane potential during ischemia) was also shown to provide better recovery of function after long-term hypothermic storage ***(89,95)***. Indeed, the combination of adenosine with lignocaine in the same cardioplegic solution, as proposed by Dobson and Jones, has been shown to dramatically enhance myocardial protection during both normothermic and hypothermic ischemia ***(95)***.

Other important electrolyte components of myocardial preservation solutions are Ca^{2+} and Mg^{2+}. As mentioned earlier, inactivation of Ca^{2+} ATPases together with activation of the Na^{+}-H^{+} exchanger during hypothermic ischemic storage allows Ca^{2+} to accumulate within the cytoplasm, resulting in Ca^{2+} overload during storage. Further activation of the Na^{+}-H^{+} exchanger on reperfusion exacerbates Ca^{2+} overload, causing activation of Ca^{2+}-dependent enzymes, which cause cell injury through a variety of actions, contracture of the myofilaments, and irreversible mitochondrial damage, culminating in cell death. Experimental studies indicate that complete omission of Ca^{2+} from preservation solution is detrimental to myocardial recovery ***(96–98)***. On the other hand, similar experimental studies demonstrate that Ca^{2+} concentrations equivalent to those of extracellular fluid are also detrimental to myocardial recovery after ischemia ***(99,100)***. Normocalcaemic concentrations appear to facilitate Ca^{2+} overload during ischemia and reperfusion. Low concentrations of Ca^{2+} in the preservation solution together with high concentrations of Mg^{2+}, however, have been shown to limit Ca^{2+} overload and improve myocardial preservation ***(100,101)***. Of the currently available commercial solutions, Celsior and STS No. 2 solution contain a low Ca^{2+} concentration in combination with a high Mg^{2+} concentration.

3.3.2. Chemical Additives

Apart from differences in electrolyte composition, preservation solutions differ with respect to chemical additives. The additives used in commercially available preservation solutions fall into one of four broad categories, although some chemicals (e.g., adenosine) may belong to more than one category. The major categories are metabolic substrates, osmotic and oncotic impermeants, antioxidants and free-radical scavengers, and acid–base buffers. Examples of chemical additives within each category are shown in **Table 2**. Experimentally at least, these additives can be shown to enhance donor organ recovery of the preservation solutions to which they have been added ***(60,102,103)***.

3.4. Novel Approaches to Myocardial Protection

Clinical studies with commercially available myocardial storage solutions indicate that they provide acceptable donor heart preservation for periods of up to 6 h. Experimental studies suggest that more prolonged periods of donor heart storage can be achieved with some storage solutions, but it is apparent from these studies that there is scope to further enhance the myocardial protection provided by these solutions. For example, Baxter and colleagues ***(81)*** demonstrated in a rat heterotopic heart transplant model that supplementation of Celsior solution with glyceryl trinitrate significantly improved myocardial preservation. In another study, Kevelaitis and colleagues ***(104)*** demonstrated in an isolated rat heart model that supplementation of Celsior with cariporide (a Na^+-H^+ exchanger inhibitor) or diazoxide (a mitochondrial K_{ATP} [mK_{ATP}] channel agonist) enhanced myocardial recovery after prolonged hypothermic storage. Interestingly, they observed that cariporide plus diazoxide produced additive benefits when Celsior solution was supplemented with both drugs.

Another potential approach to enhancing myocardial preservation is to administer treatments to the donor prior to excision of the heart. Two therapies that might be administered in this way are Na^+-H^+ exchange inhibitors and mK_{ATP} channel activators. As mentioned previously, Kevelaitis and colleagues demonstrated in an isolated rat heart model that supplementation of Celsior with cariporide (a Na^+-H^+ exchanger inhibitor) or diazoxide (a mK_{ATP} channel agonist)-enhanced myocardial recovery after prolonged hypothermic storage ***(104)***. However, there is evidence that for these therapies *optimal* benefit is seen only when the treatment is administered prior to the onset of ischemia. For example, in the Guardian Study ***(105)***, a large clinical study of patients at high risk of ischemic myocardial injury, only those patients who received the Na^+-H^+ exchange inhibitor cariporide prior to the onset of ischemia benefited from the treatment. Recently, Cropper and colleagues demonstrated in the isolated working rat heart that administration of the Na^+-H^+ exchange inhibitor cariporide produced significantly greater protection when administered prior to hypothermic storage than when added to the storage solution ***(106)***.

BMS-180448, like diazoxide, is a selective mK_{ATP} channel-opening drug. In contrast to diazoxide and other ATP-sensitive potassium channel-opening drugs, BMS-180448 is cardiac selective, such that intravenous administration is not associated with systemic hypotension ***(107)***. Intravenous administration of BMS-180448 prior to coronary ligation has been shown to reduce myocardial infarct size by approx 50% in a dog infarct model ***(107)***. This drug mimics the phenomenon of ischemic preconditioning, originally described in 1986 by Murry and colleagues ***(108)***. Our laboratory has shown that pretreatment of isolated rat hearts with ischemic preconditioning, pinacidil, diazoxide, or BMS-180448 improve cardiac function in a working rat heart model after prolonged hypothermic storage ***(109–111)***. Furthermore, combination pretreatment with cariporide and mitochondrial K_{ATP}-channel activators, produced greater protection than administration of either drug alone in the same model ***(111)***.

While these results are encouraging, they have been observed in an in vitro isolated rat heart obtained from non-brain-dead donors. We and others have shown that brain death induces transient myocardial ischemia, and thus it is possible that the process of brain death activates mK_{ATP} channels through endogenous ischemic preconditioning ***(7,112,113)***. Furthermore, there is experimental evidence that cardioplegic solutions that contain high concentrations of K^+ and Mg^+ may mediate their cardioprotection in part via activation of mK_{ATP} channels ***(101,114)***. Hence, exogenous administration of mK_{ATP} channel activators may have limited benefit in a setting where the mK_{ATP} channel is already activated by myocardial ischemia and/or cardioplegia. Indeed, our own studies on the impact of the cardioselective mK_{ATP} channel activator, BMS-180448, on myocardial preservation in a porcine brain-dead heart transplant model showed only marginal benefit from this drug when administered to the donor and no additional benefit when it was administered in combination with the Na-H exchange inhibitor cariporide ***(115)***.

4. Preservation of the Lung

Like other vascularized organs, the transplanted lung is subject to ischemia-reperfusion injury. The clinical manifestations of I/R injury can vary from asymptomatic functional and radiological abnormalities to a life-threatening syndrome of severe pulmonary edema and pulmonary hypertension. I/R injury to the lung is thought to be the major cause of primary graft failure and peri-operative mortality ***(116)***. It causes considerable postoperative morbidity ***(116)*** and is also thought to play an important pathogenetic role in chronic allograft failure (obliterative bronchiolitis syndrome) ***(117)***.

4.1. Excision of the Donor Lungs

Several techniques of donor lung excision and ex vivo preservation have been developed. These include the administration of a cold preservation solution via the pulmonary artery followed by static hypothermic storage (usually in the same preservation solution), topical cooling, donor core cooling on cardiopulmonary bypass, and ex vivo perfusion. Of these techniques, single pulmonary artery flush and static hypothermic storage is the simplest and the one most commonly used in clinical practice ***(118)***. Many variations of the single pulmonary artery flush and static storage method have been described, and the optimal method remains controversial. Controversial aspects of the single pulmonary artery flush method include the flushing conditions (use of vasodilator prostaglandins, the volume, temperature, and infusion pressure of the flush solution), the route of administration (pulmonary and/or bronchial arteries, antegrade vs retrograde), and the storage conditions (temperature, oxygenation, and state of lung inflation).

4.1.1. Flushing Conditions

Prostacyclin and related prostaglandins have been used to produce maximal vasodilatation within the pulmonary vascular bed either via prior intravenous administration ***(73–75)*** or by addition to the preservation solution ***(73,77,78)***. The primary rationale for the use of vasodilator prostaglandins is to ensure rapid and uniform distribution of the preservation solution to the lung by preventing the pulmonary arteriolar vasoconstriction that would otherwise occur in response to administration of hyperkalemic preservation solution. Other reported benefits of prostaglandin administration include inhibition of platelet aggregation, inhibition of neutrophil-mediated release of oxygen-derived free radicals, and reduction in the increased vascular permeability caused by inflammatory mediators ***(119)***. However, some experimental work has reported adverse effects of prostaglandins on donor lung preservation ***(120)***, and this may be the reason that these agents have not been adopted universally in clinical practice ***(118)***.

A survey of 112 lung transplant centers by Hopkinson and colleagues identified a wide variation in the volume of preservation solution administered to the donor at the time of pulmonary flush—from 20 to 120 mL/kg of donor body weight ***(118)***. The median volume was 60 mL/kg administered over 4 min. This infusion rate avoids excessive increases in pulmonary artery pressure. In that same survey, the authors reported considerable variation in the temperature of the perfusate and storage solution from 4 to 10°C.

4.1.2. Route of Administration of Flush/Preservation Solution

The most common route of administration of pulmonary preservation solution is antegradely via a cannula placed in the main pulmonary artery ***(118)***. Alternative routes of administration include retrograde adminstration via the left atrial appendage ***(121)*** or via the pulmonary veins either *in situ* or prior to reimplantation (on the back table) ***(122,123)***. Potential advantages of retrograde administration of pulmonary preservation solution are that it allows delivery of the solution to both the bronchial and pulmonary circulation and that pulmonary arterial constriction will not affect distribution of the solution and may actually enhance it. Furthermore, retrograde administration will flush out any thrombotic or fat emboli ***(123)***. A third route of administration is via the bronchial arteries using a cannula placed in an isolated segment of thoracic aorta ***(124)***.

4.2. Storage Conditions

Early studies of lung preservation clearly demonstrated that the collapsed lung tolerates ischemia poorly ***(125–127)***. Furthermore, these studies demonstrated that the prevention of lung collapse during harvesting and storage markedly enhances the ability of the lung to tolerate ischemic storage ***(125–127)***, but the optimal degree of lung inflation during storage is uncertain. While there is experimental evidence that hyperventilation during harvesting and hyperinflation during storage results in superior lung preservation compared with lungs stored without inflation ***(128)***, there is also evidence that hyperinflation during storage may cause barotrauma ***(129)***, increase pulmonary capillary permeability ***(130)***, and cause pulmonary edema ***(131)***. In the study of DeCampos and colleagues, optimal recovery of lung function was observed when lungs were inflated to 50% of total lung capacity during storage ***(129)***. The optimal oxygen content of the gas used to inflate the donor lung during storage is also uncertain. While high intra-alveolar oxygen concentrations permit the ischemic lung to remain metabolically active even during hypothermia ***(132,133)***, they also facilitate production of oxygen-derived free radicals both during ischemia and upon reperfusion ***(134,135)***. Perhaps because of the uncertainties mentioned above, the most common clinical practice is ventilation with an FiO_2 of between 0.3 and 0.4 during procurement and near-total inflation for storage ***(118)***.

The ideal storage temperature for lung preservation is another point of uncertainty. The most commonly used storage temperature is 4°C. Experimental studies of lung preservation at 4°C have yielded disparate findings. For example, an early study by Feeley and colleagues in a canine heart–lung transplant model suggested that 5 h of storage of the heart–lung bloc at 4°C was associated with severe physiological dysfunction and pulmonary edema with minimal evidence of cardiac dysfunction ***(136)***. In contrast, excellent recovery of lung function was demonstrated in a pig transplant model after simple storage of the donor lung at 4°C for 18 h ***(137)***. Two studies using isolated rabbit and rat lungs compared recovery of lung function after prolonged ischemic storage at temperatures ranging from 4 to 38°C. They found that optimal recovery of lung function was obtained when the lungs were stored at 10 and 12°C, respectively ***(138,139)***.

In the lung as in the heart, hypothermic inhibition of cellular ATPase activity results in cell swelling. Within the pulmonary vascular bed, endothelial cell swelling results in increased capillary permeability and pulmonary vascular resistance ***(140)***. As with other vascularized organ transplants, hypothermia-induced cell swelling can be minimized by the addition of high-molecular-weight vascular impermeants (colloids) to the perfusion or preservation fluid. The two most commonly used lung preservation solutions, Perfadex and UW solution, contain the colloidal agents hydroxyethyl starch and dextran 40, respectively.

4.3. Reperfusion

I/R injury in the lung is thought to be mediated by oxygen-derived free radicals and by activated leukocytes ***(140)***. As mentioned previously, the ischemic lung inflated with air or other oxygen-containing gas is capable of maintaining oxidative metabolism even during profound hypothermia ***(132,133)***. Indeed, several investigators have demonstrated that inflation of ischemic lungs with gas mixtures containing increased concentrations of oxygen results in increased generation of oxygen-derived free radicals and free-radical-induced lung injury even during profound hypothermic storage ***(134,135,141)***. The primary source of oxygen radical generation during oxygenated lung ischemia is likely to be activated endothelial NADPH oxidase ***(142)***.

Reperfusion of ischemic lung results in a further burst in free radical generation. In the isolated rat model, this burst appears to occur in bimodal pattern with an early peak at 30 min postreperfusion and a delayed peak at about 4 h postreperfusion ***(143)***. The late peak appeared to be mediated by activated neutrophils ***(144)***. The major brunt of the reperfusion injury is borne by the pulmonary endothelial cell. The subsequent endothelial cell injury results in vasoconstriction, platelet and leukocyte aggregation, and increased capillary permeability.

Similar approaches to the prevention of reperfusion injury have been adopted for the lung as for other organs. These include supplementation of the lung preservation solution with antioxidants ***(145,146)*** and the use of leukocyte depletion ***(147,148)***. Although these approaches appear to work well in the laboratory, their clinical application has been very limited.

One potential approach to the prevention of I/R injury that is unique to the lung is the use of inhaled NO. Interest in this approach was generated by a series of case reports in which inhaled NO was found to markedly improve lung function and pulmonary vascular resistance in patients who had developed severe I/R injury after lung transplantation ***(149,150)***. Although NO has well-characterized vasodilator, antiplatelet, and antileukocyte properties, it is itself a free radical and is able to combine with other radicals such as superoxide anion to generate even more toxic species such as peroxynitrite and higher oxides of nitrogen in combination with oxygen. Experimental and clinical studies of inhaled NO have shown conflicting results, with some investigators reporting benefit ***(151,152)*** and others reporting harm ***(153)***. A modification of the use of inhaled NO to prevent lung I/R injury is to co-administer NO with agents that directly inhibit the generation of superoxide anion—examples include superoxide dismutase and pentoxifylline ***(153,154)***. A recently reported double-blind randomized controlled study of low-dose inhaled NO (10 ppm) initiated 10 min after reperfusion in 84 lung-transplant recipients found no benefit or harm with active treatment ***(154)***, and so the benefit of prophylactic inhaled NO remains unproven.

Another consequence of pulmonary I/R injury is loss of pulmonary surfactant ***(155)***. Experimental studies of intratracheal administration of surfactant prior to lung transplant reperfusion demonstrated improved airway compliance in animals receiving surfactant compared to saline controls ***(156)***. Clinical studies of nebulized surfactant administration either alone ***(157)*** or in combination with inhaled NO *(158,159)* suggest that this may be an effective treatment for I/R injury, but controlled clinical trials are still lacking.

A nonpharmacological approach to the prevention or mitigation of reperfusion injury to the transplanted lung is the use of controlled or low-flow reperfusion. The rationale behind this approach is the prevention of stress-induced endothelial injury during the first 10–15 min of reperfusion, a period of transient increased capillary permeability ***(160)***. The beneficial effects of controlled reperfusion were initially demonstrated in an ex vivo rat lung model ***(160,161)*** and have subsequently been confirmed in a pig transplant model ***(162,163)***. In the latter studies, a leukocyte filter was also used at the time of reperfusion. Clinical application of controlled reperfusion (combined with leukocyte depletion) has been limited, but initial reports suggest that this is a promising approach ***(164,165)***.

4.4. Composition of Lung Perfusion/Preservation Solutions

The first solution to be used clinically for flush perfusion of pulmonary grafts was modified Euro-Collins solution. This choice was based on experimental studies that demonstrated better preservation of lung grafts with modified Euro-Collins solution compared with non-colloid-containing extracellular solutions such as Ringer's lactate solution or isotonic saline ***(166,167)***. The highly successful clinical application of UW solution as a flush/storage solution for intra-abdominal donor organs led to investigation of its suitability for donor lung perfusion and storage. Experimental studies demonstrated superior long-term preservation with UW solution compared with modified Euro-Collins solution ***(168,169)***, but it is unclear whether this superiority in the laboratory has translated into clinical practice ***(118)***.

As with donor heart preservation, a significant concern with the use of intracellular-based storage solutions such as UW solution and modified Euro-Collins solution for donor lung preservation is their potential to induce endothelial injury and pulmonary vasoconstriction ***(170)***. It is largely because of this concern that vasodilatory prostaglandins are commonly administered before or with pulmonary flush solutions, although the effectiveness of this treatment has been questioned ***(171,172)***. Alternative vasodilators to prostaglandins include nitric oxide donors and calcium antagonists ***(79,173)***. Both vasodilators have been shown experimentally to provide better lung preservation than prostaglandins when administered in combination with intracellular perfusion solutions ***(79,173)***. Recently, Kelly and colleagues demonstrated another potentially deleterious effect of high-K^+-containing storage solutions ***(174)***. They found that isolated rat pulmonary artery segments produced more oxygen-derived free radicals when stored in intracellular solutions compared with rings stored in extracellular solutions.

Concerns regarding the deleterious effects of the high K^+ content of intracellular storage solutions have led to renewed interest in the use of extracellular solutions for pulmonary flush and preservation. The solution that has been most extensively studied in this context is low-potassium dextran (LPD; Perfadex). As mentioned earlier, the dextran 40 in LPD acts as an oncotic agent reducing both intracellular swelling and interstitial pulmonary edema during hypothermic storage. Another potentially beneficial action of dextran 40 in the context of lung preservation is its inhibitory effect on platelet and erythrocyte aggregation, thereby minimizing microcirculatory thrombosis and endothelial cell activation within the graft ***(175,176)***. Several experimental studies have demonstrated superior lung preservation with LPD compared with Euro-Collins solution ***(170,177–179)*** or UW solution ***(170,178–180)***. Clinical studies comparing LPD with other flush solutions for lung preservation, usually Euro-Collins solution, have demonstrated equivalent or superior outcomes when the lungs were stored in LPD solution ***(181–186)***.

A number of further modifications to LPD solution have been shown experimentally to further enhance lung preservation compared with LPD solution alone. These modifications include the addition of glucose to support limited aerobic metabolism in the hypothermically stored lungs ***(187)*** and the addition of glyceryl trinitrate as a nitric oxide donor ***(188)***. It remains to be seen whether these modifications translate into better outcomes in clinical lung transplantation.

Other preservation solutions with low potassium concentration (in comparison with intracellular storage solutions) that have been assessed in lung transplantation include HTK (Bretschneider solution), Celsior, and a modified cold blood solution (Papworth or Wallwork solution). Wittwer and colleagues, using an isolated rat lung model, showed that lungs preserved in Celsior solution for 4 h demonstrated better function postreperfusion compared with lungs stored in LPD solution ***(189)***. In another study, using a rat lung transplant model, Celsior was found to produce better lung preservation than Papworth solution after 5 and 12 h of storage ***(190)***. More recently, Warnecke and colleagues used a porcine lung transplant model to compare lung preservation in Celsior, HTK, and Euro-Collins solution ***(191)***. They found that donor lung preservation was best with Celsior solution and that both HTK and Celsior provided better donor lung preservation than Euro-Collins solution. Surfactant function after reperfusion was impaired in all three treatment groups ***(191,192)***. In a large clinical study, Celsior solution and Papworth solution produced comparable clinical outcomes at 1 mo post-lung transplantation compared with Euro-Collins or UW solution ***(193)***. In the same study, the incidence of reperfusion pulmonary edema was less with the extracellular solutions, leading the authors to conclude that extracellular-type solutions were associated with better lung preservation.

As the number of centers performing lung transplantation has increased so has the variability in the choice of perfusion/preservation solutions. In the worldwide survey conducted by Hopkinson and colleagues, 77% of lung transplant centers used modified Euro-Collins solution, 13% used UW solution, and 8% used Papworth blood-based solution ***(118)***. Only one center used donor core cooling. Most centers stored the lungs in the same solution as used for flushing, although seven centers stored the lungs in isotonic saline, and only one center stored the organs in low-potassium dextran solution. A more recent survey of North American lung transplant centers demonstrated a dramatic change in the choice of perfusion/preservation solution ***(194)***. The most commonly used preservation solution in this survey was low-potassium dextran (46%), followed by UW solution (22%), modified Euro-Collins solution (18%), Celsior (12%), and Euro-Collins solution (2%)

As with other vascularized organ transplants, the ideal perfusion and preservation solution for lung transplantation is yet to be developed. Currently used solutions permit safe lung preservation for periods of 6–8 h. While this remains a very active area of research, the wide variation in animal models, perfusion solutions, and storage protocols makes comparisons between studies difficult. A major limitation of many experimental studies conducted to date is that the adverse effects of brain death and prolonged donor ventilation have not been incorporated into the study design.

4.5. Future Developments in Pulmonary Preservation

The severe shortage of suitable donor lungs has stimulated interest in the use of donor lungs from non-heart-beating donors (NHBDs). Under these circumstances the donor lung is subject to a period of obligatory warm ischemia, which exposes the lungs to a more severe I/R injury compared with lungs obtained from heart beating donors ***(194)***. On the other hand, oxygen remaining in the alveoli after circulatory arrest enables aerobic metabolism to continue for a period of time and can potential mitigate the ischemic injury ***(133)***. Experimental studies suggest that lungs obtained from NHBD animals can be successfully transplanted if the warm ischemic time is less than 2 h ***(195,196)***. These studies showed that as warm ischemic time increases beyond 2 h, the risk of primary graft failure rises dramatically. Several therapeutic strategies have been found to enhance posttransplant recovery of lungs obtained from NHBDs. These strategies include the use of inhaled NO following lung reperfusion ***(197,198)***, the addition of glyceryl trinitrate to the lung perfusate and storage solution ***(199)***, and the intravenous administration of glyceryl trinitrate prior to reperfusion ***(200)***.

Table 3
Potential Therapeutic Targets for Myocardial or Pulmonary Protection During Ischemia and Reperfusion

Target	Drugs	References
Metabolic inhibitors	2,3-butanedione monoxime	***201–203***
Nitric oxide donors	Glyceryl trinitrate	***80,81***
Endothelin antagonists	Bosentan	***204***
Ischemic preconditioning	Adenosine	***111,115***
	MitoK_{ATP} chananel agonists	
Na-H Exchanger	Cariporide	***106,115,205***
p38 MAP kinase	SP203580	***206***
NF-kB	Aspirin, Prednisolone	***207,208***
PARP	PJ34,INO-1001	***209,210***
(Additional) Anti-oxidants	Bioflavonoids, 21-aminosteroids	***211–214***
Haem oxygenase	PDTC	***208***

5. Conclusion

As greater understanding of the complex metabolic pathways involved in I/R injury has been achieved, novel targets for therapeutic intervention have been identified. **Table 3** provides a list of some of the potential metabolic pathways that are not targeted by currently employed preservation solutions. Some of these targets may be adequately addressed by further modification of current preservation solutions. Others may require separate administration of a pharmacological agent to the donor prior to the onset of ischemia or to the recipient prior to reperfusion. The integration of these novel approaches to myocardial and pulmonary protection with existing preservation strategies and the extent to which the preservation of these organs can be enhanced are likely to be active areas of laboratory and clinical research in the years to come.

References

1. Rosendale, J. D., Chabalewski, F. L., McBride, M. A., et al. (2002) Increased transplanted organs from the use of a standardized donor management protocol.[see comment]. *Am. J. Transplant.* **2(8)**, 761–768.
2. Taylor, D. O., Edwards, L. B., Mohacsi, P. J., et al. (2003) The registry of the International Society for Heart and Lung Transplantation: twentieth official adult heart transplant report—2003. *J. Heart Lung Transplant.* **22(6)**, 616–624.
3. Trulock, E. P., Edwards, L. B., Taylor, D. O., et al. (2003) The Registry of the International Society for Heart and Lung Transplantation: Twentieth Official adult lung and heart-lung transplant report—2003. *J. Heart Lung Transplant.* **22(6)**, 625–635.

4. Rosengard, B. R., Feng, S., Alfrey, E. J., et al. (2002) Report of the Crystal City meeting to maximize the use of organs recovered from the cadaver donor. *Am. J. Transplant.* **2(8)**, 701–711.
5. Zaroff, J. G., Rosengard, B. R., Armstrong, W. F., et al. (2002) Consensus conference report: maximizing use of organs recovered from the cadaver donor: cardiac recommendations, March 28–29, 2001, Crystal City, Va. *Circulation* **106(7)**, 836–841.
6. Terasaki, P. I., Cecka, J. M., Gjertson, D. W., and Takemoto, S. (1995) High survival rates of kidney transplants from spousal and living unrelated donors.[see comment]. *N. Engl. J. Med.* **333(6)**, 333–336.
7. Ryan, J. B., Hicks, M., Cropper, J. R., et al. (2003) Functional evidence of reversible ischemic injury immediately after the sympathetic storm associated with experimental brain death. *J. Heart Lung Transplant.* **22(8)**, 922–928.
8. Pratschke, J., Wilhelm, M. J., Kusaka, M., et al. (1999) Brain death and its influence on donor organ quality and outcome after transplantation. *Transplantation* **67(3)**, 343–348.
9. Finkelstein, I., Toledo-Pereyra, L. H., and Castellanos, J. (1987) Physiologic and hormonal changes in experimentally induced brain dead dogs. *Transplant. Proc.* **19(5)**, 4156–4158.
10. Macoviak, J. A., McDougall, I. R., Bayer, M. F., Brown, M., Tazelaar, H., and Stinson, E. B. (1987) Significance of thyroid dysfunction in human cardiac allograft procurement. *Transplantation* **43(6)**, 824–826.
11. Mertes, P. M., el Abassi, K., Jaboin, Y., et al. (1994) Changes in hemodynamic and metabolic parameters following induced brain death in the pig.[see comment]. *Transplantation* **58(4)**, 414–418.
12. Novitzky, D., Wicomb, W. N., Cooper, D. K., and Tjaalgard, M. A.(1987) Improved cardiac function following hormonal therapy in brain dead pigs: relevance to organ donation. *Cryobiology* **24(1)**, 1–10.
13. Bittner, H. B., Kendall, S. W., Campbell, K. A., Montine, T. J., and Van Trigt, P. (1995) A valid experimental brain death organ donor model. *J. Heart Lung Transplant.* **14(2)**, 308–317.
14. Depret, J., Teboul, J. L., Benoit, G., Mercat, A., and Richard, C. (1995) Global energetic failure in brain-dead patients. *Transplantation* **60(9)**, 966–971.
15. Wicomb, W. N., Cooper, D. K., and Novitzky, D. (1986) Impairment of renal slice function following brain death, with reversibility of injury by hormonal therapy. *Transplantation* **41(1)**, 29–33.
16. Novitzky, D., Cooper, D. K., and Reichart, B. (1987) Hemodynamic and metabolic responses to hormonal therapy in brain-dead potential organ donors. *Transplantation* **43(6)**, 852–854.
17. Howlett, T. A., Keogh, A. M., Perry, L., Touzel, R., and Rees, L. H. (1989) Anterior and posterior pituitary function in brain-stem-dead donors. A possible role for hormonal replacement therapy. *Transplantation* **47(5)**, 828–834.
18. Gramm, H. J., Meinhold, H., Bickel, U., et al. (1992) Acute endocrine failure after brain death? *Transplantation* **54(5)**, 851–857.

19. Masson, F., Thicoipe, M., Gin, H., et al. (1993) The endocrine pancreas in brain-dead donors. A prospective study in 25 patients. *Transplantation* **56(2)**, 363–367.
20. Harms, J., Isemer, F. E., and Kolenda, H. (1991) Hormonal alteration and pituitary function during course of brain-stem death in potential organ donors. *Transplant. Proc.* **23(5)**, 2614–2616.
21. Arita, K., Uozumi, T., Oki, S., Kurisu, K., Ohtani, M., and Mikami, T. (1993) The function of the hypothalamo-pituitary axis in brain dead patients. *Acta Neurochir.* **123**(1–2), 64–75.
22. Takada, M., Nadeau, K. C., Hancock, W. W., et al. (1998) Effects of explosive brain death on cytokine activation of peripheral organs in the rat. *Transplantation* **65(12)**, 1533–1542.
23. Pratschke, J., Wilhelm, M. J., Kusaka, M., et al. (2000) Accelerated rejection of renal allografts from brain-dead donors. *Ann. Surg.* **232(2),** 263–271.
24. Pienaar, H., Schwartz, I., Roncone, A., Lotz, Z., and Hickman, R. (1990) Function of kidney grafts from brain-dead donor pigs. The influence of dopamine and triiodothyronine. *Transplantation* **50(4)**, 580–582.
25. Valero, R. (2002) Donor management: one step forward.[comment]. *Am. J. Transplant.* **2(8)**, 693–694.
26. Mackersie, R. C., Bronsther, O. L., and Shackford, S. R. (1991) Organ procurement in patients with fatal head injuries. The fate of the potential donor. *Ann. Surg.* **213(2)**, 143–150.
27. Excell, L., Wride, P., and Russ, G. (2004)ANZOD Registry Report 2004. Adelaide, South Australia: The Australian & New Zealand Organ Donation Registry, pp. 44–48.
28. Marshall, R., Ahsan, N., Dhillon, S., Holman, M., and Yang, H. C. (1996) Adverse effect of donor vasopressor support on immediate and one-year kidney allograft function. *Surgery* **120(4)**, 663–666.
29. O'Brien, E. A., Bour, S. A., Marshall, R. L., Ahsan, N.m and Yang, H. C. (1996) Effect of use of vasopressors in organ donors on immediate function of renal allografts. *J. Transplant Coord.* **6(4)**, 215–216.
30. Nakatani, T., Ishikawa, Y., Kobayashi, K., and Ozawa, K. (1991) Hepatic mitochondrial redox state in hypotensive brain-dead patients and an effect of dopamine administration. *Intensive Care Med.* **17(2)**, 103–107.
31. Schneider, A., Toledo-Pereyra, L. H., Zeichner, W. D., Allaben, R., and Whitten, J. (1983) Effect of dopamine and pitressin on kidneys procured and harvested for transplantation. *Transplantation* **36(1)**, 110–111.
32. Schnuelle, P., Berger, S., de Boer, J., Persijn, G., and van der Woude, F. J. (2001) Effects of catecholamine application to brain-dead donors on graft survival in solid organ transplantation.[see comment]. *Transplantation* **72(3)**, 455–463.
33. Powner, D. J. and Darby, J. M. (2000) Management of variations in blood pressure during care of organ donors. *Prog. Transplant.* **10(1)**, 25–32.
34. Powner, D. J. and Kellum, J. A. (2000) Maintaining acid-base balance in organ donors. *Prog. Transplant.* **10(2)**, 98–105.

35. Powner, D. J., Darby, J. M., and Stuart, S. A. (2000) Recommendations for mechanical ventilation during donor care. *Prog. Transplant.* **10(1)**, 33–40.
36. Keck, T., Banafsche, R., Werner, J., Gebhard, M. M., Herfarth, C., and Klar, E. (2001) Desmopressin impairs microcirculation in donor pancreas and early graft function after experimental pancreas transplantation.[see comment]. *Transplantation* **72(2)**, 202–209.
37. Wagner, H. J. and Braunwald, E. (1956) The pressor effect of the antidiuretic principle of the posterior pituitary in orthostatic hypotension. *J. Clin. Invest.* **35**, 1412–1418.
38. Yoshioka, T., Sugimoto, H., Uenishi, M., et al. (1986) Prolonged hemodynamic maintenance by the combined administration of vasopressin and epinephrine in brain death: a clinical study. *Neurosurgery* **18(5)**, 565–567.
39. Pennefather, S. H., Bullock, R. E., Mantle, D., and Dark, J. H. (1995) Use of low dose arginine vasopressin to support brain-dead organ donors. *Transplantation* **59(1)**, 58–62.
40. Chen, J. M., Cullinane, S., Spanier, T. B., et al. (1999) Vasopressin deficiency and pressor hypersensitivity in hemodynamically unstable organ donors. *Circulation* **100(19 Suppl.)**, II244–246.
41. Manaka, D., Okamoto, R., Yokoyama, T., et al. (1992) Maintenance of liver graft viability in the state of brain death. Synergistic effects of vasopressin and epinephrine on hepatic energy metabolism in brain-dead dogs. *Transplantation* **53 (3)**, 545–550.
42. Kinoshita, Y., Yahata, K., Yoshioka, T., Onishi, S. and Sugimoto, T. (1990) Long-term renal preservation after brain death maintained with vasopressin and epinephrine. *Transplant Int.* **3(1)**, 15–18.
43. Nagareda, T., Kinoshita, Y., Tanaka, A., et al. (1989) Clinicopathological study of livers from brain-dead patients treated with a combination of vasopressin and epinephrine. *Transplantation* **47(5)**, 792–797.
44. Salim, A., Vassiliu, P., Velmahos, G. C., et al. (2001) The role of thyroid hormone administration in potential organ donors. *Arch. Surg.* **136(12)**, 1377–1380.
45. Garcia-Fages, L. C., Cabrer, C., Valero, R., and Manyalich, M. (1993) Hemodynamic and metabolic effects of substitutive triiodothyronine therapy in organ donors. *Transplant. Proc.* **25(6)**, 3038–3039.
46. Goarin, J. P., Cohen, S., Riou, B., Jet al. (1996) The effects of triiodothyronine on hemodynamic status and cardiac function in potential heart donors. *Anesth. Analgesia* **83**(1), 41–47.
47. Scheinkestel, C. D., Tuxen, D. V., Cooper, D. J., and Butt, W. (1995) Medical management of the (potential) organ donor. *Anaest. Intensive Care* **23(1)**, 51–59.
48. Meyers, C. H., D'Amico, T. A., Peterseim, D. S., et al. (1993) Effects of triiodothyronine and vasopressin on cardiac function and myocardial blood flow after brain death.[see comment]. *J. Heart Lung Transplant.* **12(1 Pt. 1)**, 68–80.
49. Taniguchi, S., Kitamura, S., Kawachi, K., Doi, Y., and Aoyama, N. (1992) Effects of hormonal supplements on the maintenance of cardiac function in potential donor patients after cerebral death. *Eur. J. Cardio-Thorac. Surg.* **6(2)**, 96–102.

50. Wheeldon, D. R., Potter, C. D., Oduro, A., Wallwork, J., and Large, S. R. (1995) Transforming the "unacceptable" donor: outcomes from the adoption of a standardized donor management technique. *J. Heart Lung Transplant.* **14(4)**, 734–742.
51. Novitzky, D., Cooper, D. K., and Reichart, B. (1987) The value of hormonal therapy in improving organ viability in the transplant donor. *Transplant. Proc.* **19(1 Pt. 3)**, 2037–2038.
52. Novitzky, D., Cooper, D. K., Morrell, D., and Isaacs, S. (1988) Change from aerobic to anaerobic metabolism after brain death, and reversal following triiodothyronine therapy. *Transplantation* **45(1)**, 32–36.
53. Rosendale, J. D., Kauffman, H. M., McBride, M. A., et al. (2003) Aggressive pharmacologic donor management results in more transplanted organs. *Transplantation* **75(4)**, 482–487.
54. Pratschke, J., Kofla, G., Wilhelm, M. J., et al. (2001) Improvements in early behavior of rat kidney allografts after treatment of the brain-dead donor. *Ann. Surg.* **234(6)**, 732–740.
55. Segel, L. D., Follette, D. M., Castellanos, L. M., Hayes, R., Baker, J. M., and Smolens, I. V. (1997) Steroid pretreatment improves graft recovery in a sheep orthotopic heart transplantation model. *J. Heart Lung Transplant.* **16(4),** 371–380.
56. Follette, D. M., Rudich, S. M., and Babcock, W. D. (1998) Improved oxygenation and increased lung donor recovery with high-dose steroid administration after brain death. *J. Heart Lung Transplant.* **17(4)**, 423–429.
57. Rosendale, J. D., Kauffman, H. M., McBride, M. A., et al. (2003) Hormonal resuscitation yields more transplanted hearts, with improved early function. *Transplantation* **75(8),** 1336–1341.
58. Wicomb, W., Cooper, D. K., Hassoulas, J., Rose, A. G., and Barnard, C. N. (1982) Orthotopic transplantation of the baboon heart after 20 to 24 hours' preservation by continuous hypothermic perfusion with an oxygenated hyperosmolar solution. *J. Thorac. Cardiovasc. Surg.* **83(1)**, 133–140.
59. Wicomb, W. N., Cooper, D. K., and Barnard, C. N. (1982) Twenty-four-hour preservation of the pig heart by a portable hypothermic perfusion system. *Transplantation* **34(5)**, 246–250.
60. Wicomb, W. N. and Collins, G. M. (1989) 24-hour rabbit heart storage with UW solution. Effects of low-flow perfusion, colloid, and shelf storage. *Transplantation* **48(1)**, 6–9.
61. Nickless, D. K., Rabinov, M., Richards, S. M., Conyers, R. A., and Rosenfeldt, F. L. (1998) Continuous perfusion improves preservation of donor rat hearts: importance of the implantation phase. *Ann. Thorac. Surg.* **65**(5), 1265–1272.
62. Jahania, M. S., Sanchez, J. A., Narayan, P., Lasley, R. D. and Mentzer, R. M., Jr. (1999) Heart preservation for transplantation: principles and strategies. *Ann. Thorac. Surg.* **68**(5), 1983–1987.
63. McCrystal, G., Pepe, S., Esmore, D. and Rosenfeldt, F. (2004) The challenge of improving donor heart prteservation. *Heart Lung Circ.***13**, 74–83.

64. Hendry, P. J., Anstadt, M. P., Plunkett, M. D., et al. (1990) Optimal temperature for preservation of donor myocardium. *Circulation* **82(5 Suppl.)**, IV306–312.
65. Shimada, Y., Yamamoto, F., Yamamoto, H., Oka, T., and Kawashima, Y. (1996) Temperature-dependent cardioprotection of exogenous substrates in long-term heart preservation with continuous perfusion: twenty-four-hour preservation of isolated rat heart with St. Thomas' Hospital solution containing glucose, insulin, and aspartate. *J. Heart Lung Transplant.* **15(5)**, 485–495.
66. Lazdunski, M., Frelin, C., and Vigne, P. (1985) The sodium/hydrogen exchange system in cardiac cells: its biochemical and pharmacological properties and its role in regulating internal concentrations of sodium and internal pH. *J. Mol. Cell. Cardiol.* **17(11)**, 1029–1042.
67. Karmazyn, M. (1999) The role of the myocardial sodium-hydrogen exchanger in mediating ischemic and reperfusion injury. From amiloride to cariporide. *Ann. NY Acad. Sci.* **874**, 326–334.
68. Verma, S., Fedak, P. W., Weisel, R. D., et al. (2002) Fundamentals of reperfusion injury for the clinical cardiologist. *Circulation* **105(20)**, 2332–2336.
69. Jordan, J. E., Zhao, Z. Q., and Vinten-Johansen, J. (1999) The role of neutrophils in myocardial injury. *Cardiovasc. Res.* **43(4)**, 860–878.
70. Rezkalla, S. H. and Kloner, R. A. (2002) No-reflow phenomenon.[see comment]. *Circulation* **105(5),** 656–662.
71. Pearl, J. M., Drinkwater, D. C., Jr., Laks, H., Stein, D. G., Capouya, E. R., and Bhuta, S. (1992) Leukocyte-depleted reperfusion of transplanted human hearts prevents ultrastructural evidence of reperfusion injury. *J. Sur. Res.* **52(4)**, 298–308.
72. Pearl, J. M., Drinkwater, D. C., Laks, H., Capouya, E. R. and Gates, R. N. (1992) Leukocyte-depleted reperfusion of transplanted human hearts: a randomized, double-blind clinical trial. *J. Heart Lung Transplant.* **11(6)**, 1082–1092.
73. Wallwork, J., Jones, K., Cavarocchi, N., Hakim, M., and Higenbottam, T. (1987) Distant procurement of organs for clinical heart-lung transplantation using a single flush technique. *Transplantation* **44(5)**, 654–658.
74. Hirt, S. W., Wahlers, T., Jurmann, M., Fieguth, H. G., Dammenhayn, L., and Haverich, A. (1992) Improvement of currently used methods for lung preservation with prostacyclin and University of Wisconsin solution. *J. Heart Lung Transplant.* **11(4 Pt. 1)**, 656–664.
75. Nawata, S., Sugi, K., Ueda, K., Nawata, K., Kaneda, Y., and Esato, K. (1996) Prostacyclin analog OP2507 prevents pulmonary arterial and airway constriction during lung preservation and reperfusion. *J. Heart Lung Transplant.* **15(5)**, 470–474.
76. Kishida, A., Kurumi, Y., and Kodama, M. (1997) Efficacy of prostaglandin I2 analog on liver grafts subjected to 30 minutes of warm ischemia. *Surg, Today* **27(11)**, 1056–1060.
77. Sanchez-Urdazpal, L., Gores, G. J., Ferguson, D. M., and Krom, R. A. (1991) Improved liver preservation with addition of iloprost to Eurocollins and University of Wisconsin storage solutions. *Transplantation* **52(6)**, 1105–1107.

78. Changani, K. K., Fuller, B. J., Bell, J. D., Taylor-Robinson, S. D., Moore, D. P., and Davidson, B. R. (1999) Improved preservation solutions for organ storage: a dynamic study of hepatic metabolism. *Transplantation* **68(3)**, 345–355.
79. Bhabra, M. S., Hopkinson, D. N., Shaw, T. E., and Hooper, T. L. (1996) Relative importance of prostaglandin/cyclic adenosine monophosphate and nitric oxide/cyclic guanosine monophosphate pathways in lung preservation. *Ann. Thorac. Surg.* **62(5)**, 1494–1499.
80. Du, Z. Y., Hicks, M., Jansz, P., Rainer, S., Spratt, P., and Macdonald, P. (1998) The nitric oxide donor, diethylamine NONOate, enhances preservation of the donor rat heart. *J. Heart Lung Transplant.* **17(11)**, 1113–1120.
81. Baxter, K., Howden, B. O., and Jablonski, P. (2001) Heart preservation with celsior solution improved by the addition of nitroglycerine. *Transplantation* **71 (10)**, 1380–1384.
82. Drinkwater, D. C., Rudis, E., Laks, H., et al. (1995) University of Wisconsin solution versus Stanford cardioplegic solution and the development of cardiac allograft vasculopathy. *J. Heart Lung Transplant.* **14(5)**, 891–896.
83. Garlicki, M. (2003) May preservation solution affect the incidence of graft vasculopathy in transplanted heart? *Ann. Transplant.* **8(1)**, 19–24.
84. Demmy, T. L., Biddle, J. S., Bennett, L. E., Walls, J. T., Schmaltz, R. A., and Curtis, J. J. (1997) Organ preservation solutions in heart transplantation—patterns of usage and related survival. *Transplantation* **63(2)**, 262–269.
85. Richens, D., Junius, F., Hill, A., Keogh, A., Macdonald, P., McGoldrick, J., and Spratt, P. (1993) Clinical study of crystalloid cardioplegia vs aspartate-enriched cardioplegia plus warm reperfusion for donor heart preservation. *Transplant. Proc.* **25(1 Pt. 2)**, 1608–1610.
86. Wildhirt, S. M., Weis, M., Schulze, C., et al. (2000) Effects of Celsior and University of Wisconsin preservation solutions on hemodynamics and endothelial function after cardiac transplantation in humans: a single-center, prospective, randomized trial. *Transplant Int.* **13 (Suppl. 1)**, S203–211.
87. Remadi, J. P., Baron, O., Roussel, J. C., et al. (2002) Myocardial preservation using Celsior solution in cardiac transplantation: early results and 5-year follow-up of a multicenter prospective study of 70 cardiac transplantations. *Ann. Thorac. Surg.* **73(5)**, 1495–1499.
88. Vega, J. D., Ochsner, J. L., Jeevanandam, V., et al. (2001) A multicenter, randomized, controlled trial of Celsior for flush and hypothermic storage of cardiac allografts. *Ann. Thorac. Surg.* **71(5)**, 1442–1447.
89. Chambers, D. J. and Hearse, D. J. (1999) Developments in cardioprotection: "polarized" arrest as an alternative to "depolarized" arrest. *Ann. Thorac. Surg.* **68(5)**, 1960–1966.
90. Suleiman, M. S., Halestrap, A. P., and Griffiths, E. J. (2001) Mitochondria: a target for myocardial protection. *Pharmacol. Ther.* **89(1)**, 29–46.
91. Yang, Q., Zhang, R. Z., Yim, A. P., and He, G. W. (2004) Histidine-tryptophan-ketoglutarate solution maximally preserves endothelium-derived hyperpolarizing

factor-mediated function during heart preservation: comparison with University of Wisconsin solution. *J. Heart Lung Transplant.* **23(3)**, 352–59.
92. Sorajja, P., Cable, D. G., and Schaff, H. V. (1997) Hypothermic storage with University of Wisconsin solution preserves endothelial and vascular smooth-muscle function. *Circulation* **96(9 Suppl.)**, II-297–303.
93. von Oppell, U. O., Pfeiffer, S., Preiss, P., Dunne, T., Zilla, P., and Reichart, B. (1990) Endothelial cell toxicity of solid-organ preservation solutions. *Ann. Thorac. Surg.* **50(6)**, 902–910.
94. Ou, R., Gavin, J. B., Esmore, D. S., and Rosenfeldt, F. L. (1999) Increased temperature reduces the protective effect of University of Wisconsin solution in the heart[see comment]. *Ann. Thorac. Surg.* **68(5)**, 1628–1635.
95. Dobson, G. P. and Jones, M. W. (2004) Adenosine and lidocaine: a new concept in nondepolarizing surgical myocardial arrest, protection, and preservation. *J. Thorac. Cardiovasc. Surg.* **127(3)**, 794–805.
96. Donnelly, A. J. and Djuric, M. (1991) Cardioplegia solutions. *Am. J. Hosp. Pharm.* **48(11)**, 2444–2460.
97. Michel, P., Hadour, G., Rodriguez, C., Chiari, P., and Ferrera, R. (2000) Evaluation of a new preservative solution for cardiac graft during hypothermia. *J. Heart Lung Transplant.* **19(11)**, 1089–1097.
98. Michel, P., Vial, R., Rodriguez, C., and Ferrera, R. (2002) A comparative study of the most widely used solutions for cardiac graft preservation during hypothermia. *J. Heart Lung Transplant.* **21**(9), 1030–1039.
99. Chen, R. H. (1996) The scientific basis for hypocalcemic cardioplegia and reperfusion in cardiac surgery. *Ann. Thorac. Surg.* **62(3)**, 910–914.
100. Fukuhiro, Y., Wowk, M., Ou, R., Rosenfeldt, F., and Pepe, S. (2000) Cardioplegic strategies for calcium control: low Ca(2+), high Mg(2+), citrate, or Na(+)/H(+) exchange inhibitor HOE-642. *Circulation* **102(19 Suppl. 3)**, III319–325.
101. McCully, J. D. and Levitsky, S. (2003) The mitochondrial K(ATP) channel and cardioprotection. *Ann. Thorac. Surg.* **75(2)**, S667–673.
102. Southard, J. H., van Gulik, T. M., Ametani, M. S., et al. (1990) Important components of the UW solution. *Transplantation* **49(2)**, 251–257.
103. Biguzas, M., Jablonski, P., Howden, B. O., et al. (1990) Evaluation of UW solution in rat kidney preservation. II. The effect of pharmacological additives. *Transplantation* **49(6)**, 1051–1055.
104. Kevelaitis, E., Oubenaissa, A., Mouas, C., Peynet, J., and Menasche, P. (2001) Ischemic preconditioning with opening of mitochondrial adenosine triphosphate-sensitive potassium channels or Na/H exchange inhibition: which is the best protective strategy for heart transplants? *J. Thorac. Cardiovasc. Surg.* **121**(1), 155–162.
105. Theroux, P., Chaitman, B. R., Danchin, N., et al. (2000) Inhibition of the sodium-hydrogen exchanger with cariporide to prevent myocardial infarction in high-risk ischemic situations. Main results of the GUARDIAN trial. Guard during ischemia against necrosis (GUARDIAN) Investigators. *Circulation* **102(25)**, 3032–3038.

106. Cropper, J. R., Hicks, M., Ryan, J. B., and Macdonald, P. S. (2003) Cardioprotection by cariporide after prolonged hypothermic storage of the isolated working rat heart. *J. Heart Lung Transplant.* **22(8)**, 929–936.
107. Grover, G. J., McCullough, J. R., D'Alonzo, A. J., Sargent, C. A., and Atwal, K. S. (1995) Cardioprotective profile of the cardiac-selective ATP-sensitive potassium channel opener BMS-180448. *Journal of Cardiovascular Pharmacology* **25(1)**, 40–50.
108. Murry, C. E., Jennings, R. B., and Reimer, K. A. (1986) Preconditioning with ischemia: a delay of lethal cell injury in ischemic myocardium. *Circulation* **74(5)**, 1124–1136.
109. Du, Z. Y., Hicks, M., Spratt, P., Mundy, J. A., and Macdonald, P. S. (1998) Cardioprotective effects of pinacidil pretreatment and lazaroid (U74500A) preservation in isolated rat hearts after 12-hour hypothermic storage. *Transplantation* **66 (2)**, 158–163.
110. Hicks, M., Du, Z. Y., Jansz, P., Rainer, S., Spratt, P., and Macdonald, P. S. (1999) ATP-sensitive potassium channel activation mimics the protective effect of ischaemic preconditioning in the rat isolated working heart after prolonged hypothermic storage. *Clin. Exp. Pharm. Physiol.* **26(1)**, 20–25.
111. Cropper, J. R., Hicks, M., Ryan, J. B., and Macdonald, P. S. (2003) Enhanced cardioprotection of the rat heart during hypothermic storage with combined Na+ - H+ exchange inhibition and ATP-dependent potassium channel activation. *J. Heart Lung Transplant.* **22(11)**, 1245–1253.
112. Pinelli, G., Mertes, P. M., Carteaux, J. P., et al. (1995) Myocardial effects of experimental acute brain death: evaluation by hemodynamic and biological studies. *Ann. Thorac. Surg.* **60(6)**, 1729–1734.
113. Halejcio-Delophont, P., Siaghy, E. M., Devaux, Y., et al. (1998) Increase in myocardial interstitial adenosine and net lactate production in brain-dead pigs: an in vivo microdialysis study. *Transplantation* **66(10)**, 1278–1284.
114. Toyoda, Y., Levitsky, S., and McCully, J. D. (2001) Opening of mitochondrial ATP-sensitive potassium channels enhances cardioplegic protection. *Ann. Thorac. Surg.* **71(4)**, 1281–1289.
115. Ryan, J. B., Hicks, M., Cropper, J. R., et al. (2003) Sodium-hydrogen exchanger inhibition, pharmacologic ischemic preconditioning, or both for extended cardiac allograft preservation. *Transplantation* **76(5)**, 766–771.
116. Thabut, G., Vinatier, I., Stern, J. B., et al. (2002) Primary graft failure following lung transplantation: predictive factors of mortality[see comment]. *Chest* **121(6)**, 1876–1882.
117. Fiser, S. M., Tribble, C. G., Long, S. M., et al. (2002) Ischemia-reperfusion injury after lung transplantation increases risk of late bronchiolitis obliterans syndrome. *Ann. Thorac. Surg.* **73(4)**, 1041–1048.
118. Hopkinson, D. N., Bhabra, M. S., and Hooper, T. L. (1998) Pulmonary graft preservation: a worldwide survey of current clinical practice. *J. Heart Lung Transplant.* **17(5)**, 525–531.
119. Novick, R. J., Reid, K. R., Denning, L., Duplan, J., Menkis, A. H., and McKenzie, F. N. (1991) Prolonged preservation of canine lung allografts: the role of prostaglandins. *Ann. Thorac. Surg.* **51(5)**, 853–859.

120. Bonser, R. S., Fragomeni, L. S., Jamieson, S. W., et al (1991) Effects of prostaglandin E1 in twelve-hour lung preservation. *J. Heart Lung Transplant.* **10(2)**, 310–316.
121. Sarsam, M. A., Yonan, N. A., Deiraniya, A. K., and Rahman, A. N. (1993) Retrograde pulmonaryplegia for lung preservation in clinical transplantation: a new technique. *J. Heart Lung Transplant.* **12(3)**, 494–498.
122. Varela, A., Cordoba, M., Serrano-Fiz, S., et al. (1997) Early lung allograft function after retrograde and antegrade preservation. *J. Thorac. Cardiovasc. Surg.* **114(6)**, 1119–1120.
123. Venuta, F., Rendina, E. A., Bufi, M., et al. (1999) Preimplantation retrograde pneumoplegia in clinical lung transplantation. [see comment]. *J. Thorac. Cardiovasc. Surg.* **118(1)**, 107–114.
124. Steen, S., Kimblad, P. O., Sjoberg, T., Lindberg, L., Ingemansson, R., and Massa, G. (1994) Safe lung preservation for twenty-four hours with Perfadex. [see comment]. *Ann. Thorac. Surg.* **57(2)**, 450–457.
125. Homatas, J., Bryant, L., and Eiseman, B. (1968) Time limits of cadaver lung viability. *J. Thorac. Cardiovasc. Surg.* **56(1)**, 132–140.
126. Veith, F. J., Sinha, S. B., Graves, J. S., Boley, S. J., and Dougherty, J. C. (1971) Ischemic tolerance of the lung. The effect of ventilation and inflation. *J. Thorac. Cardiovasc. Surg.* **61(5)**, 804–810.
127. Stevens, G. H., Sanchez, M. M., and Chappell, G. L. (1973) Enhancement of lung preservation by prevention of lung collapse. *J. Surg. Res.* **14(5)**, 400–405.
128. Puskas, J. D., Hirai, T., Christie, N., Mayer, E., Slutsky, A. S., and Patterson, G. A. (1992) Reliable thirty-hour lung preservation by donor lung hyperinflation. *J. Thorac. Cardiovasc. Surg.* **104(4)**, 1075–1083.
129. DeCampos, K. N., Keshavjee, S., Liu, M., and Slutsky, A. S. (1998) Optimal inflation volume for hypothermic preservation of rat lungs. *J. Heart Lung Transplant.* **17(6)**, 599–607.
130. Haniuda, M., Hasegawa, S., Shiraishi, T., Dresler, C. M., Cooper, J. D., and Patterson, G. A. (1996) Effects of inflation volume during lung preservation on pulmonary capillary permeability. *J. Thorac. Cardiovasc. Surg.* **112(1)**, 85–93.
131. Aoe, M., Okabayashi, K., Cooper, J. D., and Patterson, G. A. (1996) Hyperinflation of canine lung allografts during storage increases reperfusion pulmonary edema. *J. Thorac. Cardiovasc. Surg.* **112(1)**, 94–102.
132. De Leyn, P. R., Lerut, T. E., Schreinemakers, H. H., Van Raemdonck, D. E., Mubagwa, K., and Flameng, W. (1993) Effect of inflation on adenosine triphosphate catabolism and lactate production during normothermic lung ischemia. *Ann. Thorac. Surg.* **55(5)**, 1073–1079.
133. Date, H., Matsumura, A., Manchester, J. K., Cooper, J. M., Lowry, O. H., and Cooper, J. D. (1993) Changes in alveolar oxygen and carbon dioxide concentration and oxygen consumption during lung preservation. The maintenance of aerobic metabolism during lung preservation. *J. Thorac. Cardiovasc. Surg.* **105(3)**, 492–501.
134. Fisher, A. B., Dodia, C., Tan, Z. T., Ayene, I., and Eckenhoff, R. G. (1991) Oxygen-dependent lipid peroxidation during lung ischemia. *J. Clin. Invest.* **88(2)**, 674–679.

135. Haniuda, M., Dresler, C. M., Mizuta, T., Cooper, J. D., and Patterson, G. A. (1995) Free radical-mediated vascular injury in lungs preserved at moderate hypothermia. *Ann. Thorac. Surg.* **60(5)**, 1376–1381.
136. Feeley, T. W., Mihm, F. G., Downing, T. P., et al. (1985) The effect of hypothermic preservation of the heart and lungs on cardiorespiratory function following canine heart-lung transplantation. *Ann. Thorac. Surg.* **39(6)**, 558–562.
137. Muller, C., Hoffmann, H., Bittmann, I., et al. (1997) Hypothermic storage alone in lung preservation for transplantation: a metabolic, light microscopic, and functional analysis after 18 hours of preservation. *Transplantation* **63(5)**, 625–630.
138. Wang, L. S., Yoshikawa, K., Miyoshi, S., et al. (1989) The effect of ischemic time and temperature on lung preservation in a simple ex vivo rabbit model used for functional assessment. *J. Thorac. Cardiovasc. Surg.* **98(3)**, 333–342.
139. Shiraishi, T., Igisu, H., and Shirakusa, T. (1994) Effects of pH and temperature on lung preservation: a study with an isolated rat lung reperfusion model. *Ann. Thorac. Surg.* **57(3)**, 639–643.
140. Kelly, R. F. (2000) Current strategies in lung preservation. *J. Lab. Clin. Med.* **136(6)**, 427–440.
141. Du, Z. Y., Hicks, M., Winlaw, D., Spratt, P., and Macdonald, P. (1996) Ischemic preconditioning enhances donor lung preservation in the rat. *J. Heart Lung Transplant.* **15(12)**, 1258–1267.
142. Al-Mehdi, A. B., Zhao, G., Dodia, C., et al. (1998) Endothelial NADPH oxidase as the source of oxidants in lungs exposed to ischemia or high K+. *Circ. Res.* **83 (7)**, 730–737.
143. Eppinger, M. J., Jones, M. L., Deeb, G. M., Bolling, S. F., and Ward, P. A. (1995) Pattern of injury and the role of neutrophils in reperfusion injury of rat lung. *J. Surg. Res.* **58(6)**, 713–718.
144. Eppinger, M. J., Deeb, G. M., Bolling, S. F., and Ward, P. A. (1997) Mediators of ischemia-reperfusion injury of rat lung. *Am. J. Pathol.* **150(5)**, 1773–1784.
145. Nezu, K., Kushibe, K., Tojo, T., et al. (1994) Protection against lipid peroxidation induced during preservation of lungs for transplantation. *J. Heart Lung Transplant.* **13(6)**, 998–1002.
146. Du, Z., Hicks, M., Winlaw, D., Macdonald, P., and Spratt, P. (1995) Lazaroid U74500A enhances donor lung preservation in the rat transplant model. *Transplant. Proc.* **27(6)**, 3574–3577.
147. Breda, M. A., Hall, T. S., Stuart, R. S., et al. (1985) Twenty-four hour lung preservation by hypothermia and leukocyte depletion. *J. Heart Transplant.* **4(3)**, 325–329.
148. Pillai, R., Bando, K., Schueler, S., Zebly, M., Reitz, B. A., and Baumgartner, W. A. (1990) Leukocyte depletion results in excellent heart-lung function after 12 hours of storage. *Ann. Thorac. Surg.* **50(2)**, 211–214.
149. Adatia, I., Lillehei, C., Arnold, J. H., et al. (1994) Inhaled nitric oxide in the treatment of postoperative graft dysfunction after lung transplantation. *Ann. Thorac. Surg.* **57(5)**, 1311–138.

150. Macdonald, P., Mundy, J., Rogers, P., et al. (1995) Successful treatment of life-threatening acute reperfusion injury after lung transplantation with inhaled nitric oxide. *J. Thorac. Cardiovasc. Surg.* **110(3)**, 861–863.
151. Chetham, P. M., Sefton, W. D., Bridges, J. P., Stevens, T., and McMurtry, I. F. (1997) Inhaled nitric oxide pretreatment but not posttreatment attenuates ischemia-reperfusion-induced pulmonary microvascular leak. *Anesthesiology* **86(4)**, 895–902.
152. Struber, M., Harringer, W., Ernst, M., et al. (1999) Inhaled nitric oxide as a prophylactic treatment against reperfusion injury of the lung. *Thorac. Cardiovasc. Surg.* **47(3)**, 179–82.
153. Eppinger, M. J., Ward, P. A., Jones, M. L., Bolling, S. F., and Deeb, G. M. (1995) Disparate effects of nitric oxide on lung ischemia-reperfusion injury. *Ann. Thorac. Surg.* **60(5)**, 1169–1176.
154. Meade, M. O., Granton, J. T., Matte-Martyn, A., et al. (2003) A randomized trial of inhaled nitric oxide to prevent ischemia-reperfusion injury after lung transplantation.[see comment]. *Am. J. Respir. Crit. Care Med.* **167(11)**, 1483–1489.
155. Novick, R. J., Possmayer, F., Veldhuizen, R. A., Menkis, A. H., and McKenzie, F. N. (1991) Surfactant analysis and replacement therapy: a future tool of the lung transplant surgeon? *Ann. Thorac. Surg.* **52(5)**, 1194–1200.
156. Buchanan, S. A., Mauney, M. C., Parekh, V. I., et al. (1996) Intratracheal surfactant administration preserves airway compliance during lung reperfusion. *Ann. Thorac. Surg.* **62(6)**, 1617–1621.
157. Struber, M., Hirt, S. W., Cremer, J., Harringer, W., and Haverich, A. (1999) Surfactant replacement in reperfusion injury after clinical lung transplantation. *Intens. Care Med.* **25(8)**, 862–864.
158. Struber, M., Brandt, M., Cremer, J., Harringer, W., Hirt, S. W., and Haverich, A. (1996) Therapy for lung failure using nitric oxide inhalation and surfactant replacement[see comment]. *Ann. Thorac. Surg.* **61(5)**, 1543–1545.
159. Della Rocca, G., Pierconti, F., Costa, M. G., et al. (2002) Severe reperfusion lung injury after double lung transplantation [see comment]. *Cri. Care (Lond.)* **6 (3)**, 240–244.
160. Bhabra, M. S., Hopkinson, D. N., Shaw, T. E., Onwu, N., and Hooper, T. L. (1998) Controlled reperfusion protects lung grafts during a transient early increase in permeability[see comment]. *Ann. Thorac. Surg.* **65(1)**, 187–192.
161. Hopkinson, D. N., Bhabra, M. S., Odom, N. J., Bridgewater, B. J., Van Doorn, C. A., and Hooper, T. L. (1996) Controlled pressure reperfusion of rat pulmonary grafts yields improved function after twenty-four-hours' cold storage in University of Wisconsin solution. *J. Heart Lung Transplant.* **15(3)**, 283–290.
162. Halldorsson, A., Kronon, M., Allen, B. S., et al. (1998) Controlled reperfusion after lung ischemia: implications for improved function after lung transplantation. *J. Thorac. Cardiovasc. Surg.* **115(2)**, 415–425.
163. Halldorsson, A. O., Kronon, M., Allen, B. S., et al. (1998) Controlled reperfusion prevents pulmonary injury after 24 hours of lung preservation. [see comment]. *Ann. Thorac. Surg.* **66(3)**, 877–885.

164. Lick, S. D., Brown, P. S., Jr., Kurusz, M., et al. (2000) Technique of controlled reperfusion of the transplanted lung in humans [see comment]. *Ann. Thorac. Surg.* **69(3)**, 910–912.
165. Kurusz, M., Roach, J. D., Jr., Vertrees, R. A., Girouard, M. K., and Lick, S. D. (2002) Leukocyte filtration in lung transplantation. *Perfusion* **17(Suppl.)**, 63–67.
166. Kondo, Y., Turner, M. D., Cockrell, J. V., and Hardy, J. D. (1974) Ischemic tolerance of the canine autotransplanted lung. *Surgery* **76(3)**, 447–453.
167. Veith, F. J., Crane, R., Torres, M., et al. (1976) Effective preservation and transportation of lung transplants. *J. Thorac. Cardiovasc. Surg.* **72(1)**, 97–105.
168. Bresticker, M. A., LoCicero, J., 3rd, Oba, J., and Greene, R. (1992) Successful extended lung preservation with UW solution. *Transplantation* **54(5)**, 780–784.
169. Kawahara, K., Ikari, H., Hisano, H., et al. (1991) Twenty-four-hour canine lung preservation using UW solution. *Transplantation* **51(3)**, 584–587.
170. Oka, T., Puskas, J. D., Mayer, E., et al. (1991) Low-potassium UW solution for lung preservation. Comparison with regular UW, LPD, and Euro-Collins solutions. *Transplantation* **52(6)**, 984–988.
171. Sasaki, S., Yasuda, K., McCully, J. D., and LoCicero, J., 3rd (1999) Does PGE1 attenuate potassium-induced vasoconstriction in initial pulmonary artery flush on lung preservation? *J. Heart Lung Transplant.* **18(2)**, 139–142.
172. Kukkonen, S., Heikkila, L. J., Verkkala, K., Mattila, S. P., and Toivonen, H. (1995) Prostaglandin E1 or prostacyclin in Euro-Collins solution fails to improve lung preservation. *Ann. Thorac. Surg.* **60(6)**, 1617–1622.
173. Sasaki, S., Yasuda, K., McCully, J. D., and LoCicero, J., 3rd (1999) Calcium channel blocker enhances lung preservation. *J. Heart Lung Transplant.* **18(2),** 127–132.
174. Kelly, R. F., Murar, J., Hong, Z., et al. (2003) Low potassium dextran lung preservation solution reduces reactive oxygen species production. *Ann. Thorac. Surg.* **75(6)**, 1705–1710.
175. Zoucas, E., Goransson, G., and Bengmark, S. (1984) Colloid-induced changes in bleeding following liver resection in the rat. *Res. Exp. Med.* **184(4)**, 251–258.
176. Fatkin, D., Loupas, T., Low, J., and Feneley, M. (1997) Inhibition of red cell aggregation prevents spontaneous echocardiographic contrast formation in human blood. *Circulation* **96(3)**, 889–896.
177. Keshavjee, S. H., Yamazaki, F., Cardoso, P. F., McRitchie, D. I., Patterson, G. A., and Cooper, J. D. (1989) A method for safe twelve-hour pulmonary preservation. *J. Thorac. Cardiovasc. Surg.* **98(4)**, 529–534.
178. Sasaki, S., McCully, J. D., Alessandrini, F., and LoCicero, J., 3rd (1995) Impact of initial flush potassium concentration on the adequacy of lung preservation. *J. Thorac. Cardiovasc. Surg.* **109(6)**, 1090–1096.
179. Hausen, B., Beuke, M., Schroeder, F., et al. (1997) In vivo measurement of lung preservation solution efficacy: comparison of LPD, UW, EC and low K+-EC following short and extended ischemia. *Eur. J. Cardio-Thorac. Surg.* **12(5)**, 771–780.

180. Carbognani, P., Rusca, M., Solli, P., et al. (1997) Pneumocytes type II ultrastructural modifications after storage in preservation solutions for transplantation. *Eur. Surg. Res.* **29(5)**, 319–326.
181. Aziz, T. M., Pillay, T. M., Corris, P. A., et al. (2003) Perfadex for clinical lung procurement: is it an advance? *Ann. Thorac. Surg.* **75(3)**, 990–995.
182. Fischer, S., Matte-Martyn, A., De Perrot, M., et al. (2001) Low-potassium dextran preservation solution improves lung function after human lung transplantation. *J. Thorac. Cardiovasc. Surg.* **121(3)**, 594–596.
183. Muller, C., Furst, H., Reichenspurner, H., Briegel, J., Groh, J., and Reichart, B. (1999) Lung procurement by low-potassium dextran and the effect on preservation injury. Munich Lung Transplant Group. *Transplantation* **68(8)**, 1139–1143.
184. Struber, M., Wilhelmi, M., Harringer, W., et al. (2001) Flush perfusion with low potassium dextran solution improves early graft function in clinical lung transplantation. *Eur. J. Cardio-Thorac. Surg.* **19(2)**, 190–194.
185. Muller, C., Bittmann, I., Hatz, R., et al. (2002) Improvement of lung preservation—from experiment to clinical practice. *Eu. Sur. Res.* **34(1–2)**, 77–82.
186. Rabanal, J. M., Ibanez, A. M., Mons, R., et al. (2003) Influence of preservation solution on early lung function (Euro-Collins vs Perfadex) *Transplant. Proc.* **35(5)**, 1938–1939.
187. Wagner, F. M., Jamieson, S. W., Fung, J., Wolf, P., Reichenspurner, H., and Kaye, M. P. (1995) A new concept for successful long-term pulmonary preservation in a dog model. *Transplantation* **59(11)**, 1530–1536.
188. Wittwer, T., Albes, J. M., Fehrenbach, A., et al. (2003) Experimental lung preservation with Perfadex: effect of the NO-donor nitroglycerin on postischemic outcome. *J. Thorac. Cardiovasc. Surg.* **125(6)**, 1208–1216.
189. Wittwer, T., Wahlers, T., Fehrenbach, A., Elki, S. and Haverich, A. (1999) Improvement of pulmonary preservation with Celsior and Perfadex: impact of storage time on early post-ischemic lung function. *J. Heart Lung Transplant.* **18(12)**, 1198–11201.
190. Xiong, L., Legagneux, J., Wassef, M., et al. (1999) Protective effects of Celsior in lung transplantation. *J. Heart Lung Transplant.* **18(4)**, 320–327.
191. Warnecke, G., Struber, M., Hohlfeld, J. M., Niedermeyer, J., Sommer, S. P., and Haverich, A. (2002) Pulmonary preservation with Bretscheider's HTK and Celsior solution in minipigs. *Eur. J. Cardio-Thorac. Surg.* **21(6)**, 1073–1079.
192. Thabut, G., Vinatier, I., Brugiere, O., et al. (2001) Influence of preservation solution on early graft failure in clinical lung transplantation. *Am. J. Respir. Crit. Care Med.* **164(7)**, 1204–1208.
193. Levine, S. M. and Transplant/Immunology Network of the American College of Chest, P. (2004) A survey of clinical practice of lung transplantation in North America[see comment]. *Chest* **125(4)**, 1224–1238.
194. Kootstra, G. (1997) The asystolic, or non-heartbeating, donor. *Transplantation* **63(7)**, 917–921.
195. Egan, T. M., Lambert, C. J., Jr., Reddick, R., Ulicny, K. S., Jr., Keagy, B. A. and Wilcox, B. R. (1991) A strategy to increase the donor pool: use of cadaver lungs for transplantation. *Ann. Thorac. Surg.* **52(5)**, 1113–1121.

196. Aitchison, J. D., Orr, H. E., Flecknell, P. A., Kirby, J. A. and Dark, J. H. (2001) Functional assessment of non-heart-beating donor lungs: prediction of post-transplant function. *Eur. J. Cardio-Thorac. Surg.* **20(1)**, 187–194.
197. Bacha, E. A., Sellak, H., Murakami, S., et al. (1997) Inhaled nitric oxide attenuates reperfusion injury in non-heartbeating-donor lung transplantation. Paris-Sud University Lung Transplantation Group. *Transplantation* **63(10)**, 1380–1386.
198. Luh, S. P., Tsai, C. C., Shau, W. Y., et al. (2000) The effects of inhaled nitric oxide, gabexate mesilate, and retrograde flush in the lung graft from non-heart beating minipig donors. *Transplantation* **69(10)**, 2019–2027.
199. Naka, Y., Chowdhury, N. C., Liao, H., et al. (1995) Enhanced preservation of orthotopically transplanted rat lungs by nitroglycerin but not hydralazine. Requirement for graft vascular homeostasis beyond harvest vasodilation. *Circ. Res.* **76(5)**, 900–906.
200. Loehe, F., Preissler, G., Annecke, T., Bittmann, I., Jauch, K. W. and Messmer, K. (2004) Continuous infusion of nitroglycerin improves pulmonary graft function of non-heart-beating donor lungs. *Transplantation* **77(12)**, 1803–1808.
201. Siegmund, B., Klietz, T., Schwartz, P. and Piper, H. M. (1991) Temporary contractile blockade prevents hypercontracture in anoxic-reoxygenated cardiomyocytes. *Am. J. Physiol.* **260(2 Pt. 2)**, H426–435.
202. Garcia-Dorado, D., Theroux, P., Duran, J. M., et al. (1992) Selective inhibition of the contractile apparatus. A new approach to modification of infarct size, infarct composition, and infarct geometry during coronary artery occlusion and reperfusion. *Circulation* **85(3)**, 1160–1174.
203. Warnecke, G., Schulze, B., Hagl, C., Haverich, A. and Klima, U. (2002) Improved right heart function after myocardial preservation with 2,3-butanedione 2-monoxime in a porcine model of allogenic heart transplantation. *J. Thorac. Cardiovasc. Surg.* **123(1)**, 81–88.
204. Okada, K., Yamashita, C., and Okada, M. (1996) Efficacy of oxygenated University of Wisconsin solution containing endothelin-A receptor antagonist in twenty-four-hour heart preservation. *J. Heart Lung Transplant.* **15(5)**, 475–484.
205. Ryan, J. B., Hicks, M., Cropper, J. R., et al. (2003) Cariporide (HOE-642) improves cardiac allograft preservation in a porcine model of orthotopic heart transplantation. *Transplantation* **75(5)**, 625–631.
206. Hashimoto, N., Takeyoshi, I., Yoshinari, D., et al. (2002) Effects of a p38 mitogen-activated protein kinase inhibitor as an additive to Euro-Collins solution on reperfusion injury in canine lung transplantation1. *Transplantation* **74(3)**, 320–326.
207. Roberts, J. R., Rowe, P. A., and Demaine, A. G. (2002) Activation of NF-kappaB and MAP kinase cascades by hypothermic stress in endothelial cells. *Cryobiology* **44(2)**, 161–169.
208. Tsuchihashi, S., Tamaki, T., Tanaka, M., et al. (2003) Pyrrolidine dithiocarbamate provides protection against hypothermic preservation and transplantation injury in the rat liver: the role of heme oxygenase-1. *Surgery* **133(5)**, 556–567.

209. Szabo, G., Soos, P., Bahrle, S., et al. (2004) Role of poly(ADP-ribose) polymerase activation in the pathogenesis of cardiopulmonary dysfunction in a canine model of cardiopulmonary bypass. *Eur. J. Cardio-Thorac. Surg.* **25(5)**, 825–832.
210. Mangino, M. J., Ametani, M., Szabo, C., and Southard, J. H. (2004) Poly(ADP-ribose) polymerase and renal hypothermic preservation injury. *Am. J. Physiol. Renal Fluid . Electrolyte Physiol.* **286(5)**, F838–847.
211. Ahlenstiel, T., Burkhardt, G., Kohler, H., and Kuhlmann, M. K. (2003) Bioflavonoids attenuate renal proximal tubular cell injury during cold preservation in Euro-Collins and University of Wisconsin solutions. *Kidney Int.* **63(2)**, 554–563.
212. Omasa, M., Fukuse, T., Matsuoka, K., Inui, K., Hyon, S. H., and Wada, H. (2003) Effect of green tea extracted polyphenol on ischemia/reperfusion injury after cold preservation of rat lung. *Transplant. Proc.* **35(1)**, 138–139.
213. Du, Z., Hicks, M., and Macdonald, P. (1997) Enhanced preservation of the rat heart after prolonged hypothermic storage with the 21-aminosteroid compound U74500A. *Asia Pacific Heart J.* **6**, 184–189.
214. Ryan, J. B., Hicks, M., Cropper, J. R., et al. (2003) Lazaroid (U74389G)-supplemented cardioplegia: results of a double-blind, randomized, controlled trial in a porcine model of orthotopic heart transplantation. *J. Heart Lung Transplant.* **22(3)**, 347–356.

16

Pharmacological Manipulation of the Rejection Response

Peter Mark Anthony Hopkins

Summary

Immunosuppressive strategies continue to evolve, with a number of new formulations having been developed in recent years. Although acute rejection rates may have diminished, current protocols of immunosuppression for chronic organ rejection are clearly inadequate. This complication remains the primary cause of graft loss months to years after solid organ transplant. In summary, the overall goal of achieving immune tolerance remains elusive. This chapter will focus on the pharmacological manipulation of the rejection response, reviewing historical and current recommended protocols. A brief outline of potential future pathways of targeted immunosuppression is described.

Key Words: Immunosuppression; acute rejection; chronic rejection.

1. Introduction

Descriptions of solid organ transplant rejection have classically recognized three distinct categories, including hyperacute, acute, and chronic rejection *(1)*. Hyperacute rejection is mediated through the presence of preexisting circulating antidonor human leukocyte antigen (HLA) antibodies in the recipient or occurs as a consequence of inadvertent ABO blood group incompatibility. The routine pretransplant screening of recipient serum by the panel reactive antibody (PRA) test and subsequent prospective crossmatch in sensitized patients has virtually eliminated this complication *(1)*. Chronic rejection of the transplanted organ has complex immunopathogenesis including sustained T-cell activation by donor major histocompatibility complex (MHC) antigens and development of non-MHC recipient alloantibodies. This alloimmune reaction may be facilitated by the generation of adhesion molecules including vascular cell adhesion molecule (VCAM-1) and integrins on the lymphocyte cell surface *(2–5)*. Infections (particularly cytomegalovirus [CMV]) posttransplant and

From: *Methods in Molecular Biology, vol. 333: Transplantation Immunology: Methods and Protocols*
Edited by: P. Hornick and M. Rose © Humana Press Inc., Totowa, NJ

the extent of cold ischemia at the time of organ harvest may further influence the evolution to chronic allograft rejection. The histological features of chronic rejection in solid organ transplantation include fibrosis, chronic inflammation, and a number of nonimmunological cell types such as fibroblasts, smooth muscle cells, and macrophages. Current protocols of nontargeted immunosuppression for chronic rejection are clearly insufficient for prevention of this complication because it remains the primary cause of graft loss months to years post-solid organ transplant ***(6)***.

Acute rejection (AR) is an immunological process of cell-mediated inflammation of an organ recognized as foreign by the recipient. The majority of donor proteins recognized as non-self are encoded by the HLA complex ***(1)***. Recipient T-lymphocytes are the dominant effector cell and may recognize donor peptides via two pathways known as direct and indirect alloantigen recognition. Facilitating T-lymphocyte binding to antigen and MHC molecules is the T-cell receptor, which consists in part of the cluster designation (CD) determinant CD3 transmembrane complex. Direct alloantigen recognition refers to a process whereby the recipient T-cell receptor engages directly with donor HLA material expressed on a donor-derived antigen-presenting cell (APC). In indirect recognition the donor HLA molecule is processed into small peptides within the interior of a recipient APC and then placed within the groove of a recipient HLA molecule ***(7)***. Regardless of the relative contribution of each pathway in allograft rejection, T-cell activation is followed by signal transduction, gene transcription, and cytokine production, which includes interleukins (ILs), interferon (IFN)-γ, tumor necrosis factor (TNF), and transforming growth factor-β. The different patterns of lymphokine secretion emphasize distinct functional properties of each T-lymphocyte ***(8,9)***. Pharmacological manipulation of the rejection response therefore targets the following areas:

1. Production and release of cytokines from activated T-cells
2. Downregulation and inhibition of T-cell surface receptors
3. Inhibition of lymphocyte and nonimmune cell proliferation
4. Absolute T- and B-cell depletion

The majority of solid organ transplant recipients experience at least one episode of AR regardless of the immunosuppressive regimen employed. In a recently published prospective series of transbronchial lung biopsy in lung and heart–lung transplant recipients ***(10)***, only 23% of patients remained free of AR at 12 mo posttransplant. The average number of rejection episodes per patient was just over one, with a significant proportion occurring beyond 12 mo (14.5%) independent of prior rejection history. AR was most frequently observed in the first postoperative month with 26% (63 of 241) of all cases detected. Only 6.1% (28 of 462) of surveillance procedures in asymptomatic patients between 4 and 12 mo posttransplant confirmed AR. Nonetheless, AR remains an ongoing risk throughout the life of the transplanted organ. Strategies directed against rejection consist primarily of prevention through induction and maintenance immunosuppression, complemented by augmentation of immune therapy during acute episodes.

2. Prevention of Acute Rejection

2.1. Induction Therapy

Historically, induction therapy refers to antilymphocyte sera (ALS) preparations commenced peri-operatively with a view to depleting circulating T lymphocytes, thereby boosting initial regimens and inducing a state of immune tolerance. Polyclonal antilymphocyte preparations were introduced to organ transplantation in 1967 ***(11)***, with a view to supplementing existing dual immunosuppression of azathioprine and prednisone. A variety of animals have been used to generate these antibody products, including rabbit (thymoglobulin and rabbit antithymocyte globulin [RATG]) and horse (antithymocyte gammaglobulin [ATGAM] and lymphoglobulin). Polyclonal ALS target multiple T-cell surface molecules including CD2, CD3, CD4, CD8, CD25, CD40, and CD54 ***(12,13)***. Unfortunately, in the production of these antilymphocyte sera, antibodies may evolve to most T-cell lines, B cells, and nonlymphoid populations. The result is global immunosuppression with an excess risk of opportunistic infections ***(14–16)***, especially CMV, malignancy, particularly Epstein–Barr virus-induced posttransplant lymphoproliferative disease (PTLD), and bone marrow suppression with thrombocytopenia and leukopenia. In addition, transient increases in serum cytokine levels, including IL-1, IL-6, TNF, and IFN-γ, accompany first-dose infusions of ALS ***(17–19)***. Clinically, this manifests as fever and chills in the majority of recipients and sometimes nausea, diarrhea, headache, bronchospasm, and, rarely, profound hypotension. Anaphylactic reactions and serum sickness are infrequent complications and respond to cessation of the ALS infusion and high-dose steroids.

In 1981 a murine-derived monoclonal antibody (MAb) called OKT3 was introduced into protocols for the treatment of renal allograft rejection and potentially induction therapy ***(20)***. This compound specifically targeted the CD3 complex associated with the T-cell receptor expressed on all mature T lymphocytes. Binding with OKT3 is followed by opsonization and then subsequent complement-mediated and cell-mediated antibody-dependent cytolysis and destruction of T cells ***(21)***. Nonetheless, OKT3 is a pan-T-cell antibody and therefore suppresses all aspects of T-cell immunity with increased risk of CMV and PTLD posttransplant similar to polyclonal products. Similar to other ALS preparations, OKT3 administration may be complicated by a cytokine-release syndrome and, rarely, aseptic meningitis or encephalopathy ***(22,23)***. Sensitization may occur with the formation of human anti-mouse antibodies with prolonged (>10–14 d) or sequential administration *(24)*, potentially reducing clinical efficacy and causing a serum sickness syndrome. Measurement of the CD3+ peripheral blood lymphocyte count is the preferred monitoring tool for all ALS preparations. Appropriate targets are a CD3+ count of more than5% of total lymphocyte numbers or an absolute count of between 50 and 100 cells per microliter *(25)*.

Early studies demonstrated a significant benefit from induction therapy in delaying the onset of AR episodes in renal transplant recipients *(26,27)*. However, the addition of cyclosporine to immunosuppressive regimens in 1978 transformed postoperative protocols and prompted many transplant centers to scale back the routine use of cytolytic induction therapy. Subsequently, multiple studies in renal, liver, cardiac, and lung transplantation *(28–31)* have reported no significant benefit to ALS in improving graft function or survival and variable reduction in overall frequency of rejection compared with standard triple immunosuppression (cyclosporine, azathioprine, and prednisone). A recent prospective randomized trial in lung transplant recipients comparing no induction therapy with RATG showed no statistically significant difference in freedom from AR at 6 mo. A clearly higher incidence and earlier occurrence of CMV infection was observed in the ATG group *(32)*. Although the routine use of ALS is diminishing, there are certain clinical situations in which peri-operative use may be desirable. These include patients with significant renal impairment either pre- or early posttransplant as a strategy to reduce exposure to cyclosporine, those with a PRA level of greater than 5%, and patients with a positive donor crossmatch *(33)*.

An alternative approach to induction therapy is the selected neutralization of activated T lymphocytes reactive specifically against the allograft. IL-2 plays a key role in graft rejection, and IL-2 receptors (CD25) are selectively expressed on the surface of only activated T lymphocytes. Therefore, a direct approach toward targeted immunosuppression is the development of anti-CD25 MAb to competitively inhibit the binding between IL-2 and its receptor *(34)*. Basiliximab (Simulect, Novartis) and daclizumab (Zenopax, Roche) are registered chimeric human/mouse antibodies directed against the α chain (Tac subunit) of the IL-2 receptor. Comparison of induction therapy with anti-CD25 MAbs is outlined in **Table 1**. Theoretically, these agents are immunogenic, although their small murine sequences are restricted to the variable region of the immunoglobulin chain. The development of human antimouse antibodies is generally less than 1% and is not felt to be clinically relevant. Both basiliximab and dacluzimab are designed to be administered concurrently with a calcineurin inhibitor to decrease IL-2 production and provide a synergistic effect *(35–38)*. However, Cantarovich et al. have described the successful implementation of anti-CD25 MAb therapy early posttransplant to allow for a calcineurin inhibitor "holiday" in solid-organ transplant recipients with acute renal dysfunction *(39)*.

Table 1
Comparison of Anti-IL-2-Receptor (CD25) Monoclonal Antibodies

Property	Daclizumab	Basiliximab
MAb type	Humanized[a]	Chimeric
Dose	1 mg/kg iv	20 mg iv
Half-life	20 d	7 d
Regimen	5 injections: wk 0, 2, 4, 6, 8	2 injections: d 0, 4
Safety	+++	+++
Tolerability	Good	Good
Immunogenicity	Low	Low
Drug interactions	Nil	Nil

Significant depletion of T cells does not occur with CD25 MAbs because peripheral CD3 counts remain stable. The humanized nature of the antibody, along with an absence of global T-cell suppression, contributes to their excellent side-effect profile and low incidence of opportunistic infection. In a double-blind placebo-controlled multicenter trial in 260 renal transplant recipients, the incidence of biopsy confirmed that AR at 12 mo was significantly reduced when daclizumab was added to standard immunosuppression of cyclosporine, azathioprine, and prednisone (22 vs 35%; $p < 0.03$). No difference was observed in the incidence of malignancy or opportunistic infection, and graft survival was similar at 12 mo ***(40)***. Immunoprophylaxis with basiliximab in combination with azathioprine-based triple immunosuppression in liver transplant recipients has also shown increased efficacy in the prevention of AR, with no significant adverse event profile ***(37)***. Experience in cardiac transplantation with IL-2 receptor blockers and mycophenolate-based triple therapy suggests less AR and delayed onset to first rejection episode ***(41)***. A comparative analysis of OKT3, antithymocyte globulin, and daclizumab for induction immunosuppression in clinical lung transplantation shows equivalence in the prevention of early post-transplant AR and 2-yr survival ***(42)***. In conclusion, preliminary evidence supports the idea that this form of induction therapy may further aid in improving outcome post-solid-organ transplantation.

2.2. Initial Immunosuppression Early Posttransplant

Agents utilized early posttransplant exhibit additive or synergistic effects and are administered in combination to achieve multipathway inhibition of lymphocyte activation while minimizing cumulative toxicity. Recent innovations in pharmaceutical research have expanded the traditional protocols of immunosuppression used for almost 20 yr. Nonetheless, statistically significant improvement in graft function and survival has not been consistently demonstrated in

Table 2
Current Available Immunosuppressive Agents for Early Posttransplant Protocols and Their Mechanism of Action

Class of agent	Mechanism of action
Corticosteroids	Block cytokine gene transcription
Lysis of T lymphocytes	
Clacineurin inhibitors	Inhibit IL-2 gene transcription
Cyclosporine	Reduce proliferation of activated T cells
Tacrolimus	
Inhibitors of nucleotide biosynthesis	
Azathioprine	Purine analog impairs DNA synthesis
Mycophenolate mofetil	Inhibits IMPDH and B-cell proliferation
TOR inhibitors	Inhibit cyclin-dependent tyrosine kinases
Rapamycin (sirolimus)	
Everolimus (RAD)	

IL, interleukin; IMPDH, inosine monophosphate dehydrogenasde; TOR, target of rapamycin.

clinical trials of these new agents *(43)*. **Table 2** outlines the current framework for initial immunosuppression posttransplant in the prevention of the rejection response. Most transplant protocols incorporate an initial triple drug regimen consisting of prednisone or steroid equivalent, a calcineurin inhibitor, and either azathioprine or mycophenolate.

2.3. Calcineurin Inhibitors

Calcineurin blocking agents constitute the backbone of current triple immunosuppressive therapy regimens. Cyclosporine (Neoral, Novartis), introduced in 1978 *(44)*, and tacrolimus or FK506 (Prograf; Fujisawa), introduced in 1989 *(45)*, are both prodrugs that bind selectively to different intracellular proteins called immunophilins. The cyclosporine–cyclophilin and tacrolimus–FK binding protein complexes then inhibit calcineurin, a multifunctional serine threonine phosphatase enzyme that normally dephosphorylates substrates for transcription factors including nuclear factor of activated T cells, nuclear factor-κB, and c-Jun N-terminal kinase *(46)*. The result is dose-dependant inhibition of gene expression for IL-2 and other pro-inflammatory lymphokines including IL-3, IL-4, IL-5, IFN-γ, and TNF *(47)*. Cytotoxic T lymphocytes become arrested at the G_0-G_1 cell-cycle interface and are therefore unable to differentiate and proliferate. **Table 3** outlines important comparisons between the calcineurin inhibitors available in clinical practice. Side effects and toxicity common to both agents include the following:

1. Serum abnormalities: abnormal liver function tests, hyperkalemia, hypomagnesemia, hyperuricemia, renal tubular acidosis, hyperlipidemia, hyperglycemia

Table 3
Comparison of Cyclosporine and Tacrolimus

	Cyclosporine		Tacrolimus	
Chemistry	Cyclic polypeptide		Macrolide antibiotic	
Bioavailability	33%		25%	
Preparations	10-, 25-, 50-, 100-mg capsules 100 mg/mL suspension		0.5-, 1-, 5-mg capsules 5-mg, 1-mL ampules	
Initial dosage posttransplant	5–10 mg/kg/d po two divided doses, three times a day cystic fibrosis patients		0.15 mg/kg/d po two divided doses	
Terminal half-life	19 h		8.7 h	
Side-effect profile	More gingival hyperplasia, hypertension, hirsutism		More diabetes mellitus, pruritis, tremor, alopecia	
Additional immune activity	Potentially pro-proliferative, IL-6 upregulation, increased TGF-β		Antifibroproliferative activity	
Therapeutic targets	0–2 wk	300–350 ng/mL	0–6 mo	10–15 ng/mL
	3–8 wk	250–300	>6 mo	5–15 ng/mL
	2–3 mo	200–250		
	4–6 mo	180–250		
	6–12 mo	150–180		
	>12 mo	100–150		
In vitro potency	1×		50–100×[a]	

[a] Due to differences in partition coefficients and increased binding affinity of tacrolimus to FKBP.
IL, interleukin; TGF, transforming growth factor; FKBP, FK-binding protein.

2. Renal failure: acute (acute arteriolar vasoconstriction), chronic (interstitial fibrosis, glomerular sclerosis)
3. Neurotoxicity: characteristic white matter changes on computed tomography or T_2-weighted images or magnetic resonance imaging—headaches, encephalopathy, seizures, cortical blindness, quadriplegia
4. Gastrointestinal: nausea, diarrhea, constipation, vomiting
5. Other: hypertension, hemolytic–uremic syndrome

Significant inter- and intraindividual pharmacokinetic variability exists with the calcineurin inhibitors, and this contributes to their narrow therapeutic index ***(46)***. Drug monitoring is essential and is based on either enzyme-linked immunosorbent assay or high-performance liquid chromatography (HPLC) using whole blood ***(48)***. Calcineurin inhibitors display variable and temperature-dependent whole blood-to-plasma ratios. At room temperature, cyclosporine displays an equilibrium range of approx 50% bound to red blood cells, 30–40% to lipoproteins, 10% to leukocytes, and 1–6% free plasma ***(33)***. The gold standard assay is HPLC, as both drugs have multiple metabolites identified and crossreaction with MAb-based tests may be considerable ***(49)***. Cyclosporine and tacrolimus are both primarily metabolized by gut wall and the hepatic cytochrome P450-3A4 enzyme system and undergo intestinal countertransport by P-glycoprotein. Pharmacokinetic interactions are therefore common owing to modulation of cytochrome P450 enzyme activity by co-administered drugs. This includes induction of CYP3A4 enzymes and reduced calcineurin inhibitor levels with the antiepileptics including carbamazepine, phenytoin and phenobarbitol, rifabutin, rifampicin, isoniazid, and St. John's wort. Increased levels with enzyme inhibition occur with macrolide antibiotics, including erythromycin, clarithromycin and azithromycin, diltiazem, verapamil, colchicine, intravenous methylprednisolone, the oral contraceptive pill, and azoles, including itraconazole, fluconazole, and voriconazole. The pharmacokinetic behavior of both calcineurin inhibitors assumes a one-compartment model. Therapeutic monitoring has historically involved sampling a trough level just prior to the morning dose. However, calculation of the area under the curve (AUC) provides the most accurate measurement of total drug exposure, although it is clinically impractical. Cyclosporine trough concentrations (C_{min}) have displayed poor correlation with AUC in pharmacokinetic studies in liver and renal recipients, with only 34–42% of the variance in AUC explained by the C_{min}-derived regression line ***(50,51)***. Recent evidence suggests that limited sampling strategies display a high correlation coefficient with AUC, including a 2-h postdose cyclosporine assay ***(52)***. By contrast, therapeutic drug monitoring with tacrolimus suggests that C_{min} is an accurate parameter explaining 86–88% of the variance in AUC ***(53,54)***.

With lymphocyte trafficking and accumulation within the graft attenuated by calcineurin inhibitors, optimization of dosage is essential in the pharmacological manipulation of acute rejection. This clearly depends on individual side-effect profile, rejection history, time posttransplantation, and potential end-organ toxicity. Studies of AR in lung and heart–lung transplant recipients support the notion that higher blood concentrations are required in the early postoperative months ***(10,55)***.

2.4. Nucleotide-Blocking Agents

The introduction of mycophenolate mofetil (Cell Cept, Roche) into clinical practice in the early 1990s initiated a progressive decline in azathioprine usage in organ transplantation ***(56,57)***. Azathioprine (Imuran, Glaxo), a nucleoside analog, is metabolized in the liver to thio-inosine-monophosphate by hypoxanthine guanine phosphoribosyltransferase. This compound inhibits adenylic and guanylic acid production in the *de novo* purine synthesis pathway ***(58)***. Human B and T lymphocytes have immature salvage pathways and depend almost exclusively on the *de novo* pathway of purine synthesis for their replication. However, the incorporation of thio-inosine-monophosphate into DNA strands potentiates chromosomal breaks and the eventual predisposition to malignancies, especially cutaneous tumors. Mycophenolate produces reversible noncompetitive blockade of the purine pathway enzyme inosine monophosphate dehydrogenase (IMPD). The result is a significant decline in guanosine monophosphate and subsequent production of DNA via ribonucleotide reductases. Not being a nucleoside analog, mycophenolate mofetil (MMF) does not inhibit DNA repair enzymes and is theoretically less mutagenic than azathioprine. A further mechanism for the selectivity of MMF in lymphocyte inhibition is based on the two isoforms of IMPD. The type II isoform preferentially found in activated lymphocytes is inactivated more strongly by MMF than the type I IMPD in resting cells ***(59)***. **Table 4** compares the two antimetabolites. Therapeutic drug monitoring is not routinely recommended for MMF, although measurements of trough levels may help to detect underimmunosuppressed patients. Experience in kidney transplantation suggests onset of immunosuppressive effect and decreased acute rejection with trough concentrations greater than 1.0 mg/L ***(60)***. However, a study in 45 cardiac transplant recipients of combination MMF and tacrolimus showed prevention of AR episodes with C_{min} greater than 3 mg/L ***(61)***. In clinical practice, dosing of MMF is determined by the side-effect profile, which includes gastrointestinal symptoms of nausea, vomiting, anorexia, diarrhea, and myelosupression, especially leukopenia and anemia. Other rare adverse effects may include alopecia, liver dysfunction, pancreatitis, and gastritis. A randomized multicenter international trial comparing 3 g of MMF per day to 1.5–3 mg/kg of azathioprine per day in 578 cardiac transplant recipients has demonstrated a 45% reduction in mortality at 1 yr with MMF. Biopsy-proven rejection with hemodynamic compromise or graft loss at 6 mo posttransplant were significantly reduced in the

Table 4
Comparison of Azathioprine and MMF

	Azathioprine	Mycophenolate
Active metabolites	6-Mercaptopurine thio-inosine-monophosphate	Mycophenolic acid
Dosage	2–3 mg/kg/d po once per day first year, 1 mg/kg/d > 12 mo	2–3 g/d po two divided doses
Monitoring	Not required	2.0–4.5 ng/mL HPLC assay
Elimination	One compartment, expontial decay	Two compartment, enterohepatic circulation
Terminal half life	3 h	18 h
Immunosuppression	T-Cell activity	T- and B-cell activity
Drug interactions	Allopurinol—bone marrow suppression (dose reduce azathioprine 75%)	Antacids and bile acid sequestering agents reduce MMF levels; tacrolimus increases MMF levels
Other activity	—	Antiviral activity (EBV-induced B-cell lines) Inhibits glycosylation and expression of adhesion molecules Inhibits production of TGF-β Suppresses nitric oxide by iNOS Inhibits smooth muscle and fibroblast proliferation

MMF, mycophenolate mofetil; HPLC, high-performance liquid chromatography; EBV, Epstein–Barr virus; TGF, transforming growth factor; iNOS, anti-inducible nitric oxide synthase.

Table 5
Toxicity Profile of Nucleotide-Blocking Agents

		Azathioprine (%)	Mycophenolate (%)
Side effects	• Leukopeniaa	39.1	30.4
	• Abnormal LFG	12.8	9.7
	• Nausea	54.3	54.0
	• Diarrhea[a]	34.3	45.3
	• Esophagitis[a]	2.8	7.3
Malignancy	• Lymphoma	2.1	0.7
	• Other malignancy	5.2	6.2
Infections	• CMV viremia	10.0	12.1
	• CMV tissue invasive	8.7	11.4
	• Herpes simplex	14.5	20.8
	• Herpes zoster[a]	5.9	10.7
	• Aspergillus	2.1	2.1
	• Candida	17.6	18.7

[a]*p*-value for difference <0.05
LFT, Liver function test; DMV, cytomegalovirus.

MMF arm ($p = 0.045$). **Table 5** summarizes the toxicity profiles of both drugs in this clinical study ***(62)***. A similar study in 315 lung recipients reported a 12-mo survival significantly better in the MMF arm vs azathioprine (88.1% vs 79.1%; $p = 0.038$). There was no significant difference in frequency of AR at 12 mo or development of bronchiolitis obliterans syndrome in the first 3 yr posttransplant ***(63)***.

The clinical significance of MMF in inhibiting human arterial smooth muscle cell, fibroblast, and endothelial cell proliferation and the development of chronic rejection is still being evaluated. In addition, attenuation of antibody production via humoral inhibition may further reduce chronic rejection ***(59)***. Nonetheless, the Tricontinental Renal Transplant study of MMF showed no significant difference in patient survival or allograft function at 3 yr ***(64)***.

2.5. Target of Rapamycin Inhibitors

Sirolimus or rapamycin (Rapamune, Wyeth-Ayerst) is a macrolide antibiotic produced by *Streptomyces hygroscopicus* and originally discovered on Easter Island in 1975. The immunosuppressive action is mediated by binding to the FK506-binding protein (FKBP-12) and inhibiting a kinase known as mammalian target of rapamycin (TOR). Rapamycin has no effect on calcineurin phosphatase activity ***(65)***. Rather, it inhibits B- and T-lymphocyte proliferation by

Table 6
Side-Effect Profile of TOR Inhibitors

Frequent	Uncommon
Hyperlipidemia	Hypertension
Stomatitis	Increased serum creatinine
Thrombocytopenia	Dirrhea
Leukopenia	Liver inflammation
Epistaxis	Hypophosphatemia
Bacterial infections	Hypokalemia
Impaired wound healing	Intersititial pneurnonitis
Polyarthralgia	Optic neuropathy
Nausea	Distal osteitis

TOR, target of rapamycin.

blocking cytokine stimulatory signals including IL-2, IL-4, IL-6, and anti-CD28 antibodies via a serine threonine kinase called p70S6k. This results in a failure of immune effector cells to progress from the G1 to S cell-cycle interface ***(66)***. In vitro rapamycin also inhibits vascular smooth muscle cell, endothelial cell, and fibroblast proliferation induced by fibroblast growth factor, insulin-like growth factor, and platelet-derived growth factor ***(33)***. RAD or everolimus (Certican, Novartis) is a derivative of sirolimus and contains a hydroxyethyl group at position 40 to increase polarity and oral bioavailability ***(67)***. The only significant pharmacokinetic difference between these compounds pertains to half-life, which is 30 h for RAD and 62 h for sirolimus. Both TOR inhibitors display synergistic effects with calcineurin inhibitors and are being studied extensively in combination. Cyclosporine and TOR inhibitors must be administered a minimum of 2 h apart owing to complex pharmacokinetics, including inhibition of CYP3A4 and decreased P-glycoprotein intestinal countertransport of either compound. TOR inhibitors are metabolized by CYP3A4 and therefore share similar drug interactions with the calcineurin inhibitors. Clinical doses of sirolimus should target whole blood levels of 3–15 ng/mL measured by HPLC, depending on time posttransplantation ***(68,69)***. Effective RAD doses are not established, although recent reports suggest 1.5–4 mg/d have a clinically meaningful influence on AR ***(70–72)***. Potential adverse effects of TOR inhibitors are outlined in **Table 6** and in clinical practice limit dose escalation.

An open-label randomized trial of sirolimus compared with azathioprine as part of standard triple immunosuppression in 136 *de novo* cardiac transplant recipients has recently been published ***(73)***. At 6 mo the rate of biopsy-proven AR was halved in the sirolimus group (61.4% azathioprine vs 29.4% 3 mg/d and 36.2% 5 mg/d of sirloimus). A significant reduction in cardiac allograft arterial disease was also demonstrable, suggesting protection from chronic transplant vasculopathy ***(74)***. Similar results have been obtained in cardiac trials evaluating 1.5– 3 mg of RAD ***(71)***. Unfortunately, trials of RAD in lung transplantation have not shown convincing evidence of reduction in development of bronchiolitis obliterans syndrome or chronic rejection ***(75,76)***. Analysis of 24-mo data from multicenter phase III trials ***(77)*** in approx 1300 renal transplant recipients reveals that patients on 5 mg of sirolimus in addition to cyclosporine experience a significant delay in the onset and reduction in the incidence of AR compared with azathioprine ($p = 0.02$) or placebo ($p = 0.001$). Further potential roles of TOR inhibitors are in calcineurin-inhibitor-sparing regimens and weaning of corticosteroids in maintenance immunosuppression.

3. Corticosteroids in the Treatment of Acute Rejection

Corticosteroid therapy is the mainstay of treatment options for AR in solid organ transplantation. The dose of methylprednisolone employed for high-grade allograft rejection is typically 500–1000 mg/d or 10–15 mg/kg intravenously. Patients receive this as "pulse" therapy over a 3-d period, often with a continuation phase of oral prednisone or equivalent commencing at 1 mg/kg/d. This will depend on the histological features of obtained biopsy material, time post-transplantation, concurrent infection, and prior rejection history. There is also evidence in renal and cardiac transplantation of 100–200 mg/d of oral prednisone being equivalent to intravenous methylprednisolone in reversing AR ***(78,79)***. Controversy exists regarding the necessity to treat low-grade rejection scores, particularly in asymptomatic patients. In lung transplantation, minimal AR (International Society of Heart-Lung Transplantation [ISHLT] grade A_1) is detected in 22% of transbronchial lung biopsy procedures and asymptomatic in 90% of cases. In addition, the risk of surveillance A_1 lesions progressing to higher-grade rejection (ISHLT grade > A_2) or lymphocytic bronchiolitis within 3 mo is 34% ***(80)***. Nonetheless, 30% of mild rejection episodes (grade A_2) may resolve spontaneously with no initial therapy. Low grades of rejection in clinically well heart–lung patients may be poorly predictive of subsequent airway submucosal fibrosis ***(81)***. Our current policy is to treat all symptomatic low-grade biopsies with an oral steroid pulse commencing at 1 mg/kg/d and tapering by 5 mg each day. There is clinical evidence in other respiratory disease models to support that such doses are truly lymphocytolytic in nature ***(82,83)***. For asymptomatic patients, careful clinical observation is recommended, with steroid treatment reserved for those patients who show subsequent graft deterioration. Recent evidence suggests an association between multiple episodes (>2 grade A_1 biopsies) of low-grade rejection and the subsequent development of obliterative bronchiolitis in lung transplantation. Therefore, augmentation of baseline immunosuppression or a change to a more antifibroproliferative regimen may be warranted in such circumstances *(80)*.

Generally, corticosteroids form an integral part of chronic maintenance protocols, albeit at small baseline doses. A steroid-withdrawal approach to immunosuppression is certainly not universally practiced across the spectrum of solid organ transplantation. Prednisone and prednisolone have high oral bioavailability and a plasma half-life from 3 to 4 h. Prednisone undergoes hepatic metabolism to prednisolone, which is more than 90% bound to plasma proteins including albumin and cortisone-binding globulin. The therapeutic benefit of corticosteroids in acute rejection rests with their combined anti-inflammatory and immunosuppressive action. Steroids reduce the synthesis of leukotrienes and prostaglandins via inhibition of phosphodiesterase A_2. Immunosuppressive activity is multifactorial and includes:

1. Absolute T-lymphocyte depletion via induction of apoptosis
2. Inhibition of T-cell activation and proliferation via reduced cytokine gene transcription of IL-1, IL-2, IL-6, TNF, and interferon-γ
3. Reduced HLA and adhesion molecule expression
4. Inhibition of monocyte chemotaxis and migration to sites of inflammation *(33)*

4. Treatment of Persistent and Recurrent Rejection

The definition of persistent rejection in organ transplantation is histologically confirmed rejection that persists on a follow-up biopsy performed after a prior treated episode. The follow-up period varies depending on routine institutional practices, type of transplant procedure, and presence of clinical features of rejection. Recurrent rejection refers to at least three discrete episodes of rejection, not necessarily consecutive, within a defined period of time generally measured in months. **Table 7** outlines therapeutic options for patients with persistent or recurrent rejection. The management strategies include optimization of existing immunosuppressive regimens, treatment with OKT3 MAb or polyclonal ALS and changing immunosuppression to a tacrolimus- and/or MMF-based protocol. Cytolytic therapy has demonstrated efficacy in the treatment of steroid-resistant allograft rejection. A study in 18 cardiac recipients with resistant or recurrent rejection confirmed 88 and 100% efficacy, respectively, with either OKT3 5 mg/d or ATG 1.5–2.5 mg/kg/d in reversing histological findings. Throughout follow-up averaging 50 mo, there was a trend towards lower incidence of subsequent AR after ATG (25 vs 69%; $p = 0.09$) and similar incidence of infections, graft atherosclerosis, and mortality. No cases of PTLD were observed *(84)*. A randomized study in 163 renal recipients comparing ATG with equine-derived ATGAM was published in 1998. ATG had a higher rejection reversal rate than ATGAM (88 vs 76%; $p = 0.027$, primary endpoint). T-cell depletion was more significant with ATG and main-

Table 7
Therapeutic Options for Persistent or Recurrent Acute Rejection Solid Organ Transplantation

500–1000 mg intravenous methylprednisolone in association with one or more of the following:

1. Optimization of current immunosuppression:
   - Assess compliance
   - Target higher blood levels
   - Increase baseline oral prednisone dosage to 0.2 mg/kg/d
2. Alteration of maintenance triple immunosuppression:
   - Change from cyclosporine to tacrolimus
   - Convert azathiprine to MMF
   - Change route of administration: nebulized cyclosporine (in lung transplant recipients)
3. Cytolytic therapy (duration 3–14 d):
   - Polyclonal antilymphocyte sera
   - OKT3
4. Addition of or substitution with another immunosuppressive agent:
   - Methotrexate
   - Cyclophosphamide
   - TOR inhibitor (sirolimus or RAD)
   - Leflunomide (experimental)

tained more effectively at d 30 posttherapy ($p = 0.016$). Recurrent rejection at 3 mo after treatment occurred less frequently with ATG than with ATGAM (17 vs 36%; $p = 0.011$). A similar incidence of adverse events, opportunistic infection, 12-mo patient and graft survival were observed with both therapies ***(85)***. Early studies in renal transplantation confirmed the success of MMF as rescue therapy in 69% of patients with refractory rejection to ALS preparations ***(86)***. The MMF Renal Study Group evaluated 150 patients with refractory rejection and randomized them to either MMF 1.5 g twice daily or further intravenous steroids 5 mg/kg/d for 5 d. The primary efficacy variable of graft loss or death was reduced by 45% in the MMF group while the steroid cohort was twice as likely to require subsequent ALS therapy ***(87)***. Similar studies in cardiac, lung, renal, and liver transplantation evaluating tacrolimus have achieved results comparable to MMF ***(88–92)***. A study by Onsager and colleagues in thoracic organ transplant recipients showed reversal of rejection refractory to steroids and OKT3 in 73% of cases following conversion to tacrolimus from cyclosporine ***(93)***. Inhibition of IL-10 production is a critical factor in the ability of tacrolimus to reverse ongoing allograft rejection compared with cyclosporine ***(94)***. Methotrexate administered either as a single high dose (5 mg/kg) or as a supplement to maintenance immunosuppression at 7.5–22.5 mg/wk has proved successful for refractory rejection in cardiac and lung transplantation ***(95–98)***. Predictable side effects of folic acid analog therapy are mild pancytopenia and agranulocytosis. The mechanism of immunosuppression with methotrexate remains to be elucidated but is probably related to reduced intercellular adhesion molecule (ICAM)-1 expression in lymphoid tissue ***(99)***. Aerosolized cyclosporine has displayed in a dose-dependent manner some success in lung transplantation in protecting against further rejection episodes and improving graft histology ***(100,101)***. Administration consists of 300 mg of cyclosporine in 4.8 mL of propylene glycol using a jet nebulizer daily for 10–12 d, and then three times a week. A strong correlation exists between cyclosporine deposition in lung parenchyma measured by radioisotopic techniques and improvement in forced expiratory volume in 1 s. In a murine model, reversal of ongoing cardiac, kidney, and pancreas allograft rejection was achieved by rapamycin, although human studies are limited ***(102)***. Sirolimus vs MMF rescue therapy has been evaluated in 36 renal transplant patients with ongoing rejection despite steroids and 14–21 d of ALS. Reversal of renal dysfunction was observed in 96% of patients in the sirolimus group compared with 67% in the MMF group ($p = 0.03$). One-year graft and patient survival rates were similar ***(103)***. Leflunomide is a xenobiotic agent that demonstrates selective inhibition of pyrimidine synthesis. In experimental canine transplantation it has prolonged renal allograft survival when given in combination with either cyclosporine or tacrolimus ***(104,105)***.

Total lymphoid irradiation (TLI) is a potential therapy reserved for rejection refractory to all other conventional immunotherapy ***(106,107)***. TLI involves the delivery of low-dose radiotherapy in a 5- to 6-wk fractionated regimen (total dose 600–840 cGy) to lymphoid tissue in a supradiaphragmatic mantle and abdomino-pelvic inverted Y distribution. Nucleotide blocking agents are discontinued prior to initial treatment given the risks of profound bone marrow suppression. An additional disadvantage of TLI is prolonged lymphopenia with risk of opportunistic infection, especially invasive fungal and CMV infection. Mutagenesis with an excess risk of lymphoma and acute megakaryocytic leukemia have followed this modality. Trials in cardiac transplantation have found TLI to be a risk factor for transplant coronary vasculopathy ***(108)***. Although TLI has merit for the treatment of intractable AR, toxicity limits its more widespread application. Extracorporeal photochemotherapy (ECPC) or photopheresis is a relatively new immunomodulatory treatment, studied in predominately renal, cardiac, and lung transplant rejection ***(109)***. This costly technique involves the removal of recipient leukocytes using a cell separator and then irradiating an enriched lymphocyte solution with ultraviolet (UV) A light in the presence of 8-methoxypsoralen. This compound, administered orally 2 h prior, cross-links with DNA strands following UV application inducing apoptosis in activated T cells, phenotypic change to suppressor T-cell capability, and humoral inhibition ***(33)***. A typical treatment regimen involves one session per week in the first month, every 2 wk in the second and third month, and then monthly thereafter. Dall'Amico et al. have published a trial of ECPC in cardiac recipients with recurrent rejection. Only 18% of endomyocardial biopsies during 6 mo of photopheresis showed 3A/3B rejection, and a significant reduction in dosage of baseline immunosuppression was achieved ***(110)***. Depletion of circulating T lymphocytes does not occur with photopheresis, but precautions are required during the delivery of UV light to prevent retinal scarring and sunburn.

5. Future Directions in Immunosuppression and Novel Agents

Despite recent advances in immunosuppressive protocols for solid organ transplantation, acute allograft rejection remains a significant source of patient morbidity and mortality. While the field of transplantation continues to expand with new immunosuppressive formulations, the overall goal of achieving immune tolerance remains elusive. One novel avenue of investigation is the inhibition of those additional pathways critical to effective T-cell activation using monoclonal antibodies. For example, it is postulated that self-tolerance may involve the inhibition or absence of a costimulatory signal normally involved in the amplification of T-cell activity ***(111)***. Such signals may include the T-cell ligands leukocyte function antigen-1 (LFA-1), very late antigen-4, B7, VCAM-1, and ICAM-1. Therefore, interference with these molecules even in the presence of foreign or transplanted tissue may induce tolerance. An indefinite survival of cardiac allografts between fully incompatible mice strains has been documented using monoclonal antibodies to LFA-1 and ICAM-1 early posttransplant ***(112)***. Other drugs have been reported as possessing immunomodulatory properties, including pravastatin, aminoguanidine, and thalidomide, although have little clinical experience in this context ***(113)***. Finally, genetic alteration of the donor organ during procurement may ameliorate graft rejection by inducing donor-specific tolerance. Modern genetic techniques using vectors such as liposomes, adenovirus, and hyperbaric pressure to deliver molecules inhibiting donor gene expression have been employed ***(111)***.

References

1. King-Biggs, M. B. (1997) Acute pulmonary allograft rejection: mechanisms, diagnosis and management, in *Clinics in Chest Medicine* (Maurer, J. R., ed.), WB Saunders Company, London, pp. 301–310.
2. Devouassoux, G., Pison, C., Drouet, C., Pin, I., Brambilla, C., and Brambilla, E. (2001) Early lung leukocyte infiltration, HLA and adhesion molecule expression predict chronic rejection. *Transplant. Immunol.* **8**, 229–236.

3. Kauppinen, H., Soots, A., Krogerus, L., et al. (2000) Sequential analysis of adhesion molecules and their ligands in rat renal allografts during the development of chronic rejection. *Transplant. Int.* **13**, 247–254.
4. Demirci, G., Hoshino, K., and Nashan, B. (1999) Expression patterns of integrin receptors and extracellular matrix proteins in chronic rejection of human liver allografts. *Transplant. Immunol.* **7**, 229–237.
5. Von Willebrand, E., Jurcic, V., Isoniemi, H., Hayry, P., Paavonen, T., and Krogerus, L. (1997) Adhesion molecules and their ligands in chronic rejection of human renal allografts. *Transplant. Proc.* **29**, 1530–1531.
6. Charpentier, B., Hiesse, C., Durrbach, A., et al. (2000) Immunosuppression advancing in the new millenium: lessons learned from recent multicentre and single centre clinical trials. *Curr. Opin. Organ Transplant.* **5**, 249–254.
7. Game, D. S. and Lechler, R. I. (2002) Pathways of allorecognition: implications for transplantation tolerance. *Transplant. Immunol.* **10**, 101–108.
8. Mosmann, T. R. and Coffman, R. L. (1989) TH1 and TH2 cells: different patterns of lymphokine secretion lead to different functional properties. *Annu. Rev. Immunol.* **7**, 145–173.
9. Nickerson, P., Steurer, W., and Steiger, J. (1994) Cytokines and the Th1/Th2 paradigm in transplantation. *Curr. Opin. Immunol.* **6**, 757–764.
10. Hopkins, P. M., Aboyoun, C. L., Chhajed, P. N., et al. (2002) Prospective analysis of 1235 transbronchial lung biopsies in lung transplant recipients. *J. Heart Lung Transplant.* **21**, 1062–1067.
11. Starzl, T. E., Porter, K. A., and Iwasaki, Y. (1967) The use of heterologous antilymphocyte globulins in human homotransplantation in *Antilymphocyte Serum* (Wolstenholme, G. E. W., O'Connor, M., eds.), Little, Brown, Boston, p. 1.
12. Rebellato, L. M., Gross, U., and Verbanac, K. M. (1994) A comprehensive definition of the major antibody specificities in polyclonal rabbit antithymocyte globulin. *Transplantation* **57**, 685–694.
13. Bourdage, J. S. and Hamlin, D. M. (1995) Comparative polyclonal antithymocyte globulin and antilymphocyte/antilymphoblast globulin anti-CD antigen analysis by flow cytometry. *Transplantation* **59**, 1194–1200.
14. Swinnen, L. J., Costanzo-Nordin, M. R., and Fisher, S. G. (1990) Increased incidence of lymphoproliferative disorder after immunosuppression with the monoclonal antibody OKT3 in cardiac transplant recipients. *N. Engl. J. Med.* **323**, 1723–1728.
15. Kusne, S., Shapiro, R., and Fung, J. (1999) Prevention and treatment of cytomegalovirus infection in organ transplant recipients. *Transplant. Infect. Dis.* **1**, 187–203.
16. Jamil, B., Nicholls, K. M., Becker, G. J., and Walker, R. G. (2000) Influence of anti-rejection therapy on the timing of cytomegalovirus disease and other infections in renal transplant recipients. *Clin. Transplant.* **14**, 14–18.
17. Piaggio, G., Podesta, M., Pitto, A., et al. (1998) TNF-alpha, IFN-gamma and GM-CSF production by purified normal marrow CD3 cells in response to horse anti-lymphocyte and rabbit antithymocyte globulin. *Eur. J. Haematol.* **60**, 240–244.

18. Rameshwar, P. and Gascon, P. (1992) Release of interleukin-1 and interleukin-6 from human monocytes by antithymocyte globulin: requirement for de novo synthesis. *Blood* **15**, 2531–2538.
19. Oettinger, C. W., D'Souza, M., and Milton, G. V. (1996) In vitro comparison of cytokine release from antithymocyte serum and OKT3. Inhibition with soluble and microencapsulated neutralising antibodies. *Transplantation* **15**, 1690–1693.
20. Cosimi, A. B., Burton, R. C., and Colvin, R. B. (1981) Treatment of acute renal allograft rejection with OKT3 monoclonal antibody. *Transplantation* **32**, 535.
21. Bonnefoy-Berard, N. and Revillard, J.P. (1996) Mechanisms of immunosuppression induced by antithymocyte globulins and OKT3. *J. Heart Lung Transplant.* **15**, 435–442.
22. Shihab, F. S., Barry, J. M., and Norman, D. J. (1993) Encephalopathy following the use of OKT3 in renal allograft transplantation. *Transplant. Proc.* **25**, 31–34.
23. Adair, J. C., Woodley, S. L., O'Connell, J. B., Call, G. K., and Baringer, J. R. (1991) Aseptic meningitis following cardiac transplantation: clinical characteristics and relationship to immunosuppressive regimen. *Neurology* **41**, 249–252.
24. Kuus-Reichel, K., Grauer, L. S., Karavodin, L. M., Knott, C., Krusemeier, M., and Kay, N. E. (1994) Will immunogenecity limit the use, efficacy and future development of therapeutic monoclonal antibodies? *Clin. Diagn. Lab. Immunol.* **1**, 365–372.
25. Krasinskas, A. M., Kreisel, D., Acker, M. A., et al. (2002) CD3 monitoring of antithymocyte globulin therapy in thoracic organ transplantation. *Transplantation* **73**, 1339–1341.
26. Wechter, W. J., Broodie, J. A., and Morrell, R. M. (1979) Antithymocyte globulin (ATGAM) in renal allograft recipients. *Transplantation* **28**, 294–307.
27. Cosimi, A. B. (1981) The clinical value of antilymphocyte antibodies. *Transplant. Proc.* **13**, 462–468.
28. Norman, D. J., Kahana, L., Stuart, F. P., et al. (1993) A randomised clinical trial of induction therapy with OKT3 in kidney transplantation. *Transplantation* **55**, 44–50.
29. Farges, O., Ericzon, B. G., Bresson-Hadni, S., et al. (1994) A randomised trial of OKT3-based versus cyclosporine-based immunoprophylaxis after liver transplantation. Long term results of a European and Australian multicentre study. *Transplantation* **58**, 891–898.
30. Barr, M. L., Sanchez, J. A., Seche, L. A., Schulman, L. L., Smith, C. R., and Rose, E. A. (1990) Anti-CD3 monoclonal antibody induction therapy. Immunological equivalency with triple-drug therapy in heart transplantation. *Circulation* **82**, 291–294.
31. Palmer, S. M., Miralles, A. P., Lawrence, C. M., Gaynor, J. W., Davis, R. D., and Tapson, V. F. (1999) Rabbit antilymphocyte globulin decreases acute rejection after lung transplantation: results of a randomised, prospective study. *Chest* **116**, 127–133.
32. Klepetko, W., Jaksch, P., Kocher, A.A., et al. (2002) Prospective, randomised trial comparing induction therapy with daclizumab or rabbit antithymocyte glob-

uline versus no induction therapy after lung transplantation. *J. Heart Lung Transplant.* **21**, A33.
33. George, J. F. (2002) Immunosuppressive modalities, in *Heart Transplantation* (Kirklin, J. K., Young, J. B., and McGiffin, D. C., eds.), Churchill Livingstone, London, pp. 390–462.
34. Henry, M. L. and Rajab, A. (2002) The use of basiliximab in solid organ transplantation. *Expert. Opin. Pharmacother.* **3**, 1657–1663.
35. Lawen, J. G., Davies, E. A., Mourad, G., et al. (2003) Randomised double-blind study of immunoprophylaxis with basiliximab, a chimeric anti-interleukin-2 receptor monoclonal antibody, in combination with mycophenolate mofetil-containing triple therapy in renal transplantation. *Transplantation* **75**, 37–43.
36. Sollinger, H., Kaplan, B., Pescovitz, M. D., et al. (2001) Basiliximab versus antithymocyte globulin for prevention of acute renal allograft rejection. *Transplantation* **72**, 1915–1919.
37. Calmus, Y., Scheele, J. R., Gonzalez-Pinto, I., et al. (2002) Immunoprophylaxis with basiliximab, a chimeric anti-interleukin-2 receptor monoclonal antibody, in combination with azathioprine-containing triple therapy in liver transplant recipients. *Liver Transplant.* **8**, 123–131.
38. Clark, G., Walsh, G., Deshpande, P., and Koffman, G. (2002) Improved efficacy of basiliximab over antilymphocyte globulin induction therapy in paediatric renal transplantation. *Nephrol. Dial. Transplant.* **17**, 1304–1309.
39. Cantarovich, M., Metrakos, P., Giannette, N., Cecere, R., Barkun, J., and Tchervenkov, J. (2002) Anti-CD25 monoclonal antibody coverage allows for calcineurin inhibitor "holiday" in solid organ transplant patients with acute renal dysfunction. *Transplantation* **73**, 1169–1172.
40. Vincenti, F., Kirkman, R., Light, S., et al. (1998) Interleukin-2-receptor blockade with daclizumab to prevent acute rejection in renal transplantation. Daclizumab Triple Therapy Study Group. *N Engl J Med* **338**, 161–165.
41. Beniaminovitz, A., Itescu, S., Lietz, K., et al. (2000) Prevention of rejection in cardiac transplantation by blockade of the interleukin-2 receptor with a monoclonal antibody. *N. Engl. J. Med.* **342**, 613–619.
42. Brock, M.V., Borja, M. C., Ferber, L., et al. (2001) Induction therapy in lung transplantation: a prospective controlled clinical trial comparing OKT3, anti-thymocyte globulin and daclizumab. *J. Heart Lung Transplant.* **20**, 1282–1290.
43. Charpentier, B., Hiesse, C., Durrbach, A., et al. (2000) Immunosuppression advancing in the new millennium: lessons learned from recent multicentre and single centre clinical trials. *Curr. Opin. Organ. Transplant.* **5**, 249–254.
44. Calne, R. Y., White, D. J., Thiru, S., et al. (1978) Cyclosporin A in patients receiving renal allografts from cadaver donors. *Lancet* **2**, 1323–1327.
45. Todo, S., Fung, J. J., Tzakis, A., et al. (1991) One hundred ten consecutive primary orthotopic liver transplants under FK 506 in adults. *Transplant. Proc.* **23**, 1397–1402.
46. Mahalati, K. and Kahan, B.D. (2000) Advancing the art of immunosuppression with the science of pharmacology. *Curr. Opin. Organ Transplant.* **5**, 255–262.

47. Briffa, N. and Morris, R.E. (1997) New immunosuppressive regimens in lung transplantation. *Eur. Respir. J.* **10**, 2630–2637.
48. Keown, P. A. (2002) New concepts in cyclosporine monitoring. *Curr. Opin. Nephrol. Hypertens.* **11**, 619–626.
49. Tredger, J. M., Roberts, N., Sherwood, R., Higgins, G., and Keating, J. (2000) Comparison of five cyclosporin immunoassays with HPLC. *Clin. Chem. Lab. Med.* **38**, 1205–1207.
50. Barone, G., Chang, C. T., Choc, M. G., Jr., et al. (1996) The pharmacokinetics of a microemulsion formulation of cyclosporin in primary renal allograft recipients. *Transplantation* **61**, 875–880.
51. Freeman, D., Grant, D., Levy, G., et al. (1995) Pharmacokinetics of a new formulation of cyclosporin in liver transplant recipients. *Ther. Drug Monit.* **17**, 213–216.
52. Andrews, D. J. and Cramb, R. (2002) Cyclosporin: revisions in monitoring and review of current analytical methods. *Ann. Clin. Biochem.* **39**, 424–435.
53. Ihara, H., Shinkuma, D., Ichikawa, Y., Nojima, M., Nagano, S., and Ikoma, F. (1995) Intra- and interindividual variation in the pharmacokinetics of tacrolimus (FK506) in kidney transplant recipients – importance of trough levels as a practical indicator. *Int. J. Urol.* **2**, 151–155.
54. Jusko, W. J., Piekoszewski, W., Klintmalm, G. B., et al. (1995) Pharmacokinetics of tacrolimus in liver transplant recipients. *Clin. Pharmacol.* **57**, 281–290.
55. Baz, M. A., Layish, D. T., Govert, J. A., et al. (1996) Diagnostic yield of bronchoscopies after isolated lung transplantation. *Chest* **110**, 84–88.
56. Sollinger, H. W., Deierhoi, M. H., Belzer, F. O., Diethelm, A. G., and Kauffman, R. S. (1992) RS-61443—a phase I clinical trial and pilot rescue study. *Transplantation* **53**, 428–432.
57. European Mycophenolate Mofetil Cooperative Study Group. (1995) Placebo-controlled study of mycophenolate mofetil combined with cyclosporin and corticosteroids for prevention of acute rejection. *Lancet* **345**, 1321–1325.
58. Kung, L., Gourishankar, S., and Halloran, P. F. (2000) Molecular pharmacology of immunosuppressive agents in relation to their clinical use. *Curr. Opin. Organ Transplant.* **5**, 268–275.
59. Rayhill, S. C. and Sollinger, H. W. (1999) Mycophenolate mofetil: experimental and clinical experience, in *Immunosuppression in Transplantation* (Ginns, L. C., Cosimi, A. B., and Morris P., eds.), Blackwell Science, Malden, pp. 47–66.
60. Weber, L. T., Schutz, E., Lamersdorf, T., et al. (1999) Therapeutic drug monitoring of total and free mycophenolic acid (MPA) and limited sampling strategy for determination of MPA-AUC in paediatric renal transplant recipients. The German Study Group on Mycophenolate Mofetil (MMF) Therapy. *Nephrol. Dial. Transplant.* **14**, 34–35.
61. Meiser, B. M., Pfeiffer, M., Schmidt, D., et al. (1999) Combination therapy with tacrolimus and mycophenolate mofetil following cardiac transplantation: importance of mycophenolic acid therapeutic drug monitoring. *J. Heart Lung Transplant.* **18**, 143–149.

62. Mycophenolate Mofetil Investigators. (1998) A randomised active controlled trial of mycophenolate mofetil in heart transplant recipients. *Transplantation* **66**, 507–515.
63. Glanville, A. R., Corris, P. A., McNeil, K. D., and Wahlers, T., on behalf of the International MMF Lung Study Group. (2003) Mycophenolate mofetil (MMF) versus mzathioprine (AZA) in lung transplantation for the prevention of bronchiolitis obliterans syndrome (BOS): results of a 3 year international randomised trial. *J. Heart Lung Transplant.* **22**, A410.
64. Mathew, T. H. (1998) Tricontinental Mycophenolate Mofetil Renal Transplantation Study Group. A blinded long term randomised multicentre study of mycophenolate mofetil in cadaveric renal transplantation: results at three years. *Transplantation* **66**, 1450–1454.
65. Senel, F. and Kahan, B. D. (1999) New small molecule immunosuppressive agents, in *Immunosuppression in Transplantation* (Ginns, L. C., Cosimi, A. B., and Morris, P. J., eds.), Blackwell Science, Malden, pp. 67–84.
66. Ruygrok, P. N., Muller, D. W., and Serruys, P. W. (2003) Rapamycin in cardiovascular medicine. *Intern. Med. J.* **33**, 103–109.
67. Nashan, B. (2002) Review of the proliferation inhibitor everolimus. *Expert. Opin. Invest. Drugs* **11**, 1845–1857.
68. Kahan, B. D., Napoli, K. L., Kelly, P. A., et al. (2000) Therapeutic drug monitoring of sirolimus: correlations with efficacy and toxicity. *Clin. Transplant.* **14**, 97–109.
69. Kahan, B. D., Podbielski, J., Napoli, K. L., Katz, S. M., Meier-Kriesche, H. U., and Van Buren, C. T. (1998) Immunosuppressive effects and safety of a sirolimus/cyclosprine combination regimen for renal transplantation. *Transplantation* **66**, 1040–1046.
70. Kovarik, J. M., Kaplan, B., Tedesco, S. H., et al. (2002) Exposure-response relationships for everolimus in de novo kidney transplantation: defining a therapeutic range. *Transplantation* **73**, 920–925.
71. Eisen, H., Dorent, R., Mancini, D., et al. (2002) the RAD B253 Study Group. Safety and efficacy of everolimus (RAD) as part of a triple immunosuppressive regimen in de novo cardiac transplant recipients: six month analysis. *J. Heart Lung Transplant.* **21**, A1.
72. Kahan, B. D., Kaplan, B., Lorber, M. I., Winkler, M., Cambon, N., and Boger, R. S. (2001) RAD in de novo renal transplantation: comparison of three doses on the incidence and severity of acute rejection. *Transplantation* **71**, 1400–1406.
73. Keogh, A. (2002) Sirolimus immunotherapy reduces the rates of cardiac allograft rejection: 6 month results from a phase 2, open label study. *Am. J. Transplant.* **2**, 246.
74. Keogh, A. (2002) Progression of graft vessel disease in cardiac allograft recipients is significantly reduced by sirolimus immunotherapy: 6 month results from a phase 2, open label study. *Am. J. Transplant.* **2**, 246.
75. Snell, G. I., Valentine, V. G., Love, R. B., Vitulo, P., Glanville, A. R., and Pirron, U. (2003) One-year results of an international, randomised double blind study of everolimus versus azathioprine as adjunctive therapy to inhibit the decline of

pulmonary function in stable lung or heart-lung transplant recipients. *J. Heart Lung Transplant.* **22**, A411.

76. Snell, G. I., Frost, A., Glanville, A. R., et al. (2002) Results of a 1 year randomised open label multicentre study of RAD versus antilymphocyte globulin (ALG) and azathioprine in lung transplant recipients with bronchiolitis obliterans syndrome (BOS). *J. Heart Lung Transplant.* **21**, A36.
77. Kahan, B. D. (2003) Two-year results of multicentre phase III trials on the effect of the addition of sirolimus to cyclosporine based immunosuppressive regimens in renal transplantation. *Transplant. Proc.* **35**, S37–51.
78. Orta-Sibu, N., Chantler, C., Bewick, M., and Haycock, G. (1982) Comparison of high-dose intravenous methylprednisolone with low-dose oral prednisolone in acute renal allograft rejection in children. *Br. Med. J.* **285**, 258–260.
79. Park, M. H., Starling, R. C., Ratliff, N. B., et al. (1999) Oral steroid pulse without taper for the treatment of asymptomatic moderate cardiac allograft rejection. *J. Heart Lung Transplant.* **18**, 1224–1227.
80. Hopkins, P. M. A., Aboyoun, C. L., Chhajed, P. C., et al. (2002) Outcome of minimal acute rejection (grade A_1) in lung transplant recipients: the need for careful observation. *J. Heart Lung Transplant.* **21**, A144.
81. Clelland, C., Higenbottam, T., Otulana, B., et al. (1990) Histologic prognostoc indicators for the lung allografts of heart-lung transplants. *J. Heart Lung Transplant.* **9**, 177–186.
82. Tanizaki, Y., Kitani, H., Mifune, T., Mitsunobu, F., Kajimoto, K., and Sugimoto, K. (1993) Effects of glucocorticoids on humoral and cellular immunity and on airway inflammation in patients with steroid-dependant intractable asthma. *J. Asthma* **30**, 485–492.
83. Schuyler, M. R., Bondarevsky, E., Schwartz, H. J., and Schmitt, D. (1981) Corticosteroid-sensitive lymphocytes are normal in atopic asthma. *J. Allergy Clin. Immunol.* **68**, 72–78.
84. Cantarovich, M., Latter, D. A., and Loertscher, R. (1997) Treatment of steroid-resistant and recurrent acute cardiac transplant rejection with a short course of antibody therapy. *Clin. Transplant.* **11**, 316–321.
85. Gaber, A. O., First, M. R., Tesi, R. J., Gaston, R. S., Mendez, R., and Mulloy, L. L. (1998) Results of the double blind, randomised, multicentre, phase III clinical trial of thymoglobulin versus ATGAM in the treatment of acute graft rejection episodes after renal transplantation. *Transplantation* **66**, 29–37.
86. Sollinger, H. W., Deierhoi, M. H., Belzer, F. O., Diethelm, A. G., and Kauffman, R. S. (1992) RS-61443: phase I clinical trial and pilot rescue study. *Transplantation* **53**, 428–432.
87. The Mycophenolate Mofetil Renal Refractory Rejection Study Group. (1996) Mycophenolate mofetil for the treatment of refractory, acute cellular renal transplant rejection. *Transplantation* **61**, 722–729.
88. Klein, A. (1999) Tacrolimus rescue in liver transplant patients with refractory rejection or intolerance or malabsorption of cyclosporin. The US Multicentre FK506 Liver Study Group. *Liver Transplant. Surg.* **5**, 502–508.

89. Mentzer, R. M., Jahania, M. S., and Lasley, R. D. (1998) Tacrolimus as a rescue immunosuppressant after heart and lung transplantation. The US Multicentre FK506 Study Group. *Transplantation* **65**, 109–113.
90. Jordan, M. L., Naraghi, R., Shapiro, R., et al. (1997) Tacrolimus rescue therapy for renal allograft rejection – five year experience. *Transplantation* **63**, 223–228.
91. De Bonis, M., Reynolds, L., Barros, J., and Madden, B. P. (2001) Tacrolimus as a rescue immunosuppressant after heart transplantation. *Eur. J. Cardiothorac. Surg.* **19**, 690–695.
92. Wong, P., Devlin, J., Gane, E., Ramage, J., Portmann, B., and Williams, R. (1994) FK506 rescue therapy for intractable liver allograft rejection. *Transplant. Int.* **7**, S70–76.
93. Onsager, D. R., Canver, C. C., Jahania, M. S., et al. (1999) Efficacy of tacrolimus in the treatment of refractory rejection in heart and lung transplant recipients. *J. Heart Lung Transplant.* **18**, 448–455.
94. Jiang, H., Wynn, C., Pan, F., Ebbs, A., Erickson, L. M., and Kobayashi, M. (2002) Tacrolimus and cyclosporin differ in their capacity to overcome ongoing allograft rejection as a result of their differential abilities to inhibit interleukin-10 production. *Transplantation* **73**, 1808–1817.
95. Cahill, B. C., O'Rourke, M. K., Strasburg, K. A., et al. (1996) Methotrexate for lung transplant recipients with steroid-resistant acute rejection. *J. Heart Lung Transplant.* **15**, 1130–1137.
96. Ferraro, P., Carrier, M., White, M., Pelletier, G. B., and Pelletier, L. C. (1995) Antithymocyte globulin and methotrexate therapy of severe or persistent cardiac allograft rejection. *Ann. Thorac. Surg.* **60**, 372–376.
97. Ross, H. J., Gullestad, L., Pak, J., Slauson, S., Valantine, H. A., Hunt, S. A. (1997) Methotrexate or total lymphoid radiation for treatment of persistent or recurrent allograft cellular rejection: a comparative study. *J. Heart Lung Transplant.* **16**, 179–189.
98. Boettcher, H., Costard-Jackle, A., Moller, F., Hirt, S. W., and Cremer, J. (2002) Methotrexate as rescue therapy in lung transplantation. *Transplant. Proc.* **34**, 3255–3257.
99. Ciesielski, C. J., Pflug, J. J., Mei, J., and Piccinini, L. A. (1998) Methotrexate regulates ICAM-1 expression in recipients of rat cardiac allografts. *Transplant. Immunol.* **6**, 111–121.
100. Keenan, R. J., Iacono, A., Dauber, J. H., et al. (1997) Treatment of refractory acute allograft rejection with aerosolized cyclosporin in lung transplant recipients. *J. Thorac. Cardiovasc. Surg.* **113**, 335–340.
101. Iacono, A. T., Smaldone, G. C., Keenan, R. J., et al. (1997) Dose related reversal of acute lung rejection by aerosolized cyclosporin. *Am. J. Respir. Crit. Care Med.* **155**, 1690–1698.
102. Chen, H., Wu, J., Xu, D., Luo, H., and Daloze, P. M. (1993) Reversal of ongoing heart, kidney and pancreas allograft rejection and suppression of accelerated heart allograft rejection in the rat by rapamycin. *Transplantation* **56**, 661–666.

103. Hong, J. C. and Kahan, B. D. (2001) Sirolimus rescue therapy for refractory rejection in renal transplantation. *Transplantation* **71**, 1579–1584.
104. Jin, M. B., Nakayama, M., Ogata, T., et al. (2002) A novel leflunomide derivative, FK778, for immunosuppression after kidney transplantation in dogs. *Surgery* **132**, 72–79.
105. Kyles, A. E., Gregory, C. R., Griffey, S. M., Bernsteen, L., Pierce, J., and Lilja, H. S. (2003) Immunosuppression with a combination of the leflunomide analog, FK778, and microemulsified cyclosporine for renal transplantation in mongrel dogs. *Transplantation* **75**, 1128–1133.
106. Keogh, A. M., Arnold, R. H., Macdonald, P. S., Hawkins, R. C., Morgan, G. W., and Spratt, P. M. (2001) A randomised trial of tacrolimus (FK506) versus total lymphoid irradiation for the control of repetitive rejection after cardiac transplantation. *J. Heart Lung Transplant.* **20**, 1331–1334.
107. Valentine, V. G., Robbins, R. C., Wehner, J. H., Patel, H. R., Berry, G. J., and Theodore, J. (1996) Total lymphoid irradiation for refractory acute rejection in heart-lung and lung allografts. *Chest* **109**, 1184–1189.
108. Asano, M., Gundry, S. R., Razzouk, A. J., et al. (2002) Paediatric Heart Transplantation Group. Total lymphoid irradiation for refractory rejection in paediatric heart transplantation. *Ann. Thorac. Surg.* **74**, 1979–1985.
109. Dall'Amico, R. and Murer, L. (2002) Extracorporeal photochemotherapy: a new therapeutic approach for allograft rejection. *Transfus. Apheresis Sci.* **26**, 197–204.
110. Dall'Amico, R., Montini, G., Murer, L., et al. (2000) Extracorporeal photochemotherapy after cardiac transplantation: a new therapeutic approach to allograft rejection. *Int..J. Artif. Organs* **23**, 49–54.
111. Koransky, M. L. and Robbins, R. C. (2002) Additional strategies for Immunosuppression, in *Heart and Lung Transplantation* (Baumgartner, W. A., Kasper, E., Theodore, J., and Reitz, B., eds.), WB Saunders Company, London, pp. 341–351.
112. Isobe, M., Yagita, H., Okumura, K., and Ihara, A. (1992) Specific acceptance of cardiac allograft after treatment with antibodies to ICAM-1 and LFA-1. *Science* **255**, 1125–1127.
113. Ross, D. J. and Kass, R. M. (2002) Treatment of acute lung allograft rejection, in *Heart and Lung Transplantation* (Baumgartner, W. A., Kasper, E., Theodore, J., and Reitz, B., eds.), WB Saunders Company, London, pp. 333–340.

17

Experimental Models of Graft Arteriosclerosis

Behzad Soleimani and Victor C. Shi

Summary

Graft arteriosclerosis (GA) is the leading cause of mortality in long-term survivors of solid organ transplantation. Although clinical studies have suggested a multifactorial etiology, the precise mechanism of disease remains obscure. Many animal models have been developed that manifest lesions resembling those of human arteriosclerosis. These models have helped us address specific mechanistic and interventional issues but, for reasons that will be discussed, have failed to assign a unitary pathogenic mechanism to clinical GA. In this chapter we describe the commonly available experimental models of GA. We further discuss the merits and limitations of each model and outline their contribution to our understanding of the pathogenesis of the disease.

Key Words: Graft arteriosclerosis; experimental models; transplantation.

1. Introduction

Transplantation-associated GA is the major cause of cardiac allograft failure after the first postoperative year *(1)*, and it appears to be a significant problem in the long-term survival of other solid organ transplants *(2)*. Also, despite the success of immunosuppressive agents in the treatment of acute rejection (AR), there is considerable debate about whether these drugs influence the progression of GA *(3)*. Both the gross and histological features of GA differentiate it from commonly occurring native vessel arteriosclerosis. In contrast with common arteriosclerosis, the lesion associated with GA involves the artery in a concentric rather than eccenteric fashion and often involves both the epicardial and intramyocardial coronary arteries *(1)*. Lipid accumulation is less common in the early development of GA, and the tempo of the disease is faster. The cellular composition of GA lesion and the sparing of the native vessels, as well

From: *Methods in Molecular Biology, vol. 333: Transplantation Immunology: Methods and Protocols*
Edited by: P. Hornick and M. Rose © Humana Press Inc., Totowa, NJ

as the likely participation of a variety of growth factors and cytokines, suggest stimulation by an immune mechanism. However, the precise mechanism of the disease remains obscure.

There has, however, been significant progress in this area in the recent years thanks, in part at least, to the contribution made by animal models that manifest lesions resembling those of human arteriosclerosis. The first report of allograft coronary disease in an experimental animal was in a series of orthotopic cardiac allografts in dogs *(4)*. In this model allografts surviving more than 3 mo developed circumferential intimal thickening in the coronary arteries causing luminal stenosis. Subsequent to this early work by Kosek et al., many other animal models have been developed that have helped to address both mechanistic and interventional issues related to the disease.

There are two principal issues to consider in evaluating experimental models of GA: the choice of the species and the choice of the allograft. Experimental models of this disease have been described in all commonly available laboratory animals ranging from rodents to primates. Although it is generally recognized that each species offers a different perspective of the disease and confers certain advantages and disadvantages in the study of GA, the question of choice of allograft is more contentious.

The allografts hitherto described can be broadly divided into whole organ and isolated arterial grafts. In this chapter we discuss the merits and deficits of all major animal models of GA, paying particular attention to selection of species and the type of allograft used. It is important to note that the etiology of clinical GA is likely to be multifactorial, and in general terms the choice of experimental model adopted is to a great extent dictated by the nature of the question being addressed. Secondary consideration must also be given to the availability of technical expertise and personal preference.

2. Species Selection

Among laboratory animals, rodents are the most commonly used species in experimental models of GA. Availability of inbred strains with defined major and minor histocompatibility antigens allows transplantation between animals with different degrees of mismatch. Moreover, these experiments can be controlled against nonimmune mediated vascular injury such as ischemia/reperfusion injury or surgical trauma by performing isografts between inbred animals. Murine species in particular offer a large range of genetically altered strains, which can be used to investigate the role of particular gene products in GA. However, although studies based on rodent models have generated significant amounts of useful information, it must be kept in mind that there are important physiological and anatomical differences between murine species and humans *(5)*. In particular, lack of constitutive endothelial expression of major histocompatibility antigen (MHC) class II antigen, absence of neointimal lipid deposition, and resistance of rodents to native vessel arteriosclerosis are major limitations of mouse-based models of GA *(6)*. In addition, in many murine heart transplantation models, GA is generated in the context of indefinite graft survival in the absence of long-term immunosuppression *(7)*. It is conceivable that pathogenesis of GA seen in this setting may be different to that seen in clinical GA, which develops in the context of chronic immunosuppression.

Larger laboratory animals, although not as versatile in terms of availability of genetically altered strains, have some notable advantages compared to rodents. These are anatomically and physiologically closer to humans, and therefore models may be more representative of clinical GA. In addition, large animals allow multiple blood sampling, repeated biopsies, orthotopic transplantation, and in some cases serial imaging with intracoronary ultrasonography. This latter technology can facilitate assessment of progression of GA as manifested by intimal thickening in vivo and therefore allow continuous monitoring of the impact of therapeutic interventions on the disease process. The advantages of using large animals are offset by higher operative mortality and a significantly higher cost of purchase and maintenance.

Porcine models are particularly attractive, as their cardiovascular physiology and anatomy closely resemble those found in humans. There is also important homology between the immune systems of pig and human. For instance, unlike the situation in rodents, porcine coronary endothelium constitutively expresses class II antigens, a difference that may be particularly relevant given the importance of vascular endothelium in atherogenesis *(6)*.

Rabbit models also offer all the advantages of a large laboratory animal at a relatively low cost. Susceptibility of rabbits to hypercholesterolemia is well recognized and has been exploited in animal models of native vessel atherosclerosis for many years *(8)*. Studies on the role of gene therapy in prevention of GA represent one further area that has benefited from rabbit-based models *(9)*.

In contrast to lower species, a limited number of nonhuman primate models of GA have been described and characterized. Nevertheless, primates are considered to be particularly important in the study of the disease because of their close phylogenetic relationship to humans. This functional and structural homology can be exploited to evaluate novel therapeutic agents and "humanized" monoclonal antibodies (MAbs) prior to embarking on clinical trials. Susceptibility of primates to native vessel atherosclerosis is well recognized and has formed the basis of the use of these animals in atherosclerosis research *(10)*. The significant cost of purchase and maintenance of primates has, however, proved prohibitive. and the use of these species has generally been restricted to immediate preclinical evaluation of therapeutic strategies.

3. Cardiac Allograft Models

The techniques for heart transplantation in laboratory animals were described the 1960s *(11)*, and it has long been recognized that GA can be generated experimentally provided the allograft is allowed to survive for a sufficient length of time. The arterial lesions observed in these models are morphologically similar to clinical GA, comprised of concentric intimal hyperplasia affecting all epicardial and intramyocardial coronary arteries to varying degrees. The prolonged graft survival necessary to allow development of GA is generally achieved by the use of immunosuppressive agents. Introduction of immunosupressants can, however, increase the complexity of the models given that many of these agents have themselves been implicated in the pathogenesis of GA *(12,13)*. Additionally, the immunosuppressants used experimentally, such as anti-CD4 and anti-CD8 MAbs, have in general no clinical application and in some models result in permanent graft survival following only a brief period of peri-operative treatment *(14)*. This is clearly not the case in the clinical setting, and this discrepancy may have important implications when extrapolating results from these models to clinical GA. One further characteristic of these models to consider is that, as in clinical GA, the coronary artery lesions in experimental cardiac allografts are generally heterogeneous in terms of their location, distribution, and intensity **(Fig. 1)**. This is true for different regions of the same vessel, different vessels in the same graft region, and the same vessels in different grafts *(15)*. This heterogeneity in lesion distribution makes quantitative evaluation of GA severity in these models somewhat complex.

3.1. Orthotopic Heart Transplantation

In 1968, Kosek reported a series of orthotopic heart transplants in dogs *(4)*. The operation, which required the use of cardiopulmonary bypass, was performed through a left thoracotomy. Azathioprine and methylprednisolone were used as immunosuppressants to allow prolonged allograft survival. The allografts in long-term survivors developed circumferential intimal thickening in the coronary arteries, similar to clinical GA both morphologically and in terms of distribution.

Orthotopic heart transplantation has also been described in pigs *(16)* and non-human primates *(17)*, although these models have not been specifically used to address issues relevant to pathogenesis of GA. Experimental orthotopic heart transplantation has the clear advantage of simulating clinical transplantation both physiologically and anatomically. Its application in the study of GA has, however, been limited by the complexity of the procedure, the need for cardiopulmonary bypass, and significant peri-operative mortality. In addition, the operation can only be performed in higher animals, imposing substantial expense on the investigator.

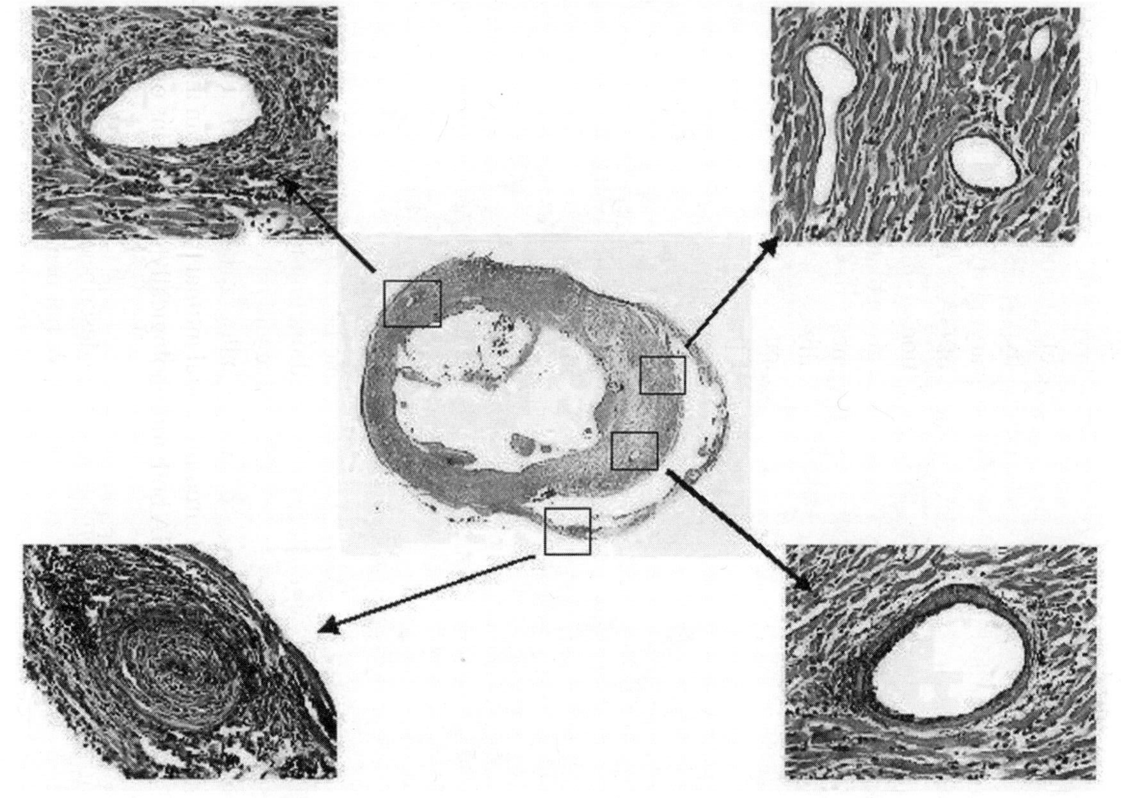

Fig. 1. Variation in GA severity among cardiac allograft vessels. The center image is a histological cross section taken from the middle portion of a 55-d mouse heart allograft (Verhoeff elastin stain, original magnification ´ 10). Four coronary arteries are enlarged from the cross section to show the diversity of intimal thickening observed within a given section of a murine heart allograft.

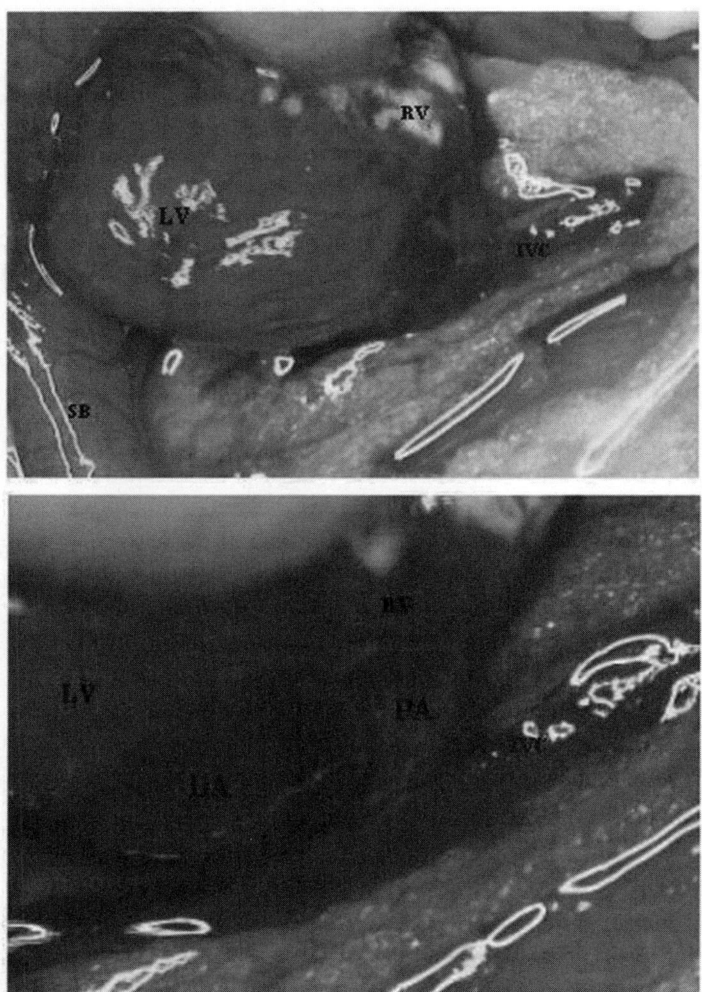

Fig. 2. Surgical photographs showing the donor heart attached to the recipient abdominal aorta and inferior vena cava. The bowel has been displaced laterally to expose the great vessels. LV, left ventricle; RV, right ventricle; PA, pulmonary artery; LA, left atrium; IVC, inferior vena cava; SB, small bowel.

3.2. Heterotopic Heart Transplantation

Intra-abdominal cardiac allografting was described by Ono and Lindsey in the 1960s ***(11)***. In this operation the donor heart is transplanted into the abdominal cavity of the recipient animal by anastomozing the donor ascending aorta and pulmonary artery to the recipient abdominal aorta and inferior vena cava, respectively **(Fig. 2)**. Heterotopically transplanted rat cardiac allografts were shown by Laden and others to develop GA, which is morphologically indistinguishable from clinical graft coronary disease provided the grafts survive long enough ***(18,19)***. This long-term survival can be achieved by exchanging grafts between strains that are disparate in non-MHC loci only ***(20,21)*** in the absence of immunosuppression or, alternatively, in MHC-mismatched transplants by the use of chronic immunosuppression ***(22)***. The versatility of this model has rendered it ideal for evaluating novel therapeutic agents ***(23–26)***. The rat model also provides abundant graft tissue for gene-expression studies. For example, these studies have demonstrated increased allograft expression of monocyte chemoattractant protein-1 in the Lewis to F-344 heart transplantation model ***(27)***. The same model has been used to demonstrate upregulation in the cardiac allograft of genes encoding interferon (IFN)-γ, interleukin(IL)-6, endothelin-1, inflammatory factor-1, and inducible nitric oxide ***(28–31)***. Other studies have shown upregulation of platelet-derived growth factor expression, which has been implicated in smooth muscle proliferation and migration into the neointima ***(32,33)***. An extension of the rat heterotopic heart model has been a retransplantation model that has been used to study the early events after transplantation. In this model, retransplantation of allografts back into the original donor strain failed to prevent GA if the grafts had resided in the primary recipient for up to 5 d; residence in the primary allogeneic recipient for less than 4 d did not result in GA in the secondary recipient ***(34)***. This indicated that the immune injury responsible for development of GA in this model occurs early after transplantation and becomes irreversible after the fifth day.

Although the technique of heterotopic heart transplantation in mice was described in the 1970s ***(35)***, it was not until recently that this model was adapted for the study of GA. The surgical technique in humans is identical to that in rats, albeit on a smaller scale. It has been shown that if cardiac allografts are exchanged between inbred strains that differ in only a single MHC locus (e.g., B10.A and B10.BR), prolonged graft survival could be achieved without the use of immunosuppression ***(36)***. In this setting intimal hyperplasia develops, affecting the coronary arteries within 30–50 d of transplantation. Since its original description, a number of variants of this model have been described that are based on the choice of strain combination and the use of immunosuppressant agents ***(7,37,38)***. These models have been used extensively to study many aspects of GA. GA has, for example, been produced in this model by transfer of alloantibodies to severe combined immune deficiency recipients of cardiac allografts ***(39)***. This important observation is generally taken as evidence that alloantibodies are necessary to promote GA. Further evidence for the role of alloantibodies came from studies on B-cell-deficient cardiac allograft recipients, which failed to generate typical intimal proliferation ***(40)***. More recently, it has been shown that the detrimental effects of alloantibodies can be averted by allograft expression of antioxidant and antiapoptotic genes and that passive transfer of alloantibody can only result in GA if it is done before allograft expression of protective genes *(7)*.

The use of blocking monoclonal antibodies has allowed identification of several key elements in the pathogenesis of GA such as adhesion molecules ***(41)***, T-cell co-stimulatory molecules *(7)*, and chemokines *(42)*. However, the main contribution of the mouse models stems from the availability of strains with targeted gene deletions. The use of knockout and transgenic strains used as cardiac allograft donors or recipients has allowed the identification of key gene products in the pathogenesis of GA. The Th1 cytokine IFN-γ has, for example, been implicated in pathogenesis of GA because IFN-γ-deficient recipients of cardiac allografts do not develop GA ***(43,44)***. Similarly targeted deletion of the transcription factor signal transducer and activation of transcription-4 resulted in attenuation of GA, possibly by promoting Th2 lymphocyte differentiation ***(45)***. In contrast, recipient's deficiencies of IL-4 or tumor necrosis factor-α receptor-1 did not diminish ***(46,47)***, and IL-10, transforming growth factor-β1, nitric oxide synthase (NOS)2, or apolipoprotein-E deficiency augmented GA ***(48–52)***.

A variant of rodent abdominal heart transplantation is cervical transplantation. In this operation the graft ascending aorta and pulmonary artery are anastomosed end-to-side to the recipient common carotid artery and external jugular vein, respectively. This approach obviates the need to breach the recipient peritoneal cavity and thus carries a lower surgical mortality. Concern, however, has been expressed about the sufficiency of flow in the recipient carotid artery to sustain the cardiac graft ***(53–55)***.

The porcine heterotopic heart transplantation model was described to allow the study of the immunological basis of GA in a large animal setting ***(6)***. Porcine species offer the advantage of having immune and cardiovascular systems similar to those of humans, with comparable susceptibility to atherosclerosis ***(56)***. Partially inbred miniature swine offer the possibility of transplantation across defined MHC barriers. There is the additional advantage of performing intracoronary ultrasonography, as the porcine coronary arteries are large enough to admit catheterization. In this model the donor heart is transplanted heterotopically in the recipient's retroperitoneal space. The donor ascending aorta and pulmonary artery are anastomosed end-to-side to the recipient infrarenal abdominal aorta and inferior vena cava, respectively. Before the anastomoses are constructed, an atrial septal defect is created and the graft mitral apparatus is disrupted to avoid left ventricular atrophy by increasing the preload. This model has been used to assess the impact of donor-specific tolerance ***(57)*** and mixed hematopoietic chimerism in the recipient ***(58)*** on the development of GA.

Cervical cardiac transplantation in the rabbit was described in the late 1970s ***(59)*** in a series of experiments in which recipients fed on a lipid-poor diet were shown to develop proliferative coronary arterial lesions typical of GA. In cholesterol-fed rabbits, arterial lesions were similarly distributed, but the majority of lesions were fatty-proliferative. It was concluded from these studies that immunological arterial injury due to allograft rejection acting in synergy with hypercholesterolemia could lead to rapidly developing arteriosclerosis. The role of hypercholesterolemia was further supported by studies in which pharmacological ***(60)*** or mechanical ***(61)*** reduction of cholesterol level diminished GA in this model. The question of the relationship between episodes of AR and development of GA was recently revisited using this model. In a study in which episodes of AR were manipulated using cyclosporine, it was shown that AR could accelerate graft vascular disease ***(62)***.

Heterotopic heart transplantation models have also been described in nonhuman primates. The technique is identical to that in other animal models ***(63)***. When cardiac allografts were exchanged between MHC class II-mismatched cynomolgus monkeys, prolonged graft survival was achieved by treatment of the recipient with humanized anti-CD154 antibody. It was shown that sustained treatment with this antibody resulted in longer median graft survival and diminished GA when compared with peri-operative dosing alone ***(63)***.

3.3. Heterotopic "Functioning" Heart Transplantation

Heterotopic cardiac allografts are physiologically "nonfunctioning" and thus may behave differently from an orthotopic heart transplant. Hemodynamic offloading of the heart in heterotopic models has been shown to lead to atrophy at organ and molecular levels ***(64)***. Although "functioning" heterotopic cardiac allografts have been described ***(64)***, these models have not been adapted for the study of GA. In the model described by Klein et al. ***(64)*** hearts are transplanted heterotopicaly using an end-to-side anastomosis between the donor's superior vena cava and the recipient's abdominal inferior vena cava. The right ventricle loads the left ventricle via a direct anastomosis of the pulmonary artery to the left atrium. The left ventricle ejects volume through an end-to-side anastomosis of the donor aorta to the recipient abdominal aorta.

4. Arterial Models

Arterial allograft models were developed as an alternative to whole-organ grafts to allow mechanistic study of GA without the complications of an immune and nonimmune response to parenchymal tissue. In contrast with the organ allograft models, the lesions seen in these models are concentric, uniform, and reproducible (**Fig. 3**). Additionally, most vessel models described to date require no immunosuppression because there is no acute destructive parenchymal rejection that would otherwise precede the emergence of GA. This is an important point because a number of immunosuppressive agents have themselves been impli-

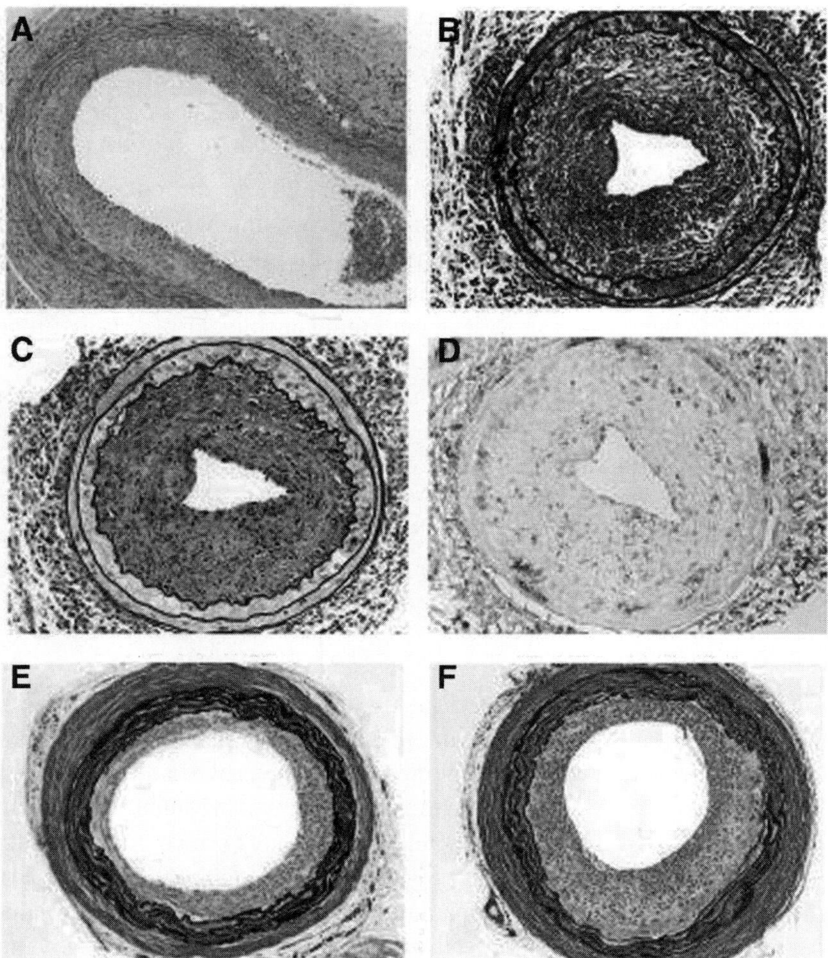

Fig. 3. Photomicrographs showing cross sections of arterial allografts. **(A)** 75-d rat aortic allograft (H&E stain, original magnification ×100). **(B–D)** 30-d mouse carotid artery allograft (original magnification ×200): **(B)** stained with Verhoeff stain (elastic lamina is stained black) delineating near-occlusive neointima, **(C)** stained for a-actin showing abundance of smooth muscle cells in the neointima, and **(D)** stained for CD45. **(E,F)** 45- and 75-d rat carotid artery allografts (original magnification ×100). Elastic lamina is stained black (Verhoeff stain), delineating the neointima. It is evident that the neointimal thickness in the rat is only moderate (nonocclusive).

cated in the pathogenesis of transplant arteriosclerosis *(3,12,13)*. Lack of immunosuppression is, however, regarded by some as a potential concern. It has, for instance, been suggested that GA seen in vessel allografts in the absence of immunosuppression may be initiated by a different mechanism from that seen in whole-organ allografts ***(65)***. Notwithstanding these concerns, and as is outlined here, arterial models of GA have helped address a number of important mechanistic and interventional issues in this disease.

4.1. Aortic Allograft Model

The rat aortic allograft was the first vessel model described for the study of GA ***(66)***. In relative terms, this is a simple procedure whereby a segment of donor descending aorta is transplanted as an interposition graft into the infrarenal descending aorta of the recipient. The model takes advantage of all the merits of isolated vessel allograft in addition to relative ease of surgery conferred by the size of rat aorta. The degree of intimal hyperplasia is, however, modest relative to the vessel diameter, in part because of the paucity of smooth muscle cells in the aortic media **(Fig. 3A)**. Also, the operation involves invasion of the peritoneal space and hence carries a higher mortality than the procedures in the neck or the groin. The rat aortic model became immediately popular after its description, particularly for evaluation of preexisting and novel agents for prevention of GA. These included cyclosporine ***(13)***, the angiotensin-converting enzyme inhibitor perindopril ***(67)***, platelet-activating factor receptor blockers ***(68)***, angiopeptin ***(69)***, mycophenolate mofetil ***(70)***, and low-molecular-weight heparin ***(71)***.

Unlike many murine vessel models, the rat aortic allograft provides abundant tissue for gene-expression studies. For example, expression of inducible NOS ***(72)*** and Fas-ligand ***(73)*** has been shown to be associated with GA.

Like the heterotopic heart model, the aortic allograft model has been extended to address the early events after transplantation by performing graft retransplantation ***(74)***. Using this modification it was possible to corroborate the notion that the vascular insult that ultimately leads to GA occurs early after transplantation and that elimination of histoincompatibility after this early phase did not alter the disease process ***(74)***.

A murine abdominal aortic model has also been described ***(75)***, which, although technically more demanding, confers the added advantage of using genetically modified strains not available in rats.

The aortic model has also been extended to larger animals. The rabbit aortic allograft model was described primarily to study cholesterol metabolism in transplanted arteries ***(76)***. The technique is similar to other vessel allograft models, albeit in a larger scale. Briefly, the donor thoracic aorta is grafted onto the recipient abdominal aorta in an end-to-side fashion to construct a bypass graft. In addition to studies on cholesterol metabolism, this model has been used to show protective roles for estrogens ***(77)*** in GA. The rabbit model of aortic transplantation has also been used to investigate the feasibility of adenovirus-mediated gene transfer to prevent GA ***(9)***.

A primate aortic model of allograft arteriosclerosis has been described specifically to study disease progression using serial intravascular ultrasound (IVUS) *(78)*. In this model, aortic allografts were transplanted below the inferior mesenteric artery of recipient rhesus monkeys. Removed and reimplanted aortic segments between renal arteries and the inferior mesenteric arteries served as control autografts. Serial postoperative IVUS studies demonstrated progressive increase in the intimal area over the 98-d observation period. Histological analysis of allografts removed at autopsy showed typical concentric intimal hyperplasia.

4.2. Carotid Artery Models

The carotid artery has been perceived to be a suitable vessel for transplantation because of a number of technical considerations. First, the operation is performed in the neck region, obviating the need to breach the peritoneum with its associated complications. Second, the common carotid artery bears no side branches, facilitating both the donor and recipient procedures. Third, the carotid artery represents a small-caliber artery, reflecting the changes in smaller sized vessels in solid organ transplants that develop arteriosclerosis. Fourth, two genetically identical grafts are available from the same donor for two comparative transplants.

In the first description of a murine carotid transplant model, a segment of donor common carotid artery was transplanted as a paratopic loop graft onto the recipient carotid artery *(79)* **(Fig. 4)**. In this model, allografts had near-occlusive intimal hyperplasia within 30 d of transplantation in the absence of immunosuppressive agents **(Fig. 3B)**. This was in contrast with preservation of normal morphology in isografts within the same time scale *(79)*. The neointima in allografts, initially composed of macrophage/monocytes and lymphocytes ($CD4^+$ and $CD8^+$), was replaced with smooth muscle cells and extracellular matrix by d 30 **(Fig. 3C,D)**.

The vascular remodeling seen in this model is morphologically similar to clinical allograft coronary disease with a smooth-muscle-rich concenteric neointima. Furthermore, the model confers uniformity and reproducibility of the neointima, which would facilitate accurate quantitative evaluation of lesion severity. Because the vessel allograft is transplanted as a loop, there was initial concern that potentially turbulent flow could cause endothelial injury and promote neointima formation. However, the absence of neointima in isografts or in allografts transplanted into certain knockout strains would suggest that turbulence alone is not a significant contributing factor in this model.

The immunological basis of GA was first addressed systematically in this model using genetically manipulated mouse strains as recipients of carotid artery allografts. It therefore became possible to decipher the relative contribution of key gene products to pathogenesis of GA. Allografts from Rag-$2^{-/-}$ recipients, for

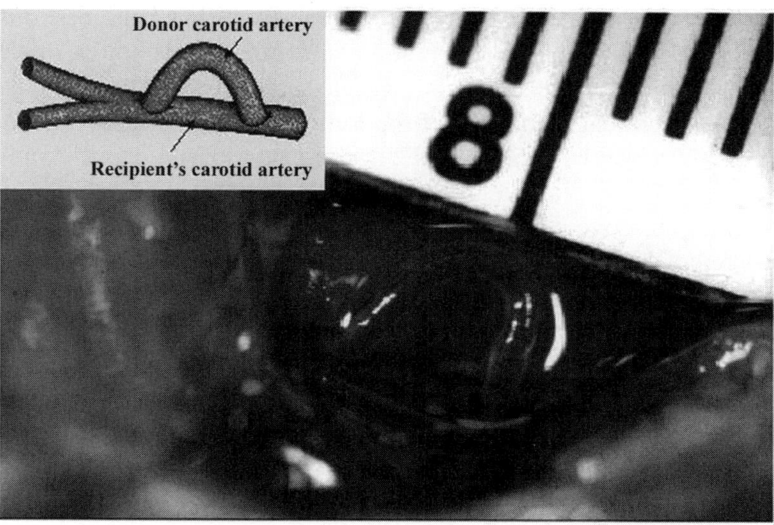

Fig. 4. Photograph of operative field showing the left carotid artery of the recipient, to which the donor artery has been sutured as a loop.

instance, which lack immunoglobulins and T-cell receptors had no neointima, indicating that GA is primarily an immune-mediated process. In addition, grafts from recipients deficient in MHC class II antigen or $CD4^+$ cells but not $CD8^+$ cells had a significantly diminished neointima *(80)*. Likewise, allografts from apoE knockout recipients had enhanced, and those from plasminogen-deficient recipients diminished, neointima formation *(81,82)*.

Using knockout strains as donors, it was then possible to demonstrate that donor expression of MHC class II but not class I was needed for GA to develop. Similarly, graft expression of intercellular adhesion molecule (ICAM)-1 but not P-selectin was shown to be necessary *(83)*.

Modifications of this model have been described in which interposition grafts were used in an attempt to reduce flow turbulence. These models use suture or cuff techniques *(84)*, adding to the complexity of the procedure. In addition, the reduced length of the interposition graft diminishes the amount of tissue available for analysis.

Carotid artery loop transplantation has also been described in rats *(85)*. The procedure is identical to that in the mouse. In this model the observation period is longer (45–75 d), and unlike the mouse carotid artery, the rat arterial lesions rarely become occlusive (**Fig. 3E,F**). However, larger vessel sizes in the rat makes the surgery easier to perform and also allow for noninvasive imaging of the graft using Doppler ultrasound *(85)*. Ultrasound imaging may allow continuous study of vascular remodeling in response to therapeutic interventions. In the LEW-to-F344 strain combination, the neointima, although rich in lymphocytes, lacked a significant smooth muscle cell component as compared with vessels seen in cardiac allografts of the same age *(85)*. Whether this discrepancy in cellularity of the neointima in different allografts is significant remains uncertain.

4.3. Femoral Artery Model

In this model, a segment of donor femoral artery is transplanted orthotopically to the recipient femoral artery *(86)*. Like the carotid artery, the rat femoral artery is a small-caliber muscular artery and therefore a suitable alternative to the aorta. The model also obviates the need to breach the peritoneal space.

An interesting observation made in this model was that in 40-d allografts, neointimal and medial smooth muscle cells were entirely of recipient origin *(87)*. The recipient origin of the neointimal cells led to the speculation that the mechanism of neointima formation may be different in vessel allografts as compared with organ allografts *(65)*. Further evidence supporting this notion came from a study using the rat aortic model, in which recolonization of allograft with recipient origin endothelial cells by the 18th postoperative day was demonstrated *(88)*. Also in this study, by postoperative day 60 the neointimal cells were noted to be of recipient origin. In contrast, in a study of long-term murine cardiac allografts *(38)*, graft endothelial and medial smooth muscle cells were shown to express donor-specific MHC class II molecules. However, the origin of neointimal smooth muscle cells was not determined in this study. It is evident from these studies that there is no clear consensus over the origin of vascular endothelial and smooth muscle cells in the remodeled arterial allograft. Nor is it established whether the origin of cellular components has any bearing toward the mechanism of vascular remodeling.

4.4. Coronary Artery Model

The isolated coronary artery transplantation model was developed in an attempt to overcome the structural differences between the coronary artery and other vessel grafts and also the heterogeneity of arterial lesions in solid organ allografts *(89)*. Like other vessel models, this model has the added advantage of not requiring the use of immunosuppression.

Technically, a segment of donor coronary artery was transplanted heterotopically into the recipient common carotid artery position. The grafts were anastomosed end-to-side to the recipient artery, and the intervening carotid artery was excised for baseline histological analysis. Allografts exhibited rapidly progressive vascular remodeling with endothelial hyperplasia, intimal fibromuscular hyperplasia, and medial necrosis.

5. Conclusions

The myriad of experimental models available for the study of GA is itself a testament to the fact that there is no single "ideal" model that can represent all aspects of what is undoubtedly a multifactorial clinical entity. The common theme in all the models described is morphological resemblance of arterial lesions in experimental allografts with lesions encountered in clinical GA. It is entirely possible that the mechanism by which this common endpoint is reached may be different in each model. It is also conceivable that the disease mechanism in each model may or may not be that which is relevant in clinical GA. This view may explain the variation in the impact of novel therapeutic strategies in various model systems and the ultimate disappointing outcome often encountered in clinical trials. This concept of model generation based on morphological outcome is, however, a consequence of the fact that clinical studies have not thus far pointed to a unitary mechanism for the disease. Until such time that clinical studies can focus our attention on relevant pathways of the disease, we are obliged to address each potential mechanism by adopting a different model. Therefore, potentially relevant early events can be targeted by using models that do not require immunosuppression such as vessel models, and later more chronic events can be addressed by adopting organ-based models. However, neither approach can unequivocally define the mechanisms that are both necessary and sufficient to produce clinical GA, and therapeutic strategies based on these models must be regarded as tentative until verified in clinical trials.

6. Technical Procedures

6.1. Surgical Technique: Murine Heterotopic Heart (35)

6.1.1. Donor Procedure

1. The animal is anesthetized and fixed in supine position.
2. A midline thoraco-abdominal incision is made exposing the heart and the entire length of aorta and inferior vena cava (IVC).
3. After injecting 5 mL of heparinized saline, the inferior vena cava is divided followed by division of the superior vena cava.
4. The ascending aorta and the main pulmonary artery are then divided allowing ligation of all pulmonary veins *en bloc*.
5. The allograft is then stored in heparinized saline on ice.

6.1.2. Recipient Procedure

1. The animal is anesthetized and fixed in supine position.
2. The operation is performed under an operating microscope (×16 magnification).
3. A Gable type rooftop incision is made, allowing access to the abdomen.
4. The bowel is displaced laterally to expose the infrarenal aorta and the IVC.

5. Lumbar vein and arteries are identified and cauterized. The aorta and the IVC are then clamped above and below, exposing a 1-cm infrarenal segment of the great vessels.
6. The donor ascending aorta is anastomosed end-to-side using 10-0 nylon to the recipient aorta.
7. The donor pulmonary artery is anastomosed end-to-side to the recipient IVC using 10-0 nylon suture.
8. The clamps are removed, allowing perfusion of the graft and commencement of sinus rhythm.

6.2. Surgical Technique: Murine Carotid Artery Model (79)

6.2.1. Donor Procedure

1. The donor animal is fixed in a supine position with its neck extended.
2. Following a midline incision in the neck the cleidomastoid muscles are resected. Both the left and right carotid arteries are fully dissected from the arch to the bifurcation and removed.
3. Harvested arteries are washed with heparinized saline and preserved in isotonic saline at room temperature until grafted into two recipient animals.

6.2.2. Recipient Procedure

1. The recipient animal is then fixed in a supine position with its neck extended.
2. A midline incision is made on the ventral surface of the neck from the suprasternal notch to the chin.
3. The left cleidomastoid muscle is resected. The left carotid artery is dissected from the bifurcation in the distal end toward the proximal end as far as technically possible.
4. The artery is then occluded with two microvascular clamps, one at each end, and two longitudinal arteriotomies (0.5–0.6 mm) are made with a fine (30-gauge) needle and scissors.
5. The graft is then transplanted paratopically into the recipient with an end-to-side anastomosis with an 11/0 continuous nylon suture under ×16–25 magnification.
6. Before the distal anastomosis is constructed, the proximal clamp is released to flush away residual blood inside the lumen. Both clamps are released after the two anastomoses are completed. At this point prominent pulsations should be visible in both the transplanted loop and the native vessel. If there are no pulsations or they are diminished within a few minutes of restoration of blood flow, thrombosis at the anastomosis is assumed and the procedure is terminated and considered a surgical failure.
7. If there are vigorous pulsations in the transplanted vessel, the skin incision is closed.

6.3. Surgical Technique: Rat Aortic Model (66)

6.3.1. Donor Operation

1. A midline abdominal incision is made and the bowel is retracted to the right.
2. A segment of aorta between the renal arteries and its bifurcation is separated from the vena cava.

3. Following injection of 0.5 mL of saline solution containing 50 U of heparin into the inferior vena cava, the segment of aorta is removed.

6.3.2. Recipient Operation

1. A midline incision is made from the xiphoid to the pelvis, and the abdominal walls are retracted.
2. The bowel is wrapped in saline-solution-moistened gauze and displaced to the animal's right.
3. The infrarenal aorta is dissected free and mobilized as far as possible, between the renal arteries proximally and the bifurcation distally.
4. All of the small branches of this segment are cut with the fine-tip cautery.
5. The proximal and distal portions of the aorta are clamped, and the intervening segment is resected.
6. The donor aorta is placed in the orthotopic position, and the anastomosis is performed using interrupted 10-0 nylon suture.

References

1. Billingham, M. E. (1987) Graft coronary disease: the lesions and the patients. *Transplant. Proc.* **19**, 19.
2. Hayry, P., Paavonen, T., Mennander, A., Ustinov, J., Raisanen, A., and Lemstrom, K. (1993) Pathophysiology of allograft arteriosclerosis. *Transplant. Proc.* **25**, 2070.
3. Meiser, B. M., Billingham, M. E., and Morris, R. E. (1991) Effects of cyclosporin, FK506, and rapamycin on graft-vessel disease [see comments]. *Lancet* **338**, 1297.
4. Kosek, J. C., Hurley, E. J., and Lower, R. R. (1968) Histopathology of orthotopic canine cardiac homografts. *Lab. Invest.* **19**, 97.
5. Muller, D. W., Ellis, S. G., and Topol, E. J. (1992) Experimental models of coronary artery restenosis [published erratum appears in *J. Am. Coll.Cardiol.*1992 **19(7)**,1678]. *J. Am. Coll. Cardiol.* **19**, 418.
6. Madsen, J. C., Sachs, D. H., Fallon, J. T., and Weissman, N. J. (1996) Cardiac allograft vasculopathy in partially inbred miniature swine. I. Time course, pathology, and dependence on immune mechanisms. *J. Thorac. Cardiovasc. Surg.* **111**, 1230.
7. Hancock, W. W., Buelow, R., Sayegh, M. H., and Turka, L. A. (1998) Antibody-induced transplant arteriosclerosis is prevented by graft expression of anti-oxidant and anti-apoptotic genes. *Nat. Med.* **4**, 1392.
8. Besterman, E. M. (1970) Experimental coronary atherosclerosis in rabbits. *Atherosclerosis* **12**, 75.
9. Mehra, M. R., Stapleton, D. D., Cook, J. L., et al. (1996) Adenovirus-mediated in vivo gene transfer in a rabbit model of allograft vasculopathy. *J. Heart Lung Transplant.* **15**, 51.
10. Vesselinovitch, D. (1988) Animal models and the study of atherosclerosis. *Arch. Pathol. Lab. Med.* **112**, 1011.

11. Ono, K., and Lindsey, E. S. (1969) Improved technique of heart transplantation in rats. *J. Thorac. Cardiovasc. Surg.* **57**, 225.
12. Arai, S., Teramoto, S., and Senoo, Y. (1992) The impact of FK506 on graft coronary disease of rat cardiac allograft—a comparison with cyclosporine. *J. Heart Lung Transplant.* **11**, 757.
13. Mennander, A., Tiisala, S. Paavonen, T. Halttunen, J., and Hayry, P. (1991) Chronic rejection of rat aortic allograft. II. Administration of cyclosporin induces accelerated allograft arteriosclerosis. *Transplant. Int.* **4**, 173.
14. Russell, P. S., Chase, C. M., Winn, H. J., and Colvin, R. B. (1994) Coronary atherosclerosis in transplanted mouse hearts. I. Time course and immunogenetic and immunopathological considerations. *Am. J. Pathol.* **144**, 260.
15. Armstrong, A. T., Strauch, A. R., Starling, R. C., Sedmak, D. D., and Orosz, C. G. (1997) Morphometric analysis of neointimal formation in murine cardiac allografts. *Transplantation* **63**, 941.
16. Cullum, P. A., Baum, M., Clarke, A., Wemyss-Gorman, P. B., Howard, E., and McClelland, R. M. (1970) Orthotopic transplantation of the pig heart. *Thorax* **25**, 744.
17. Pennock, J. L., Reitz, B. A., Bieber, C. P., et al. (1981) Survival of primates following orthotopic cardiac transplantation treated with total lymphoid irradiation and chemical immune suppression. *Transplantation* **32**, 467.
18. Laden, A. M. and Sinclair, R. A. (1971) Thickening of arterial intima in rat cardiac allografts. A light and electron microscopic study. *Am. J. Pathol.* **63**, 69.
19. Lurie, K. G., Billingham, M. E., Jamieson, S. W., Harrison, D. C., and Reitz, B. A. (1981) Pathogenesis and prevention of graft arteriosclerosis in an experimental heart transplant model. *Transplantation* **31**, 41.
20. Laden, A. M. (1972) The effects of treatment on the arterial lesions of rat and rabbit cardiac allografts. *Transplantation* **13**, 281.
21. Adams, D. H., Tilney, N. L., Collins, Jr., J. J., and Karnovsky, M. J. (1992) Experimental graft arteriosclerosis. I. The Lewis-to-F-344 allograft model. *Transplantation* **53**, 1115.
22. Hosenpud, J. D., Boyle, T. M., Hensler, H., Sanford, G., and Khanna, A. K. (2000) The relationship between acute rejection and chronic rejection is highly dependent on specific MHC matching: a multi-strain rat heterotopic heart transplant study. *Transplantation* **69**, 2173.
23. Hachida, M., Lu, H., Zhang, X., et al. (1999) Inhibitory effect of triptolide on platelet derived growth factor-A and coronary arteriosclerosis after heart transplantation. *Transplant. Proc.* **31**, 2719.
24. Hachida, M., Zhang, X. L., Lu, H., Hoshi, H., and Koyanagi, H. (1999) Late multiglycosidorum tripterygium treatment ameliorates established graft coronary arteriosclerosis after heart transplantation in the rat. *Transplant. Proc.* **31**, 2020.
25. Zhang, X., Hachida, M., Lu, H., Hoshi, H., and Koyanagi, H. (1999) Effect of 15-deoxyspergualine on coronary arteriosclerosis and platelet-derived growth factor-A mRNA expression in the transplanted heart. *Transplant. Proc* **31**, 1706.

26. Teranishi, K., Poston, R. S., Reitz, B. A., and Robbins, R. C. (1998) Oral delivery of low molecular weight heparin in rat cardiac allografts. *Transplant. Proc.* **30**, 996.
27. Russell, M. E., Adams, D. H., Wyner, L. R., Yamashita, Y., Halnon, N. J., and Karnovsky, M. J. (1993) Early and persistent induction of monocyte chemoattractant protein 1 in rat cardiac allografts. *Proc. Natl. Acad. Sci. USA* **90**, 6086.
28. Russell, M. E., Wallace, A. F., Hancock, W. W., et al. (1995) Upregulation of cytokines associated with macrophage activation in the Lewis-to-F344 rat transplantation model of chronic cardiac rejection. *Transplantation* **59**, 572.
29. Watschinger, B., Sayegh, M. H., Hancock, W. W., and Russell, M. E. (1995) Up-regulation of endothelin-1 mRNA and peptide expression in rat cardiac allografts with rejection and arteriosclerosis. *Am. J. Pathol.* **146**, 1065.
30. Utans, U., Arceci, R. J., Yamashita, Y., and Russell, M. E. (1995) Cloning and characterization of allograft inflammatory factor-1: a novel macrophage factor identified in rat cardiac allografts with chronic rejection. *J. Clin. Invest.* **95**, 2954.
31. Russell, M. E., Wallace, A. F., Wyner, L. R., Newell, J. B., and Karnovsky, M. J. (1995) Upregulation and modulation of inducible nitric oxide synthase in rat cardiac allografts with chronic rejection and transplant arteriosclerosis. *Circulation* **92**, 457.
32. Hachida, M., Zhang, X., Lu, H., et al. (1998) Association between the degree of platelet-derived growth factor-A chain mRNA expression and coronary arteriosclerosis in the transplanted heart. *Heart Vessels* **13**, 24.
33. Ito, H., Hamano, K., Gohra, H., et al. (1998) Coronary arteriosclerosis did not occur in the transplanted hearts of tolerance-induced rats, analysis from platelet-derived growth factor expression. *Transplant. Proc.* **30**, 3871.
34. Izutani, H., Miyagawa, S., Shirakura, R., et al. (1995) Evidence that graft coronary arteriosclerosis begins in the early phase after transplantation and progresses without chronic immunoreaction. Histopathological analysis using a retransplantation model. *Transplantation* **60**, 1073.
35. Corry, R. J., Winn, H. J., and Russell, P. S. (1973) Heart transplantation in congenic strains of mice. *Transplant. Proc.* **5**, 733.
36. Ardehali, A., Billingsley, A., Laks, H., Drinkwater, Jr., D. C., Sorensen, T. J., and Drake, T. A. (1993) Experimental cardiac allograft vasculopathy in mice. *J. Heart Lung Transplant.* **12**, 730.
37. Hirozane, T., Matsumori, A., Furukawa, Y., and Sasayama, S. (1995) Experimental graft coronary artery disease in a murine heterotopic cardiac transplant model. *Circulation* **91**, 386.
38. Hasegawa, S., Becker, G., Nagano, H., Libby, P., and Mitchell, R. N. (1998) Pattern of graft- and host-specific MHC class II expression in long-term murine cardiac allografts: origin of inflammatory and vascular wall cells. *Am. J. Pathol.* **153**, 69.
39. Russell, P. S., Chase, C. M., Winn, H. J., and Colvin, R. B. (1994) Coronary atherosclerosis in transplanted mouse hearts. II. Importance of humoral immunity. *J. Immunol.* **152**, 5135.

40. Russell, P. S., Chase, C. M., and Colvin, R. B. (1997) Alloantibody- and T cell-mediated immunity in the pathogenesis of transplant arteriosclerosis: lack of progression to sclerotic lesions in B cell-deficient mice. *Transplantation* **64**, 1531.
41. Russell, P. S., Chase, C. M., and Colvin, R. B. (1995) Coronary atherosclerosis in transplanted mouse hearts. IV Effects of treatment with monoclonal antibodies to intercellular adhesion molecule-1 and leukocyte function-associated antigen-1. *Transplantation* **60**, 724.
42. Gao, W., Topham, P. S., King, J. A., et al. (2000) Targeting of the chemokine receptor CCR1 suppresses development of acute and chronic cardiac allograft rejection. *J. Clin. Invest.* **105**, 35.
43. Nagano, H., Mitchell, R. N., Taylor, M. K., Hasegawa, S., Tilney, N. L., and Libby, P. (1997) Interferon-gamma deficiency prevents coronary arteriosclerosis but not myocardial rejection in transplanted mouse hearts. *J. Clin. Invest.* **100**, 550.
44. Raisanen-Sokolowski, A., Glysing-Jensen, T., Koglin, J., and Russell, M. E. (1998) Reduced transplant arteriosclerosis in murine cardiac allografts placed in interferon-gamma knockout recipients. *Am. J. Pathol.* **152**, 359.
45. Koglin, J., Glysing-Jensen, T., Gadiraju, S., and Russell, M. E. (2000) Attenuated cardiac allograft vasculopathy in mice with targeted deletion of the transcription factor STAT4. *Circulation* **101**, 1034.
46. Nagano, H., Tilney, N. L., Stinn, J. L., et al. (1999) Deficiencies of IL-4 or TNF-alpha receptor-1 do not diminish graft arteriosclerosis in cardiac allografts. *Transplant. Proc.* **31**, 152.
47. Mottram, P. L., Raisanen-Sokolowski, A., Glysing-Jensen, T., Stein-Oakley, A. N., and Russell, M. E. (1998) Cardiac allografts from IL-4 knockout recipients: assessment of transplant arteriosclerosis and peripheral tolerance. *J. Immunol.* **161**, 602.
48. Raisanen-Sokolowski, A., Glysing-Jensen, T., and Russell, M. E. (1998) Leukocyte-suppressing influences of interleukin (IL)-10 in cardiac allografts: insights from IL-10 knockout mice. *Am. J. Pathol.* **153**, 1491.
49. Furukawa, Y., Becker, G., Stinn, J. L., Shimizu, K., Libby, P., and Mitchell, R. N. (1999) Interleukin-10 (IL-10) augments allograft arterial disease: paradoxical effects of IL-10 in vivo. *Am. J. Pathol.* **155**, 1929.
50. Koglin, J., Glysing-Jensen, T., Raisanen-Sokolowski, A., and Russell, M. E. (1998) Immune sources of transforming growth factor-beta1 reduce transplant arteriosclerosis: insight derived from a knockout mouse model. *Circ Res* **83**, 652.
51. Koglin, J., Glysing-Jensen, T., Mudgett, J. S., and Russell, M. E. (1998) NOS2 mediates opposing effects in models of acute and chronic cardiac rejection: insights from NOS2-knockout mice. *Am. J. Pathol.* **153**, 1371.
52. Russell, P. S., Chase, C. M., and Colvin, R. B. (1996) Accelerated atheromatous lesions in mouse hearts transplanted to apolipoprotein-E-deficient recipients. *Am. J. Pathol.* **149**, 91.
53. Tomita, Y., Zhang, Q. W., Yoshikawa, M., Uchida, T., Nomoto, K., and Yasui, H. (1997) Improved technique of heterotopic cervical heart transplantation in mice. *Transplantation* **64**, 1598.

54. Chen, Z. H. (1991) A technique of cervical heterotopic heart transplantation in mice. *Transplantation* **52**, 1099.
55. Matsuura, A., Abe, T., and Yasuura, K. (1991) Simplified mouse cervical heart transplantation using a cuff technique. *Transplantation* **51**, 896.
56. Fuster, V., Badimon, L., Badimon, J. J., Ip, J. H., and Chesebro, J. H. (1991) The porcine model for the understanding of thrombogenesis and atherogenesis. *Mayo Clin. Proc.* **66**, 818.
57. Madsen, J. C., Yamada, K., Allan, J. S., et al. (1998) Transplantation tolerance prevents cardiac allograft vasculopathy in major histocompatibility complex class I-disparate miniature swine. *Transplantation* **65**, 304.
58. Schwarze, M. L., Menard, M. T., Fuchimoto, Y., et al. (2000) Mixed hematopoietic chimerism induces long-term tolerance to cardiac allografts in miniature swine. *Ann. Thorac. Surg.* **70**, 131.
59. Alonso, D. R., Starek, P. K., and Minick, C. R. (1977) Studies on the pathogenesis of atheroarteriosclerosis induced in rabbit cardiac allografts by the synergy of graft rejection and hypercholesterolemia. *Am. J. Pathol.* **87**, 415.
60. Ogawa, N., Koyama, I., Shibata, T., et al. (1996) Pravastatin prevents the progression of accelerated coronary artery disease after heart transplantation in a rabbit model. *Transplant. Int.* **9**, S226.
61. Esper, E., Glagov, S., Karp, R. B., et al. (1997) Role of hypercholesterolemia in accelerated transplant coronary vasculopathy: results of surgical therapy with partial ileal bypass in rabbits undergoing heterotopic heart transplantation. *J. Heart Lung Transplant.* **16**, 420.
62. Nakagawa, T., Sukhova, G. K., Rabkin, E., Winters, G. L., Schoen, F. J., and Libby, P. (1995) Acute rejection accelerates graft coronary disease in transplanted rabbit hearts. *Circulation* **92**, 987.
63. Pierson, R. N., 3rd, Chang, A. C., Blum, M. G., et al. (1999) Prolongation of primate cardiac allograft survival by treatment with ANTI-CD40 ligand (CD154) antibody. *Transplantation* **68**, 1800.
64. Klein, I., Hong, C., and Schreiber, S. S. (1990) Cardiac atrophy in the heterotopically transplanted rat heart: in vitro protein synthesis. *J. Mol. Cell. Cardiol.* **22**, 461.
65. Orosz, C. G. (2000) Considerations regarding the contributions of B cells to chronic allograft rejection in experimental animal models. *J. Heart Lung Transplant.* **19**, 634.
66. Halttunen, J., Partanen, T., Leszczynski, D., Rinta, K., and Hayry, P. (1990) Rat aortic allografts: a model for chronic vascular rejection. *Transplant. Proc.* **22**, 125.
67. Michel, J. B., Plissonnier, D., and Bruneval, P. (1992) Effect of perindopril on the immune arterial wall remodeling in the rat model of arterial graft rejection. *Am. J. Med.* **92,** 39S.
68. Raisanen, A., Mennander, A., Ustinov, J., Paavonen, T., and Hayry, P. (1993) Effect of platelet-activating factor (PAF) receptor blockers on smooth muscle cell replication in vitro and allograft arteriosclerosis in vivo. *Transplant. Int.* **6**, 251.

69. Raisanen-Sokolowski, A., Mennander, A., Ustinov, J., Paavonen, T., and Hayry, P. (1993) Chronic rejection in rat aortic allograft: mechanism of angiopeptin (BIM 23014C) inhibition on vascular smooth muscle cell proliferation in chronic rejection. *Transplant. Proc.* **25**, 944.
70. Raisanen-Sokolowski, A., Myllarniemi, M., and Hayry, P. (1994) Effect of mycophenolate mofetil on allograft arteriosclerosis (chronic rejection). *Transplant. Proc.* **26**, 3225.
71. Akyurek, M. L., Larsson, E., Funa, K., Wanders, A., Kaijser, M., and Fellstrom, B. C. (1995) Experimental transplant arteriosclerosis: inhibition by angiopeptin and low molecular weight heparin derivatives. *Transplant. Proc.* **27**, 3555.
72. Akyurek, L. M., Fellstrom, B. C., Yan, Z. Q., Hansson, G. K., Funa, K., and Larsson, E. (1996) Inducible and endothelial nitric oxide synthase expression during development of transplant arteriosclerosis in rat aortic grafts. *Am. J. Pathol.* **149**, 1981.
73. Akyurek, L. M., Johnsson, C., Lange, D., et al. (1998) Tolerance induction ameliorates allograft vasculopathy in rat aortic transplants. Influence of Fas-mediated apoptosis. *J. Clin. Invest.* **101**, 2889.
74. Mennander, A. and Hayry, P. (1996) Reversibility of allograft arteriosclerosis after retransplantation to donor strain. *Transplantation* **62**, 526.
75. Koulack, J., McAlister, V. C., Giacomantonio, C. A., Bitter-Suermann, H., MacDonald, A. S., and Lee, T. D. (1995) Development of a mouse aortic transplant model of chronic rejection. *Microsurgery* **16**, 110.
76. Hjelms, E. and Stender. S. (1992) Accelerated cholesterol accumulation in homologous arterial transplants in cholesterol-fed rabbits. A surgical model to study transplantation atherosclerosis. *Arterioscler. Thromb.* **12**, 771.
77. Jacobsson, J., Cheng, L., Lyke, K., et al. (1992) Effect of estradiol on accelerated atherosclerosis in rabbit heterotopic aortic allografts. *J. Heart Lung Transplant.* **11**, 1188.
78. Gummert, J. F., Ikonen, T., Briffa, N., et al. (1998) A new large-animal model for research of graft vascular disease. *Transplant. Proc.* **30**, 4023.
79. Shi, C., Russell, M. E., Bianchi, C., Newell, J. B., and Haber, E. (1994) Murine model of accelerated transplant arteriosclerosis. *Circ. Res.* **75**, 199.
80. Shi, C., Lee, W. S., He, Q., et al. (1996) Immunologic basis of transplant-associated arteriosclerosis. *Proc. Natl. Acad. Sci. USA* **93**, 4051.
81. Shi, C., Lee, W. S., Russell, M. E., et al. (1997) Hypercholesterolemia exacerbates transplant arteriosclerosis via increased neointimal smooth muscle cell accumulation: studies in apolipoprotein E knockout mice. *Circulation* **96**, 2722.
82. Moons, L., Shi, C., Ploplis, V., et al. (1998) Reduced transplant arteriosclerosis in plasminogen-deficient mice. *J. Clin. Invest.* **102**, 1788.
83. Shi, C., Feinberg, M. W., Zhang, D., et al. (1999) Donor MHC and adhesion molecules in transplant arteriosclerosis. *J. Clin. Invest.* **103**, 469.
84. Dietrich, H., Hu, Y., Zou, Y., et al. (2000) Mouse model of transplant arteriosclerosis: role of intercellular adhesion molecule-1. *Arterioscler. Thromb. Vasc. Biol.* **20**, 343.

85. Hancock, W. W., Shi, C., Picard, M. H., Bianchi, C., and Russell, M. E. (1995) LEW-to-F344 carotid artery allografts: analysis of a rat model of posttransplant vascular injury involving cell-mediated and humoral responses. *Transplantation* **60**, 1565.
86. Gregory, C. R., Huie, P., Shorthouse, R., et al. (1993) Treatment with rapamycin blocks arterial intimal thickening following mechanical and alloimmune injury. *Transplant. Proc.* **25**, 120.
87. Brazelton, T. R., Adams, B., Shorthouse, R., and Morris, R. E. (1999) Chronic rejection: the result of uncontrolled remodelling of graft tissue by recipient mesenchymal cells? Data from two rodent models and the effects of immunosuppressive therapies. *Inflamm. Res.* **48**, S134.
88. Plissonnier, D., Nochy, D., Poncet, P., et al. (1995) Sequential immunological targeting of chronic experimental arterial allograft. *Transplantation* **60**, 414.
89. Tixier, D. B., Czer, L. S., Fishbein, M. C., et al. (1996) Isolated coronary artery transplantation in pigs: a new model to study transplantation arteriosclerosis and humoral rejection. *J. Heart Lung Transplant.* **15**, 919.

Index